Natural Products with Pharmaceutical Activities

Natural Products with Pharmaceutical Activities

Natural Products with Pharmaceutical Activities

Guest Editors

Sokcheon Pak
Soo Liang Ooi

MDPI

Basel • Beijing • Wuhan • Barcelona • Belgrade • Novi Sad • Cluj • Manchester

Guest Editors
Sokcheon Pak
School of Dentistry and Medical Sciences
Charles Sturt University
Bathurst, NSW
Australia

Soo Liang Ooi
School of Dentistry and Medical Sciences
Charles Sturt University
Bathurst, NSW
Australia

Editorial Office
MDPI AG
Grosspeteranlage 5
4052 Basel, Switzerland

This is a reprint of the Special Issue, published open access by the journal *Molecules* (ISSN 1420-3049), freely accessible at: https://www.mdpi.com/journal/molecules/special_issues/O1TP4FZ98W.

For citation purposes, cite each article independently as indicated on the article page online and as indicated below:

Lastname, A.A.; Lastname, B.B. Article Title. *Journal Name* **Year**, *Volume Number*, Page Range.

ISBN 978-3-7258-6490-4 (Hbk)
ISBN 978-3-7258-6491-1 (PDF)
https://doi.org/10.3390/books978-3-7258-6491-1

Contents

About the Editors

Sokcheon Pak

Sok Cheon Pak has taught and conducted research at Charles Sturt University in Australia since 2007. His expertise lies in the field of complementary medicine, and he is recognized nationally and internationally through ongoing external research collaborations. His research interests centre on introducing evidence-based approaches to complementary medicine, supported by laboratory-based investigations that utilize modern medical technologies to clarify the mechanisms and therapeutic rationale of natural health products. Over recent years, his principal research focus has shifted to nutraceuticals with clinically relevant applications, particularly Rice Bran Arabinoxylan Compound (RBAC). He currently leads research examining the effects of RBAC on immune health and quality of life in cancer patients, as well as related investigations into gut microbiota and other natural therapeutic compounds. His work aims to provide credible, translational evidence for the effective integration of nutraceuticals into clinical practice.

Soo Liang Ooi

Soo Liang Ooi is a practising nutritionist and naturopath with clinical experience in Australia and Singapore. He holds a Bachelor of Health Science degree from Charles Sturt University, a Master of Business Administration degree from the National University of Singapore, and a Master of Mathematics degree from the University of Waterloo in Canada. Soo Liang completed his Doctor of Philosophy (PhD) in investigating the immunomodulating properties of rice bran arabinoxylan compound and its effects on the quality of life of cancer patients at Charles Sturt University in 2024. His research interests include evidence-based complementary medicine, nutritional medicine, naturopathy, herbal medicine, meditation, and integrative cancer therapies. As an avid academic writer, Soo Liang has published extensively in major peer-reviewed scholarly journals. He was nominated for the prestigious Elsevier Atlas award in 2017 for his work on "Transcendental meditation for lowering blood pressure: An overview of systematic reviews and meta-analyses". He is also a co-editor of several academic books, including *Health Benefits of Meditation, Nutraceuticals in Immune Function* and *Modified Rice Bran Arabinoxylan—Therapeutic Applications in Cancer and Other Diseases.*

Preface

With the rise of multidrug resistance, emerging diseases, and the growing need for novel therapeutic agents, natural products play a crucial role in pharmaceutical research. Exploring bioactive compounds from natural sources offers vast potential for discovering new treatments for diseases. Natural products promise to improve human health, with anti-inflammatory, anticancer, and antimicrobial properties, as well as cardiovascular, neuroprotective, and immunomodulatory effects. However, the identification, isolation, and optimization of these active compounds, along with their mechanisms of action, remain challenging. The Special Issue "Natural Products with Pharmaceutical Activities" in the journal *Molecules* aims to highlight research exploring the pharmaceutical potential of natural compounds, especially studies that emphasise novel extraction methods, structure–activity relationships, mechanisms of action, and clinical potential. Launched on 29 October 2024 and closed on 1 July 2025, this Special Issue attracted 27 submissions from researchers worldwide. The submissions include original research articles and reviews focusing on the identification, isolation, structural characterization, and pharmacological evaluation of bioactive compounds from natural sources. After rigorous peer review, only 13 articles were published. This Reprint is an anthology of promising research on natural products with enormous potential for pharmaceutical advancement. We thank all the authors for their invaluable contributions to this Reprint. Their insights, experimental findings, and critical analyses have enriched this reprint, fostering a deeper understanding of the therapeutic potential locked within nature's abundant offerings. It is through their tireless efforts that we are able to present a diverse and multidimensional exploration of natural products, offering new avenues for healthcare professionals, researchers, and enthusiasts to harness their power.

Sokcheon Pak and Soo Liang Ooi
Guest Editors

molecules

MDPI

Editorial

Natural Products with Pharmaceutical Activities

Soo Liang Ooi and Sok Cheon Pak *

School of Dentistry and Medical Sciences, Charles Sturt University, Panorama Avenue, Bathurst, NSW 2795, Australia; sooi@csu.edu.au
* Correspondence: spak@csu.edu.au

1. Introduction

Natural products are bioactive molecules or compounds derived from natural sources that can be harnessed to develop therapeutic agents. Despite competition with synthetic molecules and biologics, drug discovery and development based on natural products remains a mainstay [1]. In recent years, advances in analytical chemistry, omics technologies, computational modelling, bioinformatics, automation, and artificial intelligence have accelerated the identification, characterisation, and pharmacological evaluation of bioactive natural compounds [2–5]. These developments have deepened our understanding of the mechanisms underlying the therapeutic effects of natural products and expanded their potential applications in modern medicine [6].

Despite these advancements, significant knowledge gaps and challenges remain—particularly in translating traditional ethnopharmacological knowledge and preclinical findings into clinically validated pharmaceutical agents [7]. Specifically, complex metabolites in plant- and marine-based natural products collectively contribute to their pharmacological properties, but hurdles still exist in the extraction and isolation of bioactive compounds for drug development [8]. Studying the pharmacokinetics of natural products to improve compound stability and bioavailability is also problematic due to the presence of multiple, diverse active compounds in their extracts [9]. In recent years, nanoparticle-based technology has shown tremendous potential in maximising drug delivery to ensure stability and bioavailability [10]. However, translational progress from the laboratory to viable production is often hindered by the complex interplay of regulatory and commercialisation hurdles [7].

The increasing demand for medicinal and aromatic plants from the pharmaceutical and cosmetic industries also intensifies their production, increasing the risk of overexploiting natural resources. Sustainable practices have become a necessity to ensure long-term economic, social, and environmental viability [11]. Sustainability in the natural product development life cycle includes harnessing bio-waste as a source of pharmacological compound discovery, developing sustainable methods for large-scale production, and eco-friendly and circular waste management [12–15]. However, with the predominant focus on the research and development of well-known compounds from medicinal and edible plants or food sources, many other promising natural product candidates have been left unexplored [16].

This Special Issue on "Natural Products with Pharmaceutical Activities" was conceived to address some of these knowledge gaps by showcasing current research and comprehensive reviews that explore natural compounds from diverse biological sources. The contributions highlight that, in addition to traditional medicinal plants, sustainable industrial byproducts and unconventional natural materials are promising resources for

 https://doi.org/10.3390/molecules30234557

drug discovery. Novel approaches to the extraction, delivery, and production of natural pharmaceutical agents are also explored.

A total of thirteen papers, comprising eight original research articles and five reviews, were accepted after rigorous peer review. Collectively, these works demonstrate the growing integration of sustainability, innovation, and multidisciplinary approaches in natural product research.

2. An Overview of the Published Articles

2.1. Medicinal Plant Sources

Medicinal plants remain one of the most essential foundations for discovering new pharmaceutical agents; several papers in this Special Issue are dedicated to investigating these plants or their isolated bioactive compounds.

1′-Acetoxychavicol acetate (ACA) is a natural compound derived from the rhizomes of the Zingiberaceae family. Moriwaki et al. investigated the molecular mechanisms by which ACA inhibits the NF-κB signalling pathway in human lung adenocarcinoma A549 cells. The results showed that ACA lowered tumour necrosis factor (TNF)-α-induced NF-κB signalling pathway activity, which led to decreased intercellular adhesion molecule-1 (ICAM-1) expression by selectively downregulating the expression of the TNF receptor-associated factor protein (TRAF2) via the ubiquitin–proteasome system. In addition, ACA was also found to suppress the transcriptional process of NF-κB directly. The findings support ACA as a potential natural product candidate with anti-inflammatory and anticancer properties.

Naidoo and Khathi investigated the hepatoprotective properties of gossypetin, a natural flavonoid isolated from the calyx and flowers of Roselle (*Hibiscus sabdariffa*), in a pre-diabetic murine model. Gossypetin treatment significantly ($p < 0.05$) reduced liver triglycerides, liver weights, and plasma sterol regulatory binding element regulatory protein-1c, and improved liver antioxidant enzyme levels, compared to the pre-diabetic control. Decreased lipid droplet accumulation and improved tissue integrity were also observed in liver histology. The effects were found to be similar to those of metformin treatment. Notably, gossypetin was found to offer greater hepatoprotective effects in mice in the absence of dietary intervention.

Salvia guevarae is a species of flowering plant belonging to the Lamiaceae family, native to South America. Commonly cultivated for ornamental purposes, the species is also used in herbal remedies in folk medicine. Torres-Medicis et al. studied the antiproliferative and anti-inflammatory activities of nine neo-clerodane-type diterpenoids isolated from the dichloromethane extract of *S. guevarae* Bedolla & Zamudio leaves in vitro. Specifically, guevarain B and 6α-hydroxy patagonol acetonide showed moderate activity against the K562 human leukaemia cell line, whereas 2-oxo-patagonal, 6α-hydroxy patagonol acetonide, and 7α-acetoxy-ent-clerodan-3,13-dien-18,19:16,15-diolide inhibited nitric oxide production in RAW 264.7 macrophages.

Kanak et al. conducted a literature review on the application of Alchemilla species for skin health and dermatological disorders. Commonly known as lady's mantle, Alchemilla is a genus of perennial herbaceous plants in the family Rosaceae. The review found that *Alchemilla* spp. exhibit antioxidant, anti-inflammatory, antimicrobial, and wound-healing activities. Extracts of Alchemilla plants were successfully used to treat dermatological issues including skin rashes, acne, stretch marks, eczema, psoriasis, and wrinkles. Nevertheless, more research is still needed to identify the most potent species or varieties, develop efficient extraction methods, and investigate efficacy in human application with appropriate formulations.

Sacha inchi (*Plukenetia volubilis*) is a plant native to South America that is renowned as a natural source of unsaturated fatty acids with enormous economic potential. Redjeki et al. reviewed the bioactivity, extraction methods, and encapsulation techniques of sacha inchi oil to inform nutraceutical and pharmaceutical development. The oil is rich in omega-3, omega-6, and omega-9, tocopherols, phytosterols, and polyphenols with bioactive activities including antioxidant, anti-inflammatory, antiproliferative, and neuroprotective effects beneficial to cardiovascular health. The stability of sacha inchi oil was a significant concern, with many current research studies discussing optimised extraction approaches and advanced microencapsulation techniques to enhance the efficacy of sacha inchi oil in application. Human research, especially clinical studies, remains lacking and is needed to validate the therapeutic benefits of the oil.

Polyscias fruticosa, commonly known as Ming aralia or "Vietnamese ginseng", is used in traditional medicine in Southeast Asia for the treatment of a variety of conditions, such as fatigue, asthma, metabolic disorders, inflammation, and neurodegenerative diseases. A review by Śliwińska and Tomiczak offered a synthesis of the current understanding of the biotechnological methods, phytochemical diversity, and pharmacological activities of *P. fruticosa*. The review showed that *P. fruticosa* exhibits a complex phytochemical profile comprising triterpenoid saponins, flavonoids, phenolic acids, sterols, polyacetylenes, and fatty acid derivatives, with preclinical models demonstrating anti-inflammatory, antidiabetic, antiasthmatic, neuroprotective, and antiresorptive activities. Suspension cultures derived from callus tissues of *P. fruticosa* demonstrated biosynthetic competence for various classes of secondary metabolites, including triterpenoid saponins and phenolic compounds. Hence, the plant could be a promising alternative sustainable source of Araliaceae-type saponins for future pharmaceutical applications.

Pharmacokinetics software is increasingly being used in drug research to shorten development time and achieve cost savings. Silva et al. leveraged a range of computational tools to predict the pharmacological properties of withanolides, identified as a promising antineoplastic drug lead. Withanolides are naturally occurring C-28 ergostane steroidal lactones, commonly isolated from nightshade plants (Solanaceae family). This in silico study predicted their good oral absorption, low toxicity, and CYP3A4 metabolism with no inhibition of other P450 cytochromes; they were also unable to cross the blood–brain barrier. The molecules were predicted to show low inhibition of pharmacokinetic transporters and a high probability of nuclear receptor interactions, although they showed significant signs of aquatic ecotoxicity. Withanolides may therefore possess viability for oral drug development.

2.2. Sustainable Use of Bio-Wastes

Sustainability and circular use of resources are key emerging trends in natural product research.

Li et al. addressed environmental sustainability by exploring the potential use of *Cucumaria frondosa* tentacles, a waste product of the sea cucumber industry, as a natural antioxidant and anti-fatigue alternative. They found that the hydrolysates obtained through protease hydrolysis exhibited significant antioxidant capacity. The product was not toxic to mice and enhanced their exhaustive swimming time, significantly increased ($p < 0.01$) blood glucose and liver glycogen levels, reduced fatigue-related metabolites ($p < 0.05$), and elevated superoxide dismutase and glutathione peroxidase levels ($p < 0.05$). These findings support the potential utilisation of *Cucumaria frondosa* tentacles as a natural source of anti-fatigue products.

Xanthohumol is a prenylated chalcone found in hops (*Humulus lupulus*) and byproducts of beer production. Dlugosz et al. reviewed its mechanisms of action and therapeutic potential for the prevention of selected neurodegenerative diseases, including Alzheimer's disease, Parkinson's disease, and amyotrophic lateral sclerosis. Experimental evidence suggests that xanthohumol possesses potent antioxidant capabilities, beneficial for protecting neurons from oxidative damage, and could also alleviate neuroinflammation by inhibiting NF-κB, TNF-α, and IL-1β and reduce the chronic activation of microglia and astrocytes to prevent neuronal damage. Xanthohumol further influences the Nrf2/ARE neuroprotective pathway to enhance neuronal resilience, sustains neuronal energy metabolism by maintaining ATP production, and positively impacts synaptic plasticity, supporting memory enhancement; it could therefore have medical applications in the prevention and treatment of neurodegenerative diseases.

Roșcan et al. explored the potential of using plant waste, specifically from species such as red raspberry (*Rubus idaeus*) and cherry trees (*Prunus avium, Prunus serotina*, and *Prunus cerasus*), as a natural source of pharmaceutical agents. They found that plant waste from *R. idaeus, P. serotina, P. avium*, and *P. cerasus* contained complex bioactive compounds such as flavonoids, flavonols, tannins, cyanogenic glycosides, vitamins, aldehydes, and phenolic acids that exhibited pharmacological and pro-health properties, including antibacterial, antitumour, antidiabetic, anti-carcinogenic, neuroprotective, anti-inflammatory, antioxidant, and cardioprotective effects. A range of available extraction methods, from conventional ethanol extraction to more environmentally friendly solutions such as subcritical water extraction and supercritical CO_2 extraction, were found in the literature. Also observed was an affinity for chromatographic methods for the isolation and purification of target compounds from the four plant sources, making them potentially valuable sources for numerous cosmetic, pharmaceutical, and food applications.

Xanthan gum is a biopolymer produced through the fermentation of sugars by the bacteria *Xanthomonas campestris*. Xanthan gum has extensive industrial applications and possesses many beneficial pharmaceutical properties. It is a non-toxic, biodegradable, and biocompatible substance that exhibits high viscosity and stability under a wide range of pH and temperature, and can thus be used as an excipient in many drug delivery systems, including sustained- or controlled-release formulations. Jonuskiene et al. investigated the use of renewable alternative carbon sources in the production of xanthan gum to replace sucrose and glucose and reduce environmental burden. The study demonstrated that L-glutamic acid was a suitable source for 72 h bacterial fermentation, yielding the highest production. However, other renewable natural resources, including avocado hydrolysates and lemon peels, could also achieve high xanthan gum yields with only 24 h of fermentation and exhibited the highest antioxidant activity. Thus, these renewable resources could be used to improve the sustainability of xanthan gum production.

2.3. Diverse Natural Sources

The remaining two papers broaden the scope of natural product research beyond traditional plant-based systems.

To manage foodborne illnesses caused by pathogens such as *Salmonella enterica* and *Escherichia coli*, Maione et al. assessed the viability of phenyllactic acid produced by lactic acid bacteria as an anti-microbial agent in vitro, which was found to be non-toxic to intestinal cells and effective in inhibiting biofilm formation and bacterial planktonic growth, with minimum inhibitory concentrations ranging from 2 to 2.75 mg/mL. Experimenting with real food, the application of phenyllactic acid to minced beef significantly ($p < 0.05$) lowered microbial populations compared to controls. It was also found that phenyllactic acid has the potential to prevent intestinal bacterial colonisation, making it a promising agent not only for controlling microbial contamination in food processing but also for making the intestinal microenvironment less hospitable for harmful bacteria.

Amber is a type of organic gemstone formed from the fossilisation of ancient tree resin. Yodweerapong et al. examined the T cell inhibition activities of kujigamberol, a dinorlabdane compound isolated from amber mined from the Kuji region of Japan. This compound was found to lower IFN-γ production and IL-2 mRNA expression in murine lymphoma BW5147 T-cell and cytotoxic T-cell line CTLL-2. Kujigamberol also reduced nuclear factor of activated T cell (NFAT)-dependent transcription in human embryonic kidney 293 T cells and suppressed T-cell activities through interfering with the binding of NFATc2 to the IFN-γ and IL-2 promoters. Hence, it could be a potential lead for immunosuppressive agents.

3. Conclusions

The studies published in this Special Issue collectively showcase the remarkable diversity of natural sources for pharmaceutical discovery, ranging from traditional medicinal plants and sustainable industrial byproducts to rare materials like amber.

They reflect the ongoing global commitment to unlocking nature's pharmacological potential while embracing sustainability, biotechnological innovation, and interdisciplinary collaboration. Together, these contributions reinforce that natural product research remains a vibrant, evolving field that continues to offer promising leads for the development of novel therapeutics addressing modern health challenges.

Author Contributions: Conceptualization, S.L.O. and S.C.P.; writing—original draft preparation, S.L.O.; writing—review and editing, S.C.P. All authors have read and agreed to the published version of the manuscript.

Conflicts of Interest: The authors declare no conflict of interest.

List of Contributions:

1. Dlugosz, A.; Blaszak, B.; Czarnecki, D.; Szulc, J. Mechanism of action and therapeutic potential of xanthohumol in prevention of selected neurodegenerative diseases. *Molecules* **2025**, *30*, 694. https://doi.org/10.3390/molecules30030694.
2. Jonuskiene, I.; Davicijonaite, E.; Vaskeviciute, M.; Kala, I.; Stankeviciene, R.; Kantminiene, K.; Tumosiene, I. Sustainable production and antioxidant activity of bacterial xanthan gum. *Molecules* **2025**, *30*, 2734. https://doi.org/10.3390/molecules30132734.
3. Kanak, S.; Krzeminska, B.; Berecka-Rycerz, A.; Kopec, M.; Dos Santos Szewczyk, K. Harnessing the power of Alchemilla: A natural solution for skin health and dermatological disorders. *Molecules* **2025**, *30*, 1861. https://doi.org/10.3390/molecules30081861.
4. Li, M.; Chen, J.; Wang, Q.; Liu, C.; Song, W.; Sun, L. Characteristics, antioxidant activity stability, and anti-fatigue activity of hydrolysates from *Cucumaria frondosa* tentacles. *Molecules* **2025**, *30*, 889. https://doi.org/10.3390/molecules30040889.
5. Maione, A.; Buonanno, A.; Imparato, M.; Maglione, G.; Rossetti, C.; Montone, A.M.I.; Guida, M.; Galdiero, E.; Zinno, P. Antibacterial and antibiofilm efficacy of phenyllactic acid against foodborne pathogens Salmonella enterica serotype derby and *Escherichia coli* O26. *Molecules* **2025**, *30*, 1738. https://doi.org/10.3390/molecules30081738.
6. Moriwaki, C.; Takahashi, S.; Thi Vu, N.; Miyake, Y.; Kataoka, T. 1′-acetoxychavicol acetate selectively downregulates tumor necrosis factor receptor-associated factor 2 (TRAF2) expression. *Molecules* **2025**, *30*, 1243. https://doi.org/10.3390/molecules30061243.
7. Naidoo, K.; Khathi, A. Investigating the effects of Gossypetin on liver health in diet-induced pre-diabetic male Sprague Dawley rats. *Molecules* **2025**, *30*, 1834. https://doi.org/10.3390/molecules30081834.
8. Redjeki, S.G.; Hulwana, A.F.; Aulia, R.N.; Maya, I.; Chaerunisaa, A.Y.; Sriwidodo, S. Sacha Inchi (*Plukenetia volubilis*): Potential bioactivity, extraction methods, and microencapsulation techniques. *Molecules* **2025**, *30*, 160. https://doi.org/10.3390/molecules30010160.
9. Roșcan, A.G.; Ifrim, I.-L.; Patriciu, O.-I.; Fînaru, A.-L. Exploring the therapeutic value of some vegetative parts of Rubus and Prunus: A literature review on bioactive profiles and their pharmaceutical and cosmetic interest. *Molecules* **2025**, *30*, 3144. https://doi.org/10.3390/molecules30153144.

10. Silva, G.; Marques, A.M.; Sampaio, A.L.F. Anticancer effects of Withanolides: In silico prediction of pharmacological properties. *Molecules* **2025**, *30*, 2457. https://doi.org/10.3390/molecules30112457.
11. Śliwińska, A.A.; Tomiczak, K. Advancing the potential of *Polyscias fruticosa* as a source of bioactive compounds: Biotechnological and pharmacological perspectives. *Molecules* **2025**, *30*, 3460. https://doi.org/10.3390/molecules30173460.
12. Torres-Medicis, J.P.; Bustos-Brito, C.; Quijano, L.; Bedolla-Garcia, B.Y.; Zamudio, S.; Ramirez-Apan, T.; Martinez-Otero, D.; Esquivel, B. The antiproliferative activity and no inhibition of neo-clerodane diterpenoids from Salvia guevarae in raw 264.7 macrophages. *Molecules* **2025**, *30*, 1628. https://dor.org/10.3390/molecules30071628.
13. Yodweerapong, T.; Ueno, Y.; Yamaguchi, R.; Yarangsee, P.; Kimura, K.I.; Kataoka, T. Kujigamberol inhibits IFN-gamma and IL-2 mRNA expression and NFATc2 binding to their promoters in response to a phorbol ester and ionomycin stimulation. *Molecules* **2025**, *30*, 2214. https://doi.org/10.3390/molecules30102214.

References

1. Butler, M.S.; Capon, R.J.; Blaskovich, M.A.T.; Henderson, I.R. Natural product-derived compounds in clinical trials and drug approvals. *Nat. Prod. Rep.* **2025**. [CrossRef] [PubMed]
2. Del Carratore, F.; Breitling, R. Engineering microbiomes for natural product discovery and production. In *Natural Product Reports*; The Royal Society of Chemistry: London, UK, 2025.
3. Gagare, S.; Patil, P.; Jain, A. Natural product-inspired strategies towards the discovery of novel bioactive molecules. *Future J. Pharm. Sci.* **2024**, *10*, 55. [CrossRef]
4. Zhai, L.; Hao, B.; Dammer, E.B.; Xu, Z. Editorial: Mechanism study of bioactive molecules using omics technology. *Front. Cell Dev. Biol.* **2025**, *13*, 1720475. [CrossRef] [PubMed]
5. Dzobo, K. The role of natural products as sources of therapeutic agents for innovative drug discovery. *Compr. Pharmacol.* **2022**, *2*, 408–422.
6. Safe, S. Natural products as anticancer agents and enhancing their efficacy by a mechanism-based precision approach. *Explor. Drug Sci.* **2024**, *2*, 408–427. [CrossRef]
7. Loh, J.S.; Low, C.Y.; Low, W.P.; Ng, Y.L.; Mak, W.Q.; Stella Tan, L.K.; Chan, H.H.; Ong, Y.S.; Cheah, S.K.A.; Albert, E.L.; et al. Traversing the Valley of Death for nanotechnology-based natural products: Strategies and insights from pharmaceutical stakeholders. *Drug Deliv. Transl. Res.* **2025**, *15*, 4126–4140. [CrossRef] [PubMed]
8. Ahmad, M.; Tahir, M.; Hong, Z.; Zia, M.A.; Rafeeq, H.; Ahmad, M.S.; Rehman, S.U.; Sun, J. Plant and marine-derived natural products: Sustainable pathways for future drug discovery and therapeutic development. *Front. Pharmacol.* **2024**, *15*, 1497668. [CrossRef] [PubMed]
9. Asano, T. Investigating the pharmacokinetics of natural products: Challenges and advances in bioavailability. *J. Pharmacogn. Nat. Prod.* **2024**, *10*, 326.
10. Cahyani, D.M.; Mubarok, A.S.; Hariawan, B.S.; Amalina, I.; Drake, P.; Parumasivam, T.; Sahu, R.K.; Rijal, M.A.S.; Sari, R.; Miatmoko, A. Nanoparticle tools for maximizing oral drug delivery. *Braz. J. Med. Biol. Res.* **2025**, *58*, e14459. [CrossRef] [PubMed]
11. Marcelino, S.; Hamdane, S.; Gaspar, P.D.; Paço, A. Sustainable agricultural practices for the production of medicinal and aromatic plants: Evidence and recommendations. *Sustainability* **2023**, *15*, 14095. [CrossRef]
12. Taesuwan, S.; Jirarattanarangsri, W.; Wangtueai, S.; Hussain, M.A.; Ranadheera, S.; Ajlouni, S.; Zubairu, I.K.; Naumovski, N.; Phimolsiripol, Y. Unexplored opportunities of utilizing food waste in food product development for cardiovascular health. *Curr. Nutr. Rep.* **2024**, *13*, 896–913. [CrossRef] [PubMed]
13. Martins, A.M.; Marto, J.M. A sustainable life cycle for cosmetics: From design and development to post-use phase. *Sustain. Chem. Pharm.* **2023**, *35*, 101178. [CrossRef]
14. Pourmadadi, M.; Aslani, A.; Holghoomi, R.; Fathi-karkan, S.; Rahdar, A.; Kharaba, Z.; Pandey, S. Harnessing bio-waste for biomedical applications: A new horizon in sustainable healthcare. *Eur. J. Med. Chem. Rep.* **2024**, *12*, 100234. [CrossRef]

15. Sapkota, B.; Pariatamby, A. Pharmaceutical waste management system—Are the current techniques sustainable, eco-friendly and circular? A review. *Waste Manag.* **2023**, *168*, 83–97. [CrossRef] [PubMed]
16. Mikropoulou, E.V.; Basdeki, A.; Halabalaki, M. Metabolism and bioavailability aspects of natural products of plant origin using mass spectrometry-based and metabolomic approaches. *Nat. Prod. Rep.* **2025**. [CrossRef] [PubMed]

molecules

MDPI

Article

1′-Acetoxychavicol Acetate Selectively Downregulates Tumor Necrosis Factor Receptor-Associated Factor 2 (TRAF2) Expression

Chihiro Moriwaki [1], Shingo Takahashi [1], Nhat Thi Vu [1], Yasunobu Miyake [2] and Takao Kataoka [1,3,*]

1 Department of Applied Biology, Kyoto Institute of Technology, Matsugasaki, Sakyo-ku, Kyoto 606-8585, Japan
2 Division of Molecular and Cellular Immunoscience, Department of Biomolecular Sciences, Faculty of Medicine, Saga University, Nabeshima, Saga 849-8501, Japan
3 Biomedical Research Center, Kyoto Institute of Technology, Matsugasaki, Sakyo-ku, Kyoto 606-8585, Japan
* Correspondence: takao.kataoka@kit.ac.jp

Abstract: 1′-Acetoxychavicol acetate (ACA) is a natural compound derived from rhizomes of the Zingiberaceae family that suppresses the nuclear factor κB (NF-κB) signaling pathway; however, the underlying mechanisms remain unclear. Therefore, the present study investigated the molecular mechanisms by which ACA inhibits the NF-κB signaling pathway in human lung adenocarcinoma A549 cells. The results obtained showed ACA decreased tumor necrosis factor (TNF)-α-induced intercellular adhesion molecule-1 (ICAM-1) expression in A549 cells. It also inhibited TNF-α-induced ICAM-1 mRNA expression and ICAM-1 promoter-driven and NF-κB-responsive luciferase reporter activities. Furthermore, the TNF-α-induced degradation of the inhibitor of NF-κB α protein in the NF-κB signaling pathway was suppressed by ACA. Although ACA did not affect TNF receptor 1, TNF receptor-associated death domain, or receptor-interacting protein kinase 1 protein expression, it selectively downregulated TNF receptor-associated factor 2 (TRAF2) protein expression. The proteasome inhibitor MG-132, but not inhibitors of caspases or lysosomal degradation, attenuated ACA-induced reductions in TRAF2 expression. ACA also downregulated TRAF2 protein expression in human fibrosarcoma HT-1080 cells. This is the first study to demonstrate that ACA selectively downregulates TRAF2 protein expression.

Keywords: 1′-acetoxychavicol acetate; TRAF2; TNF-α; NF-κB; ICAM-1; proteasome

1. Introduction

Pro-inflammatory cytokines are secreted predominantly by macrophages at sites of inflammation [1,2]. Pro-inflammatory cytokines up-regulate the expression of adhesion molecules, such as intercellular adhesion molecule-1 (ICAM-1) in various cell types, including endothelial, epithelial, immune, and tumor cells [3]. In vascular endothelial cells, ICAM-1 plays an essential role in the recruitment of circulating leukocytes and their transmigration from the interior of blood vessels to extravascular sites of inflammation [4,5]. ICAM-1 expression is also upregulated in several cancers, such as lung and colorectal cancers, and is associated with their malignancy, metastasis, and poor prognosis [6,7]. ICAM-1 expression is mainly regulated by the transcription nuclear factor κB (NF-κB) [8,9].

Tumor necrosis factor α (TNF-α) is one of the pro-inflammatory cytokines, and interacts with two cell-surface receptors: TNF receptors 1 and 2 [10]. TNF-α has been implicated in the pathogenesis of inflammatory diseases and in the promotion and progression of cancer [11,12]. TNF receptor 1 is ubiquitously expressed, whereas TNF receptor 2 is more restrictedly expressed [13,14]. TNF receptor 1 contains a death domain (DD), and interacts with multiple adaptor proteins, including TNF receptor-associated death domain (TRADD), receptor-interacting protein kinase 1 (RIPK1), and TNF receptor-associated factor (TRAF2), leading to the formation of the TNF receptor 1 signaling complex [12–14]. The TNF receptor 1 signaling complex is required for the activation of the inhibitor of NF-κB (IκB) kinase complex, which converts IκBα to its phosphorylated form [15,16]. Phosphorylated IκBα is immediately ubiquitinated and degraded by the proteasome, allowing for the release of sequestered NF-κB heterodimers into the cytoplasm and their nuclear translocation [17,18]. The NF-κB heterodimers induce the transcription of many genes, such as those regulating inflammation, tumor promotion and metastasis [19,20].

1′-Acetoxychavicol acetate (ACA) (Figure 1A) is a natural compound derived from plants of the Zingiberaceae family (e.g., *Alpinia galanga*), which are used as a spice and in folk medicine [21,22]. ACA exerts various biological effects, including anticancer and anti-inflammatory activities [21,22]. Related to anti-inflammatory activity, ACA has been reported to inhibit the lipopolysaccharide (LPS)-induced expression of inducible nitric oxide synthase and cyclooxygenase 2 in murine macrophage cell line RAW264 cells and mouse peritoneal macrophages [23–26]. Previous studies also reported that ACA inhibited IκBα degradation and the subsequent NF-κB signaling pathway in macrophages [23,24,26–28]. In several human cancer cell lines, ACA prevented the activation of NF-κB, which was activated constitutively or by the addition of inflammatory and carcinogenic agents [29–31] and in vivo tumor models [32,33]. However, the mechanisms of action of ACA on the NF-κB signaling pathway remain unclear.

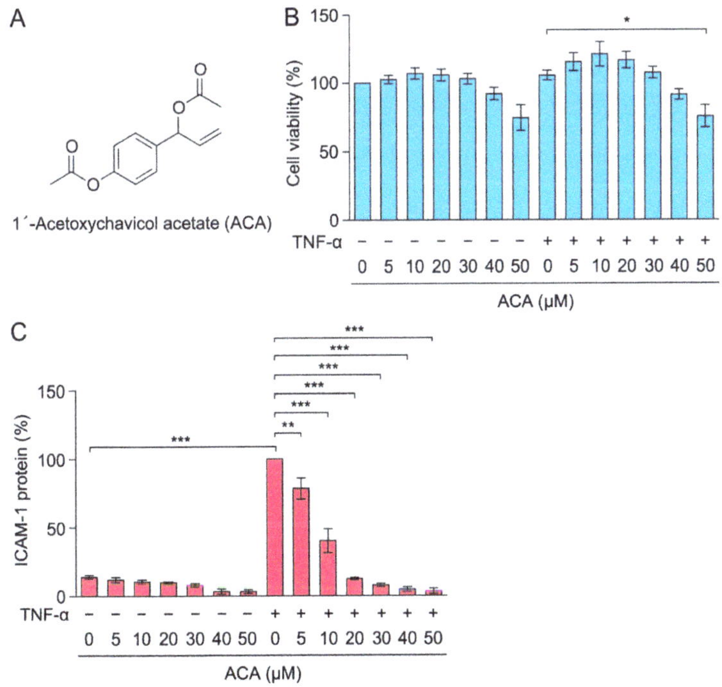

Figure 1. *Cont.*

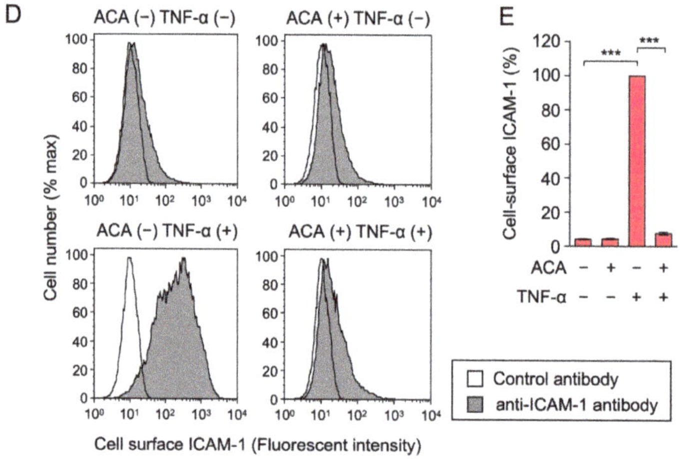

Figure 1. ACA inhibited TNF-α-induced ICAM-1 expression in A549 cells. (**A**) Structure of 1′-acetoxychavicol acetate (ACA). (**B**,**C**) A549 cells were preincubated with ACA for 1 h and then incubated with (+) or without (−) TNF-α (2.5 ng/mL) for 6 h in the presence or absence of ACA. Cell viability (%) is shown as the mean ± standard error of three independent experiments (**B**). Cell-ELISA was used to measure the amount of the ICAM-1 protein. ICAM-1 protein (%) is shown as the mean ± standard error of three independent experiments (**C**). (**D**,**E**) A549 cells were preincubated with (+) or without (−) ACA for 1 h, and were then incubated with (+) or without (−) TNF-α (2.5 ng/mL) in the presence (+) or absence (−) of ACA (30 μM). Cells were stained with a control antibody (white area) and an anti-ICAM-1 antibody (gray area) followed by a fluorescent secondary antibody, and were then analyzed by flow cytometry. Representative histograms are shown (**D**). Cell-surface ICAM-1 (%) is shown as the mean ± standard error of three independent experiments (**E**). * $p < 0.05$, ** $p < 0.01$, and *** $p < 0.001$.

To search anti-inflammatory and anticancer agents, we established a screening system to monitor the NF-κB-dependent expression of cell-surface ICAM-1 upon stimulation with pro-inflammatory cytokines in human lung adenocarcinoma A549 cells and human vascular endothelial cells [34]. During our screening, ACA was identified as a natural compound that inhibits TNF-α-induced ICAM-1 expression in A549 cells. Therefore, further investigations were conducted to elucidate the mechanisms by which ACA inhibits the NF-κB signaling pathway. In the present study, ACA was found to selectively downregulate the expression of TRAF2 among the components of the TNF receptor 1 signaling complex.

2. Results

2.1. ACA Inhibited TNF-α-Induced ICAM-1 Protein Expression in A549 Cells

Human lung adenocarcinoma A549 cells were preincubated with ACA for 1 h, and were then incubated with or without TNF-α for 6 h. Cell viability was assessed by 3-(4,5-dimetylthiazol-2-yl)-2,5-diphenyltetrazolium bromide (MTT)-reducing activity. ACA did not markedly affect the viability of A549 cells at concentrations up to 40 μM (Figure 1B).

ICAM-1 protein expression was evaluated by a cell enzyme-linked immunosorbent assay (cell-ELISA). ACA was found to inhibit TNF-α-induced ICAM-1 protein expression in a dose-dependent manner and basal level at concentrations higher than 20 μM (Figure 1C). The results of the flow cytometry analysis confirmed that ACA at 30 μM inhibited TNF-α-induced cell-surface ICAM-1 expression to the unstimulated level (Figure 1D,E). These results show that ACA inhibited TNF-α-induced ICAM-1 expression at concentrations that did not affect cell viability.

Following preincubation with ACA for 1 h, A549 cells were incubated with or without TNF-α for 24 and 48 h and then subjected to the MTT assay to assess cell viability. The results obtained showed that cell viability was reduced by ACA at concentrations higher than 20 μM for 24 h or 48 h (Figure 2A,B). Therefore, ACA reduced the viability of A549 cells more effectively when they were incubated for longer periods of time, which may be related to its anticancer activity.

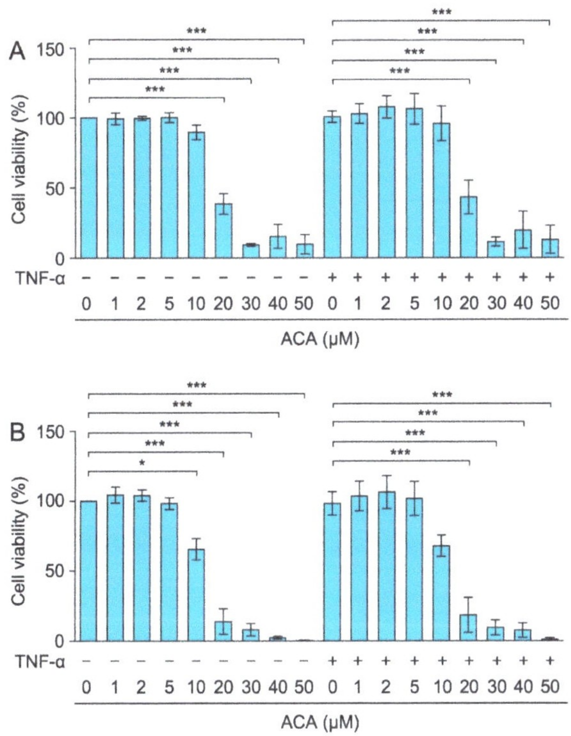

Figure 2. Effect of ACA on the viability of A549 cells for longer periods of time. (**A**,**B**) A549 cells were preincubated with ACA for 1 h and then incubated with (+) or without (−) TNF-α (2.5 ng/mL) for 24 h (**A**) and 48 h (**B**) in the presence or absence of ACA. Cell viability (%) is shown as the mean ± standard error of three independent experiments. * $p < 0.05$ and *** $p < 0.001$.

2.2. Glutathione and N-Acetyl-L-Cysteine (NAC) Did Not Reverse the Inhibitory Activity of ACA on TNF-α-Induced ICAM-1 Expression

Glutathione and NAC are often used as antioxidants that suppress reactive oxygen species (ROS). ACA has been shown to increase ROS generation in cancer cells, and glutathione and NAC suppressed the reduction in cell viability caused by ACA [35–39]. Therefore, we examined the abilities of glutathione and NAC to reverse the inhibitory effects of ACA on TNF-α-induced ICAM-1 expression. A549 cells were preincubated with glutathione and NAC for 1 h, followed by an incubation with ACA for 1 h, and were then stimulated with TNF-α for 6 h. Neither glutathione nor NAC at concentrations up to 10 mM affected the inhibitory activity of ACA on TNF-α-induced ICAM-1 expression (Figure 3A,B). Thus, these data suggested that the inhibitory activity of ACA on TNF-α-induced ICAM-1 expression was not due to ROS generation.

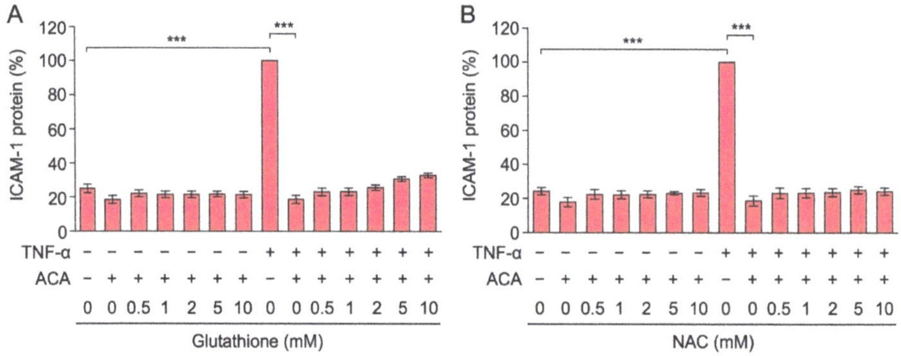

Figure 3. Glutathione and NAC did not reverse the inhibitory effect of ACA on TNF-α-induced ICAM-1 expression. (**A**,**B**) A549 cells were preincubated with glutathione (**A**) and NAC (**B**) for 1 h, and were then incubated with (+) or without (−) ACA (40 μM) for 1 h, followed by an incubation with (+) or without (−) TNF-α (2.5 ng/mL) for 6 h in the presence of compounds. The amount of the ICAM-1 protein was measured by cell-ELISA. ICAM-1 protein (%) is shown as the mean ± standard error of three independent experiments. *** $p < 0.001$.

2.3. ACA Inhibited TNF-α-Induced ICAM-1 mRNA Expression in A549 Cells

To investigate the effects of ACA on TNF-α-induced ICAM-1 expression at the mRNA level, total RNA was extracted and analyzed by reverse-transcriptase real-time PCR. TNF-α up-regulated the expression of ICAM-1 mRNA within 2 h (Figure 4A). ACA inhibited the TNF-α-induced expression of ICAM-1 mRNA in a dose-dependent manner and to the basal level at concentrations higher than 20 μM (Figure 4A).

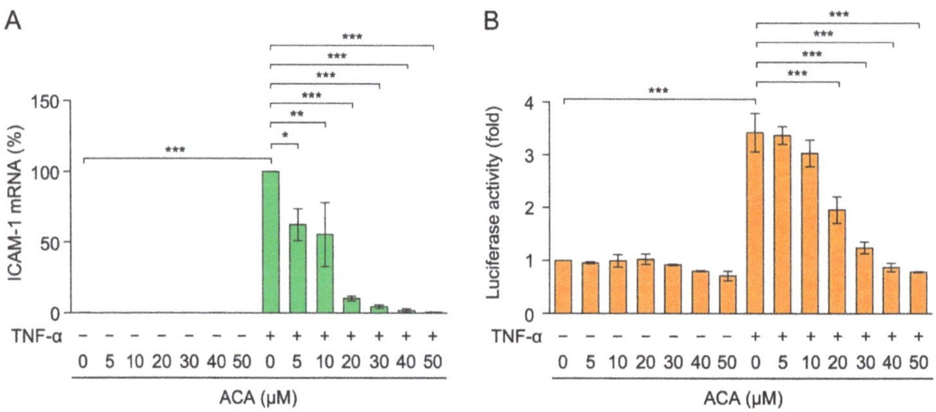

Figure 4. ACA inhibited TNF-α-induced ICAM-1 mRNA expression in A549 cells. (**A**) A549 cells were preincubated with ACA for 1 h, and were then incubated with (+) or without (−) TNF-α (2.5 ng/mL) for 2 h in the presence or absence of ACA. Real-time PCR was used to measure the amount of mRNA. ICAM-1 mRNA expression was normalized to β-actin mRNA expression. ICAM-1 mRNA (%) is shown as the mean ± standard error of four independent experiments. (**B**) A549 cells were transiently transfected with reporter plasmids encoding ICAM-1 promoter-driven firefly luciferase, together with a reporter plasmid encoding CMV promoter-driven *Renilla* luciferase for 24 h. Transfected A549 cells were preincubated with ACA for 1 h, and were then incubated with (+) or without (−) TNF-α (2.5 ng/mL) for 2.5 h in the presence or absence of ACA. Firefly luciferase activity was normalized to *Renilla* luciferase activity. Luciferase activity (fold) is shown as the mean ± standard error of three independent experiments. * $p < 0.05$, ** $p < 0.01$, and *** $p < 0.001$.

The luciferase reporter driven by the ICAM-1 promoter (−1604 to +40) was used to evaluate the effects of ACA on ICAM-1 transcription. A549 cells were transfected with an expression vector encoding the ICAM-1 promoter-driven firefly luciferase reporter. TNF-α up-regulated ICAM-1 promoter-driven luciferase activity within 2.5 h (Figure 4B). ACA decreased TNF-α-induced luciferase activity at concentrations higher than 20 μM (Figure 4B). These results indicate that ACA inhibited TNF-α-induced ICAM-1 expression at the transcriptional level.

2.4. ACA Inhibited the TNF-α-Induced NF-κB Signaling Pathway in A549 Cells

TNF-α-induced ICAM-1 transcription is mainly up-regulated by NF-κB transcription factors [8,9]. When the NF-κB luciferase reporter containing two copies of κB sites was used, TNF-α increased NF-κB-responsive luciferase reporter activity to a level similar to that of the ICAM-1 promoter-driven luciferase reporter (Figure 5A). ACA reduced TNF-α-induced NF-κB-responsive luciferase activity at concentrations higher than 20 μM (Figure 5A). These results demonstrate that ACA inhibited TNF-α-induced NF-κB-dependent transcription.

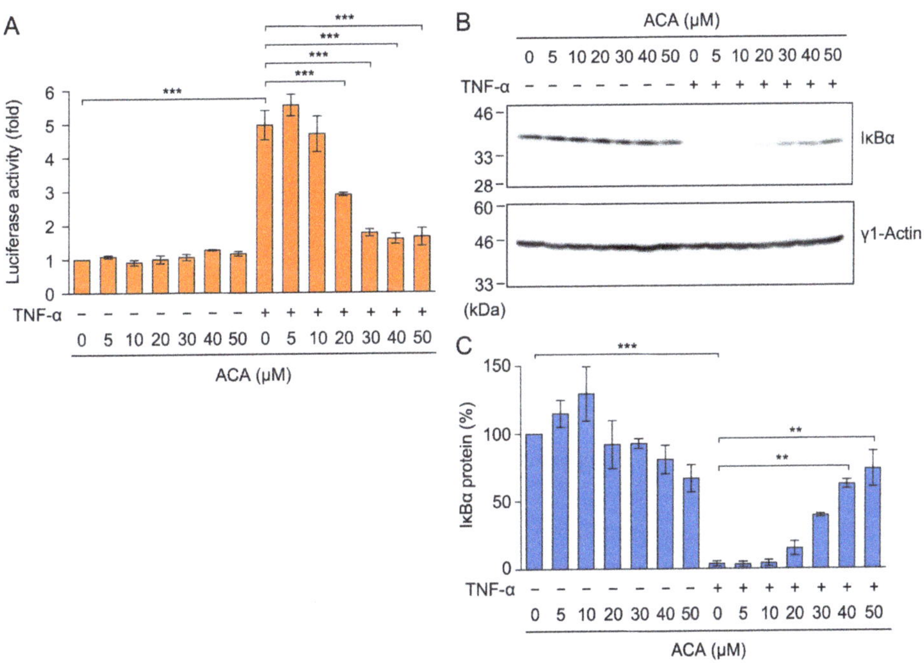

Figure 5. ACA inhibited the TNF-α-induced NF-κB signaling pathway in A549 cells. (**A**) A549 cells were transiently transfected with reporter plasmids encoding NF-κB-responsive firefly luciferase, together with a reporter plasmid encoding CMV promoter-driven *Renilla* luciferase for 24 h. Transfected A549 cells were preincubated with ACA for 1 h, and were then incubated with (+) or without (−) TNF-α (2.5 ng/mL) for 2.5 h in the presence or absence of ACA. Firefly luciferase activity was normalized to *Renilla* luciferase activity. Luciferase activity (fold) is shown as the mean ± standard error of three independent experiments. (**B**,**C**) A549 cells were preincubated with ACA for 1 h, and were then incubated with (+) or without (−) TNF-α (2.5 ng/mL) for 15 min in the presence or absence of ACA. Western blotting was performed to analyze cell lysates. Representative blots of IκBα and γ1-actin expression are shown (**B**). The amount of the γ1-actin protein was used to normalize the amount of the IκBα protein. IκBα protein (%) is shown as the mean ± standard error of three independent experiments (**C**). ** $p < 0.01$ and *** $p < 0.001$. Original blots are shown in Figures S1–S4.

NF-κB transcription factors are associated with the IκBα protein in the cytosol, and a TNF-α stimulation has been shown to induce the proteasome-dependent degradation of the IκBα protein [17,18]. In A549 cells, TNF-α induced the degradation of the IκBα protein within 15 min (Figure 5B,C). ACA inhibited the TNF-α-induced degradation of the IκBα protein in a dose-dependent manner (Figure 5B,C). These results show that ACA inhibited the TNF-α-induced NF-κB signaling pathway.

2.5. ACA Selectively Downregulated the Expression of TRAF2 in A549 Cells

TNF receptor 1 is responsible for the TNF-α-induced NF-κB signaling pathway in A549 cells because these cells express TNF receptor 1, but not TNF receptor 2 [40]. When A549 cells were exposed to ACA for 1 h, the amount of the TNF receptor 1 protein in cell lysates was not markedly decreased by ACA (Figure 6A,B).

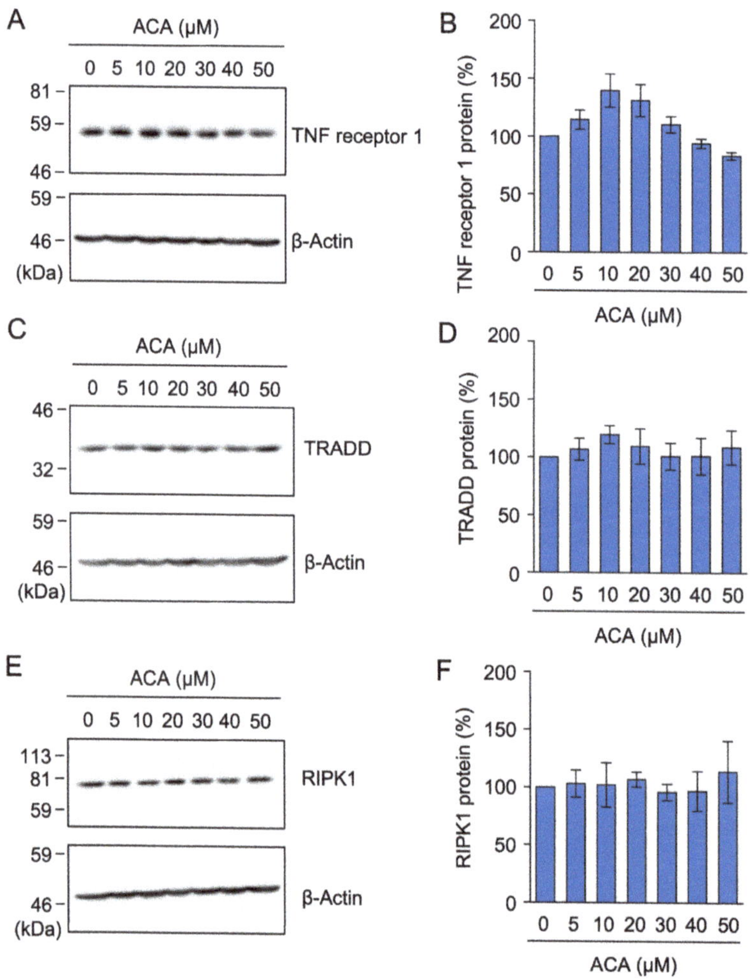

Figure 6. *Cont.*

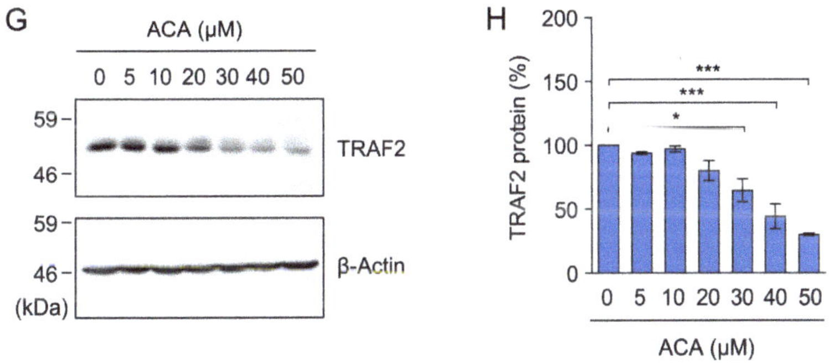

Figure 6. ACA did not affect the expression of the TNF receptor 1, TRADD, or RIPK1 protein, but reduced the expression of the TRAF2 protein in A549 cells. (**A–H**) A549 cells were incubated with the indicated concentrations of ACA for 1 h. Cytoplasmic fractions were prepared as cell lysates using 1% Triton X-100. A Western blotting analysis of cell lysates was then performed. Representative blots for the expression of TNF receptor 1, TRADD, RIPK1, TRAF2, and β-actin are shown (**A**,**C**,**E**,**G**). The amount of the β-actin protein was used to normalize the amount of each test protein. TNF receptor 1 protein (%), TRADD protein (%), RIPK1 protein (%), and TRAF2 protein (%) are shown as the mean ± standard error of three independent experiments (**B**,**D**,**F**,**H**). * $p < 0.05$ and *** $p < 0.001$. Original blots are shown in Figures S5–S20.

In response to a TNF-α stimulation, TNF receptor 1 has been shown to form a membrane-bound complex to trigger the NF-κB signaling pathway by recruiting TRADD, RIPK1, and TRAF2 [12–14]. To investigate the effects of ACA on the expression of components of the TNF receptor 1 complex, A549 cells were incubated with ACA for 1 h, cytoplasmic fractions were prepared as cell lysates using 1% Triton X-100, and these lysates were analyzed by Western blotting. ACA at concentrations up to 50 μM did not markedly affect TRADD or RIPK1 protein expression (Figure 6C–F). In contrast, ACA at 30–50 μM reduced TRAF2 protein expression (Figure 6G,H). These results showed that among the components of the TNF receptor 1 complex, ACA selectively reduced TRAF2 protein expression.

2.6. ACA Decreased the Amount of the TRAF2 Protein in Whole-Cell Lysates of A549 Cells

To further confirm the effects of ACA on TRAF2 protein expression, A549 cells were incubated with ACA for 1 h, and whole-cell lysates were prepared using 1% SDS lysis buffer. In whole-cell lysates, ACA reduced TRAF2 protein expression in a dose-dependent manner (Figure 7A,B). To clarify whether ACA promoted the translocation of the TRAF2 protein from cytoplasmic fractions to nuclear fractions, we lysed A549 cells using 1% Triton X-100 lysis buffer and separated them into cytoplasmic fractions and nuclear fractions containing nuclei and insoluble materials. A treatment with ACA for 1 h did not significantly affect the amount of the TRAF2 protein in nuclear fractions, while it decreased that in cytoplasmic fractions (Figure 7C–E). Therefore, these results showed that ACA promoted the downregulation of TRAF2 protein expression in whole-cell lysates.

2.7. ACA Promoted the Proteasomal Degradation of TRAF2 in A549 Cells

We previously reported that the treatment with the translation inhibitor cycloheximide for 1 h did not decrease TRAF2 protein expression in A549 cells [40]. Based on this finding, we herein investigated whether ACA promoted the proteolytic degradation of the TRAF2 protein using cellular proteolysis inhibitors, i.e., the caspase inhibitor Z-VAD-FMK, the proteasome inhibitor MG-132, and the vacuolar-type H^+-ATPase inhibitor bafilomycin A_1, which inhibits lysosomal degradation. MG-132 selectively reversed the reduction in the

TRAF2 protein in ACA-treated A549 cells, whereas Z-VAD-FMK and bafilomycin A_1 did not (Figure 8A,B).

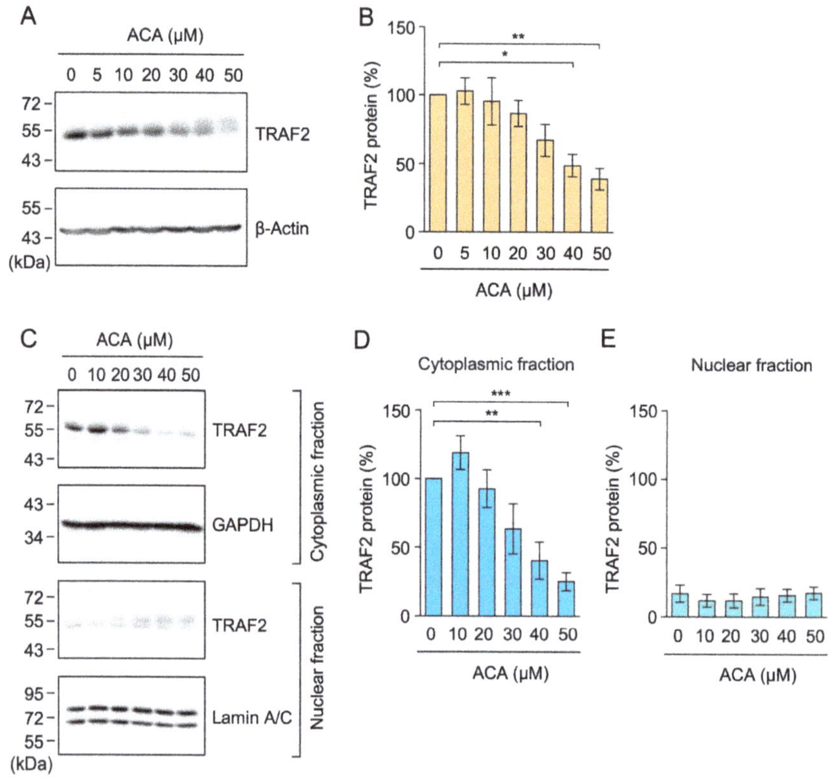

Figure 7. ACA decreased the amount of the TRAF2 protein in whole-cell lysates of A549 cells. (**A**,**B**) A549 cells were incubated with the indicated concentrations of ACA for 1 h. Western blotting was conducted to analyze whole-cell lysates prepared using 1% SDS. Representative blots for the expression of TRAF2 and β-actin are shown (**A**). The amount of the β-actin protein was used to normalize the amount of the TRAF2 protein. TRAF2 protein (%) is shown as the mean ± standard error of four independent experiments (**B**). (**C**–**E**) A549 cells were incubated with the indicated concentrations of ACA for 1 h. Western blotting was conducted to analyze cytoplasmic and nuclear fractions. Representative blots for the expression of TRAF2, GAPDH, and lamin A/C are shown (**C**). The amount of the GAPDH and lamin A/C proteins was used to normalize the amount of TRAF2 protein. TRAF2 protein (%) in cytoplasmic fractions (**D**) and nuclear fractions (**E**) is shown as the mean ± standard error of three independent experiments. * $p < 0.05$, ** $p < 0.01$, and *** $p < 0.001$. Original blots are shown in Figures S21–S32.

A previous study reported that ACA increased proteasome activity by activating protein kinase A in rat pheochromocytoma PC-12 cells [41]. Therefore, we investigated whether ACA increased proteasome activity in A549 cells. A549 cells were pretreated with or without the protein kinase A inhibitor H-89 for 1 h, and were then treated with ACA for 1 h. In contrast to PC-12 cells, chymotrypsin-like activity and trypsin-like activity were not markedly affected by the presence of ACA and/or H-89 in A549 cells (Figure 8C,D). These results indicate that ACA did not increase the global proteasome activity in A549 cells. Taken together, it appears that ACA affects the ubiquitination process of the TRAF2 protein prior to proteasomal degradation.

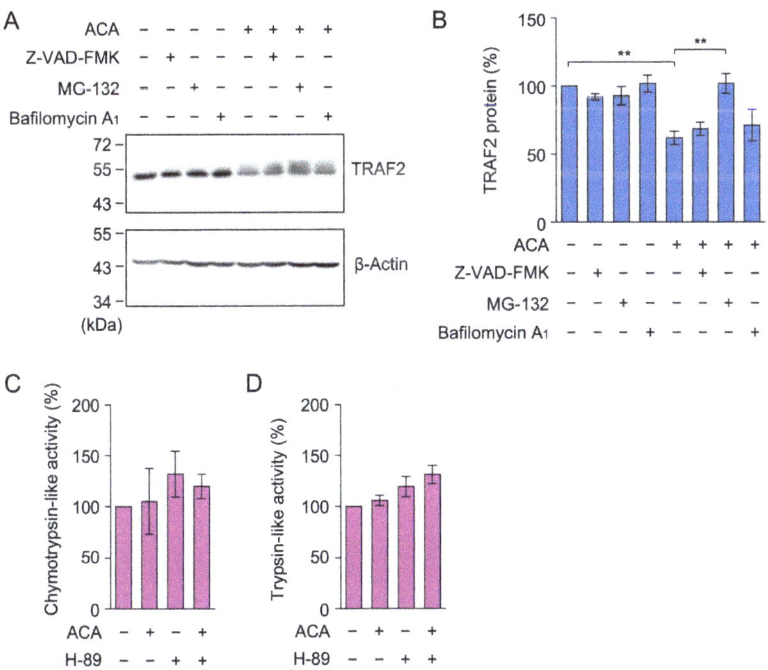

Figure 8. ACA promoted the proteasomal degradation of TRAF2 in A549 cells. (**A**,**B**) A549 cells were preincubated with (+) or without (−) Z-VAD-FMK, MG-132, and bafilomycin A_1 for 1 h, and were then incubated with (+) or without (−) ACA for 1 h (40 μM) in the presence of Z-VAD-FMK (20 μM), MG-132 (20 μM), and bafilomycin A_1 (100 nM). Western blotting was used to analyze whole-cell lysates. Representative blots for the expression of TRAF2 and β-actin are shown (**A**). The amount of the β-actin protein was used to normalize the amount of the TRAF2 protein. TRAF2 protein (%) is shown as the mean ± standard error of three independent experiments (**B**). ** $p < 0.01$. Original blots are shown in Figures S33–S36. (**C**,**D**) A549 cells were preincubated with (+) or without (−) H-89 (10 μM) for 1 h, and were then incubated with (+) or without (−) ACA (50 μM) for 1 h at the indicated concentrations. Chymotrypsin-like activity (%) (**C**) and trypsin-like activity (%) (**D**) are shown as the mean ± standard error of three independent experiments. No significant differences were observed in Figure 8C,D.

2.8. ACA Inhibited the TNF-α-Induced NF-κB Signaling Pathway in HT-1080 Cells

Human fibrosarcoma HT-1080 cells are responsive to TNF-α, which induces the activation of the NF-κB signaling pathway [42]. HT-1080 cells were used as an additional cell line to generalize the inhibitory activity of ACA on the TNF-α-dependent NF-κB signaling pathway. ACA decreased the viability of HT-1080 cells during a 3-h incubation at concentrations higher than 30 μM (Figure 9A). HT-1080 cells were treated with ACA for 1 h and were then stimulated with TNF-α for 15 min. TNF-α strongly induced the degradation of the IκBα protein (Figure 9B,C). ACA inhibited TNF-α-induced IκBα degradation at concentrations higher than 20 μM (Figure 9B,C). These results indicate that ACA inhibited the TNF-α-induced NF-κB signaling pathway in HT-1080 cells.

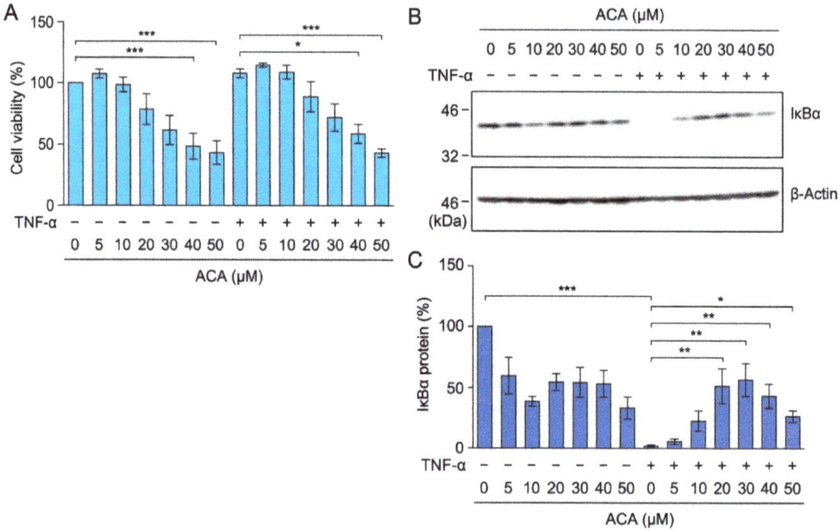

Figure 9. ACA inhibited TNF-α-induced IκBα degradation in HT-1080 cells. (**A**) HT-1080 cells were preincubated with ACA for 1 h, and were then incubated with (+) or without (−) TNF-α (2.5 ng/mL) for 2 h in the presence (+) or absence (−) of ACA. Cell viability (%) is shown as the mean ± standard error of three independent experiments. (**B**,**C**) HT-1080 cells were preincubated with ACA for 1 h, and were then incubated with (+) or without (−) TNF-α (2.5 ng/mL) for 15 min in the presence (+) or absence (−) of ACA. Western blotting was performed to analyze whole-cell lysates. Representative blots for the expression of IκBα and β-actin are shown (**B**). The amount of the IκBα protein was normalized to the amount of the β-actin protein. IκBα protein (%) is shown as the mean ± standard error of three independent experiments (**C**). * $p < 0.05$, ** $p < 0.01$, and *** $p < 0.001$. Original blots are shown in Figures S37–S40.

2.9. ACA Downregulated TRAF2 Protein Expression in HT-1080 Cells

Further investigations were performed to examine the effects of ACA on TRAF2 protein expression in HT-1080 cells. ACA markedly reduced TRAF2 protein expression at concentrations higher than 10 μM (Figure 10A,B). These results show that ACA reduced TRAF2 protein expression in HT-1080 cells at concentrations that did not affect cell viability.

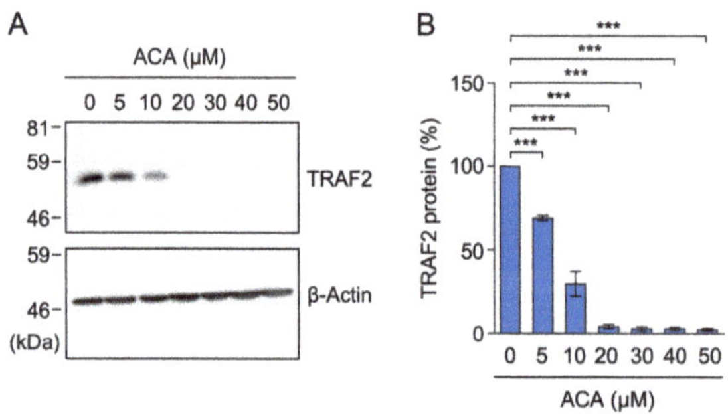

Figure 10. ACA downregulated the expression of TRAF2 in HT-1080 cells. (**A**,**B**) HT-1080 cells were incubated with ACA for 1 h. Western blotting was performed to analyze cell lysates. Representative blots for the expression of TRAF2 and β-actin are shown (**A**). The amount of the β-actin protein was used to normalize the amount of the TRAF2 protein. TRAF2 protein (%) is shown as the mean ± standard error of three independent experiments (**B**). *** $p < 0.001$. Original blots are shown in Figures S41–S44.

3. Discussion

ACA has been reported to inhibit the degradation of the IκBα protein and the subsequent NF-κB signaling pathway [23,24,26–33]; however, the underlying mechanisms remain unclear. In the present study, we found that ACA selectively downregulated TRAF2 protein expression without affecting the TNF receptor 1, TRADD, or RIPK1 protein. We also showed that ACA promoted the proteasomal degradation of the TRAF2 protein. These results reveal a novel biological activity for ACA, namely, the targeting of the TRAF2 protein. The potential mechanism by which ACA affects the TNF-α-induced NF-κB signaling pathway is shown in Figure 11.

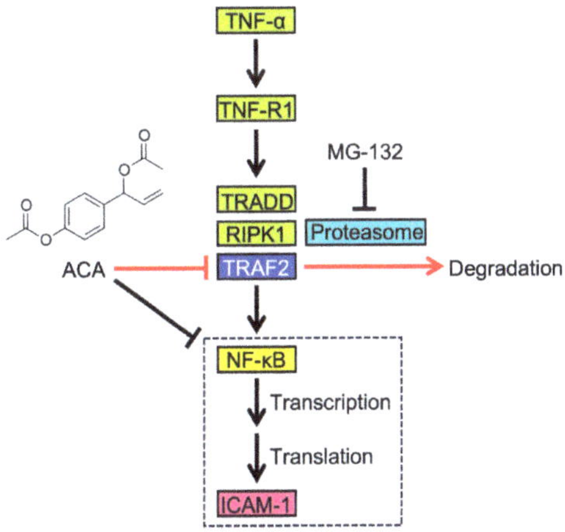

Figure 11. Proposed mechanism by which ACA affects the TNF-α-induced NF-κB pathway and ICAM-1 expression. Upon binding to TNF-α, TNF-R1 recruits TRADD, RIPK1, and TRAF2, which are required for the activation of NF-κB. NF-κB translocates to the nucleus and promotes the transcription of ICAM-1 as one of its target genes. ICAM-1 mRNA is then used to synthesize its translated product, which is transported to the cell surface. As an initial step in TNF-α-induced ICAM-1 expression, ACA downregulates TRAF2 expression through proteasome-dependent degradation. Luciferase reporter and quantitative PCR assays suggest that ACA inhibits the transcriptional process of NF-κB in addition to its effects on TRAF2.

ACA was previously shown to decrease cell viability and induce cell death in human breast cancer cells, mouse Ehrlich ascites tumor cells, and human leukemia HL-60 cells [35–39]. ACA increased ROS generation in cancer cells [35–39]. Furthermore, NAC or glutathione ethyl ester reversed the decrease in cell viability and the increase in cell death induced by ACA [35–39]. Consistent with these findings, ACA decreased cellular glutathione levels [35,38,39]. Therefore, these studies indicate that ACA inhibited tumor cell viability and induced cell death by affecting the intracellular ROS level.

ROS inactivate or activate the NF-κB signaling pathway in a cell context-dependent manner [43,44]. NAC and glutathione can be used as radical scavengers to inhibit the generation of ROS. In the NF-κB signaling pathway, many natural and synthetic compounds are known to bind the cysteine residues of essential proteins (i.e., IκB kinases and NF-κB subunits) and thereby inhibit their biological activities [34,45–47]. In addition to radical scavengers, NAC and glutathione can also be used to antagonize the binding of thiol-reactive compounds to their target proteins. To investigate whether the inhibitor activity of ACA is attributed to its binding of cellular proteins in a thiol-dependent manner or its promotion of ROS generation, NAC and glutathione were used as blocking agents. However, the addition of NAC or glutathione did not prevent TNF-α-induced ICAM-1 expression. Therefore, ACA appeared to inhibit NF-κB-dependent gene expression in a manner independent of the intracellular ROS levels or direct binding to cysteine residues of target proteins.

The NF-κB signaling pathway is activated by various stimuli, including pro-inflammatory cytokines and Toll-like receptor (TLR) ligands [2,48,49]. These stimuli trigger distinct sets of adaptor proteins required for the activation of the IκB kinase complex [12–14,48,49]. ACA has been reported to inhibit LPS (the TLR4 ligand)-induced IκB degradation in mouse RAW264.7 cells [23,26], LPS-induced IκB degradation in mouse bone marrow-derived macrophages and human monocytic THP-1 cells [28], and RANKL-induced IκB phosphorylation and degradation in RAW264.7 cells [27]. In the present study, we showed that ACA inhibited TNF-α-induced IκB degradation in A549 cells and HT-1080 cells. ACA also inhibited constitutively activated IκB phosphorylation and degradation in various human cancer cell lines [29,30]. The phosphorylation of IκB kinase α and β was decreased by ACA in human oral cancer cells [33]. Collectively, these findings suggest that ACA prevents the early process required for the activation of IκB kinase. However, it is currently unclear whether ACA inhibits a common step upstream of the activation of IκB kinase required for each signaling pathway.

Dose-dependent experiments were performed to examine the effects of ACA on ICAM-1 protein expression, ICAM-1 mRNA expression, ICAM-1 promoter-driven and NF-κB-dependent luciferase reporters, and TRAF2 protein expression. ACA almost completely inhibited TNF-α-induced ICAM-1 expression at the protein and mRNA levels at concentrations higher than 20 μM. Furthermore, ICAM-1 promoter-driven and NF-κB-dependent luciferase activities were decreased to unstimulated levels by ACA at concentrations higher than 30 μM. In the NF-κB pathway, ACA decreased TRAF2 protein expression and inhibited IκBα protein degradation in a dose-dependent manner at 20–50 μM. Therefore, ACA inhibited the NF-κB signaling pathway at the initial targets, while also suppressing downstream processes involved in transcription (Figure 11).

We demonstrated that a treatment with the translation inhibitor cycloheximide for 1 h did not affect TRAF2, TRADD, or RIPK1 protein amounts in A549 cells [40], indicating that these proteins are relatively stable in A549 cells. ACA selectively downregulated TRAF2 protein expression without affecting TNF receptor 1, TRADD, or RIPK1 protein amounts in cytoplasmic fractions. In whole-cell lysates prepared by 1% SDS lysis buffer, ACA decreased the amount of the TRAF2 protein. The presence of some TRAF2 protein in the nuclear fractions is consistent with previous findings showing the presence of TRAF2 in the cytoplasm and nucleus in different cell types [50–52] and the sequestration of TRAF2 in stress granules as insoluble materials [53,54].

The TRAF2 protein is ubiquitinated and subsequently undergoes proteasomal degradation [55–57] and lysosomal degradation [58,59]. The decrease in TRAF2 protein expression induced by ACA was reversed by the proteasome inhibitor MG-132, but not by the vacuolar-type H^+-ATPase inhibitor bafilomycin A_1, which blocks lysosomal proteolysis. ACA has been shown to increase proteasome activity by activating protein kinase A in rat pheochromocytoma PC12 cells [41]. In contrast to PC-12 cells, chymotrypsin-like and trypsin-like proteasome activities were not increased by ACA in the presence or absence of the protein kinase A inhibitor H-89 in A549 cells. Therefore, the ACA-induced downregulation of TRAF2 protein expression was not due to a global increase in proteasome activity. Thus, it seems most likely that ACA affects the ubiquitination process of the TRAF2 protein.

The TRAF family of proteins consists of seven members (TRAF1 to TRAF7) in mammals, and possesses conserved domains: the N-terminal RING domain (except TRAF1), the zinc finger domain, and the TRAF domain (except TRAF7) [60,61]. The RING domain is characterized by E3 ubiquitin ligases and is responsible for catalytic activity, while the

TRAF domain is divided into the TRAF-N domain and the TRAF-C domain, which are associated with receptors and adaptor proteins [60]. The TRAF2 protein has been shown to undergo ubiquitination mediated by Siah2, c-IAP1, and FBXL2 as the E3 ubiquitin ligase or its subunit [55,56,62,63], whereas ubiquitin-specific proteinase 19 (USP19) and USP48, as the deubiquitinating enzymes, stabilize the TRAF2 protein [57,64]. Therefore, in addition to constitutive transcription and translation, the cellular level of the TRAF2 protein is regulated by the overall balance of multiple E3 ubiquitin ligases and deubiquitinating enzymes. Further experiments are needed to clarify whether ACA promotes the ubiquitination of the TRAF2 protein.

Previous studies reported that ACA exhibited anti-inflammatory activities toward allergic and anaphylactic reactions, as well as anticancer activity toward various tumor cells, such as colorectal carcinoma cells, multiple myeloma cells, and breast carcinoma cells [21,22]. Regarding TRAF2, somatic mutations in TRAF2 have been detected in diffuse large B-cell lymphoma [65]; the knockdown of TRAF2 suppressed the proliferation of human breast carcinoma cells [66,67], and liquidambaric acid inhibited colon carcinoma cells by directly targeting TRAF2 [68]. Collectively, these findings indicate the potential of TRAF2 as a target for anticancer drugs. The ablation of TRAF2 has been shown to reduce the TNF-dependent cytotoxicity threshold, thereby augmenting the susceptibility of tumors to immunotherapy mediated by $CD8^+$ T cells [69]. Therefore, the downregulation of TRAF2 expression by ACA is promising as an anticancer agent.

4. Materials and Methods

4.1. Cell Culture

Human lung adenocarcinoma A549 cells (JCRB0076) and human fibrosarcoma HT-1080 cells (JCRB9113) were obtained from the National Institutes of Biomedical Innovation, Health and Nutrition JCRB Cell Bank (Osaka, Japan). Both cell lines were cultured with an RPMI 1640 medium (Thermo Fisher Scientific, Gland Island, NY, USA) containing fetal calf serum (Sigma-Aldrich, St. Louis, MO, USA), which was inactivated by a treatment at 56 °C for 30 min, and penicillin–streptomycin mixed solution (stabilized) (Nacalai Tesque, Kyoto, Japan).

4.2. Reagents

ACA (LKT Laboratories, Inc., St. Paul, MN, USA), bafilomycin A_1 (Cayman Chemical, Ann Arbor, MI, USA), glutathione (Nacalai Tesque), H-89 (Abcam, Waltham, MA, USA), NAC (Nacalai Tesque), Z-Leu-Leu-Leu-H (MG-132) (Peptide Institute, Osaka, Japan), and Z-Val-Ala-Asp(OMe)-CH_2F (Z-VAD-FMK) (Peptide Institute, Osaka, Japan) were obtained from commercial suppliers. Recombinant human TNF-α was provided by Dainippon Pharmaceutical Co., Ltd. (Osaka, Japan).

4.3. Antibodies

Primary mouse antibodies reactive to β-actin (A5441; Sigma-Aldrich, St. Louis, MO, USA), GAPDH (sc-32233; Santa Cruz Biotechnology, Dallas, TX, USA), γ1-actin (012-27823; FUJIFILM Wako Pure Chemical Corporation, Osaka, Japan), ICAM-1 (clone number: 15.2) (C167; Leinco Technologies, Inc., St. Louis, MO, USA), IκBα (610690; BD Biosciences, San Jose, CA, USA), lamin A/C (sc-376248; Santa Cruz Biotechnology), RIPK1 (610458; BD Biosciences), TNF-R1 (sc-8436; Santa Cruz Biotechnology), TRADD (610572; BD Biosciences), and TRAF2 (sc-136999; Santa Cruz Biotechnology), and a control mouse antibody (clone number: MOPC-21) (400101; BioLegend, San Diego, CA, USA), were used. A peroxidase-conjugated anti-mouse IgG(H+L) antibody (115-035-146; Jackson ImmunoResearch Laboratories, West Grove, PA, USA) and a phycoerythrin-conjugated anti-mouse IgG antibody (115-115-164; Jackson ImmunoResearch) were used as secondary antibodies.

4.4. Plasmids

A pGL4.22[luc2CP/Puro] vector encoding the ICAM-1 promoter (−1604 to +40) [70], an NF-κB-responsive firefly luciferase reporter vector [63], and a pCR3 expression vector containing cytomegalovirus promoter-driven *Renilla* luciferase were used in reporter assays. The NF-κB-responsive firefly luciferase reporter is under the control of two copies of κB sequences from the Igκ enhancer [71].

4.5. Measurement of Cell Viability

Cell viability was evaluated by using the MTT assay as previously described [72,73]. Absorbance at 570 nm was measured by an iMark™ microplate reader (Bio-Rad Laboratories, Hercules, CA, USA).

4.6. Measurement of ICAM-1 Expression

ICAM-1 expression was evaluated using cell-ELISA as previously described [72,73]. A549 cells were treated with an anti-ICAM-1 antibody (clone number: 15.2) as the primary antibody and a peroxidase-conjugated anti-mouse IgG antibody as the secondary antibody. Absorbance at 450 nm was measured by the iMark™ microplate reader.

4.7. Flow Cytometry

Flow cytometry was performed as previously described [74]. A549 cells were stained with the anti-ICAM-1 antibody (clone number: 15.2) or an isotype control antibody (clone number: MOPC-12) and then with a phycoerythrin-labeled secondary antibody, followed by an analysis using FACSCalibur (BD Biosciences) and FlowJo software version 8.5.1 (Tomy Digital Biology, Tokyo, Japan).

4.8. Measurement of mRNA Expression

Sepasol®-RNA I Super G (Nacalai Tesque), ReverTra Ace® (TOYOBO, Osaka, Japan), and TB Green® Premix Ex Taq™ II (Tli RNase H Plus) (Takara Bio, Kusatsu, Japan) were obtained from commercial suppliers. The primers for human ICAM-1 (148 bp) [75] and β-actin (143 bp) [76] were previously described. Real-time PCR conditions using Thermal Cycler Dice® Real-Time System Lite (Takara Bio) were described in another study [72,73]. The amount of mRNA expression was calculated based on primer-specific standard curves.

4.9. Luciferase Reporter Assay

HilyMax transfection reagent (Dojindo Laboratories, Kumamoto, Japan) was used for the transfection of luciferase reporter plasmids. The preparation of cell lysates and the measurement of firefly and *Renilla* luciferase activities were performed as previously reported [72]. Relative light units were measured by Lumitester C-110 (Kikkoman Biochemifa, Tokyo, Japan). Firefly luciferase activity was normalized by *Renilla* luciferase activity.

4.10. Preparation of Cell Lysates and Whole-Cell Lysates

Cells were washed with PBS and lyzed on ice for 15 min with Triton X-100 lysis buffer, consisting of 50 mM Tris-HCl (pH 7.4), 1% Triton X-100, 2 mM dithiothreitol, 2 mM sodium vanadate, and cOmplete™ protease inhibitor cocktail (Sigma-Aldrich). After centrifugation (15,300× *g*, 5 min), cytoplasmic fractions were collected as supernatants. Precipitates were washed with Triton X-100 lysis buffer and further treated with sonication to prepare nuclear fractions. To prepare whole-cell lysates, cells were washed with PBS and then treated with Triton X-100 lysis buffer or SDS lysis buffer, consisting of 50 mM Tris-HCl (pH 7.4), 1% SDS, 2 mM dithiothreitol, 2 mM sodium vanadate, and 2 mM PMSF, and further treated with sonication. Protein concentrations were measured by Protein Assay CBB solution (5×) (Nacalai Tesque).

4.11. Western Blotting

Cell lysates or whole-cell lysates were analyzed by Western blotting as previously described [72,73]. Images of Western blots were captured using an Amersham Imager 680 (GE Healthcare Japan, Tokyo, Japan). Membranes were treated with a stripping solution (Fujifilm Wako Pure Chemical Corporation) and were then subjected to additional Western blotting using anti-β-actin, γ1-actin, GAPDH, and lamin A/C antibodies. The intensity of protein bands was measured using ImageQuantTL software toolbox version 7.0.1.0 (GE Healthcare Japan). The amounts of target proteins were normalized by that of β-actin, γ1-actin, GAPDH, and lamin A/C.

4.12. Proteasome Assay

Proteasome activities were measured using the proteasome-Glo™ Chymotrypsin-Like Cell-based Assay (G8660) (Promega, Madison, MI, USA) and the Proteasome-Glo™ Trypsin-Like Cell-based Assay (G8760) (Promega). Cells were washed twice with PBS and were then suspended in PBS. The cell suspension was incubated with the proteasome assay mixture for 10 min. Relative light units were measured using Lumitester C-110.

4.13. Statistical Analysis

Experiments were independently repeated at least three times for a quantitative analysis. The number of experiments was described in each figure caption. Means ± standard errors were calculated from at least three independent experiments. Data were analyzed statistically by a one-way ANOVA followed by Tukey's test (KaleidaGraph software version 4.5.1.; Hulinks, Tokyo, Japan).

5. Conclusions

ACA is a major ingredient of plants in the Zingiberaceae family used as a spice and in folk medicine. The present results revealed the novel biological activity of ACA, which downregulates the expression of the TRAF2 protein via the ubiquitin–proteasome system. TRAF2 is one of the components of the TNF receptor 1 complex and regulates the NF-κB signaling pathway. Previous studies showed that ACA inhibited the NF-κB signaling pathway induced by various inflammatory stimuli, and the constitutive activation of NF-κB in in vitro cancer cell lines in in vivo tumor models. These findings indicate the potential of ACA as an anti-inflammatory and anticancer drug. Further studies are needed to elucidate the comprehensive molecular mechanisms by which ACA inhibits the NF-κB signaling pathway induced by various agents, including pro-inflammatory cytokines and the TLR ligands.

Supplementary Materials: The following supporting information can be downloaded at: https://www.mdpi.com/article/10.3390/molecules30061243/s1, Figure S1: Original blots in Figure 5B; Figure S2: Original blots (1) in Figure 5C; Figure S3: Original blots (2) in Figure 5C; Figure S4: Original blots (3) in Figure 5C; Figure S5: Original blots in Figure 6A; Figure S6: Original blots (1) in Figure 6B; Figure S7: Original blots (2) in Figure 6B; Figure S8: Original blots (3) in Figure 6B; Figure S9: Original blots in Figure 6C; Figure S10: Original blots (1) in Figure 6D; Figure S11: Original blots (2) in Figure 6D; Figure S12: Original blots (3) in Figure 6D; Figure S13: Original blots in Figure 6E; Figure S14: Original blots (1) in Figure 6F; Figure S15: Original blots (2) in Figure 6F; Figure S16: Original blots (3) in Figure 6F; Figure S17: Original blots in Figure 6G; Figure S18: Original blots (1) in Figure 6H; Figure S19: Original blots (2) in Figure 6H; Figure S20: Original blots (3) in Figure 6H; Figure S21: Original blots in Figure 7A; Figure S22: Original blots (1) in Figure 7B; Figure S23: Original blots (3) in Figure 7B; Figure S24: Original blots (3) in Figure 7B; Figure S25: Original blots (4) in Figure 7B; Figure S26: Original blots in Figure 7C; Figure S27: Original blots (1) in Figure 7D; Figure S28: Original blots (2) in Figure 7D; Figure S29: Original blots (3) in Figure 7D; Figure S30: Original blots (1) in Figure 7E; Figure S31: Original blots (2) in Figure 7E; Figure S32: Original blots (3) in Figure 7E; Figure S33: Original blots in Figure 8A; Figure S34: Original blots (1) in Figure 8B; Figure S35: Original blots (2) in Figure 8B; Figure S36: Original blots (3) in Figure 8B; Figure S37: Original blots in Figure 9B; Figure S38: Original blots (1) in Figure 9C; Figure S39: Original blots (2) in Figure 9C; Figure S40: Original blots (3) in Figure 9C; Figure S41: Original blots in Figure 10A; Figure S42: Original blots (1) in Figure 10B; Figure S43: Original blots (2) in Figure 10B; Figure S44: Original blots (3) in Figure 10B.

Author Contributions: Conceptualization, C.M., S.T., N.T.V., Y.M. and T.K.; formal analysis, C.M., S.T., N.T.V. and Y.M.; investigation, C.M., S.T., N.T.V. and Y.M.; writing—original draft preparation, T.K.; writing—review and editing, Y.M. and T.K.; visualization, C.M., S.T., N.T.V., Y.M. and T.K.; supervision, T.K.; funding acquisition, T.K. All authors have read and agreed to the published version of the manuscript.

Funding: This work was supported in part by the Japan Society for the Promotion of Science (JSPS) KAKENHI Grant number 19H02885 (to T.K.).

Institutional Review Board Statement: Not applicable.

Informed Consent Statement: Not applicable.

Data Availability Statement: Data will be made available upon reasonable request.

Conflicts of Interest: The authors declare no conflicts of interest.

References

1. Shapouri-Moghaddam, A.; Mohammadian, S.; Vazini, H.; Taghadosi, M.; Esmaeili, S.A.; Mardani, F.; Seifi, B.; Mohammadi, A.; Afshari, J.T.; Sahebkar, A. Macrophage plasticity, polarization, and function in health and disease. *J. Cell Physiol.* **2018**, *233*, 6425–6440. [CrossRef] [PubMed]
2. Wang, T.; He, C. Pro-inflammatory cytokines: The link between obesity and osteoarthritis. *Cytokine Growth Factor Rev.* **2018**, *44*, 38–50. [CrossRef] [PubMed]
3. Bui, T.M.; Wiesolek, H.L.; Sumagin, R. ICAM-1: A master regulator of cellular responses in inflammation, injury resolution, and tumorigenesis. *J. Leukoc. Biol.* **2020**, *108*, 787–799. [CrossRef] [PubMed]
4. Gerhardt, T.; Ley, K. Monocyte trafficking across the vessel wall. *Cardiovasc. Res.* **2015**, *107*, 321–330. [CrossRef]
5. Vestweber, D. How leukocytes cross the vascular endothelium. *Nat. Rev. Immunol.* **2015**, *15*, 692–704. [CrossRef]
6. Harjunpää, H.; Llort Asens, M.; Guenther, C.; Fagerholm, S.C. Cell adhesion molecules and their roles and regulation in the immune and tumor microenvironment. *Front. Immunol.* **2019**, *10*, 1078. [CrossRef]
7. Qiu, Z.; Wang, Y.; Zhang, Z.; Qin, R.; Peng, Y.; Tang, W.; Xi, Y.; Tian, G.; Zhang, Y. Roles of intercellular cell adhesion molecule-1 (ICAM-1) in colorectal cancer: Expression, functions, prognosis, tumorigenesis, polymorphisms and therapeutic implications. *Front. Oncol.* **2022**, *12*, 1052672. [CrossRef]
8. Zhong, L.; Simard, M.J.; Huot, J. Endothelial microRNAs regulating the NF-κB pathway and cell adhesion molecules during inflammation. *FASEB J.* **2018**, *32*, 4070–4084. [CrossRef]
9. Singh, M.; Thakur, M.; Mishra, M.; Yadav, M.; Vibhuti, R.; Memon, A.M.; Nagda, G.; Dwivedi, V.P.; Dakal, T.C.; Yadav, V. Gene regulation of intracellular adhesion molecule-1 (ICAM-1): A molecule with multiple functions. *Immunol. Lett.* **2021**, *240*, 123–136. [CrossRef]
10. Wallach, D. The tumor necrosis factor family: Family conventions and private idiosyncrasies. *Cold Spring Harb. Perspect. Biol.* **2018**, *10*, a028431. [CrossRef]
11. Ham, B.; Fernandez, M.C.; D'Costa, Z.; Brodt, P. The diverse roles of the TNF axis in cancer progression and metastasis. *Trends Cancer Res.* **2016**, *11*, 1–27. [PubMed]
12. Kalliolias, G.D.; Ivashkiv, L.B. TNF biology, pathogenic mechanisms and emerging therapeutic strategies. *Nat. Rev. Rheumatol.* **2016**, *12*, 49–62. [CrossRef] [PubMed]

be present in compound **4**, as in the case of **2**. The carbon signals at δ_C 200.0, 121.4, and 173.6 were assigned to C-2, C-3, and C-4 of this chromophore. These facts led us to establish the structure of compound **4** as 2-oxo-patagonol, as depicted in Figure 1. The absolute configuration of **4** was established as 5*R*, 8*R*, 9*S*, and 10*R* via a comparison between the theoretical and experimental ECD data (Figure 10).

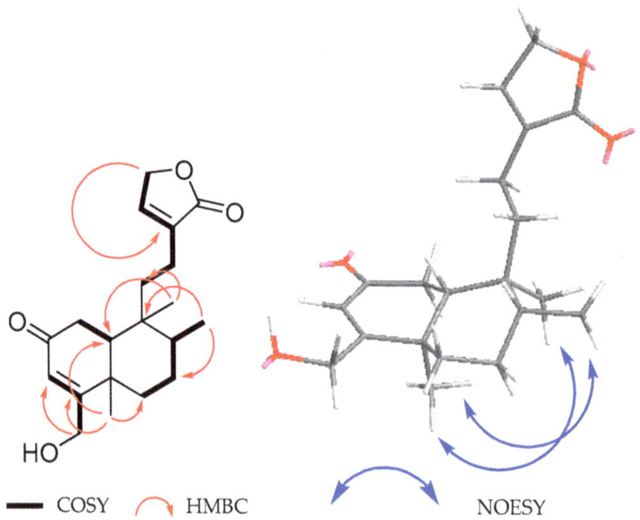

Figure 9. Selected COSY, HMBC, and NOESY correlations for **4**.

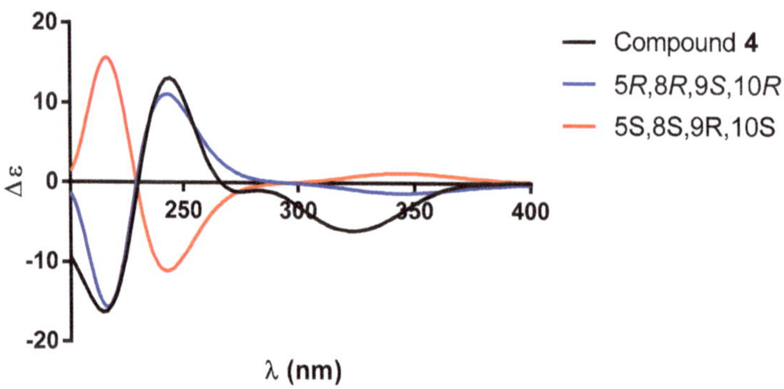

Figure 10. Comparison between the experimental (black line) and calculated ECD spectra for enantiomers (5*R*, 8*R*, 9*S*, 10*R*)-**4** (blue line) and (5*S*, 8*S*, 9*R*, 10*S*)-**4** (red line).

Diterpenoid **5**, $C_{20}H_{28}O_5$ (HR-DART-MS), had similar IR and NMR spectral data to those of **4**, except for the presence of multiple signals at δ_H 3.83 in the ^{1}H NMR spectrum of **5** (Table 3), ascribed to the hydrogen atom geminal to the hydroxyl group attached to C-6. The ^{13}C NMR spectrum of **5** supports the presence of this oxygenated function since a signal was observed at δ_C 73.8, ascribed to C-6. In agreement with the presence of a ketone carbonyl at C-2, the signals of an ABC system were observed in the ^{1}H NMR spectrum at δ_H 2.54 (dd, *J* = 17.8, 13.9 Hz), 2.37 (dd, *J* = 17.8, 3.4 Hz), and 1.91 (dd, *J* = 13.9, 3.6 Hz) (Table 3). The AB part was ascribed to the hydrogen atoms of the C-1 methylene and the C part to the β-*axial* H-10. The rest of the spectrum was similar to that obtained for 2-oxo-patagonol (**4**). As in the case of the previously described diterpenoids **2–4**, the absolute configuration of **5** was established via ECD spectroscopy. Figure 11 shows a

13. Wajant, H.; Siegmund, D. TNFR1 and TNFR2 in the control of the life and death balance of macrophages. *Front. Cell Dev. Biol.* **2019**, *7*, 91. [CrossRef] [PubMed]
14. Atretkhany, K.S.N.; Gogoleva, V.S.; Drutskaya, M.S.; Nedospasov, S.A. Distinct modes of TNF signaling through its two receptors in health and disease. *J. Leukoc. Biol.* **2020**, *107*, 893–905. [CrossRef]
15. Scheidereit, C. IκB kinase complexes: Gateways to NF-κB activation and transcription. *Oncogene* **2006**, *25*, 6685–6705. [CrossRef]
16. Hayden, M.S.; Ghosh, S. Shared principles in NF-κB signaling. *Cell* **2008**, *132*, 344–362. [CrossRef]
17. Bhoj, V.G.; Chen, Z.J. Ubiquitylation in innate and adaptive immunity. *Nature* **2009**, *458*, 430–437. [CrossRef]
18. Sasaki, K.; Iwai, K. Roles of linear ubiquitinylation, a crucial regulator of NF-κB and cell death, in the immune system. *Immunol. Rev.* **2015**, *266*, 175–189. [CrossRef]
19. Puar, Y.R.; Shanmugam, M.K.; Fan, L.; Arfuso, F.; Sethi, G.; Tergaonkar, V. Evidence for the involvement of the master transcription factor NF-κB in cancer initiation and progression. *Biomedicines* **2018**, *6*, 82. [CrossRef]
20. Guo, Q.; Jin, Y.; Chen, X.; Ye, X.; Shen, X.; Lin, M.; Zeng, C.; Zhou, T.; Zhang, J. NF-κB in biology and targeted therapy: New insights and translational implications. *Signal Transduct. Target Ther.* **2024**, *9*, 53. [CrossRef]
21. Chouni, A.; Paul, S. A review on phytochemical and pharmacological potential of Alpinia galanga. *Pharmacogn. J.* **2018**, *10*, 9–15. [CrossRef]
22. Kojima-Yuasa, A.; Matsui-Yuasa, I. Pharmacological effects of 1′-acetoxychavicol acetate, a major constituent in the rhizomes of *Alpinia galanga* and *Alpinia conchigera*. *J. Med. Food* **2020**, *23*, 465–475. [CrossRef] [PubMed]
23. Ohata, T.; Fukuda, K.; Murakami, A.; Ohigashi, H.; Sugimura, T.; Wakabayashi, K. Inhibition by 1′-acetoxychavicol acetate of lipopolysaccharide- and interferon-γ-induced nitric oxide production through suppression of inducible nitric oxide synthase gene expression in RAW264 cells. *Carcinogenesis* **1998**, *19*, 1007–1012. [CrossRef] [PubMed]
24. Murakami, A.; Matsumoto, K.; Koshimizu, K.; Ohigashi, H. Effects of selected food factors with chemopreventive properties on combined lipopolysaccharide- and interferon-γ-induced IκB degradation in RAW264.7 macrophages. *Cancer Lett.* **2003**, *195*, 17–25. [CrossRef]
25. Ando, S.; Matsuda, H.; Morikawa, T.; Yoshikawa, M. 1′S-1′-Acetoxychavicol acetate as a new type inhibitor of interferon-β production in lipopolysaccharide-activated mouse peritoneal macrophages. *Bioorg. Med. Chem.* **2005**, *13*, 3289–3294. [CrossRef]
26. Murakami, A.; Shigemori, T.; Ohigashi, H. Zingiberaceous and citrus constituents, 1′-acetoxychavicol acetate, zerumbone, auraptene, and nobiletin, suppress lipopolysaccharide-induced cyclooxygenase-2 expression in RAW264.7 murine macrophages through different modes of action. *J. Nutr.* **2005**, *135*, 2987S–2992S. [CrossRef]
27. Ichikawa, H.; Murakami, A.; Aggarwal, B.B. 1′-Acetoxychavicol acetate inhibits RANKL-induced osteoclastic differentiation of RAW 264.7 monocytic cells by suppressing nuclear factor-κB activation. *Mol. Cancer Res.* **2006**, *4*, 275–281. [CrossRef]
28. Ong, G.H.; Ori, D.; Kawasaki, T.; Kawai, T. Inhibition of lipopolysaccharide-induced inflammatory responses by 1′-acetoxychavicol acetate. *Genes Cells* **2022**, *27*, 482–492. [CrossRef]
29. Ichikawa, H.; Takada, Y.; Murakami, A.; Aggarwal, B.B. Identification of a novel blocker of IκBα kinase that enhances cellular apoptosis and inhibits cellular invasion through suppression of NF-κB-regulated gene products. *J. Immunol.* **2005**, *174*, 7383–7392. [CrossRef]
30. Ito, K.; Nakazato, T.; Xian, M.J.; Yamada, T.; Hozumi, N.; Murakami, A.; Ohigashi, H.; Ikeda, Y.; Kizaki, M. 1′-Acetoxychavicol acetate is a novel nuclear factor κB inhibitor with significant activity against multiple myeloma in vitro and in vivo. *Cancer Res.* **2005**, *65*, 4417–4424. [CrossRef]
31. Misawa, T.; Dodo, K.; Ishikawa, M.; Hashimoto, Y.; Sagawa, M.; Kizaki, M.; Aoyama, H. Structure-activity relationships of benzhydrol derivatives based on 1′-acetoxychavicol acetate (ACA) and their inhibitory activities on multiple myeloma cell growth via inactivation of the NF-κB pathway. *Bioorg. Med. Chem.* **2015**, *23*, 2241–2246. [CrossRef] [PubMed]
32. Batra, V.; Syed, Z.; Gill, J.N.; Coburn, M.A.; Adegboyega, P.; DiGiovanni, J.; Mathis, J.M.; Shi, R.; Clifford, J.L.; Kleiner-Hancock, H.E. Effects of the tropical ginger compound, 1′-acetoxychavicol acetate, against tumor promotion in K5.Stat3C transgenic mice. *J. Exp. Clin. Cancer Res.* **2012**, *31*, 57. [CrossRef] [PubMed]
33. In, L.L.; Arshad, N.M.; Ibrahim, H.; Azmi, M.N.; Awang, K.; Nagoor, N.H. 1′-Acetoxychavicol acetate inhibits growth of human oral carcinoma xenograft in mice and potentiates cisplatin effect via proinflammatory microenvironment alterations. *BMC Complement. Altern. Med.* **2012**, *12*, 179. [CrossRef]
34. Kataoka, T. Chemical biology of inflammatory cytokine signaling. *J. Antibiot.* **2009**, *62*, 655–667. [CrossRef] [PubMed]
35. Moffatt, J.; Kennedy, D.O.; Kojima, A.; Hasuma, T.; Yano, Y.; Otani, S.; Murakami, A.; Koshimizu, K.; Ohigashi, H.; Matsui-Yuasa, I. Involvement of protein tyrosine phosphorylation and reduction of cellular sulfhydryl groups in cell death induced by 1′-acetoxychavicol acetate in Ehrlich ascites tumor cells. *Chem. Biol. Interact.* **2002**, *139*, 215–230. [CrossRef]
36. Campbell, C.T.; Prince, M.; Landry, G.M.; Kha, V.; Kleiner, H.E. Pro-apoptotic effects of 1′-acetoxychavicol acetate in human breast carcinoma cells. *Toxicol. Lett.* **2007**, *173*, 151–160. [CrossRef]

37. Unahara, Y.; Kojima-Yuasa, A.; Higashida, M.; Kennedy, D.O.; Murakami, A.; Ohigashi, H.; Matsui-Yuasa, I. Cellular thiol status-dependent inhibition of tumor cell growth via modulation of p27(kip1) translocation and retinoblastoma protein phosphorylation by 1′-acetoxychavicol acetate. *Amino Acids* **2007**, *33*, 469–476. [CrossRef]
38. Higashida, M.; Xu, S.; Kojima-Yuasa, A.; Kennedy, D.O.; Murakami, A.; Ohigashi, H.; Matsui-Yuasa, I. 1′-Acetoxychavicol acetate-induced cytotoxicity is accompanied by a rapid and drastic modulation of glutathione metabolism. *Amino Acids* **2009**, *36*, 107–113. [CrossRef]
39. Xu, S.; Kojima-Yuasa, A.; Azuma, H.; Kennedy, D.O.; Konishi, Y.; Matsui-Yuasa, I. Comparison of glutathione reductase activity and the intracellular glutathione reducing effects of 13 derivatives of 1′-acetoxychavicol acetate in Ehrlich ascites tumor cells. *Chem. Biol. Interact.* **2010**, *185*, 235–240. [CrossRef]
40. Ogura, H.; Tsukumo, Y.; Sugimoto, H.; Igarashi, M.; Nagai, K.; Kataoka, T. Ectodomain shedding of TNF receptor 1 induced by protein synthesis inhibitors regulates TNF-α-mediated activation of NF-κB and caspase-8. *Exp. Cell Res.* **2008**, *314*, 1406–1414. [CrossRef]
41. Yaku, K.; Matsui-Yuasa, I.; Kojima-Yuasa, A. 1′-Acetoxychavicol acetate increases proteasome activity by activating cAMP-PKA signaling. *Planta Med.* **2018**, *84*, 153–159. [CrossRef] [PubMed]
42. Fukuhara, S.; Tanigaki, R.; Kimura, K.; Kataoka, T. Kujigamberol interferes with pro-inflammatory cytokine-induced expression of and *N*-glycan modifications to cell adhesion molecules at different stages in human umbilical vein endothelial cells. *Int. Immunopharmacol.* **2018**, *62*, 313–325. [CrossRef] [PubMed]
43. Nakajima, S.; Kitamura, M. Bidirectional regulation of NF-κB by reactive oxygen species: A role of unfolded protein response. *Free Radical Biol. Med.* **2013**, *65*, 162–174. [CrossRef] [PubMed]
44. Lingappan, K. NF-κB oxidative stress. *Curr. Opin. Toxicol.* **2018**, *7*, 81–86. [CrossRef]
45. Gilmore, T.D.; Herscovitch, M. Inhibitors of NF-κB signaling: 785 and counting. *Oncogene* **2006**, *25*, 6887–6899. [CrossRef]
46. Pande, V.; Sousa, S.F.; Ramos, M.J. Direct covalent modification as a strategy to inhibit nuclear factor-kappa B. *Curr. Med. Chem.* **2009**, *16*, 4261–4273. [CrossRef]
47. Zhang, J.; Zhang, R.; Li, W.; Ma, X.C.; Qiu, F.; Sun, C.P. IκB kinase β (IKKβ): Structure, transduction mechanism, biological function, and discovery of its inhibitors. *Int. J. Biol. Sci.* **2023**, *19*, 4181–4203. [CrossRef]
48. Kawai, T.; Akira, S. Toll-like receptors and their crosstalk with other innate receptors in infection and immunity. *Immunity* **2011**, *34*, 637–650. [CrossRef]
49. Cohen, P. The TLR and IL-1 signaling network at a glance. *J. Cell Sci.* **2014**, *127*, 2383–2390.
50. Min, W.; Bradley, J.R.; Galbraith, J.J.; Jones, S.J.; Ledgerwood, E.C.; Pober, J.S. The N-terminal domains target TNF receptor-associated factor-2 to the nucleus and display transcriptional regulatory activity. *J. Immunol.* **1998**, *161*, 319–324. [CrossRef]
51. Thakar, N.Y.; Ovchinnikov, D.A.; Hastie, M.L.; Kobe, B.; Gorman, J.J.; Wolvetang, E.J. TRAF2 recruitment via T61 in CD30 drives NFκB activation and enhances hESC survival and proliferation. *Mol. Biol. Cell* **2015**, *26*, 993–1006. [CrossRef] [PubMed]
52. El Hokayem, J.; Brittain IV, G.C.; Nawaz, Z.; Bethea, J.R. Tumor necrosis factor receptor associated factors (TRAFs) 2 and 3 form a transcriptional complex with phosho-RNA polymerase II and p65 in CD40 ligand activated Neuro2a cells. *Mol. Neurobiol.* **2017**, *54*, 1301–1313. [CrossRef] [PubMed]
53. Kim, W.J.; Back, S.H.; Kim, V.; Ryu, I.; Jang, S.K. Sequestration of TRAF2 into stress granules interrupts tumor necrosis factor signaling under stress conditions. *Mol. Cell. Biol.* **2005**, *25*, 2450–2462. [CrossRef]
54. Kim, W.J.; Kim, J.H.; Jang, S.K. Anti-inflammatory lipid mediator 15d-PGJ2 inhibits translation through inactivation of eIF4A. *EMBO J.* **2007**, *26*, 5020–5032. [CrossRef] [PubMed]
55. Habelhah, H.; Frew, I.J.; Laine, A.; Janes, P.W.; Relaix, F.; Sassoon, D.; Bowtell, D.D.L.; Ronai, Z. Stress-induced decrease in TRAF2 stability is mediated by Siah2. *EMBO J.* **2002**, *21*, 5756–5765. [CrossRef]
56. Li, X.; Yang, Y.; Ashwell, J.D. TNF-RII and c-IAP1 mediate ubiquitination and degradation of TRAF2. *Nature* **2002**, *416*, 345–349. [CrossRef]
57. Dhingra, R.; Rabinovich-Nikitin, I.; Rothman, S.; Guberman, M.; Gang, H.; Margulets, V.; Jassal, D.S.; Alagarsamy, K.N.; Dhingra, S.; Ripoll, C.V.; et al. Proteasomal degradation of TRAF2 mediates mitochondrial dysfunction in doxorubicin-cardiomyopathy. *Circulation* **2022**, *146*, 934–954. [CrossRef]
58. Vince, J.E.; Chau, D.; Callus, B.; Wong, W.W.L.; Hawkins, C.J.; Schneider, P.; McKinlay, M.; Benetatos, C.A.; Condon, S.M.; Chunduru, S.K.; et al. TWEAK-FN14 signaling induces lysosomal degradation of a cIAP1-TRAF2 complex to sensitize tumor cells to TNFα. *J. Cell Biol.* **2008**, *182*, 171–184. [CrossRef]
59. Li, L.; Soetandyo, N.; Wang, Q.; Ye, Y. The zinc finger protein A20 targets TRAF2 to the lysosomes for degradation. *Biochim. Biophys. Acta* **2009**, *1793*, 346–353. [CrossRef]
60. Park, H.H. Structure of TRAF Family: Current understanding of receptor recognition. *Front. Immunol.* **2018**, *9*, 1999. [CrossRef]
61. Arkee, T.; Bishop, G.A. TRAF family molecules in T cells: Multiple receptors and functions. *J. Leukoc. Biol.* **2020**, *107*, 907–915. [CrossRef] [PubMed]

62. Chen, B.B.; Coon, T.A.; Glasser, J.R.; McVerry, B.J.; Zhao, J.; Zhao, Y.; Zou, C.; Ellis, B.; Sciurba, F.C.; Zhang, Y.; et al. A combinatorial F box protein directed pathway controls TRAF adaptor stability to regulate inflammation. *Nat. Immunol.* **2013**, *14*, 470–479. [CrossRef] [PubMed]
63. Mallampalli, R.K.; Coon, T.A.; Glasser, J.R.; Wang, C.; Dunn, S.R.; Weathington, N.M.; Zhao, J.; Zou, C.; Zhao, Y.; Chen, B.B. Targeting F box protein Fbxo3 to control cytokine-driven inflammation. *J. Immunol.* **2013**, *191*, 5247–5255. [CrossRef] [PubMed]
64. Li, S.; Wang, D.; Zhao, J.; Weathington, N.M.; Shang, D.; Zhao, Y. The deubiquitinating enzyme USP48 stabilizes TRAF2 and reduces E-cadherin-mediated adherens junctions. *FASEB J.* **2018**, *32*, 230–242. [CrossRef]
65. Compagno, M.; Lim, W.K.; Grunn, A.; Nandula, S.V.; Brahmachary, M.; Shen, Q.; Bertoni, F.; Ponzoni, M.; Scandurra, M.; Califano, A.; et al. Mutations of multiple genes cause deregulation of NF-κB in diffuse large B-cell lymphoma. *Nature* **2009**, *459*, 717–721. [CrossRef]
66. Sun, L.L.; Wang, J.; Zhao, Z.J.; Liu, N.; Wang, A.L.; Ren, H.Y.; Yang, F.; Diao, K.X.; Fu, W.N.; Wan, E.H.; et al. Suppressive role of miR-502-5p in breast cancer via downregulation of TRAF2. *Oncol. Rep.* **2014**, *31*, 2085–2092. [CrossRef]
67. Peramuhendige, P.; Marino, S.; Bishop, R.T.; de Ridder, D.; Khogeer, A.; Baldini, I.; Capulli, M.; Rucci, N.; Idris, A.I. TRAF2 in osteotropic breast cancer cells enhances skeletal tumour growth and promotes osteolysis. *Sci. Rep.* **2018**, *8*, 39. [CrossRef]
68. Yan, R.; Zhu, H.; Huang, P.; Yang, M.; Shen, M.; Pan, Y.; Zhang, C.; Zhou, X.; Li, H.; Ke, X.; et al. Liquidambaric acid inhibits Wnt/β-catenin signaling and colon cancer via targeting TNF receptor-associated factor 2. *Cell Rep.* **2022**, *38*, 110319. [CrossRef]
69. Vredevoogd, D.W.; Kuilman, T.; Ligtenberg, M.A.; Boshuizen, J.; Stecker, K.E.; de Bruijn, B.; Krijgsman, O.; Huang, X.; Kenski, J.C.N.; Lacroix, R.; et al. Augmenting immunotherapy impact by lowering tumor TNF cytotoxicity threshold. *Cell* **2019**, *178*, 585–599. [CrossRef]
70. Vo, N.T.; Kusagawa, E.; Nakano, K.; Moriwaki, C.; Miyake, Y.; Haruyama, S.; Fukuhara, S.; Nguyen, N.T.; Dang, P.H.; Nguyen, M.T.T.; et al. Biological evaluation of alkyl triphenylphosphonium ostruthin derivatives as potential anti-inflammatory agents targeting the nuclear factor κB signaling pathway in human lung adenocarcinoma A549 cells. *BioChem* **2021**, *1*, 107–121. [CrossRef]
71. Dohrman, A.; Kataoka, T.; Cuenin, S.; Russell, J.Q.; Tschopp, J.; Budd, R.C. Cellular FLIP (long form) regulates CD8$^+$ T cell activation through caspase-8-dependent NF-κB activation. *J. Immunol.* **2005**, *174*, 5270–5278. [CrossRef] [PubMed]
72. Vu, Q.V.; Baba, K.; Sakaki, S.; Kawaguchi, K.; Hirano, H.; Osada, H.; Kataoka, T. Alantolactone derivatives inhibit the tumor necrosis factor α-induced nuclear factor κB pathway by a different mechanism from alantolactone. *Eur. J. Pharmacol.* **2024**, *969*, 176458. [CrossRef] [PubMed]
73. Vu, Q.V.; Vu, N.T.; Baba, K.; Sasaki, S.; Tamura, R.; Morimoto, K.; Hirano, H.; Osada, H.; Kataoka, T. Porphyrin derivatives inhibit tumor necrosis factor α-induced gene expression and reduce the expression and increase the cross-linked forms of cellular components of the nuclear factor κB signaling pathway. *Eur. J. Pharmacol.* **2024**, *977*, 176747. [CrossRef] [PubMed]
74. Vo, N.T.; Sasaki, S.; Miyake, Y.; Nguyen, N.T.; Dang, P.H.; Nguyen, M.T.T.; Kataoka, T. α-Conidendrin inhibits the expression of intercellular adhesion molecule-1 induced by tumor necrosis factor-α in human lung adenocarcinoma A549 cells. *Eur. J. Pharmacol.* **2021**, *890*, 173651. [CrossRef]
75. Wan, M.; Liu, J.; Ouyang, X. Nucleotide-binding oligomerization domain 1 regulates *Porphyromonas gingivalis*-induced vascular cell adhesion molecule 1 and intercellular adhesion molecule 1 expression in endothelial cells through NF-κB pathway. *J. Periodontal. Res.* **2015**, *50*, 189–196. [CrossRef]
76. Zhang, Y.; Lian, F.; Zhu, Y.; Xia, M.; Wang, Q.; Ling, W.; Wang, X.D. Cyanidin-3-*O*-*β*-glucoside inhibits LPS-induced expression of inflammatory mediators through decreasing IκBα phosphorylation in THP-1 cells. *Inflamm. Res.* **2010**, *59*, 723–730. [CrossRef]

molecules

MDPI

Article

Investigating the Effects of Gossypetin on Liver Health in Diet-Induced Pre-Diabetic Male Sprague Dawley Rats

Karishma Naidoo * and Andile Khathi

Department of Human Physiology, School of Laboratory Medicine and Medical Sciences, College of Health Sciences, University of KwaZulu-Natal, Durban 4000, South Africa; khathia@ukzn.ac.za
* Correspondence: karishma280199@gmail.com; Tel.: +27-31-260-7132

Abstract: The rising prevalence of non-alcoholic fatty liver disease among patients with type 2 diabetes mellitus has emerged as a global health challenge. Gossypetin (GTIN) is a natural flavonoid which has recently demonstrated antihyperglycaemic, antioxidant, and anti-inflammatory effects. Despite these findings, no studies have investigated its effects on liver health in the pre-diabetic state. Hence, this study aimed to investigate the effects of GTIN on liver health in diet-induced pre-diabetic male rats in the presence and absence of dietary intervention and to compare these effects with those of metformin (MET). Following 20 weeks of pre-diabetes induction, the animals were divided into six groups ($n = 6$) as follows: non-pre-diabetic (NPD) control, pre-diabetic (PD) control, and PD groups treated with GTIN (15 mg/kg body weight (bw)) or metformin (500 mg/kg bw) on either a normal diet or a high-fat, high-carbohydrate diet for 12 weeks. The results showed that the PD group had significantly higher liver triglycerides (TAG), liver weights, sterol regulatory binding element regulatory protein-1c (SREBP-1c), malondialdehyde (MDA) levels, and liver injury enzyme levels, along with decreased liver superoxide dismutase (SOD) activity, glutathione peroxidase (GPx) activity, and plasma bilirubin levels in comparison to NPD. Histologically, there was an increased lipid droplet accumulation and structural disarray in the PD group. GTIN treatment significantly reduced liver TAGs, liver weights, and plasma SREBP-1c levels, as well as improved liver SOD and GPx activity while decreasing liver MDA levels and liver injury enzymes in comparison to the PD control. Notably, GTIN treatment increased plasma bilirubin levels. Liver histology in the GTIN-treated groups revealed decreased lipid droplet accumulation and improved tissue integrity. Similar results were observed for the liver parameters in the MET-treated groups. The findings of this study may suggest that GTIN and MET exhibit therapeutic effects on liver health in diet-induced pre-diabetes in both the presence and absence of diet intervention. Dietary intervention may confer beneficial effects on liver health, with the most favorable therapeutic outcomes observed through a combination of treatment with dietary intervention. Additionally, GTIN may exhibit greater hepatoprotective effects than MET in rats without dietary intervention.

Keywords: gossypetin; NAFLD; liver injury; flavonoids; steatosis; high-caloric diets

1. Introduction

The chronic intake of unhealthy diets coupled with sedentary lifestyles contribute to the development of diabetes and associated liver complications such as non-alcoholic fatty liver disease (NAFLD) [1]. Pre-diabetes precedes the onset of overt type 2 diabetes mellitus (T2DM), with previous studies showing that around 70% of untreated pre-diabetic individuals progress to T2DM [2,3]. Insulin resistance and hyperinsulinemia associated with pre-diabetes contribute to the development of liver complications [4]. Insulin resistance promotes increased liver triglyceride accumulation by disrupting the ability of insulin to suppress adipose tissue lipolysis [5]. Hyperinsulinemia, elevated glucose, and free fatty acid flux into the liver upregulates hepatic de novo lipogenesis through steroid regulatory elementary binding protein-1c [6]. The accumulation of lipids in the liver contributes to hepatic insulin resistance and the development of NAFLD [7]. This triggers a cascade of oxidative and inflammatory events which leads to liver damage [7]. Moreover, it has been shown that liver injury marker levels which include alanine transaminase and aspartate transaminase were significantly higher in the pre-diabetic state [8]. Histopathological changes observed in NAFLD include lipid droplet accumulation, inflammation, and lobular disarray [9]. This condition may not only disrupt the normal functioning of the liver but can also create a feedback loop in which liver impairment further exacerbates the pre-diabetic state [10].

The main approaches to the management of diabetes-associated liver dysfunction include a combination of dietary and pharmacological intervention [11,12]. There has been low patient compliance with lifestyle modifications due to the challenges of maintaining long-term dietary change and exercise [13,14]. Metformin is primarily used as a first-line treatment for T2DM and has been shown to improve liver health in the diabetic state [15]. However, there have been some challenges with the current drugs under investigation, which include inconsistent findings and a lack of evidence supporting their effectiveness in humans [16]. Thus, there is a need to identify compounds which are effective in treating diabetic liver complications in the presence and absence of dietary modifications. Flavonoids found in plant sources have been shown to improve T2DM and associated liver complications through their multifactorial effects, low toxicity, and vast availability [17,18]. Gossypetin (GTIN) is a naturally occurring flavonoid that serves as a structural analog of quercetin with an additional hydroxyl group [19]. This compound has been isolated from the calyx and flowers of *Hibiscus sabdariffa* [20]. Previous studies have highlighted GTIN for its potent antioxidant and anti-inflammatory properties [21, 22]. Recent studies have demonstrated that GTIN improves glucose homeostasis and cardiovascular function in the pre-diabetic state [23,24]. Despite these current findings, no studies have explored the effects of GTIN on liver health in the pre-diabetic state. Hence, this study aimed to investigate the effects of GTIN on liver health in both the presence and absence of dietary intervention in a diet-induced pre-diabetic male rat model and to compare these effects with those of metformin. The oral dose of 15 mg/kg GTIN was selected to be used in our study based on previous studies, demonstrating its efficacy and safety within the 10–20 mg/kg range [25,26]. The 500 mg/kg dose of MET was selected due to its established therapeutic benefits and minimal adverse effects [4,27].

2. Results

2.1. Liver Triglycerides and Liver Weights

Liver triglyceride levels and liver weights were measured to assess the extent of lipid accumulation and liver enlargement. A one-way ANOVA showed significant differences in liver TAG levels ($F (5, 30) = 68.11$, $p < 0.0001$) and liver weights ($F (5, 30) = 78.87$, $p < 0.0001$) between the groups. Post hoc comparisons showed (Figure 1) that the pre-diabetic (PD) control group exhibited significantly ($p < 0.05$) higher liver TAG levels and liver weights in comparison to the non-pre-diabetic (NPD) group. However, the PD animals receiving gossypetin with a normal diet (GTIN+ND) and a high-fat, high-carbohydrate diet (GTIN+HFHC) exhibited significantly ($p < 0.05$) lower liver TAG levels and liver weights in comparison to the PD control. Similar results ($p < 0.05$) were observed in the PD animals receiving metformin with a normal diet (MET+ND) and high-fat, high-carbohydrate diet (MET+HFHC) for liver TAG levels and liver weights. A two-way ANOVA revealed that both treatment (F (1, 20) = 45.16, $p < 0.0001$) and diet (F (1, 20) = 67.03, $p < 0.0001$) exhibited significant main effects on liver TAGs. Similarly, significant main effects of treatment (F (1, 20) = 18.08, $p < 0.0004$) and diet (F (1, 20) = 79.37, $p < 0.0001$) were observed for liver weight. There was a significant interaction between treatment and diet on liver TAG (F (1, 20) = 10.73, $p = 0.0038$). However, there was no significant interaction between treatment and diet on liver weight (F (1, 20) = 3.76, $p = 0.0667$). Post hoc comparisons showed that GTIN treatment (GTIN+HFHC) resulted in significantly ($p < 0.05$) lower liver TAG levels and liver weights in comparison to MET treatment (MET+HFHC). Animals on an ND (GTIN+ND and MET+ND) exhibited significantly ($p < 0.05$) lower levels of both parameters in comparison to those on a HFHC diet (GTIN+HFHC and MET+HFHC).

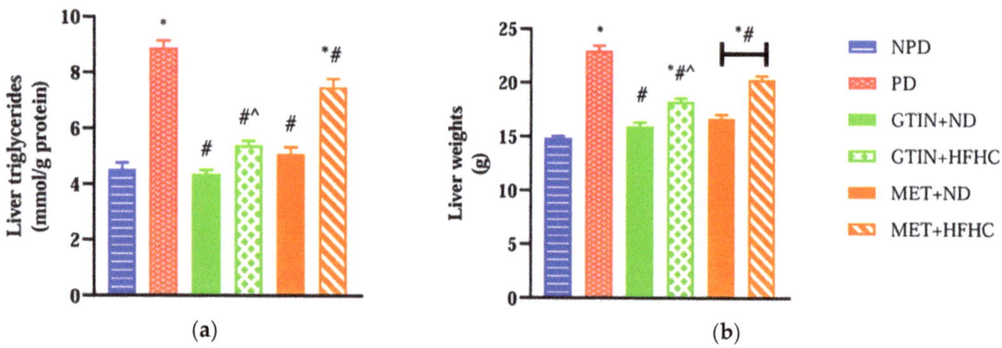

Figure 1. The effects of GTIN on (**a**) liver TAG levels and (**b**) liver weights in rats in both the presence and absence of dietary intervention at week 32 of the experimental period ($n = 6$, per group). Values are presented as mean ± SEM. * = $p < 0.05$ denotes comparison with the non-pre-diabetic control (NPD); # = $p < 0.05$ denotes comparison with the pre-diabetic control (PD); ^ = $p < 0.05$ denotes comparison with the metformin + high-fat, high-carbohydrate (MET+HFHC) group.

2.2. *Plasma SREBP-1c Levels*

Plasma SREBP-1c levels were measured to assess the regulation of lipogenesis in the liver. A one-way ANOVA showed significant differences (F (5, 30) = 74.47, $p < 0.0001$) in plasma SREBP-1c levels between the groups. Post hoc comparisons showed (Figure 2) that the PD control group exhibited significantly ($p < 0.05$) higher plasma SREBP-1c levels in comparison to the NPD group. However, the GTIN+ND and GTIN+HFHC groups exhibited significantly ($p < 0.05$) lower plasma SREBP-1c levels in comparison to the PD control. Similar results ($p < 0.05$) were observed for plasma SREBP-1c levels in the MET+ND and MET+HFHC groups. A two-way ANOVA revealed that both treatment (F (1, 20) = 24.86, $p < 0.0001$) and diet (F (1, 20) = 223.30, $p < 0.0001$) exhibited significant main effects on plasma SREBP-1c levels. There was a significant (F (1, 20) = 10.74, $p = 0.0038$) interaction between treatment and diet on plasma SREBP-1c levels. Post hoc comparisons showed that GTIN treatment (GTIN+ND) resulted in significantly ($p < 0.05$) lower plasma SREBP-1c levels in comparison to MET treatment (MET+ND). Animals on an ND (GTIN+ND and MET+ND) exhibited significantly ($p < 0.05$) lower levels of this parameter in comparison to those on a HFHC diet (GTIN+HFHC and MET+HFHC).

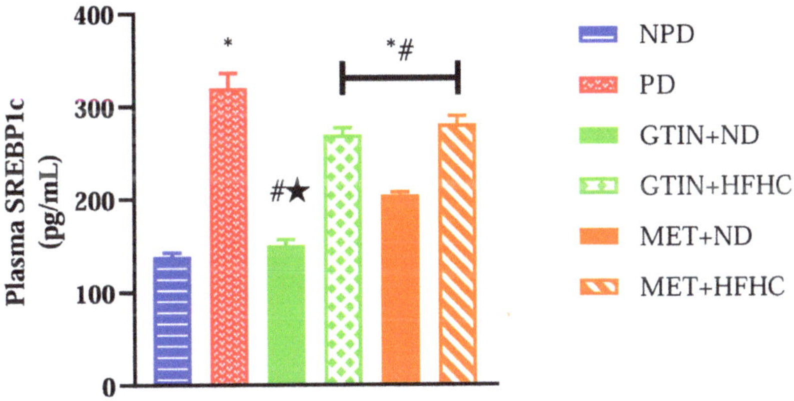

Figure 2. The effects of GTIN on plasma SREBP-1c levels in rats in both the presence and absence of dietary intervention at week 32 of the experimental period ($n = 6$, per group). Values are presented as mean ± SEM. * = $p < 0.05$ denotes comparison with the non-pre-diabetic control (NPD); # = $p < 0.05$ denotes comparison with the pre-diabetic control (PD); ★ = $p < 0.05$ denotes comparison with the metformin + normal diet (MET+ND) group.

2.3. Liver Oxidative Status

Liver oxidative status was assessed by measuring MDA levels for lipid peroxidation and SOD and GPx activities for enzymatic antioxidant defense. A one-way ANOVA showed significant differences in liver MDA (F (5, 30) = 14.44, $p < 0.0001$), SOD activity (F (5, 30) = 211.50, $p < 0.0001$), and Gpx activity (F (5, 30) = 29.17, $p < 0.0001$) between the groups. Post hoc comparisons showed (Figure 3) that the PD control group exhibited significantly ($p < 0.05$) higher liver MDA levels with reduced SOD and GPx activity in comparison to the NPD group. However, the GTIN+ND and GTIN+HFHC groups exhibited significantly ($p < 0.05$) lower liver MDA levels with improved SOD and GPx activity in comparison to the PD control. Similar results ($p < 0.05$) were observed for liver MDA levels and Gpx activity in the MET+ND and MET+HFHC groups. The MET+ND group showed significantly ($p < 0.05$) higher liver Gpx activity in comparison to the PD control.

A two-way ANOVA revealed that both treatment (F (1, 20) = 10.51, $p < 0.0041$) and diet (F (1, 20) = 34.04, $p < 0.0001$) exhibited significant main effects on liver MDA levels. Similarly, both treatment (F (1, 20) = 252.90, $p < 0.0001$) and diet (F (1, 20) = 138.50, $p < 0.0001$) exhibited significant main effects on liver SOD activity. Furthermore, both treatment (F (1, 20) = 10.59, $p = 0.0040$) and diet (F (1, 20) = 21.54, $p = 0.0002$) exhibited significant main effects on liver Gpx activity. There was no significant (*F (1, 20)* = 0.42, $p = 0.5242$) interaction between treatment and diet on liver MDA levels. However, there was a significant interaction between treatment and diet on liver SOD activity (F (1, 20) = 1.05, $p = 0.3174$) and Gpx activity (F (1, 20) = 4.54, $p = 0.0457$). Post hoc comparisons showed that GTIN treatment (GTIN+ND and GTIN+HFHC) resulted in significantly ($p < 0.05$) higher liver SOD activity in comparison to MET treatment (MET+ND and MET+HFHC). Additionally, GTIN treatment (GTIN+HFHC) resulted in significantly ($p < 0.05$) higher liver Gpx activity in comparison to MET treatment (MET+HFHC). Animals on an ND (GTIN+ND and MET+ND) exhibited significantly ($p < 0.05$) lower liver MDA levels and higher SOD activity in comparison to those on a HFHC diet (GTIN+HFHC and MET+HFHC).

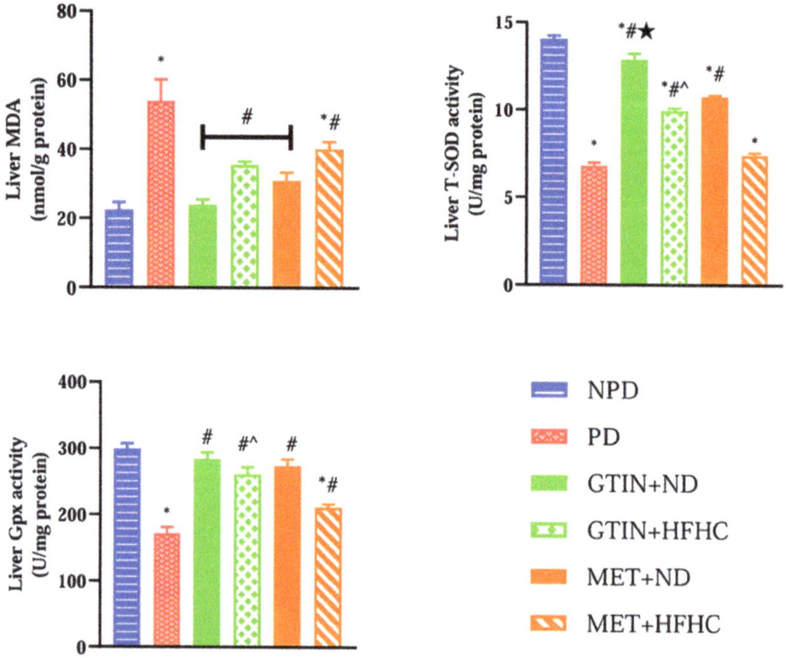

Figure 3. The effects of GTIN on liver oxidative status in rats in both the presence and absence of dietary intervention at week 32 of the experimental period ($n = 6$, per group). Values are presented as mean ± SEM. * = $p < 0.05$ denotes comparison with the non-pre-diabetic control (NPD); # = $p < 0.05$ denotes comparison with the pre-diabetic control (PD); ★ = $p < 0.05$ denotes comparison with the metformin + normal diet (MET+ND) group; ^ = $p < 0.05$ denotes comparison with the metformin+ high-fat, high-carbohydrate (MET+HFHC) group.

2.4. Plasma Liver Injury Enzymes

Plasma aspartate transaminase (AST) and alanine transaminase (ALT) were measured to assess liver function and injury. A one-way ANOVA showed significant differences in plasma AST (F (5, 30) = 59.97, $p < 0.0001$) and ALT (F (5, 30) = 122.50, $p < 0.0001$) levels between the groups. Post hoc comparisons showed (Figure 4) that the PD control group exhibited significantly ($p < 0.05$) higher plasma AST and ALT levels in comparison to the NPD group. However, the GTIN+ND and GTIN+HFHC groups exhibited significantly ($p < 0.05$) lower plasma AST and ALT levels in comparison to the PD control. Similar results ($p < 0.05$) were observed for plasma AST and ALT levels in the MET+ND and MET+HFHC groups. A two-way ANOVA revealed that both treatment (F (1, 20) = 33.80, $p < 0.0001$) and diet (F (1, 20) = 105.60, $p < 0.0001$) exhibited significant main effects on plasma AST levels. Similarly, both treatment (F (1, 20) = 27.82, $p < 0.0001$) and diet (F (1, 20) = 79.67, $p < 0.0001$) exhibited significant main effects on plasma ALT levels. There was a significant (F (1, 20) = 14.33, $p = 0.0012$) interaction between treatment and diet on plasma AST levels. However, there was no significant (F (1, 20) = 3.33, $p = 0.0829$) interaction between treatment and diet on plasma ALT levels. Post hoc comparisons showed that GTIN treatment (GTIN+HFHC) resulted in significantly ($p < 0.05$) lower plasma AST and ALT levels in comparison to MET treatment (MET+HFHC). Animals on an ND (GTIN+ND and MET+ND) exhibited significantly ($p < 0.05$) lower levels of both these parameters in comparison to those on a HFHC diet (GTIN+HFHC and MET+HFHC).

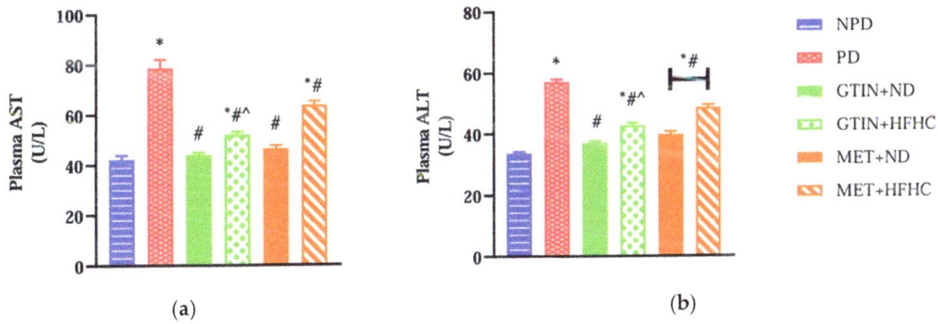

Figure 4. The effects of GTIN on plasma (**a**) AST and (**b**) ALT levels in rats in both the presence and absence of dietary intervention at week 32 of the experimental period ($n = 6$, per group). Values are presented as mean ± SEM. * = $p < 0.05$ denotes comparison with the non-pre-diabetic control (NPD); # = $p < 0.05$ denotes comparison with the pre-diabetic control (PD); ^ = $p < 0.05$ denotes comparison with the metformin + high-fat, high-carbohydrate (MET+HFHC) group.

2.5. Plasma Bilirubin

Plasma bilirubin levels were measured to assess liver function and antioxidant status in the pre-diabetic state. A one-way ANOVA showed significant (F (5, 30) = 62.93, $p < 0.0001$) differences in plasma bilirubin levels between the groups. Post hoc comparisons showed (Figure 5) that the PD control group exhibited significantly ($p < 0.05$) lower plasma bilirubin levels in comparison to the NPD group. However, the GTIN+ND and GTIN+HFHC groups exhibited significantly ($p < 0.05$) higher plasma bilirubin in comparison to the PD control. Similar results ($p < 0.05$) were observed for plasma bilirubin levels in the MET+ND and MET+HFHC groups. A two-way ANOVA revealed that both treatment (F (1, 20) = 14.85, $p < 0.0010$) and diet (F (1, 20) = 51.21, $p < 0.0001$) exhibited significant main effects on plasma bilirubin levels. There was a significant (F (1, 20) = 4.85, $p = 0.0396$) interaction between treatment and diet on plasma bilirubin levels. Post hoc comparisons showed that GTIN treatment (GTIN+HFHC) resulted in significantly ($p < 0.05$) higher plasma bilirubin levels in comparison to MET treatment (MET+HFHC). Animals on an ND (GTIN+ND and MET+ND) exhibited significantly ($p < 0.05$) higher levels of this parameter in comparison to those on a HFHC diet (GTIN+HFHC and MET+HFHC).

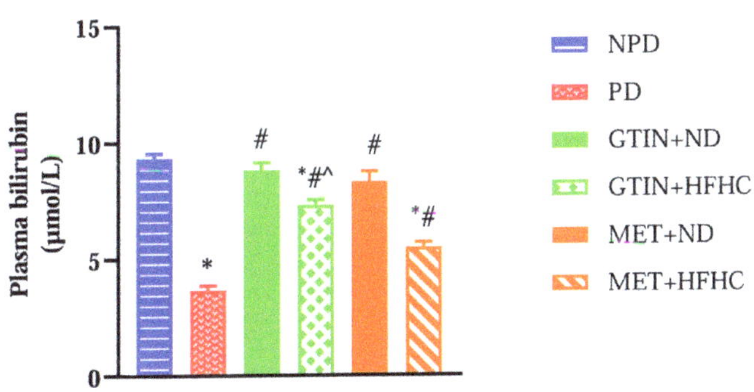

Figure 5. The effects of GTIN on plasma bilirubin levels in rats in both the presence and absence of dietary intervention at week 32 of the experimental period ($n = 6$, per group). Values are presented as mean ± SEM. * = $p < 0.05$ denotes comparison with the non-pre-diabetic control (NPD); # = $p < 0.05$ denotes comparison with the pre-diabetic control (PD); ^ = $p < 0.05$ denotes comparison with the metformin + high-fat, high-carbohydrate (MET+HFHC) group.

2.6. Liver Histology

Liver histology was measured to assess liver architecture and cellular damage. The results (Figure 6B) showed increased lipid droplet accumulation, hepatocyte nucleus displacement, disturbed sinusoidal space, and hepatocyte plate arrangement in the PD group in comparison to the NPD group. There was no remarkable difference in the number of binucleated hepatocytes in the PD group in comparison to the NPD group. The GTIN+ND (Figure 6C) and GTIN+HFHC (Figure 6D) groups showed a decrease in lipid droplet accumulation and hepatocyte nucleus displacement, as well as improved sinusoidal space and hepatocyte arrangement in comparison to the PD group. Similar results were observed in the MET+ND (Figure 6E) and MET+HFHC (Figure 6F). There was no remarkable difference in the number of binucleated hepatocytes in the treatment groups (GTIN+ND, GTIN+HFHC, MET+ND, MET+HFHC) in comparison to the PD group. The histopathological scores for each parameter are shown in Table 1. For each histological parameter, the scores were the same for all animals within each group.

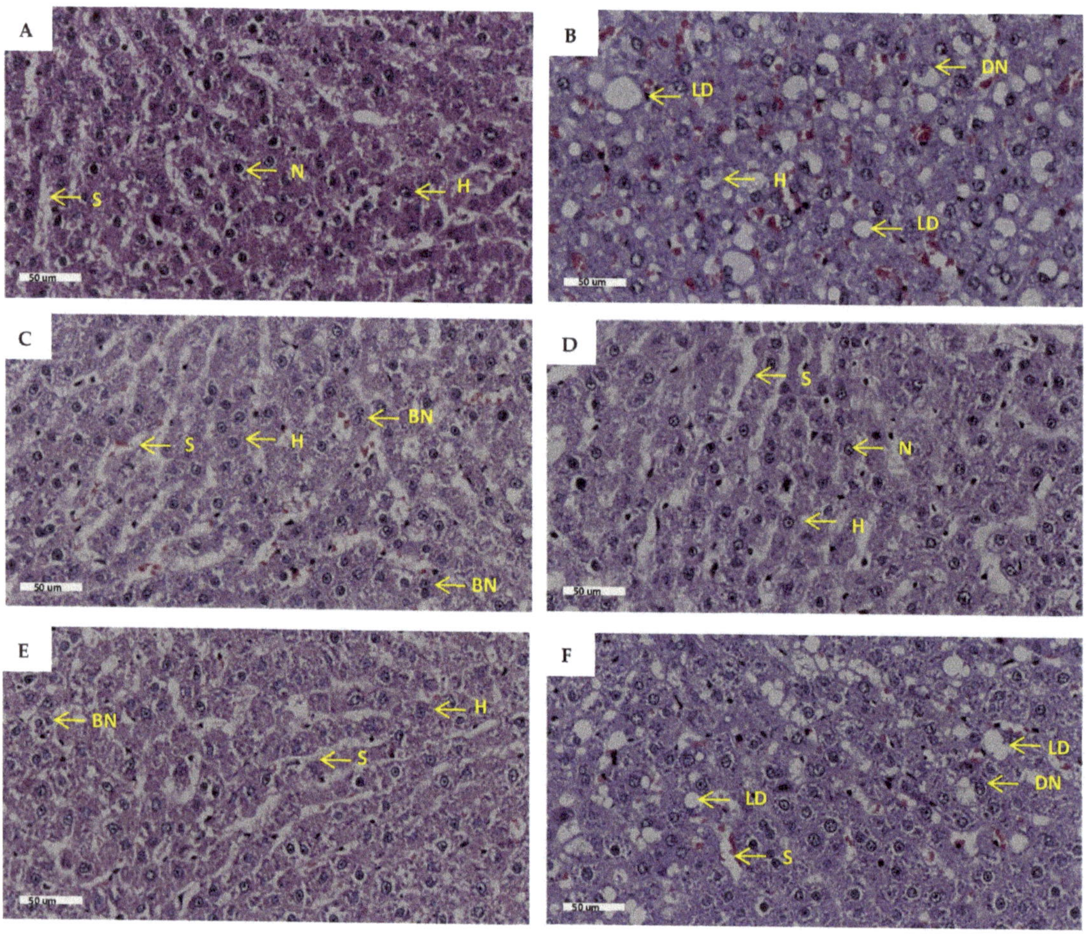

Figure 6. The effects of GTIN on liver histopathology in rats in both the presence and absence of dietary intervention at week 32 of the experimental period (n = 2, per group). Hematoxylin and eosin stain (H&E), magnification 40×, scale bar length = 50 μm. (**A**) NPD group; (**B**) PD group; (**C**) GTIN+ND group; (**D**) GTIN+HFHC group; (**E**) MET+ND group; (**F**) MET+HFHC group. BN = binuclear; DN= displaced nucleus; H = hepatocyte; LD = lipid droplet; N= nucleus; S = sinusoid.

Table 1. Histopathological scoring of liver tissue at week 32 of the experimental period (n = 2, per group).

Groups	Lipid Droplets	Nuclei Displacement	Sinusoid Arrangement	Hepatocyte Plate Arrangement	Binuclear Hepatocytes
NPD	0	0	0	0	1
PD	3	2	3	3	1
GTIN+ND	1	1	1	1	1
GTIN+HFHC	1	1	1	1	1
MET+ND	1	1	1	1	1
MET+HFHC	2	1	2	2	1

3. Discussion

Excess glucose influx into the liver triggers the activation of lipogenic transcription factor SREBP-1c, which drives de novo lipogenesis and leads to increased TAG accumulation [28]. In this study, the liver TAG levels, liver weights, and plasma SREBP-1c levels were significantly higher in the PD group in comparison to the NPD group. The development of NAFLD has been associated with unhealthy dietary patterns characterized by high saturated fat and carbohydrate content along with a low intake of fruits and vegetables [29]. Additionally, fructose has been identified as a key factor in the development of NAFLD in humans and rodents [30]. The high-fat, high-carbohydrate (HFHC) diet and fructose-supplemented water used to induce pre-diabetes in our study may have promoted insulin resistance contributing to hyperinsulinemia and elevated glucose levels, as previously reported [31]. This may have led to increased liver TAG accumulation through increased adipose tissue lipolysis and hepatic lipogenesis via SREBP-1c in the PD group. The increased liver weights may have been attributed to the accumulation of TAGs in the liver, which is a key feature of NAFLD.

However, both GTIN-treated groups exhibited significantly lower liver TAG levels, liver weights, and plasma SREBP-1c levels in comparison to the PD control. A recent study showed that the administration of 15 mg/kg body weight (bw) of GTIN promoted weight loss and improved insulin sensitivity by reducing ghrelin levels and caloric intake [23]. Additionally, another study found that the administration of 20 mg/kg bw of GTIN to mice on a methionine–choline-deficient diet for 4 weeks reduced hepatic lipid accumulation by inhibiting lipogenic pathways and promoting β-oxidation [25]. They also found that GTIN attenuates hepatic lipid accumulation by promoting AMP-activated protein kinase (AMPK) activation [25]. Therefore, in our study, we speculate that GTIN may have reduced liver TAG accumulation by improving insulin sensitivity, promoting β-oxidation, and inhibiting lipogenic pathways, as evidenced by the low plasma SREBP1c levels in the GTIN-treated groups. The decreased liver TAG levels may have led to a decrease in liver weight. Similar results were observed for liver TAG levels, liver weights, and plasma SREBP-1c levels in MET-treated groups. Studies have shown that MET was effective in reducing intrahepatic lipid accumulation [32,33]. In skeletal muscle, MET has been reported to activate AMPK, which increases glucose transporter-4 translocation and improves glucose uptake [34,35]. This has shown to reduce insulin resistance, ultimately leading to a reduction in SREBP-1c activation, hepatic steatosis, and liver weight [36].

Animals maintained on a normal diet exhibited significantly lower levels of liver TAGs, liver weights, and plasma SREBP-1c levels in comparison to those on the HFHC diet. Our findings corroborated a previous study which showed that the consumption of a HFHC diet consisting of 30% fat and 55% carbohydrate for 10 weeks promoted increased de novo lipogenesis [37]. Another study showed that mice fed a high-fat diet (HFD) composed of 42% fat and 42.7% carbohydrates for 3 months significantly increased liver weight [38]. Additionally, a study showed that the consumption of a HFD composed of 60% fats for 2 weeks significantly increased liver TAG levels [39]. A significant interaction between treatment and diet was observed for liver TAG levels and plasma SREBP-1c concentrations, whereas no significant interaction was observed for liver weight. These findings may suggest that the therapeutic effects of treatment on liver TAG and SREBP-1c levels may be enhanced when combined with dietary intervention. Furthermore, GTIN treatment exhibited significantly lower liver TAG levels and liver weights in comparison to MET in HFHC-fed animals. GTIN treatment also exhibited significantly lower plasma SREBP-1c levels than MET in animals on a normal diet. These findings may suggest that GTIN exerts greater therapeutic effects on liver TAGs, liver weights, and SREBP-1c levels than MET treatment, particularly in animals without dietary intervention.

Reactive oxygen species (ROS) are generated from various endogenous and exogenous sources, including mitochondrial respiration, enzymatic reactions, and environmental factors [40]. The body utilizes enzymatic and non-enzymatic antioxidant systems to counteract the harmful effects of ROS production [40]. Enzymatic antioxidants include SOD, GPx, and catalase, while non-enzymatic antioxidants include glutathione, vitamin C, vitamin E, and bilirubin, among others [40]. In the pre-diabetic state, liver MDA levels, which are a by-product of lipid peroxidation, were significantly higher in comparison to the control group [41,42]. Insulin resistance associated with NAFLD increases the flow of free fatty acids (FFAs) into the liver which triggers β-oxidation to manage the excess lipids [43]. Mitochondria adapt to lipid accumulation in hepatocytes by increasing β-oxidation [40]. However, increased substrate delivery to the electron transport chain (ETC) leads to increased ROS production [40]. In NAFLD, elevated ROS levels not only promote lipid peroxidation but also deplete antioxidant molecules and impair antioxidant enzyme activity [44]. Patients with NAFLD exhibit a diminished antioxidant capacity in hepatocytes, as evidenced by a significant decrease in enzymatic antioxidants such as SOD, GPx, and catalase [44]. Moreover, oxidative stress plays a pivotal role in the progression from simple steatosis to NASH [45]. In this study, the liver MDA levels were significantly higher in the PD group in comparison to the NPD group. This was further accompanied by significantly lower liver SOD and Gpx activity. This may suggest increased hepatic lipid peroxidation and decreased enzymatic antioxidant activity in the liver during the pre-diabetic state.

However, both GTIN-treated groups showed significantly lower liver MDA levels in comparison to the PD control. This was further accompanied by significantly increased liver SOD and Gpx activity. Flavonoids are natural antioxidants present in the human diet and have gained attention as promising treatment options for NAFLD due to their potent antioxidant effects and safety profile [46,47]. Their therapeutic effects on oxidative stress have been attributed to the activation of AMPK signaling and the nuclear factor erythroid 2-related factor 2 (Nrf2) pathways [48]. AMPK signaling reduces ROS production, while Nrf2 activation promotes the upregulation of GPx and catalase [49]. A recent study showed that the administration of 20 mg/kg bw of GTIN for 4 weeks directly reduces oxidative stress in the liver rather than upregulating Nrf2-dependent antioxidant responses [25]. However, another study showed that the oral administration of 30 mg/kg bw of GTIN for 3 days upregulated SOD expression by increasing the nuclear translocation of Nrf2 [50]. The observed improvement on liver SOD and GPx activity in the GTIN-treated groups of our study may have been due to the longer treatment duration of 12 weeks as compared to the 4-week treatment period reported in the previous study [25]. Similar results were observed for liver MDA levels and SOD activity in the MET-treated groups, while the MET+ND showed comparable Gpx activity. Our study's results corroborated previous studies showing that MET alleviates oxidative stress in the liver by enhancing the activity of SOD and GPx in a high-fat diet-fed rat model [51,52].

Animals maintained on a normal diet exhibited significantly lower levels of liver MDA as well as higher activities of SOD and GPx in comparison to those on the HFHC diet. The results of this study corroborated a previous study which showed that consumption of a diet containing 44.3% fat and 20% fructose for 4 weeks resulted in increased liver MDA levels and decreased SOD and Gpx activity [53]. Interestingly, a significant interaction between diet and treatment was observed for liver Gpx activities despite small differences in mean values. There was no significant interaction detected for liver MDA and SOD activity. These findings suggest that the most pronounced reductions in liver Gpx activities may be achieved through a combination of pharmacological and dietary intervention. The lack of interaction between treatment and diet on liver MDA levels and SOD activity may suggest that the effects of treatment are not influenced by diet. Furthermore, GTIN treatment demonstrated significantly higher SOD activity in comparison to MET in rats fed a normal diet and HFHC diet. Additionally, GTIN exhibited significantly higher GPx activity in comparison to MET in HFHC-fed animals. This may suggest that GTIN treatment exerts greater beneficial effects than MET on liver SOD and GPx activity in rats without dietary intervention.

Under normal physiological conditions, ALT and AST are enzymes found in hepatocytes [54]. The increased levels of AST and ALT in circulation serve as a marker for liver injury, since these enzymes are released when hepatocytes are damaged [54]. Studies have shown increased plasma ALT and AST levels in the progression of NAFLD [55,56]. Liver injury is driven by insulin resistance, oxidative stress, and inflammation, all of which have been associated with high-caloric diets [57]. Hepatic fatty acid accumulation during insulin resistance enhances β-oxidation, which increases ROS production and promotes oxidative stress [58]. This damages cell membranes of hepatocytes, which leads to liver tissue injury [58]. In this study, the plasma AST and ALT levels were significantly higher in the PD control group in comparison to the NPD group. This may suggest that diet-induced pre-diabetes damages hepatocytes, and this may have been due to hepatic FFA accumulation and lipid peroxidation, as seen in the PD group. However, both GTIN-treated groups showed significantly lower plasma AST and ALT levels in comparison to the PD control. Our results corroborated two recent studies which showed that GTIN administration reduced liver injury [25,50]. In our study, GTIN may have reduced liver damage due to its ability to regulate lipid metabolism and mitigate oxidative stress [25]. Similar results were observed for plasma AST and ALT levels in the MET-treated groups. Previous studies have shown that MET reduces liver injury by enhancing insulin sensitivity and decreasing hepatic lipid accumulation through activation of the AMPK pathway [15,59].

Animals maintained on a normal diet exhibited significantly lower levels of plasma AST and ALT levels in comparison to those on the HFHC diet. Our findings corroborated a previous study which has shown that consumption of a HFD composed of 49% fat for 8 weeks promoted significantly elevated plasma AST and ALT levels [60]. Another study showed that the consumption of a high-carbohydrate diet composed of 80% carbohydrates also promoted an increase in plasma AST and ALT levels [61]. A significant interaction between diet and treatment was observed for plasma AST levels, whereas no significant interaction was detected for plasma ALT levels. These findings may suggest that dietary intervention enhances the beneficial effects of treatment on plasma AST levels. The lack of interaction between treatment and diet on plasma ALT may suggest that the effects of treatment are not influenced by diet. Furthermore, GTIN treatment exhibited significantly lower plasma AST and ALT levels in comparison to MET in HFHC-fed animals. This may suggest that GTIN treatment exerts greater beneficial effects than MET on plasma AST and ALT levels in rats without dietary intervention.

Bilirubin is formed in the reticuloendothelial cells of the liver, spleen, and bone marrow through the breakdown of heme [62]. Studies have shown that bilirubin exerts potent antioxidant, anti-inflammatory, and cytoprotective effects in T2DM, hepatic steatosis, and cardiovascular diseases [63,64]. In this study, the plasma bilirubin levels were significantly lower in the PD control in comparison to the NPD group. This study's results corroborated previous studies which have shown similar results in the pre-diabetic state [4,65]. Plasma bilirubin levels have been shown to be inversely associated with T2DM and NAFLD [66,67]. Bilirubin has been explored for its therapeutic effects in managing NAFLD in T2DM due to a lack of approved pharmacological treatments [68]. Bilirubin has been shown to enhance insulin sensitivity in diet-induced obese mice by suppressing endoplasmic reticulum stress and chronic inflammation in adipose tissue and the liver [69]. Furthermore, a previous study showed that bilirubin was more effective in protecting against lipid peroxidation than glutathione [70]. Notably, plasma bilirubin contributes to the total antioxidant capacity of the blood [71]. In this study, both GTIN-treated groups exhibited significantly higher plasma bilirubin levels in comparison to the PD control. The increased plasma bilirubin may have contributed to the reduction in hepatic oxidative stress. These findings suggest that GTIN may contribute to improved liver health by enhancing antioxidant plasma bilirubin levels. Similar results were observed for plasma bilirubin levels in the MET-treated groups. This study's results corroborated a previous study showing elevated plasma bilirubin levels after MET administration [65]. Notably, animals maintained on a normal diet exhibited significantly higher plasma bilirubin levels in comparison to those on the HFHC diet. Our findings corroborated a previous study which has shown that plasma bilirubin decreased after consumption of a HFD [72]. A significant interaction between diet and treatment was observed for plasma bilirubin levels. This may suggest that the effects of pharmacological treatment on plasma bilirubin levels may be enhanced when combined with dietary intervention. Furthermore, GTIN treatment exhibited significantly higher plasma bilirubin levels in comparison to MET in HFHC-fed animals. This may suggest that GTIN treatment exerts greater beneficial effects than MET on plasma bilirubin in rats without dietary intervention.

Under normal physiological conditions, the liver is composed of hexagonal lobules with hepatocytes arranged in radial plates around the central vein [73]. Sinusoids are located between hepatocytes and facilitate the exchange of nutrients and waste [73]. Macrovesicular steatosis is a key histological feature of NAFLD and has been observed in the pre-diabetic state [65,74]. The accumulation of fat in hepatocytes displaces the nucleus to the periphery and lipid-laden hepatocytes reduce sinusoidal space in NAFLD [75]. High-caloric diets and insulin resistance promotes increased hepatic FFA influx, which contributes to hepatic steatosis [43]. In this study, the PD group exhibited notable features such as increased lipid droplet accumulation, the displacement of hepatocyte nuclei, disturbed sinusoidal space, and hepatocyte plate arrangement in comparison to the NPD group. The increased intrahepatic TAG accumulation seen in the PD group may have contributed to the macrovesicular steatosis present histologically. Furthermore, the hepatocyte plate arrangement may have been disrupted due to fat deposition, leading to disarray within the liver lobules. However, both GTIN-treated groups showed reductions in lipid droplet accumulation, displaced hepatocyte nuclei, and improved sinusoidal space and hepatocyte arrangement in comparison to the PD group. These improvements may have been attributed to the antilipidaemic, antioxidant, and anti-inflammatory properties of GTIN [21,22]. Additionally, the MET+ND and MET+HFHC groups showed similar histological improvements as the GTIN-treated groups. However, the MET+HFHC group showed increased lipid droplet accumulation, reduced sinusoidal space, and moderate disruption to hepatocyte plate arrangement in comparison to the MET+ND group. The HFHC diet may have limited the ability of MET to effectively reduce hepatic lipid accumulation [5]. There was no remarkable difference in the number of binucleated hepatocytes among all six groups, which may suggest that hepatocyte regeneration may be occurring at similar rates.

This study highlights the potential of GTIN as an effective compound for ameliorating liver complications associated with the pre-diabetic state. The results demonstrated that GTIN administration in the presence and absence of dietary intervention significantly improved liver TAG levels, liver weights, plasma SREBP-1c, and bilirubin levels in comparison to the PD group. Additionally, GTIN administration reduced liver MDA levels and increased liver SOD and Gpx activity. It also decreased liver injury, demonstrated by reduced plasma AST and ALT levels. Moreover, GTIN improved liver histology by reducing steatosis and restoring liver architecture in comparison to the PD group. The effects of GTIN on liver parameters were comparable to MET treatment. Moreover, dietary intervention may positively influence liver health in pre-diabetes. However, the combination of pharmacological and dietary intervention may exhibit greater therapeutic outcomes on liver health than when used independently. Notably, GTIN may exert greater protective effects than MET in rats without dietary intervention.

4. Materials and Methods

4.1. Chemicals and Drugs

The chemicals employed were of analytical grade and sourced from standard commercial suppliers (Merck chemicals (PTY) Ltd., Wadeville, Gauteng, South Africa). Gossypetin was purchased from INDOFINE Chemical Company (Hillsborough, NJ, USA). Metformin was purchased from Sigma-Aldrich (St. Louis, MI, USA).

4.2. Animals and Housing

The study involved 36 male Sprague Dawley rats (150–180 g), which were bred and kept in the Biomedical Research Unit (BRU) at the University of KwaZulu-Natal (UKZN), Westville campus. Under standard laboratory conditions, the animals were housed at a constant temperature of 22 ± 2 °C, a carbon dioxide (CO_2) content of <5000 p.m, relative humidity of 55 ± 5%, and a 12 h light/dark cycle (lights on at 07:00). Noise levels were kept under 65 decibels. Food and water were provided ad libitum to all animals. All animal experiments and handling were approved by the Animal Research Ethics Committee of the University of KwaZulu-Natal (ethics number: AREC/0000495/2022). Pain and discomfort were closely monitored in accordance with the humane endpoint criteria outlined by the UKZN Institutional Animal Ethics Committee. The rats were housed in well-ventilated polycarbonate plastic cages (Techniplast, Labotec, Midrand, South Africa). Before the experimental diet (high fat high carbohydrate) was introduced, the rats were allowed to acclimatize to their new environment while consuming a standard rat diet (Meadow Feeds, Lanseria, South Africa) and tap water for 1 week [31].

4.3. Induction of Pre-Diabetes

The animals were randomly distributed into two groups based on diet (Figure 7) as follows: group 1 (n = 6) and group 2 (n = 30). The induction of experimental pre-diabetes in the animals was carried out using the protocol outlined by Luvuno et al. [31]. Group 1 animals were given a standard rat diet and tap water, while group 2 animals received a high-fat, high-carbohydrate (HFHC) diet (AVI Products (Pty) Ltd., Waterfall, Johannesburg, South Africa) supplemented with 15% fructose-enriched water to induce pre-diabetes for 20 weeks. The HFHC diet was composed of 55% carbohydrates, 30% fats, and 15% proteins of the total energy content [31]. Following 20 weeks, the animals were assessed for pre-diabetes using the American Diabetes Association criteria [76]. Animals with a fasting blood glucose concentration of 5.6 to 6.9 mmol/L and a 2 h oral glucose tolerance test glucose concentration of 7.8 to 11.0 mmol/L were classified as the pre-diabetic group. The animals on the standard diet were also assessed at week 20 to confirm normoglycemia and were categorized as the non-pre-diabetic group. To measure glucose concentration, blood was collected using the tail-prick method [77]. Glucose levels were assessed using a OneTouch Select glucometer (LifeScan, Mosta, Malta). Blood samples were taken at week 20 and every 4 weeks during the treatment period to monitor changes in glucose levels. The sample size was selected based on similar studies and power analysis to ensure adequate statistical power while ensuring animal welfare [65,78].

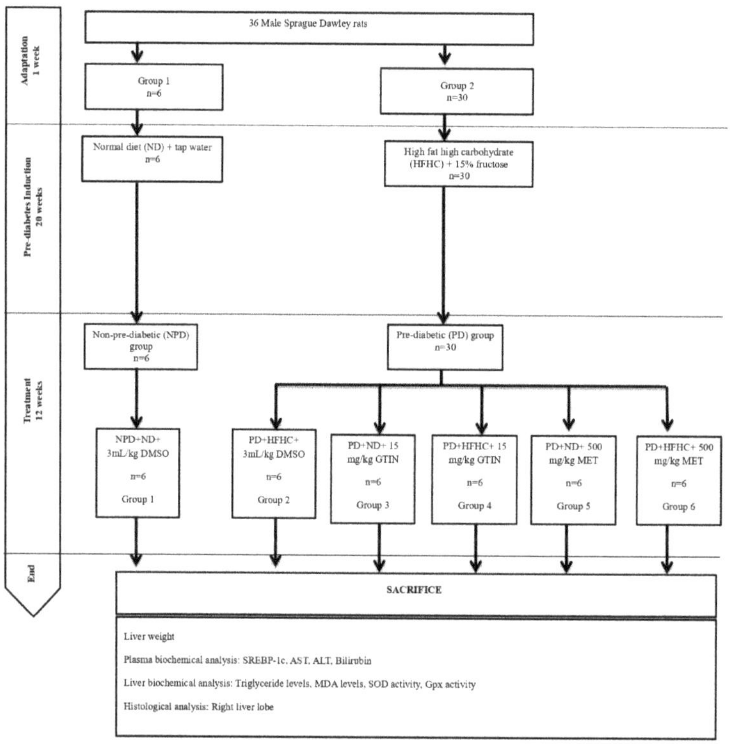

Figure 7. Layout of experimental design and grouping.

4.4. Experimental Design and Treatment

Following the induction of pre-diabetes, the pre-diabetic group (n = 30) was randomly subdivided into five groups (Groups 2 to 6), each group comprising six animals each. The pre-diabetic animals either continued the HFHC diet or changed to a normal standard diet (ND) while receiving either 15 mg/kg body weight (b.w) gossypetin (GTIN) or 500 mg/kg bw metformin (MET) orally once every third day at 9:00 a.m. for 12 weeks. The doses of 15 mg/kg GTIN and 500 mg/kg MET were selected based on previous studies, demonstrating their effectiveness in similar pre-diabetic rat models [4,23]. The non-pre-diabetic control (NPD, Group 1) animals were continuously fed on a normal diet (ND). The pre-diabetic control (PD, Group 2) group consisted of untreated pre-diabetic rats that were continuously fed a HFHC diet. Group 3 (GTIN+ND) animals were changed to the ND and received

GTIN, whereas Group 4 (GTIN+HFHC) animals remained on the HFHC diet and received GTIN. Group 5 (MET+ND) animals were changed to the ND and were given MET, while Group 6 (MET+HFHC) animals continued on the HFHC diet and received MET. In all treatment groups, the drugs were dissolved in 3 mL/kg of diluted dimethyl sulfoxide (DMSO) (prepared as 2 mL DMSO in 19 mL normal saline, p.o). To ensure consistency and control for any potential effects of the vehicle, the control groups were also administered the same dose of DMSO without any dissolved drug. We have used 10% DMSO as a vehicle, as it has proven to dissolve organic compounds based on previous studies in our laboratory [79,80]. The amount of DMSO administered was 3 mL/kg every third day. We have selected this volume based on the recommended safe volume to be administered to rodents [81].

4.5. *Blood Collection and Tissue Harvesting*

At the end of week 32 of the experimental period, all animals were anesthetized for 3 min with Isofor (100 mg/kg bw) (Safeline Pharmaceuticals (Pty) Ltd., Roodeport, South Africa) using a gas anesthetic chamber (BRU, UKZN, Durban, South Africa). After the animals were anesthetized, blood was obtained via cardiac puncture and placed into pre-cooled heparinized containers. The blood samples were centrifuged (Eppendorf centrifuge 5403, Germany) at 4 °C, at 503× *g* for 15 min to obtain plasma. Each plasma sample was transferred into Eppendorf tubes and stored in a Bio Ultra freezer (Snijers Scientific, Tilburg, The Netherlands) until ready for biochemical analysis. The liver was removed, weighed, and rinsed with a cold normal saline solution. The left lobe was immediately snap-frozen in liquid nitrogen and stored at −80 °C in a BioUltra freezer (Snijers Scientific, Tilburg, The Netherlands) for biochemical analysis, while the right lobe was preserved in 10% formalin buffer for histopathological examination.

4.6. *Biochemical Analysis*

At the end of week 32 of the experimental period, various biochemical parameters were assessed.

4.6.1. Plasma Biochemical Analysis

Plasma aspartate transaminase (AST), alanine transaminase (ALT), and bilirubin levels were analyzed with IDEXX Catalyst One Chemistry Analyzer (IDEXX Laboratories Inc. Westbrook, ME, USA). Plasma sterol regulatory element binding protein 1c (SREBP-1c) levels were measured using the relevant ELISA kit (catalog no.: EKC39725) according to the manufacturer's instructions (Biomatik USA, LLC, Wilmington, DE, USA) (Supplementary Materials S1). The absorbance was measured at 450 nm using the Spectrostar Nanospectrophotometer (BMG Labtech, Ortenberg, Germany).

4.6.2. Liver Biochemical Analysis

Liver tissue samples and the homogenate medium used for determining liver triglycerides levels, superoxide dismutase, and glutathione peroxidase activity were prepared according to the manufacturer's instructions (Elabscience Biotechnology Co., Ltd., Houston, TX, USA). Briefly, 20 mg of liver tissue was harvested for each assay. The tissue was washed with ice-cold phosphate-buffered saline (PBS, 0.01 M, pH 7.4) and then homogenized on ice in 180 μL of PBS. The homogenate was centrifuged at 10,000× *g* for 10 min at 4 °C. The supernatant was collected and kept on ice for immediate analysis or stored at −80 °C for later use.

Liver triglyceride (TAG) levels were quantified using the triglyceride colorimetric assay kit (GPO-PAP method, catalog no.: E-BC-K238) according to the manufacturer's instructions (Elabscience Biotechnology Co., Ltd., Houston, TX, USA) (Supplementary

Materials S2). The activity of superoxide dismutase (SOD) was determined using the total superoxide dismutase (T-SOD) activity assay kit (WST-1 method, catalog no.: E-BC-K020-M) according to the manufacturer's instructions (Supplementary Materials S3). The activity of glutathione peroxidase (Gpx) was measured using the glutathione peroxidase (GSH-Px) activity assay kit (catalog no.: E-BC-K096-S) (Supplementary Materials S4). The Spectrostar Nanospectrophotometer (BMG Labtech, Ortenberg, Germany) was used to measure the absorbance for TAG at 510 nm, SOD at 450 nm, and GPx at 412 nm.

4.7. MDA Assay

The liver malondialdehyde (MDA) concentration was quantified following a previously established laboratory protocol [82]. Briefly, 50 mg of liver tissue was homogenized in 500 μL of 0.2% phosphoric acid. The homogenate was centrifuged at 400× *g* for 10 min. Thereafter, 400 μL of the homogenate was combined with 400 μL of 2% phosphoric acid and then divided into two glass tubes, each receiving equal volumes of the solution. Then, 200 μL of 7% phosphoric acid was added to both tubes, followed by the addition of 400 μL of thiobarbituric acid (TBA)/butylated hydroxytoluene (BHT) solution to the sample tube and 400 μL of 3 mM hydrochloric acid (HCl) to the blank tube. To adjust the pH to 1.5, 200 μL of 1 M HCl was added to both tubes. The tubes were heated at 100 °C for 15 min and allowed to cool to room temperature. After cooling, 1.5 mL of butanol was added, the solution was vortexed for 1 min for thorough mixing, and then allowed to settle until two phases could be distinguished. The upper butanol phase was transferred to Eppendorf tubes and centrifuged at 13,200× *g* for 6 min. The samples were aliquoted into a 96-well microtiter plate in triplicate, and the absorbance was measured at 532 nm (reference 600 nm) using a Spectrostar Nanospectrophotometer (BMG Labtech, Ortenberg, Germany). The absorbance from these wavelengths was used to calculate the concentration of MDA using Beer's Law as follows: MDA concentration = Average Absorbance/Absorption coefficient (156 nm) [82].

4.8. Histological Analysis

A histological examination of the liver was performed on two randomly selected animals per group, following a previously documented protocol [83]. Following removal from the animals, liver tissues were immediately fixed in 10% formalin buffer. The samples were dehydrated with alcohol and embedded in paraffin wax. A microtome was used to slice 5 μm sections of liver tissue, which were then stained with hematoxylin and eosin (H&E). The processed tissue sections were visualized and captured with a Leica SCN400 scanner and analyzed using Aperio ImageScope software (version 12.4.6; Leica Biosystems, Buffalo Grove, IL, USA).

Lipid droplet scores were assigned using the Brunt method [84] as follows: Grade 0: none; Grade 1: <33% hepatocytes affected; Grade 2: 33–66% hepatocytes affected; Grade 3: >66% hepatocytes affected.

Nuclei displacement scores were assigned as follows: Grade 0: none; Grade 1: 1–24% displaced nuclei; Grade 2: 25–50% displaced nuclei; Grade 3: >50% displaced nuclei.

Sinusoid disruption scores were assigned as follows: Grade 0: normal well-defined sinusoids; Grade 1: mild changes with some sinusoidal dilation but no significant loss; Grade 2: moderate disruption with sinusoidal dilation and focal areas of loss; Grade 3: severe disruption with large loss of sinusoidal space.

Hepatocyte plate arrangement scores were assigned as follows: Grade 0: radial plate arrangement; Grade 1: mild disruption where some plates are irregular but general organization is maintained; Grade 2: moderate disruption where plates are disorganized with gaps; Grade 3: severe disruption with no clear plate formation.

Binuclear hepatocyte scores were assigned as follows: Grade 0: none; Grade 1: <5% binucleated hepatocytes; Grade 2: 5–20% binucleated hepatocytes; Grade 3: >20% binucleated hepatocytes.

4.9. Statistical Analysis

Data were presented as the mean ± standard error of the mean (SEM). The Shapiro–Wilk test was used to evaluate the normality of the data and Bartlett's test was used to test for homogeneity of variance. A one-way analysis of variance (ANOVA) was used to compare differences among all groups for the dependent variable. An ordinary two-way ANOVA was conducted on the GTIN+ND, GTIN+HFHC, MET+ND, and MET+HFHC groups. This analysis assessed the effects of two factors, namely diet (ND vs. HFHC) and treatment (GTIN vs. MET) on the dependent variable. Post hoc comparisons were made using the Tukey test via GraphPad Prism 5 software. Statistical significance was determined at a value of $p < 0.05$.

5. Limitations and Future Recommendations

A limitation of this study was the restricted sample size for histological analysis, as only two animals per group were examined due to logistical constraints and shortages of laboratory supplies. Additionally, while lipid peroxidation and antioxidant activity were assessed, only selected markers were measured. Future studies should investigate a broader range of oxidative stress markers and antioxidant enzymes. Quantitative histological analysis should also be conducted on a larger sample size, and control animals without DMSO should be included in future studies.

6. Conclusions

Taken together, GTIN may serve as an effective candidate for managing liver complications in the pre-diabetic state in the presence and absence of dietary modification. This was evidenced by reduced liver TAGs, liver weights, and plasma SREBP-1c levels in the GTIN-treated animals. It also reduced liver MDA levels and injury while improving plasma bilirubin levels, SOD activity, Gpx activity, and liver histology. Similar results were observed for the liver parameters in the MET-treated groups. The findings of this study may suggest that GTIN and MET have beneficial effects on liver health in diet-induced pre-diabetes, with the best outcomes achieved when treatment and dietary intervention are used in conjugation. Notably, GTIN offers greater protective effects in comparison to MET, particularly in rats without dietary intervention.

Supplementary Materials: The following supporting information can be downloaded at: https://www.mdpi.com/article/10.3390/molecules30081834/s1, Supplementary Materials S1: Protocol for SREBP-1c assay. Supplementary Materials S2: Protocol for triglyceride assay. Supplementary Materials S3: Protocol for superoxide dismutase activity assay. Supplementary Materials S4: Protocol for glutathione peroxidase activity assay.

Author Contributions: Conceptualization, K.N. and A.K.; methodology, K.N.; software, K.N.; validation, K.N. and A.K.; formal analysis, K.N.; investigation, K.N.; resources, K.N.; data curation, K.N.; writing—original draft preparation, K.N.; writing—review and editing, K.N.; visualization, K.N.; supervision, A.K.; project administration, K.N.; funding acquisition, A.K. All authors have read and agreed to the published version of the manuscript.

Funding: This research was funded by the National Research Foundation; grant number: UID 140586.

Institutional Review Board Statement: The animal study protocol was approved by the Institutional Animal Research Ethics Committee of University of KwaZulu-Natal UKZN (protocol code AREC/0000495/2022 and date of approval: 13 February 2023).

Informed Consent Statement: Not applicable.

Data Availability Statement: The data presented in this study are available upon request from the corresponding author.

Acknowledgments: The authors acknowledge the technicians from the physiology department for laboratory assistance, as well as the UKZN Biomedical Resource Unit (BRU) personnel for their technical assistance.

Conflicts of Interest: The authors declare no conflicts of interest. The funders had no role in the design of the study; in the collection, analyses, or interpretation of data; in the writing of the manuscript; or in the decision to publish the results.

References

1. Mourouti, N.; Mavrogianni, C.; Mouratidou, T.; Liatis, S.; Valve, P.; Rurik, I.; Torzsa, P.; Cardon, G.; Bazdarska, Y.; Iotova, V.; et al. The Association of Lifestyle Patterns with Prediabetes in Adults from Families at High Risk for Type 2 Diabetes in Europe: The Feel4Diabetes Study. *Nutrients* **2023**, *15*, 3155. [CrossRef] [PubMed]
2. Khan, R.M.M.; Chua, Z.J.Y.; Tan, J.C.; Yang, Y.; Liao, Z.; Zhao, Y. From Pre-Diabetes to Diabetes: Diagnosis, Treatments and Translational Research. *Medicina* **2019**, *55*, 546. [CrossRef]
3. Hostalek, U. Global epidemiology of prediabetes—Present and future perspectives. *Clin. Diabetes Endocrinol.* **2019**, *5*, 5. [CrossRef]
4. Gamede, M.; Mabuza, L.; Ngubane, P.; Khathi, A. Plant-derived oleanolic acid ameliorates markers associated with non-alcoholic fatty liver disease in a diet-induced pre-diabetes rat model. *Diabetes Metab. Syndr. Obes.* **2019**, *12*, 1953–1962. [CrossRef]
5. Chen, Z.; Yu, R.; Xiong, Y.; Du, F.; Zhu, S. A vicious circle between insulin resistance and inflammation in nonalcoholic fatty liver disease. *Lipids Health Dis.* **2017**, *16*, 203. [CrossRef]
6. Smith, G.I.; Shankaran, M.; Yoshino, M.; Schweitzer, G.G.; Chondronikola, M.; Beals, J.W.; Okunade, A.L.; Patterson, B.W.; Nyangau, E.; Field, T.; et al. Insulin resistance drives hepatic de novo lipogenesis in nonalcoholic fatty liver disease. *J. Clin. Investig.* **2020**, *130*, 1453–1460. [CrossRef]
7. Marušić, M.; Paić, M.; Knobloch, M.; Liberati Pršo, A.-M. NAFLD, insulin resistance, and diabetes mellitus type 2. *Can. J. Gastroenterol. Hepatol.* **2021**, *2021*, 6613827. [CrossRef] [PubMed]
8. Sharma, A.K. Metamorphic Changes of Liver Enzymes in Prediabetic Young Adult Subjects. *J. Med. Sci. Clin. Res.* **2018**, *6*, 1208–1214. [CrossRef]
9. Tamaki, N.; Ajmera, V.; Loomba, R. Non-invasive methods for imaging hepatic steatosis and their clinical importance in NAFLD. *Nat. Rev. Endocrinol.* **2022**, *18*, 55–66. [CrossRef]
10. Jung, I.; Koo, D.-J.; Lee, W.-Y. Insulin Resistance, Non-Alcoholic Fatty Liver Disease and Type 2 Diabetes Mellitus: Clinical and Experimental Perspective. *Diabetes Metab. J.* **2024**, *48*, 327–339. [CrossRef]
11. Mazzotti, A.; Caletti, M.T.; Marchignoli, F.; Forlani, G.; Marchesini, G. Which treatment for type 2 diabetes associated with non-alcoholic fatty liver disease? *Dig. Liver Dis.* **2017**, *49*, 235–240. [CrossRef] [PubMed]
12. Lin, C.-Y.; Adhikary, P.; Cheng, K. Cellular protein markers, therapeutics, and drug delivery strategies in the treatment of diabetes-associated liver fibrosis. *Adv. Drug Deliv. Rev.* **2021**, *174*, 127–139. [CrossRef]
13. Shibayama, K.; Furushima, C.; Saka, M.; Sakamoto, T.; Takahashi, H. Barriers to lifestyle modification in patients with non-alcoholic fatty liver disease: A scoping review. *J. Rural Med.* **2024**, *19*, 1–9. [CrossRef] [PubMed]
14. Parry, S.A.; Hodson, L. Managing NAFLD in Type 2 Diabetes: The Effect of Lifestyle Interventions, a Narrative Review. *Adv. Ther.* **2020**, *37*, 1381–1406. [CrossRef]
15. Perazza, F.; Leoni, L.; Colosimo, S.; Musio, A.; Bocedi, G.; D'Avino, M.; Agnelli, G.; Nicastri, A.; Rossetti, C.; Sacilotto, F.; et al. Metformin and the Liver: Unlocking the Full Therapeutic Potential. *Metabolites* **2024**, *14*, 186. [CrossRef]
16. Genua, I.; Cusi, K. Pharmacological Approaches to Nonalcoholic Fatty Liver Disease: Current and Future Therapies. *Diabetes Spectr.* **2024**, *37*, 48–58. [CrossRef] [PubMed]
17. Bell, W.; Jennings, A.; Thompson, A.S.; Bondonno, N.P.; Tresserra-Rimbau, A.; Kühn, T.; Cassidy, A. A flavonoid-rich diet is associated with lower risk and improved imaging biomarkers of nonalcoholic fatty liver disease: A prospective cohort study. *Am. J. Clin. Nutr.* **2024**, *120*, 1325–1334. [CrossRef]
18. Yi, X.; Dong, M.; Guo, N.; Tian, J.; Lei, P.; Wang, S.; Yang, Y.; Shi, Y. Flavonoids improve type 2 diabetes mellitus and its complications: A review. *Front. Nutr.* **2023**, *10*, 1192131. [CrossRef]
19. Lee, M.S.; Tsai, C.W.; Wang, C.P.; Chen, J.H.; Lin, H.H. Anti-prostate cancer potential of gossypetin via inducing apoptotic and autophagic cell death. *Mol. Carcinog.* **2017**, *56*, 2578–2592. [CrossRef]
20. Huang, K.; Liu, Z.; Kim, M.-O.; Kim, K.-R. Anticancer effects of gossypetin from Hibiscus sabdariffa in oral squamous cell carcinoma. *J. Appl. Oral Sci.* **2023**, *31*, e20230243. [CrossRef]

21. Proença, C.; Rufino, A.T.; Santos, I.; Albuquerque, H.M.; Silva, A.M.; Fernandes, E.; Ferreira de Oliveira, J.M.P. Gossypetin is a novel modulator of inflammatory cytokine production and a suppressor of osteosarcoma cell growth. *Antioxidants* **2023**, *12*, 1744. [CrossRef] [PubMed]
22. Lin, H.-H. In vitro and in vivo atheroprotective effects of gossypetin against endothelial cell injury by induction of autophagy. *Chem. Res. Toxicol.* **2015**, *28*, 202–215. [CrossRef] [PubMed]
23. Naidoo, K.; Khathi, A. Effects of Gossypetin on Glucose Homeostasis in Diet-Induced Pre-Diabetic Rats. *Molecules* **2024**, *29*, 4410. [CrossRef] [PubMed]
24. Naidoo, K.; Khathi, A. Investigating the Effects of Gossypetin on Cardiovascular Function in Diet-Induced Pre-Diabetic Male Sprague Dawley Rats. *Int. J. Mol. Sci.* **2024**, *25*, 12105. [CrossRef]
25. Oh, E.; Lee, J.; Cho, S.; Kim, S.W.; Jo, K.W.; Shin, W.S.; Gwak, S.H.; Ha, J.; Jeon, S.Y.; Park, J.-H. Gossypetin prevents the progression of nonalcoholic steatohepatitis by regulating oxidative stress and AMP-activated protein kinase. *Mol. Pharmacol.* **2023**, *104*, 214–229. [CrossRef]
26. Gulsheen; Kumar, A.; Sharma, A. Antianxiety and antidepressant activity guided isolation and characterization of gossypetin from Hibiscus sabdariffa Linn. calyces. *J. Biol. Act. Prod. Nat.* **2019**, *9*, 205–214. [CrossRef]
27. Meng, X.-M.; Ma, X.-X.; Tian, Y.-L.; Jiang, Q.; Wang, L.-L.; Shi, R.; Ding, L.; Pang, S.-G. Metformin improves the glucose and lipid metabolism via influencing the level of serum total bile acids in rats with streptozotocin-induced type 2 diabetes mellitus. *Eur. Rev. Med. Pharmacol. Sci.* **2017**, *21*, 2232–2237.
28. Li, N.; Li, X.; Ding, Y.; Liu, X.; Diggle, K.; Kisseleva, T.; Brenner, D.A. SREBP Regulation of Lipid Metabolism in Liver Disease, and Therapeutic Strategies. *Biomedicines* **2023**, *11*, 3280. [CrossRef]
29. Vancells Lujan, P.; Viñas Esmel, E.; Sacanella Meseguer, E. Overview of Non-Alcoholic Fatty Liver Disease (NAFLD) and the Role of Sugary Food Consumption and Other Dietary Components in Its Development. *Nutrients* **2021**, *13*, 1442. [CrossRef]
30. Yu, S.; Li, C.; Ji, G.; Zhang, L. The contribution of dietary fructose to non-alcoholic fatty liver disease. *Front. Pharmacol.* **2021**, *12*, 783393. [CrossRef]
31. Luvuno, M.; Mabandla, M.; Khathi, A. Voluntary ingestion of a high-fat high-carbohydrate diet: A model for prediabetes. *PONTE Int. Sci. Res. J.* **2018**, *74*, 119–143.
32. Yasmin, T.; Rahman, M.M.; Khan, F.; Kabir, F.; Nahar, K.; Lasker, S.; Islam, M.D.; Hossain, M.M.; Hasan, R.; Rana, S.; et al. Metformin treatment reverses high fat diet- induced non-alcoholic fatty liver diseases and dyslipidemia by stimulating multiple antioxidant and anti-inflammatory pathways. *Biochem. Biophys. Rep.* **2021**, *28*, 101168. [CrossRef]
33. Zhang, D.; Ma, Y.; Liu, J.; Deng, Y.; Zhou, B.; Wen, Y.; Li, M.; Wen, D.; Ying, Y.; Luo, S. Metformin alleviates hepatic steatosis and insulin resistance in a mouse model of high-fat diet-induced nonalcoholic fatty liver disease by promoting transcription factor EB-dependent autophagy. *Front. Pharmacol.* **2021**, *12*, 689111. [CrossRef]
34. Herman, R.; Kravos, N.A.; Jensterle, M.; Janež, A.; Dolžan, V. Metformin and insulin resistance: A review of the underlying mechanisms behind changes in GLUT4-mediated glucose transport. *Int. J. Mol. Sci.* **2022**, *23*, 1264. [CrossRef] [PubMed]
35. Song, Y.; Liu, Z.; Zhu, X.; Hao, C.; Hao, W.; Wu, S.; Yang, J.; Lu, X.; Jin, C. Metformin alleviates the cognitive impairment caused by aluminum by improving energy metabolism disorders in mice. *Biochem. Pharmacol.* **2022**, *202*, 115140. [CrossRef]
36. Esquejo, R.M.; Salatto, C.T.; Delmore, J.; Albuquerque, B.; Reyes, A.; Shi, Y.; Moccia, R.; Cokorinos, E.; Peloquin, M.; Monetti, M. Activation of liver AMPK with PF-06409577 corrects NAFLD and lowers cholesterol in rodent and primate preclinical models. *EBioMedicine* **2018**, *31*, 122–132. [CrossRef]
37. Swarbrick, M.M.; Stanhope, K.L.; Elliott, S.S.; Graham, J.L.; Krauss, R.M.; Christiansen, M.P.; Griffen, S.C.; Keim, N.L.; Havel, P.J. Consumption of fructose-sweetened beverages for 10 weeks increases postprandial triacylglycerol and apolipoprotein-B concentrations in overweight and obese women. *Br. J. Nutr.* **2008**, *100*, 947–952. [CrossRef]
38. VanSaun, M.N.; Lee, I.K.; Washington, M.K.; Matrisian, L.; Gorden, D.L. High fat diet induced hepatic steatosis establishes a permissive microenvironment for colorectal metastases and promotes primary dysplasia in a murine model. *Am. J. Pathol.* **2009**, *175*, 355–364. [CrossRef] [PubMed]
39. St-Amand, R.; Ngo Sock, É.T.; Quinn, S.; Lavoie, J.M.; St-Pierre, D.H. Two weeks of western diet disrupts liver molecular markers of cholesterol metabolism in rats. *Lipids Health Dis.* **2020**, *19*, 192. [CrossRef]
40. Afzal, S.; Abdul Manap, A.S.; Attiq, A.; Albokhadaim, I.; Kandeel, M.; Alhojaily, S.M. From imbalance to impairment: The central role of reactive oxygen species in oxidative stress-induced disorders and therapeutic exploration. *Front. Pharmacol.* **2023**, *14*, 1269581. [CrossRef]
41. Mulla, I.G.; Anjankar, A.; Pratinidhi, S.A.; Lambe, S.D.; Agrawal, S.V. Oxidative Stress in Prediabetic Young Adults. *Cureus* **2024**, *16*, e62504. [CrossRef] [PubMed]
42. Saghir, F.S.; Ibrahim, F.S.; Amom, Z.; Othman, L. The Role of Oxidative Stress and Inflammation in Prediabetes: A Review. *Malays. J. Med. Health Sci.* **2023**, *19*, 326–331. [CrossRef]

43. Tanase, D.M.; Gosav, E.M.; Costea, C.F.; Ciocoiu, M.; Lacatusu, C.M.; Maranduca, M.A.; Ouatu, A.; Floria, M. The Intricate Relationship between Type 2 Diabetes Mellitus (T2DM), Insulin Resistance (IR), and Nonalcoholic Fatty Liver Disease (NAFLD). *J. Diabetes Res.* **2020**, *2020*, 3920196. [CrossRef] [PubMed]
44. Gonzalez, A.; Huerta-Salgado, C.; Orozco-Aguilar, J.; Aguirre, F.; Tacchi, F.; Simon, F.; Cabello-Verrugio, C. Role of oxidative stress in hepatic and extrahepatic dysfunctions during nonalcoholic fatty liver disease (NAFLD). *Oxidative Med. Cell Longev.* **2020**, *2020*, 1617805. [CrossRef]
45. Chen, Z.; Tian, R.; She, Z.; Cai, J.; Li, H. Role of oxidative stress in the pathogenesis of nonalcoholic fatty liver disease. *Free Radic. Biol. Med.* **2020**, *152*, 116–141. [CrossRef] [PubMed]
46. Tan, P.; Jin, L.; Qin, X.; He, B. Natural flavonoids: Potential therapeutic strategies for non-alcoholic fatty liver disease. *Front. Pharmacol.* **2022**, *13*, 1005312. [CrossRef]
47. Liao, Y.; Lv, F.; Quan, T.; Wang, C.; Li, J. Flavonoids in natural products for the therapy of liver diseases: Progress and future opportunities. *Front. Pharmacol.* **2024**, *15*, 1485065. [CrossRef]
48. Zhou, G.; Myers, R.; Li, Y.; Chen, Y.; Shen, X.; Fenyk-Melody, J.; Wu, M.; Ventre, J.; Doebber, T.; Fujii, N.; et al. Role of AMP-activated protein kinase in mechanism of metformin action. *J. Clin. Investig.* **2001**, *108*, 1167–1174. [CrossRef]
49. Petsouki, E.; Cabrera, S.N.S.; Heiss, E.H. AMPK and NRF2: Interactive players in the same team for cellular homeostasis? *Free Radic. Biol. Med.* **2022**, *190*, 75–93. [CrossRef]
50. Khan, A.; Manna, K.; Das, D.K.; Kesh, S.B.; Sinha, M.; Das, U.; Biswas, S.; Sengupta, A.; Sikder, K.; Datta, S. Gossypetin ameliorates ionizing radiation-induced oxidative stress in mice liver—A molecular approach. *Free Radic. Res.* **2015**, *49*, 1173–1186. [CrossRef]
51. Conde de la Rosa, L.; Vrenken, T.E.; Buist-Homan, M.; Faber, K.N.; Moshage, H. Metformin protects primary rat hepatocytes against oxidative stress-induced apoptosis. *Pharmacol. Res. Perspect.* **2015**, *3*, e00125. [CrossRef] [PubMed]
52. Cahova, M.; Palenickova, E.; Dankova, H.; Sticova, E.; Burian, M.; Drahota, Z.; Cervinkova, Z.; Kucera, O.; Gladkova, C.; Stopka, P. Metformin prevents ischemia reperfusion-induced oxidative stress in the fatty liver by attenuation of reactive oxygen species formation. *Am. J. Physiol. Gastrointest. Liver Physiol.* **2015**, *309*, G100–G111. [CrossRef] [PubMed]
53. Jarukamjorn, K.; Jearapong, N.; Pimson, C.; Chatuphonprasert, W. A High-Fat, High-Fructose Diet Induces Antioxidant Imbalance and Increases the Risk and Progression of Nonalcoholic Fatty Liver Disease in Mice. *Scientifica* **2016**, *2016*, 5029414. [CrossRef] [PubMed]
54. Lala, V.; Zubair, M.; Minter, D. *Liver Function Tests*; StatPearls: St. Petersburg, FL, USA, 2023.
55. Sogabe, M.; Okahisa, T.; Kurihara, T.; Takehara, M.; Kagemoto, K.; Okazaki, J.; Kida, Y.; Hirao, A.; Tanaka, H.; Tomonari, T. Differences among patients with and without nonalcoholic fatty liver disease having elevated alanine aminotransferase levels at various stages of metabolic syndrome. *PLoS ONE* **2020**, *15*, e0238388. [CrossRef]
56. Lahmi, A.; Oryan, S.; Eidi, A.; Rohani, A.H. Comparative effects of thymol and vitamin E on nonalcoholic fatty liver disease in male Wistar rats. *Braz. J. Biol.* **2023**, *84*, e268781. [CrossRef]
57. Yang, K.; Chen, J.; Zhang, T.; Yuan, X.; Ge, A.; Wang, S.; Xu, H.; Zeng, L.; Ge, J. Efficacy and safety of dietary polyphenol supplementation in the treatment of non-alcoholic fatty liver disease: A systematic review and meta-analysis. *Front. Immunol.* **2022**, *13*, 949746. [CrossRef]
58. Ma, Y.; Lee, G.; Heo, S.Y.; Roh, Y.S. Oxidative Stress Is a Key Modulator in the Development of Nonalcoholic Fatty Liver Disease. *Antioxidants* **2021**, *11*, 91. [CrossRef]
59. Xie, F.; Zhong, Y.; Wang, D.; So, K.F.; Xiao, J.; Lv, Y. Metformin protects against ethanol-induced liver triglyceride accumulation by the LKB1/AMPK/ACC pathway. *Mol. Biol. Rep.* **2022**, *49*, 7837–7848. [CrossRef]
60. Lasker, S.; Rahman, M.M.; Parvez, F.; Zamila, M.; Miah, P.; Nahar, K.; Kabir, F.; Sharmin, S.B.; Subhan, N.; Ahsan, G.U.; et al. High-fat diet-induced metabolic syndrome and oxidative stress in obese rats are ameliorated by yogurt supplementation. *Sci. Rep.* **2019**, *9*, 20026. [CrossRef]
61. Gao, Y.; Hua, R.; Peng, K.; Yin, Y.; Zeng, C.; Guo, Y.; Wang, Y.; Li, L.; Li, X.; Qiu, Y.; et al. High-starchy carbohydrate diet aggravates NAFLD by increasing fatty acids influx mediated by NOX2. *Food Sci. Hum. Wellness* **2023**, *12*, 1081–1101. [CrossRef]
62. Guerra Ruiz, A.R.; Crespo, J.; López Martínez, R.M.; Iruzubieta, P.; Casals Mercadal, G.; Lalana Garcés, M.; Lavin, B.; Morales Ruiz, M. Measurement and clinical usefulness of bilirubin in liver disease. *Adv. Lab. Med.* **2021**, *2*, 352–372. [CrossRef]
63. Ramírez-Mejía, M.M.; Castillo-Castañeda, S.M.; Pal, S.C.; Qi, X.; Méndez-Sánchez, N. The Multifaceted Role of Bilirubin in Liver Disease: A Literature Review. *J. Clin. Transl. Hepatol.* **2024**, *12*, 939–948. [CrossRef]
64. Jayanti, S.; Dalla Verde, C.; Tiribelli, C.; Gazzin, S. Inflammation, dopaminergic brain and bilirubin. *Int. J. Mol. Sci.* **2023**, *24*, 11478. [CrossRef] [PubMed]
65. Mabuza, L.P.; Gamede, M.W.; Maikoo, S.; Booysen, I.N.; Nguban, P.S.; Khathi, A. Hepatoprotective Effects of a Ruthenium(II) Schiff Base Complex in Rats with Diet-Induced Prediabetes. *Curr. Ther. Res.* **2019**, *91*, 66–72. [CrossRef] [PubMed]
66. Yang, M.; Ni, C.; Chang, B.; Jiang, Z.; Zhu, Y.; Tang, Y.; Li, Z.; Li, C.; Li, B. Association between serum total bilirubin levels and the risk of type 2 diabetes mellitus. *Diabetes Res. Clin. Pract.* **2019**, *152*, 23–28. [CrossRef]

67. Wei, Y.; Liu, C.; Lai, F.; Dong, S.; Chen, H.; Chen, L.; Shi, L.; Zhu, F.; Zhang, C.; Lv, X. Associations between serum total bilirubin, obesity and type 2 diabetes. *Diabetol. Metab. Syndr.* **2021**, *13*, 143. [CrossRef] [PubMed]
68. Hinds, T.D., Jr.; Creeden, J.F.; Gordon, D.M.; Stec, D.F.; Donald, M.C.; Stec, D.E. Bilirubin nanoparticles reduce diet-induced hepatic steatosis, improve fat utilization, and increase plasma β-hydroxybutyrate. *Front. Pharmacol.* **2020**, *11*, 594574. [CrossRef]
69. Dong, H.; Huang, H.; Yun, X.; Kim, D.-s.; Yue, Y.; Wu, H.; Sutter, A.; Chavin, K.D.; Otterbein, L.E.; Adams, D.B.; et al. Bilirubin Increases Insulin Sensitivity in Leptin-Receptor Deficient and Diet-Induced Obese Mice Through Suppression of ER Stress and Chronic Inflammation. *Endocrinology* **2014**, *155*, 818–828. [CrossRef]
70. Vítek, L. The role of bilirubin in diabetes, metabolic syndrome, and cardiovascular diseases. *Front. Pharmacol.* **2012**, *3*, 55. [CrossRef]
71. Žiberna, L.; Jenko-Pražnikar, Z.; Petelin, A. Serum bilirubin levels in overweight and obese individuals: The importance of anti-inflammatory and antioxidant responses. *Antioxidants* **2021**, *10*, 1352. [CrossRef]
72. Pallister, T.; Jackson, M.; Martin, T.; Glastonbury, C.; Jennings, A.; Beaumont, M.; Mohney, R.; Small, K.; MacGregor, A.; Steves, C. Untangling the relationship between diet and visceral fat mass through blood metabolomics and gut microbiome profiling. *Int. J. Obes.* **2017**, *41*, 1106–1113. [CrossRef]
73. Trefts, E.; Gannon, M.; Wasserman, D.H. The liver. *Curr. Biol.* **2017**, *27*, R1147–R1151. [CrossRef] [PubMed]
74. Brown, G.T.; Kleiner, D.E. Histopathology of nonalcoholic fatty liver disease and nonalcoholic steatohepatitis. *Metabolism* **2016**, *65*, 1080–1086. [CrossRef] [PubMed]
75. Leow, W.Q.; Chan, A.W.; Mendoza, P.G.L.; Lo, R.; Yap, K.; Kim, H. Non-alcoholic fatty liver disease: The pathologist's perspective. *Clin. Mol. Hepatol.* **2023**, *29*, S302–S318. [CrossRef]
76. Association, A.D. 2. Classification and diagnosis of diabetes: Standards of care in diabetes—2023. *Diabetes Care* **2023**, *46*, S19–S40.
77. Lee, G.; Goosens, K.A. Sampling blood from the lateral tail vein of the rat. *J. Vis. Exp.* **2015**, *99*, 52766.
78. Siboto, A.; Akinnuga, A.M.; Khumalo, B.N.; Ismail, M.B.; Booysen, I.N.; Sibiya, N.H.; Ngubane, P.S.; Khathi, A. The effects of a [3 + 1] oxo-free rhenium (V) compound with uracil-derived ligands on selected parameters of glucose homeostasis in diet-induced pre-diabetic rats. *Obes. Med.* **2020**, *19*, 100258. [CrossRef]
79. Gamede, M.; Mabuza, L.; Ngubane, P.; Khathi, A. Plant-derived oleanolic acid ameliorates markers of subclinical inflammation and innate immunity activation in diet-induced pre-diabetic rats. *Ther. Adv. Endocrinol. Metab.* **2020**, *11*, 2042018820935771. [CrossRef]
80. Khumalo, B.; Siboto, A.; Akinnuga, A.M.; Sibiya, N.; Khathi, A.; Ngubane, P.S. Momordica balsamina improves glucose handling in a diet-induced prediabetic rat model. *PLoS ONE* **2023**, *18*, e0295498. [CrossRef]
81. Jones-Bolin, S. Guidelines for the care and use of laboratory animals in biomedical research. *Curr. Protoc. Pharmacol.* **2012**, *59*, A.4B.1–A.4B.9. [CrossRef]
82. Mkhwanazi, B.N.; Serumula, M.R.; Myburg, R.B.; Van Heerden, F.R.; Musabayane, C.T. Antioxidant effects of maslinic acid in livers, hearts and kidneys of streptozotocin-induced diabetic rats: Effects on kidney function. *Ren. Fail.* **2014**, *36*, 419–431. [CrossRef] [PubMed]
83. Mzimela, N.C.; Ngubane, P.S.; Khathi, A. The changes in immune cell concentration during the progression of pre-diabetes to type 2 diabetes in a high-fat high-carbohydrate diet-induced pre-diabetic rat model. *Autoimmunity* **2019**, *52*, 27–36. [CrossRef] [PubMed]
84. Santiago-Rolón, A.; Purcell, D.; Rosado, K.; Toro, D.H. A Comparison of Brunt's Criteria, the Non-Alcoholic Fatty Liver Disease Activity Score (NAS), and a Proposed NAS Scoring that Includes Fibrosis in Non-Alcoholic Fatty Liver Disease Staging. *Puerto Rico Health Sci. J.* **2015**, *34*, 189–194.

molecules

MDPI

Article

The Antiproliferative Activity and NO Inhibition of *Neo*-Clerodane Diterpenoids from *Salvia guevarae* in RAW 264.7 Macrophages

Juan Pablo Torres-Médicis [1], Celia Bustos-Brito [1], Leovigildo Quijano [1], Brenda Y. Bedolla-García [2], Sergio Zamudio [3], Teresa Ramírez-Apan [1], Diego Martínez-Otero [1] and Baldomero Esquivel [1,*]

[1] Instituto de Química, Universidad Nacional Autónoma de México, Circuito Exterior, Ciudad Universitaria, Ciudad de México 04510, Mexico; quijano@unam.mx (L.Q.); diegomtz@unam.mx (D.M.-O.)
[2] Instituto de Ecología, A.C., Centro Regional del Bajío, Apartado Postal 386, Pátzcuaro 61600, Mexico; brenda.bedolla@inecol.mx
[3] Independent Researcher, Apartado Postal 392, Pátzcuaro 61600, Mexico
* Correspondence: baldo@unam.mx

Abstract: In this study, nine *neo*-clerodane-type diterpenoids (**1–9**) were isolated from the dichloromethane extract of *Salvia guevarae* Bedolla & Zamudio leaves. Compounds **1–6** were new natural products, and **7–9** were acetone artifacts. In addition, four *neo*-clerodanes diterpenoids (**10–13**) previously described from different sources and six triterpenoids—identified as 3β,20,25-trihydroxylupane, oleanolic acid, 3β-*O*-acetyl-oleanolic acid, ursolic acid, 3β-*O*-acetyl-betulinic acid, and 3β,28-*O*-diacetyl-betulin—were isolated. Additionally, five flavonoids were also isolated from the methanol extract: quercetin-3-*O*-β-xylopyranosyl-(1 → 2)-β-galactopyranoside, taxifolin-7-*O*-β-glucopyranoside, naringenin-7-*O*-β-glucopyranoside, a mixture of 2*R* and 2*S* eriodictyol-7-*O*-β-glucopyranoside, caffeic acid, the methyl ester of rosmarinic acid, and rosmarinic acid. The structure of the isolated compounds was established by spectroscopic means, mainly ^{1}H and ^{13}C NMR, including 1D and 2D homo- and heteronuclear experiments. The absolute configuration of **1** and **10** was ascertained via an X-ray analysis, and that of the other compounds via ECD. The antiproliferative activity of some diterpenoids was determined using the sulforhodamine B method, where guevarain B (**2**) and 6α-hydroxy-patagonol acetonide (**7**) showed moderate activity against the K562 line, with IC_{50} (μM) = 33.1 ± 1.3 and 39.8 ± 1.5, respectively. The NO inhibition in RAW 264.7 macrophage activity was also determined for some compounds, where 2-oxo-patagonal (**6**), 6α-hydroxy-patagonol acetonide (**7**), and 7α-acetoxy-*ent*-clerodan-3,13-dien-18,19:16,15-diolide (**10**) were proven to be active, with IC_{50} (μM) of 26.4 ± 0.4, 17.3 ± 0.5, and 13.7 ± 2.0, respectively. The chemotaxonomy of *Salvia guevarae* is also discussed.

Keywords: *Salvia guevarae*; *neo*-clerodanes diterpenoids; RAW 264.7 macrophages

1. Introduction

Salvia L. (Lamiaceae) is one of the most species-rich genera of angiosperm plants, with about 1000 species with a sub-cosmopolitan distribution [1]. Recent taxonomic and phylogenetic analyses have led to the organization of the genus into 11 subgenera [2], with the subgenera *Audibertia* and *Calosphace* being endemic to the American continents. With a biogeographic distribution ranging from North America to Central America, the Caribbean, and South America, the subgenus *Calosphace*, with an estimated 550 species, is the most diverse, comprising 55% of the whole genus. The *Salvia* species growing in Mexico mainly belong to this subgenus. With an estimated 312 species, with 57% of species from the subgenus *Calosphace* and 31% from the subgenus Mundial, *Salvia* is the most species-rich genus in Mexico, which is considered, due to this diversity and an estimated endemism of 82%, the center of the origin and diversification of this subgenus [3]. Several *Salvia* species are widely cultured in gardens around the world and in Mexico and profusely used as medicinal plants for different ailments including gastrointestinal, nervous system, gynecological, and folk illnesses [4].

From systematic phytochemical studies on Mexican *Salvia* species, starting in 1984, diterpenoids have been found to be the most diversified secondary metabolites. Diterpenoids with *neo*-clerodane-type (sometimes also referred to as *ent*-clerodanes) [5] and abietane-type skeletons are the most frequently isolated, although pimarane-, totarane-, and recently labdane-type diterpenoids [6] have also been described from some members of the genus. Several rearranged scaffolds derived mainly from the *neo*-clerodane type and, to a lesser extent, the abietane- and pimarane-type skeletons, have also frequently been described, highlighting the chemical features of Mexican *Salvia* species. The distribution of these types of compounds, in some cases, parallels that of the botanical classification proposed by Epling, as in the case of sections *Erythrostachys*, *Fulgentes*, *Angulatae*, *Tomentellae*, and *Scorodonia*. Another interesting result is that the distribution of diterpenoids in species of the subgenus *Calosphace* differs markedly from that found in species from Europe and Asia, from which mainly abietane and abietane-derived diterpenoids have been isolated. The presence of diterpenoids in the genus *Salvia* is, therefore, of chemo-systematic relevance [7].

As a result of intensive botanical field work during the past three decades all over the country, the number of *Salvia spp.* has constantly grown in Mexico, with several new species being described, all belonging to the subgenus *Calosphace*. Since 2007, 62 new species have been described, some of which have been classified up to the taxonomic section rank [5]. *Salvia guevarae* Bedolla & Zamudio was recently described and determined to be a new botanical species [8]. The morphology of this species, with its red markedly ventricose corollas with short lips, allowed it to be classified in section *Holwaya* (Ramamoorthy) [9] and suggests its close relation to *S. involucrata* and *S. puberula*. Recently, we described the diterpenoid content of the newly described *S. carranzae* Bedolla & Zamudio, which led us to propose that this species is closely related to those classified in section *Erythrostachys* (Epling) [7]. In this study, we report on the phytochemical analysis of *S. guevarae*, supporting its inclusion in section *Holwaya*, and evaluate the biological activity of some isolated secondary metabolites. The dichloromethane and methanol extracts of this species were thoroughly analyzed using chromatographic techniques to afford nine not previously described *neo*-clerodane-type diterpenoids, with three of them being acetone artifacts, four *neo*-clerodane diterpenoids, six triterpenoids, and eight polyphenolic compounds, already known. Their antiproliferative activities against human cancer cell cultures and capacity for the inhibition of nitric oxide (NO) production in RAW 264.7 macrophages were also evaluated.

2. Results and Discussion

2.1. Characterization

The leaves and flowers of *S. guevarae* afforded, after dichloromethane extraction and thorough chromatographic purification, 13 *neo*-clerodane derivatives (**1–13**) (Figure 1). Compounds **1–6** are undescribed *neo*-clerodane diterpenoids with structures related to those of patagonol (**14**) and patagonal (**15**), two *neo*-clerodane diterpenoids previously isolated from a liana collected from the Surinam rainforest, tentatively identified as a *Casimirella* species [10]. Diterpenoids **7–9** are artifacts obtained, most likely, via a reaction with acetone, used in the purification process, and products **10–13** are previously known compounds isolated from several sources. The structural elucidation of all the isolated compounds was carried out via spectroscopic and chemical methods and a comparison with literature data.

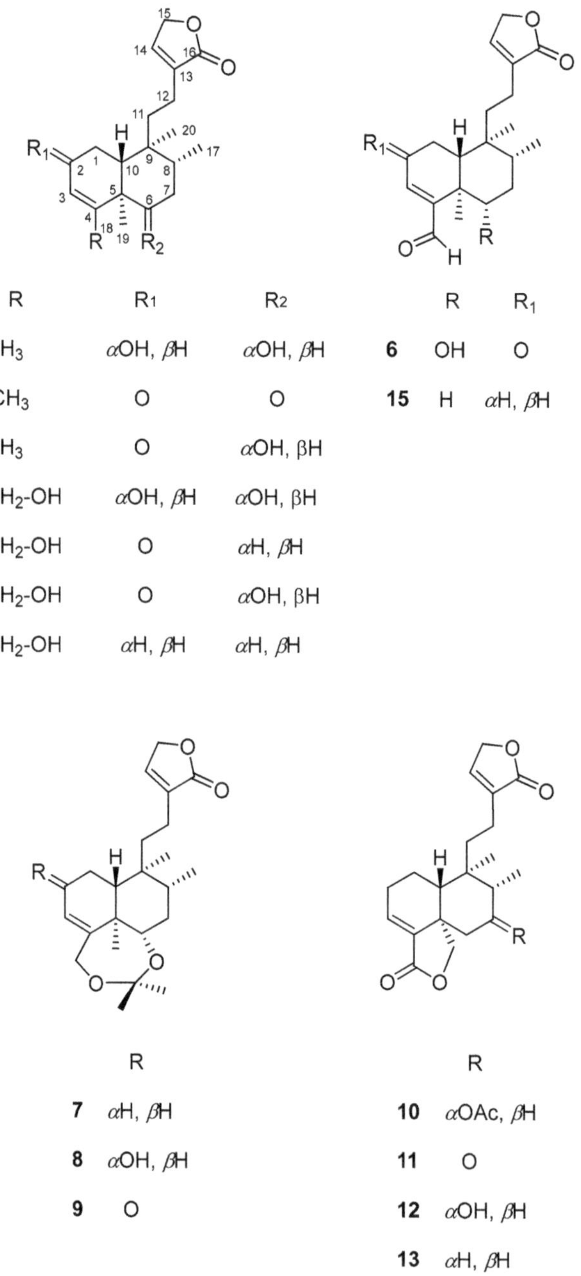

	R	R1	R2
1	CH_3	αOH, βH	αOH, βH
1a	CH_3	O	O
2	CH_3	O	αOH, βH
3	CH_2-OH	αOH, βH	αOH, βH
4	CH_2-OH	O	αH, βH
5	CH_2-OH	O	αOH, βH
14	CH_2-OH	αH, βH	αH, βH

	R	R_1
6	OH	O
15	H	αH, βH

	R
7	αH, βH
8	αOH, βH
9	O

	R
10	αOAc, βH
11	O
12	αOH, βH
13	αH, βH

Figure 1. Compounds isolated from *S. guevarae*.

Compound **1** was the major component and was isolated as a crystalline solid at mp 136–138 °C. The HR-DART-MS showed a *pseudo*-molecular ion $[M + H - H_2O]^+$ at m/z 317.2103 (calculated for $C_{20}H_{30}O_4 + H - H_2O$, 317.2117) consistent with the molecular formula $C_{20}H_{30}O_4$ minus the loss of an H_2O molecule from the molecular ion. Its IR spectrum exhibited characteristic absorptions for α,β-unsaturated-γ-lactone function (1755 cm^{-1}), hydroxyl groups (3606 cm^{-1}), and double bounds (1654, 1602 cm^{-1}). The UV spectrum [MeOH, λ_{max} (log ε) 207 (6.32) nm] was consistent with these assignments.

In the ^{1}H NMR spectrum of **1** (Table 1), signals of an α-substituted butenolide were observed at C-12. A quintet at δ_H 7.41 (J = 1.7 Hz) was assigned to the vinylic H-14 coupled with two methylene groups with signals at δ_H 4.79 and 2.14/2.05 due to CH_2-15 and CH_2-12, respectively, and with similar ^3J and ^4J coupling constant values to those of H-14 and H-12, according to their COSY spectra (Table 1, Figure 2). The ^{13}C NMR spectrum of **1** (Table 1) supports the above assumption, since the corresponding signals of C-13, C-14, C-15, and C-16 were observed at δ_C 134.3, 146.2, 71.0, and 174.7, respectively, which is in accordance with the results obtained from the HSQC and HMBC experiments (Figure 2). The presence of an α-substituted butenolide group is a frequent feature in *neo*-clerodane-type diterpenoids isolated from *Salvia* species [9] and is present in all diterpenoids (**1**–**13**) isolated from *S. guevarae*.

Table 1. NMR data (700 MHz) of **1** and **2**.

	1 [a]			**2** [b]		
Position	δ_C	**Type**	δ_H, **Multiplicity (*J* in Hz)**	δ_C	**Type**	δ_H, **Multiplicity (*J* in Hz)**
1	29.2	CH_2	1.94, ddd (12.6, 7.0, 1.4) 1.49, td (12.6, 10.1)	34.4	CH_2	2.48, dd (17.8, 13.9) 2.32, dd (17.8, 3.6)
2	69.1	CH	4.13, m	199.7	C	
3	127.9	CH	5.19, brs	126.5	CH	5.72, brs
4	146.7	C		172.8	C	
5	45.2	C		45.5	C	
6	75.3	CH	3.48, dt (9.5, 5.6)	73.5	CH	3.70, dd (11.1, 4.8)
7	38.7	CH_2	1.57, m	37.9	CH_2	1.69 ddd(13.0, 4.7, 3.7) 1.62, ddd (13.0, 12.4, 11.1)
8	35.2	CH	1.70, m	34.4	CH	1.73, m
9	38.8	C		38.7	C	
10	45.4	CH	1.35, dd (12.6, 1.4)	44.9	CH	1.88, dd (13.9, 3.6)
11	36.8	CH_2	1.62, ddd (14.6, 12.7, 5.1) 1.55, m	35.0	CH_2	1.58, m 1.47, ddd (14.6, 13.0, 4.9)
12	19.4	CH_2	2.14, m 2.05, m	18.7	CH_2	2.16, m 2.00, m
13	134.3	C		134.3	C	
14	146.2	CH	7.41, p (1.7) *	144.0	CH	7.09, p (1.7) *
15	71.0	CH_2	4.79, q (1.8)	70.4	CH_2	4.76, p (1.7)
16	174.7	C		174.3	C	
17	16.0	CH_3	0.84, d (6.8)	15.5	CH_3	0.89, d (6.8)
18	22.6	CH_3	1.84, dd (1.6, 1.7)	23.0	CH_3	2.14, d (1.3)
19	15.6	CH_3	1.06, s	13.6	CH_3	1.12, s
20	18.3	CH_3	0.75, s	17.4	CH_3	0.84, s
2 OH			3.6, d (6.1)			
6 OH			3.39, d (5.6)			

[a] $(CD_3)_2CO$; [b] $CDCl_3$; * ^4J.

The other relevant signals observed in the ^{1}H NMR spectrum of **1** (Table 1) included a broad singlet at δ_H 5.19, which was ascribed to the vinylic H-3, and multiple signals at δ_H 4.13, assigned to the allylic proton H-2, geminal to the hydroxyl group at the C-2 position.

In the COSY spectrum of **1** (Figure 2), cross peaks of correlation were observed between the H-2 signal (δ_H 4.13) with H-3 (δ_H 5.19); a three-proton signal at δ_H 1.84; and the hydrogens of a methylene group at δ_H 1.94 (ddd, J = 12.6, 7.0, 1.4 Hz) and 1.49 (td, J = 12.6, 10.1 Hz), which were ascribed to the vinylic CH_3-18 and to H-1 *equatorial* and H-1 *axial*, respectively. All other relevant COSY interactions are depicted in Figure 2.

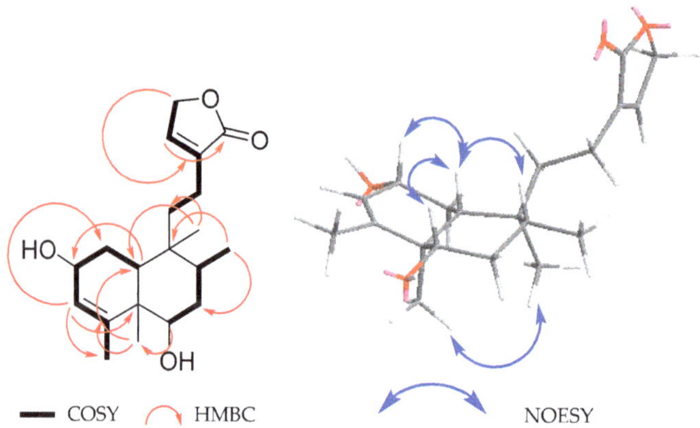

Figure 2. Selected COSY, HMBC, and NOESY correlations for **1**.

The ^{1}H NMR spectrum of **1** (Table 1) also exhibited the signal for a second hydrogen atom geminal to a hydroxyl group, which was observed at δ_H 3.48 (dt, J = 9.5, 5.6 Hz). The multiplicity and the coupling constant values led us to propose that the hydroxyl group is located at the C-6 position with an α *equatorial* orientation. Signals due to characteristic C-17, C-19, and C-20 methyl groups of a *neo*-clerodane-type diterpenoid were also observed at δ_H 0.84 (d, J = 6.8 Hz), 1.06 (s), and 0.75 (s), respectively. Finally, a doublet of doublets at δ_H 1.35 (J = 12.6, 1.4 Hz), ascribed to the β-*axially* oriented H-10, coupled with the methylene signals of -CH_2-1 at δ_H 1.94 (ddd, J = 12.6, 7.0, 1.4 Hz)/1.49, td (J = 12.6, 10.1 Hz), was also observed in the ^{1}H NMR spectrum of **1** (Table 1). These facts, in combination with the chemical shifts observed for C-17 and C-20 in the ^{13}C NMR spectrum of **1** (Table 1), indicated a *trans* fusion of A/B rings, which is the most frequently observed for the *neo*-clerodane diterpenoids hitherto isolated from *Salvia* spp. [5]. All other signals in the ^{13}C NMR spectrum of **1** (Table 1) agreed with the proposed structure, and all connectivities were confirmed with the aid of the HMBC spectrum (Figure 2).

The NOESY spectrum supports relative stereochemistry since it showed NOE correlations between the β-*axially* oriented H-10 and H-2 (Figure 2), indicating that the latter must also be β-*axially* oriented; therefore, the C-2 hydroxyl group must be α-*equatorially* oriented. On the other hand, the cross peaks of correlation between H-10 and H-8 established that the C-17 methyl group was also α-*equatorially* oriented. The NOE effect observed between the C-19 and C-20 methyl groups indicated that both were cofacial [10], as shown in Figure 1. Therefore, compound **1** corresponds to a new *neo*-clerodane compound that we named guevarain A.

The absolute configuration of guevarain A was established via an X-ray diffraction analysis. Guevarain A was crystallized as a monohydrate in the monoclinic P2(1) space group, and the absolute configuration was determined to have the following parameters: Flack(x), −0.02(3); Hooft(y), −0.02(2); and Parsons(z), −0.019(16). This configuration confirms the assignment of the crystal model as well as the configuration of the chiral carbon atoms as being 2*R*, 5*R*, 6*S*, 8*R*, 9*S*, and 10*R*. The molecular structure was shown in Figure 3, and the crystallographic details are presented in the Supplementary Materials

(Table S1). Figure 4 shows the crystalline packing, where three discrete hydrogen bonds described as $D_1^1(2)$ were found, labeled as a, c, and d, where one water molecule participate as donor (c, d) and one (a) as an acceptor. An eight-membered one-dimensional chain, described as $C_1^1(8)$ in terms of graph set descriptors, labeled as b, formed through the O-H fragments of compound **1**. The hydrogen bond distances and angles corresponding to guevarain A (**1**) are shown in the Supplementary Materials (Table S2).

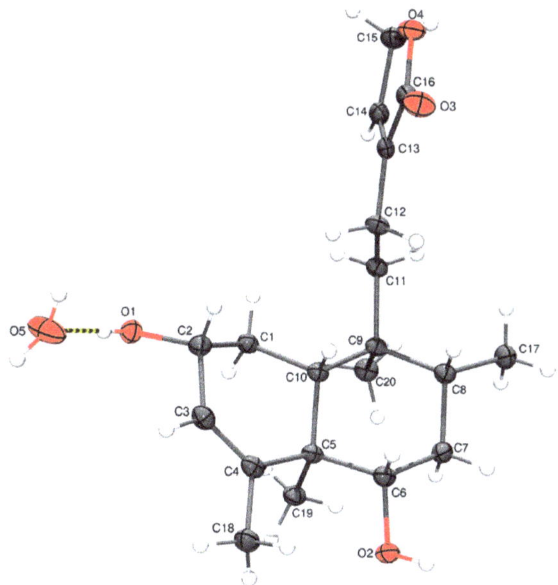

Figure 3. The molecular structure of compound **1**. The thermal ellipsoids are set at 50% of the probability level.

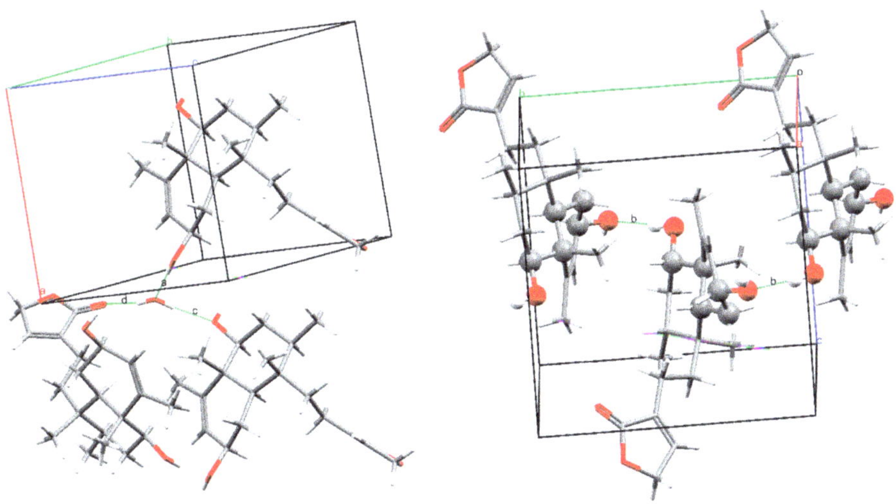

Discrete hydrogen bonds in compound **1**

One-dimensional eight-membered chain formed by hydrogen bonds

Figure 4. Hydrogen bonds in the packing structure found in compound **1**.

Diterpenoid **2**, $C_{20}H_{28}O_4$, (HR-DART-MS), showed a similar IR spectrum to that of guevarain A (**1**), except for the presence of an intense band at 1644 cm^{-1} due to an α,β-unsaturated carbonyl group, also supported by the UV spectrum, since a λ_{max} at 239.8 nm (log ε = 4.07) was observed. The ^1H and ^{13}C NMR spectra of **2** (Table 1) confirmed the presence of a C2-C3-C4 α,β-unsaturated ketone, given that a broad singlet at δ_H 5.72, ascribed to the vinylic H-3, was found to be coupled to a three-proton doublet at δ_H 2.14 (J = 1.3 Hz), assigned to C-18 vinylic methyl, in the ^1H NMR spectrum. Signals for C-2 carbonyl, C-3:C-4 double bond, and C-18 methyl were observed at δ_C 199.7, 126.5, 172.8, and 23.0, respectively, in the ^{13}C NMR spectrum. All these assignments were supported by COSY and HMBC spectra (Figure 5).

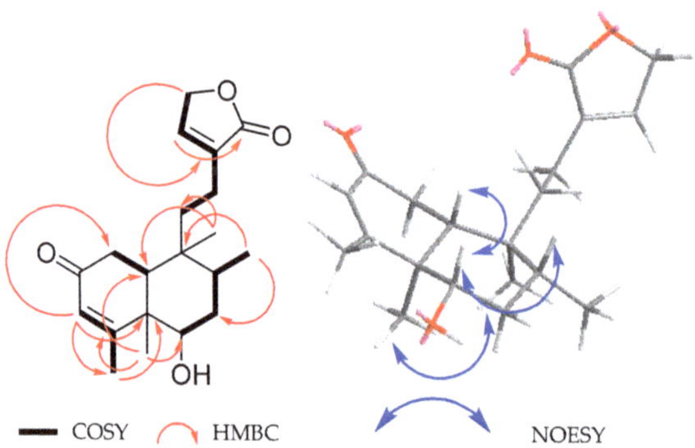

Figure 5. Selected COSY, HMBC, and NOESY correlations for **2**.

The signal for the hydrogen geminal to the hydroxyl group at C-6 in compound **2** was observed at δ_H 3.70 (J = 11.1, 4.8 Hz), similarly to that of **1**. The main difference in the ^1H NMR spectrum was in the signals associated with the presence of a carbonyl group at C-2. Thus, in the COSY spectrum of compound **2** (Figure 5), the CH_2-1 signals at δ_H 2.48 (J = 17.8, 13.9 Hz) and 2.32 (J = 17.8, 3.5 Hz) showed couplings only with the doublet of doublets at δ_H 1.88 (J = 13.9, 3.6 Hz) ascribed to the β-*axially* oriented H-10. The characteristic signals of the methyl groups of a *neo*-clerodane skeleton were observed at δ_H 0.89 (d, J = 6.8 Hz), 1.12 (s), and 0.84 (s) and ascribed to CH_3-17, CH_3-19, and CH_3-20, respectively. The ^{13}C NMR data (Table 1) agree with the proposed structure for compound **2**. All NMR assignments for diterpenoid **2** were confirmed with the aid of HMBC (Figure 5) and HSQC spectra.

The relative configuration depicted in **2** was established with the aid of a NOESY spectrum (Figure 5), since cross peaks of correlation were observed between the β-*axially* oriented H-10 and H-6, indicating cofacial orientations for these protons. On the other hand, the signal for H-6 showed NOE with multiple signals at δ_H 1.73, ascribed to H-8, also β-*axially* oriented.

Based on the previous discussion, the structure of compound **2** was established as the oxidation product of the secondary OH group at C-2 of guevarain A (**1**) and named guevarain B (**2**). The absolute configuration of guevarain B was established via a comparison of the experimental ECD spectrum and the enantiomeric calculated spectra [11]. Figure 6 indicates that the absolute configuration of this diterpenoid corresponds to the 5*R*, 6*S*, 8*R*, 9*S*, 10*R* enantiomer.

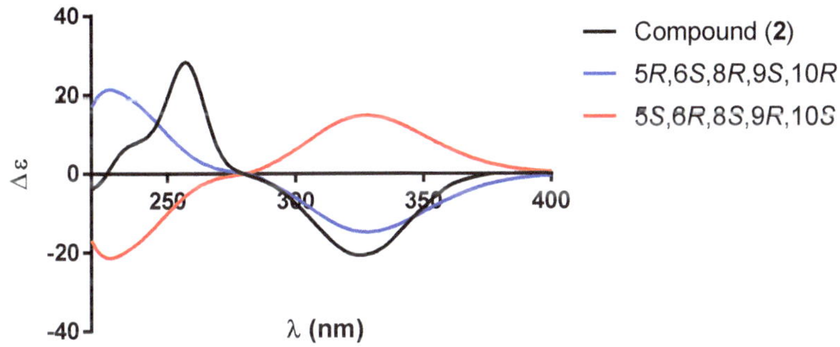

Figure 6. Comparison between the experimental (black line) and calculated ECD spectra for enantiomers (5*R*,6*S*,8*R*,9*S*,10*R*)-**2** (blue line) and (5*S*,6*R*,8*S*,9*R*,10*S*)-**2** (red line).

The treatment of guevarain A (**1**) with pyridinium chlorochromate (PCC) in CH_2Cl_2 afforded a mixture of two reaction products. The main product (44.7% yield) was identical in all aspects to guevarain B (**2**), thus confirming the proposed structure for compound **2**. Structure **1a** was assigned to the minor product (21.8% yield) based on its spectroscopic properties. The ^{1}H NMR spectrum of **1a** (Table 2) lacked the signals for the geminal protons of the hydroxyl groups at C-2 and C-6 observed in guevarain A (**1**), while the ^{13}C NMR spectrum (Table 2) displayed two carbonyls due to the C-2 and C-6 ketone groups at δ_C 197.8 and 210.7, respectively, thus confirming oxidation at the C-2 and C-6 positions.

Table 2. NMR data of **1a** and **3**.

	1a [a]			**3** [b]		
Position	δ_C	**Type**	δ_H, **Multiplicity (*J* in Hz)**	δ_C	**Type**	δ_H, **Multiplicity (*J* in Hz)**
1	34.2	CH_2	2.53, dd (17.0, 14.3) 2.39, dd (17.0, 3.1)	28.9	CH_2	2.02, ddt (12.5, 6.8, 1.3) 1.57, td (12.3, 10.3)
2	197.8	C		69.5	CH	4.23, m
3	127.9	CH	5.82, brs	129.6	CH	5.56, brs
4	167.2	C		149.4	C	
5	55.4	C		45.6	C	
6	210.7	C		75.9	CH	3.58, m
7	43.7	CH_2	2.85, dd (12.7, 12.6) 2.19, dd (12.7, 4.0)	37.20	CH_2	1.64, m
8	40.5	CH	2.13, m	35.9	CH	1.76, m
9	39.3	C		39.2	C	
10	48.2	CH	2.25, dd (14.2, 3.2)	45.6	CH	1.40, brd (12.3)
11	35.4	CH_2	1.68, ddd (14.2, 12.7, 4.2) 1.53, ddd (14.6, 12.7, 4.9)	37.2	CH_2	1.68, ddd (13.7, 12.3, 4.9) 1.61, m
12	19.1	CH_2	2.14, m 2.00, m	19.7	CH_2	2.21, m 2.18, m
13	133.8	C		134.7	C	
14	144.5	CH	7.10, p (1.6) *	147.4	CH	7.36, p (1.5) *
15	70.3	CH_2	4.76, q (1.8)	72.1	CH_2	4.82, q (1.7)
16	174.1	C		176.8	C	
17	16.2	CH_3	1.01, d (6.6)	16.0	CH_3	0.89, d (6.8)
18	21.4	CH_3	2.17, d (1.3)	65.5	CH_2	4.08, d (13.5) 4.23, brd (13.5)
19	18.4	CH_3	1.51, s	16.5	CH_3	1.13, s
20	17.9	CH_3	1.06, s	18.6	CH_3	0.79, s

[a] 500 MHz, [b] $CDCl_3$, 700 MHz; CD_3OD; * ^4J.

The structure of compound **3** was deduced mainly from the ^{1}H NMR spectrum and MS. The molecular formula $C_{20}H_{30}O_5$ was established via HR-DART-MS, indicating an index of hydrogen deficiency $\Omega = 6$. The three degrees of unsaturation can be readily explained by the presence of the butenolide moiety at C-12.

The ^{1}H NMR of compound **3** (Table 2) was like that of compound **1**, with the main differences being the lack of a vinylic methyl signal and the presence of two AB doublets at δ_H 4.08 and 4.23 (J = 13.5 Hz), coupled with the vinylic hydrogen broad singlet at δ_H 5.56 (H-3), which in turn was found to be coupled with overlapping multiple signals at δ_H 4.23 (H-2), in accordance with the COSY spectrum (Figure 7). These facts, in addition to their chemical shifts, led us to ascribe these signals to the C-18 methylene protons and the geminal hydrogen to the hydroxyl group at C-2. The H-2 signal, in turn, showed cross peaks of correlation with two methylene protons at δ_H 2.02 (ddt, J = 12.5, 6.8, 1.3 Hz) and 1.57 (td, J = 12.5, 10.3 Hz) due to H-1 *equatorial* and H-1 *axial*, respectively. A β-*axially* oriented H-10 appeared at δ_H 1.40 (brd, J = 10.3 Hz) and the hydrogen atom geminal to the hydroxyl group at C-6 appeared at δ_H 3.58 as multiple signals similarly to that in guevarain A (**1**).

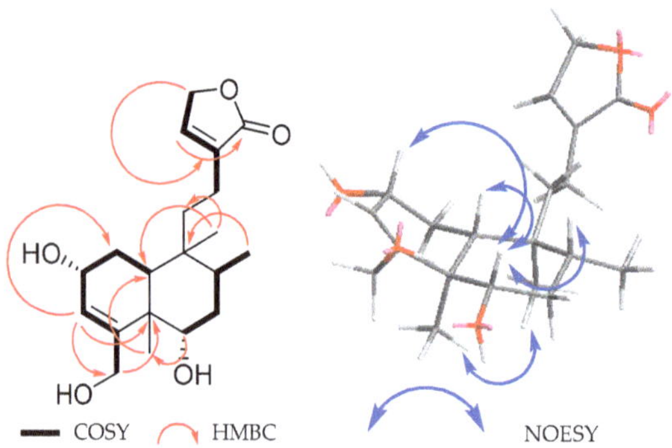

Figure 7. Selected COSY, HMBC, and NOESY correlations for **3**.

The relative configuration of **3** was established based on NOE interactions (Figure 7). In the NOESY spectrum, the β-*axially* oriented H-10 signal showed cross peaks of correlation with H-2 and H-6, while H-6 showed correlation with H-8, indicating that H-10, H-2, H-6, and H-8 were cofacial. On the other hand, the C-19 methyl hydrogens exhibited NOE with the C-20 methyl group, thus indicating that they were on the same face of the molecule. Based on all the above data, the structure of compound **3** was established as the 18-hydroxy derivative of compound **1**, a structure closely related to that of patagonol (**14**); thus, it was named 2α,6α-dihydroxy-patagonol. The absolute configuration of **3** was established as 2*R*, 5*R*, 6*S*, 8*R*, 9*S*, and 10*R* based on the comparison between the theoretical (blue and red lines) and experimental (black line, Figure 8) ECD curves.

The structure of diterpenoid **4** was closely related to that of compound **3**, mainly deduced from its NMR data. The ^{1}H NMR spectrum (Table 3) displayed a broad singlet at δ_H 6.10 due to the vinylic H-3, which showed cross peaks of correlation in the COSY spectrum (Figure 9) with the C-18 allylic methylene signals at δ_H 4.40 (dd, J = 17.6, 1.8 Hz) and 4.35 (dd, J = 17.6, 1.8 Hz). An ABC system was observed at δ_H 2.44 (dd, J = 17.8, 13.5 Hz), 2.37 (dd, J = 17.8, 4.3 Hz), and 1.98 (dd, J = 13.5, 4.3 Hz), while the AB part of this system corresponds to the hydrogen atoms of the CH_2-1, and the C part is ascribed to the β-*axial* H-10. The COSY spectrum of **4** (Figure 9) supports these assignments since the expected cross peaks of correlation were observed. In the ^{1}H NMR spectrum of **4**, despite being similar to that of compound **3**, the lack of an additional hydrogen atom geminal to a hydroxyl function indicated that **4** was devoid of the secondary hydroxyl group at C-6 present in **3**.

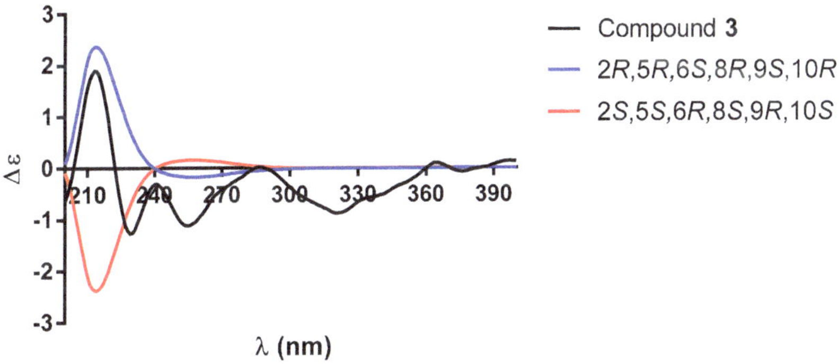

Figure 8. Comparison between the experimental (black line) and calculated ECD spectra for enantiomers (2*R*, 5*R*, 6*S*, 8*R*, 9*S*, 10*R*)-**3** (blue line) and (2*S*, 5*S*, 6*R*, 8*S*, 9*R*, 10*S*)-**3** (red line).

Table 3. NMR data (500 MHz, $CDCl_3$) of **4** and **5**.

		4			5	
Position	δ_C	**Type**	δ_H, **Multiplicity (*J* in Hz)**	δ_C	**Type**	δ_H, **Multiplicity (*J* in Hz)**
1	35.3	CH_2	2.44, dd (17.8, 13.5) 2.37, dd (17.8, 4.3)	34.7	CH_2	2.54, dd (17.8, 13.9) 2.37, dd (17.8, 3.4)
2	200.1	C		200.2	C	
3	121.4	CH	6.10, br s	125.4	CH	5.97, br s
4	173.6	C		170.6	C	
5	39.2,	C		35.0	C	
6	34.6	CH_2	1.57, m 1.45, m	73.8	CH	3.83, dd (8.7, 6.9)
7	26.7	CH_2	1.53, m	37.0	CH_2	1.63, m
8	36.2	CH	1.58, m			1.55, m
9	38.9	C		34.5	CH	1.70, m
10	45.8	CH	1.98, dd (13.5, 4.3)	45.1	CH	1.91, dd (13.9, 3.6)
11	35.1	CH_2	1.54, m	35.0	CH_2	2.51, ddd (13.7, 12.3, 4.9) 1.49, m
12	18.9	CH_2	2.21, m 2.04, m	18.8	CH_2	2.13, m 1.96, m
13	134.4	C		134.2	C	
14	143.9	CH	7.09, q (1.7)	144.2	CH	7.10, p (1.4)
15	70.4	CH_2	4.77, m	70.4	CH_2	477, q (1.7)
16	173.6	C		170.6	C	
17	15.8	CH_3	0.87, d (6.4)	14.8	CH_3	0.91, d (6.4)
18	60.6	CH_2	4.40, dd (17.6, 1.8) 4.35, dd (17.6, 1.8)	65.1	CH_2	4.51, d (15.0) 4.37, br d (15.0)
19	19.6	CH_3	1.20, s	17.6	CH_3	1.22, s
20	17.9	CH_3	0.85, s	15.5	CH_3	0.85, s

On the other hand, the ^{13}C NMR spectrum (Table 3) indicated the presence of three methyl, seven methylene (including two bonded to oxygen), and four methine (two of them of olefinic nature) groups and six fully substituted carbons (including two carbonyls, two sp^2 olefins, and two fully substituted sp^3 carbons). The UV spectrum exhibited two absorption maxima at λ_{max} 218 nm (log ε = 3.65) and 235.4 nm (log ε = 3.52), indicating that in addition to the α,β-unsaturated-γ-lactone, an α,β-unsaturated ketone must

comparison between the experimental and theoretical ECD spectra that led us to establish that the absolute configuration of **5** was 5*R*, 6*S*, 8*R*, 9*S*, and 10*R*, as depicted. Based on all the above data, compound **5** was identified as a patagonol (**14**) derivative named 2-oxo-6α-hydroxy-patagonol.

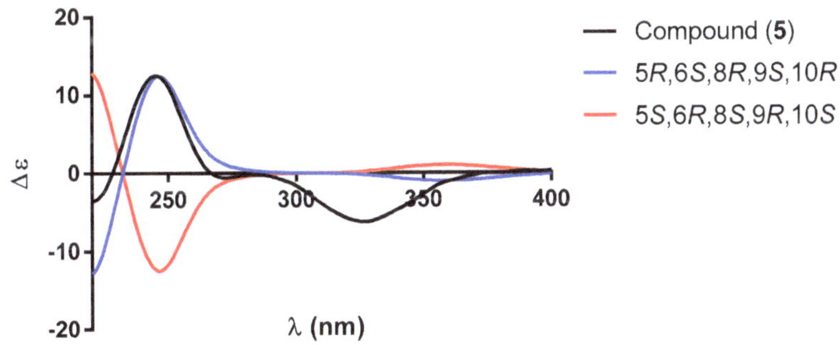

Figure 11. Comparison between the experimental (black line) and calculated ECD spectra for enantiomers (5*R*, 6*S*, 8*R*, 9*S*, 10*R*)-**5** (blue line) and (5*S*, 6*R*, 8*S*, 9*R*, 10*S*)-**5** (red line).

Compound **6** was isolated as a white powder at mp 48–50 °C. The UV spectrum showed two absorption maxima at λ_{max} 217 (log ε = 3.93) and 233 nm (log ε 3.86), thus indicating the presence of chromophores similar to those present in compounds **4** and **5**. The IR spectrum of compound **6** was similar to those of 2-oxo-patagonol (**4**) and 2-oxo-6α-hydroxy-patagonol (**5**), although the intensity of the band at 1676 cm^{-1} ascribed to the α,β-unsaturated ketone was higher, indicating the presence of an additional conjugated carbonyl group. This carbonyl group was part of an aldehyde moiety, since in the ^{13}C NMR spectrum of **6** (Table 4), a signal at δ_C 197.5 was observed, which correlated in the HSQC spectrum with a signal at δ_H 9.75 (Table 4). These facts indicated that the diterpenoid **6** was closely related to patagonal (**15**), a diterpenoid isolated together with patagonol (**14**) from the *Casimirella* species [10]. Another relevant signal observed in the ^1H NMR spectrum of **6** was a doublet of doublets at δ_H 3.75 (J = 11.1, 4.7 Hz), which was ascribed to the hydrogen atom geminal to a secondary hydroxyl group located at C-6. The coupling constants, J = 11.1, 4.7 Hz, indicated that the hydroxyl was *equatorially* oriented. Based on the previous discussion, the diterpenoid **6** was identified as 6α-hydroxy-patagonal. The absolute configuration of 6α-hydroxy-patagonal (**6**) was also established via ECD. Figure 12 shows a comparison between the experimental and calculated ECD spectra that led us to the conclusion that compound **6** possessed the same absolute configuration as diterpenoids **1–5**.

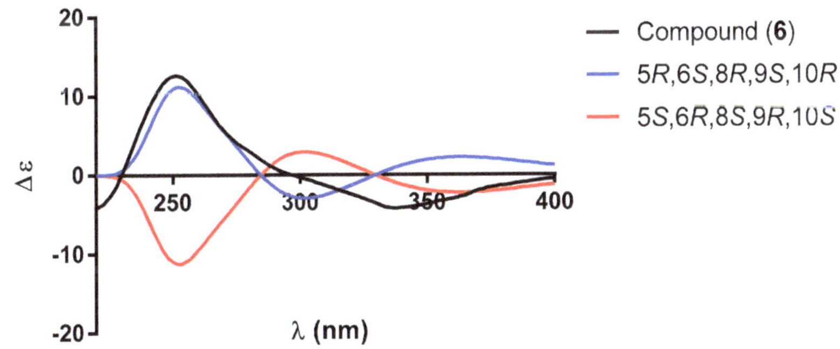

Figure 12. Comparison between the experimental (black line) and calculated ECD spectra for enantiomers (5*R*, 6*S*, 8*R*, 9*S*, 10*R*)−**6** (blue line) and (5*S*, 6*R*, 8*S*, 9*R*, 10*S*)−**6** (red line).

Table 4. NMR data (500 MHz, $CDCl_3$) of **6**.

	6				6		
Position	δ_C	Type	δ_H (J in Hz)	Position	δ_C	Type	δ_H (J in Hz)
1	35.3	CH_2	2.65 dd (18.1, 14.1) 2.56, dd (18.1, 3.6)	11	35	CH_2	1.62, m 1.51, ddd (14.7, 12.8, 4.8)
2	199.9	C					
3	141.1	CH	6.43, br s	12	18.7	CH_2	2.18, tdd (12.9, 4.3, 2.0) 1.97, m
4	163.8	C		13	134.1	C	
5	45.8	C		14	144.1	CH	7.10, br s
6	72.1	CH	3.75, dd (11.1, 4.7)	15	70.4	CH_2	4.77, q (2.1)
7	35.5	CH_2	177, ddd (13.3, 4.8, 3.0) 1.65, m	16	174.2	C	
				17	15.6	CH_3	0.84, d (6.6)
8	34.2	CH	1.71, m	18	197.5	CH	9.75, s
9	38.6	C		19	15.2	CH_3	1.13, s
10	44.8	CH	1.95, dd (14.1, 3.5)	20	17.1	CH_3	0.78, s
				6-OH			4.63, s

The treatment of 2α,6α-dihydroxy-patagonol (**3**) with PCC afforded, after 24 h of stirring at room temperature, a mixture of compounds identical in all aspects to **5** (10.9% yield) and **6** (31.4% yield), thus confirming the proposed structure for these diterpenoids.

Compounds **7–9** exhibited similar ^{1}H and ^{13}C NMR spectra to those of **3** and **5** (see the experimental section). In addition to the signals that indicated their *neo*-clerodane nature, the ^{13}C NMR spectra of **7–9** displayed signals of quaternary carbons at δ_C 101.1, 101.3, and 101.6, respectively. These signals, in addition to the signals of two additional methyl groups, in the range of 23.9–24.9, indicated the presence of an acetonide group in compounds **7–9**. Their ^{1}H NMR spectra support the presence of the acetonide group since, besides the characteristic methyl groups of a *neo*-clerodane-type diterpenoid, the signals of two additional methyl groups at δ_H 1.34–1.37 were observed. The HMBC spectra of **7–9** showed correlation cross peaks between the C-18 methylene hydrogens (δ_H 3.65–4.59) and H-6 (δ_H 3.58–3.75), with the quaternary carbons (δ_C 100.1–100.6) indicating that the acetonide was formed between the OH groups at the C-18 and C-6 positions. Acetonides **7–9** must have formed during the chromatographic purification since acetone was used as an eluent. An inspection of the Dreiding models of compounds **7–9** and the precursor diols indicated that the formation of the acetonide is highly favored. That the plausible precursor diols for acetonides **8** and **9** are 2α,6α-dihydroxy-patagonol (**3**) and 2-oxo-6α-hydroxy-patagonol (**5**) was proven via the treatment of 2α,6α-dihydroxy-patagonol (**3**) with anhydrous acetone in the presence of anhydrous $CuSO_4$, yielding **8**, and further oxidation of **8** with PCC in dichloromethane, affording compound **9**. While the diols **3** and **5** were obtained from the DCM extract of *S. guevarae*, the precursor of **7** (6α-hydroxy-patagonol) was not isolated; thus, we considered that it was present in the crude extract in small quantities. Based on the previous discussion, acetonides **7–9** should be considered acetone artifacts, instead of natural products.

Compound **10** was isolated as colorless crystals at mp 182-184 °C and identified as 7α-acetoxy-*ent*-clerodan-3,13-dien-18,19:16,15-diolide based mainly on its NMR data. Diterpenoid **10** was previously isolated from a population of *Salvia melissodora* Lag. [12] collected in the State of San Luis Potosí, Mexico. The undescribed high-resolution NMR and DART-MS data are recorded in the experimental section. On the other hand, in this study, we report the X-ray analysis of **10** since the absolute configuration of this diterpenoid was not established in its original description. The molecular structure of **10** is shown in Figure 13, and the crystallographic details are presented in the Supplementary Materials (Table S1). Compound **10** was crystallized in the orthorhombic P2(1)2(1)2(1) space group, and its absolute structure parameters—Flack(x), 0.01(5); Hooft(y), 0.00(5); and Parsons(z), 0.00(3)—confirm the assignment of the crystal model as well as the configuration of the chiral carbon atoms as being 5*S*, 7*R*, 8*S*, 9*R*, and 10*R*.

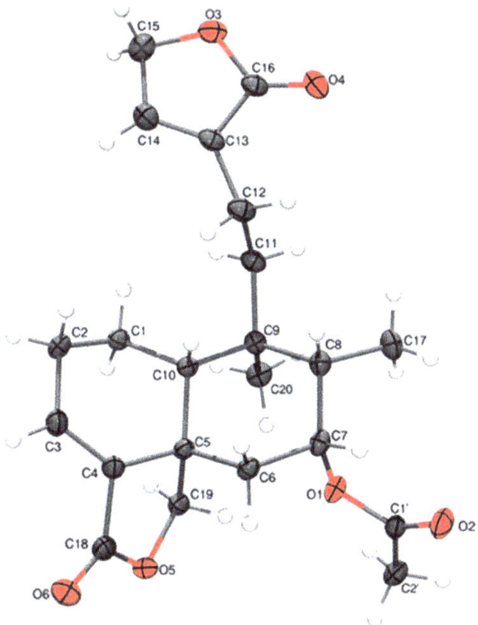

Figure 13. The molecular structure of compound **10**. The thermal ellipsoids are set at 50% of the probability level.

While products **11** and **12** have previously been obtained from *S. melissodora* and identified as 7-keto-*ent*-clerodan-3,13-dien-18,19:16,15-diolide and 7α-hydroxy-*ent*-clerodan-3,13-dien-18,19:16,15-diolide, respectively [12], compound **13** was identical in all aspect to mkapwanin, previously isolated from *Dodonea angustifolia* (Sapindaceae) [13]. The absolute configuration of these diterpenoids, as depicted in **11–13**, was established via a comparison of their experimental ECD spectra with theoretically calculated curves (see Supplemental Figure S61 and Figure S62, and S63). The undescribed high-resolution NMR and DART-MS data are recorded in the experimental section.

In addition to the previously described *neo*-clerodane diterpenoids, six already known triterpenoids were isolated from the DCM extract of *S. guevarae*, identified as 3β,20,25-trihydroxylupane [14], oleanolic acid [15], 3β-*O*-acetyl-oleanolic acid [16], ursolic acid [17], 3β-*O*-acetyl-betulinic acid [18], and 3β,28-*O*-diacetyl-betulin [19].

Chromatographic purification of the methanol extract of *S. guevarae* afforded several previously described phenolic compounds identified via spectroscopic and spectrometric methods and a comparison with literature data: quercetin-3-*O*-β-xylopyranosil-(1 → 2)-β-galactopyranoside, taxifolin-7-*O*-β-glucopyranoside, naringenin 7-*O*-β-glucopyranoside, a mixture of 2*R* and 2*S* eriodictyol-7-*O*-β-glucopyranoside, caffeic acid, the methyl ester of rosmarinic acid, and rosmarinic acid. Quercetin-3-*O*-β-xylopyranosil-(1 → 2)-β-galactopyranoside was originally isolated from the horseradish *Amoracia rusticana* (Brassicaceae) [20]; white clover *Trifolium repens* (Fabaceae) [21]; *Asclepias syriaca* (Asclepidaceae) [22]; *Prunus padus* (Rosaceae) [23]; and recently, *Elaeagnus umbellata* (Elaeagnaceae) [24]. Taxifolin-7-*O*-β-glucopyranoside was isolated for the first time from *Podocar-*

pus nivalis (Podocarpaceae) [25] and from species belonging to different plant families including Pinaceae [26–28], Rosaceae, and Lamiaceae [29]. While the herbal drugs *Crataegus pentagyna* (Rosaceae) (*Crataegi folium cum flore*) [30] and *Lysimachia patungensis* (Primulaceae) are natural sources of naringenin 7-*O*-β-glucopyranoside, a mixture of diastereomers (2*R*) and (2*S*)-eriodictyol 7-*O*-β-D-glucopyranoside was isolated from the parasitic plant *Balanophora involucrata* (Balanophoraceae) [31]. Caffeic acid is a widely distributed compound and has been reported in several *Salvia spp.* [32–34]. Rosmarinic acid is an ester of caffeic acid and 3,4-dihydroxyphenyllactic acid, commonly found in members of the Lamiaceae family, and exhibits a wide range of biological activities, such as antioxidant, antibacterial, antiviral, and anti-inflammatory activities [35]. The methyl ester of rosmarinic acid is also widely distributed in genera of the Lamiaceae family such as *Salvia* and *Melissa* [36].

2.2. Biological Activity

2.2.1. Antiproliferative Activity

The Lamiaceae and Euphorbiaceae families are a rich source of diterpenoids with promising anticancer activity. In the Lamiaceae family, although several abietane- and icetexane-type diterpenoids exhibited interesting antiproliferative activity in different cancer cell lines, some *trans*-clerodane diterpenoids also have demonstrated interesting cytotoxic activity [37]. Therefore, we evaluated the antiproliferative activity of some of the diterpenoids isolated from *S. guevarae* against a panel of six human cancer cell lines: U251 (glioblastoma), PC-3 (prostate cancer), K562 (chronic myelogenous leukemia), HCT-15 (colon cancer), MCF-7 (breast cancer), and SKLU-1 (lung adenocarcinoma). The cell line COS-7 (monkey kidney) was used for an evaluation of the cytotoxicity in a normal cell line. The results of the primary screening of the crude DCM extract at 25 ppm and diterpenoids **1–3**,**1a**, **3**, and **5–11** at 25 μM are included in Table S3. Significant inhibition of the K562 cell line was observed for the crude DCM extract, with 96.6%, and no significant cytotoxicity was observed in the other cancer cell lines of the panel. Guevarain B (**2**) and the acetonide of 6α-hydroxy-patagonol (**7**) showed only moderate, although selective, activity against K562, with 43.3 and 46.9% inhibition, respectively, being non-cytotoxic to normal cell line COS-7 and the rest of the panel. Weak cytotoxic activity against K562 was observed for 6α-hydroxy-patagonal (**6**) (34.7%) and compound **10** (31.7%). Compound **1a** and 6α-hydroxy-patagonal (**6**) also exhibited weak activity against U251 (35.2%) and PC-3 (38.1%), respectively. Only diterpenoid **10** proved to be weakly cytotoxic against COS-7 (30.6%). Table 5 shows the results of the IC_{50} of guevarain B (**2**) and the acetonide of 6α-hydroxy-patagonol (**7**) against the chronic myelogenous leukemia K562 cell line compared with that of Adriamycin.

Table 5. IC_{50} (μM) values of the antiproliferative activity for compounds **2** and **7** against K562.

Compounds	IC_{50}
2	33.1 ± 1.3
7	39.8 ± 1.5
Adriamycin	0.2 ± 0.0

2.2.2. Anti-Inflammatory Activity Due to the Inhibition of NO Production in RAW 264.7 Macrophage Cells

Terpenoids have been widely studied due to their great structural diversity and the wide range of biological activities they have exhibited, among which an anti-inflammatory effect can be listed. Diterpenes belonging to different molecular arrangements, including labdane-, kaurane-, pimarane-, and clerodane-type diterpenoids, have been shown to have interesting anti-inflammatory effects in different experimental models, among them the inhibition of NO release in lipopolysaccharide-stimulated RAW 264.7 macrophage cells [38]. Based on these backgrounds, the evaluation of the anti-inflammatory effect of some of the diterpenes obtained from *S. guevarae* was carried out through the quantification of the release of NO via nitrite formation, through the Griess reaction, in stimulated RAW 264.7 macrophages. The induction of NO was promoted using *E. coli* lipopolysaccharide at 1 μg/mL (*E. coli*, serotype 055 B5, Sigma). Table S4 shows the results obtained for diterpenoids **1–3**, **5–7**, and **9–10**. Aminoguanidine and celecoxib, at a concentration of 100 μM, were used as standards. Cell viability was evaluated via the MTT method. It is important to mention that none of the evaluated diterpenes generated nitrites in the supernatant, which indicates that they do not induce the formation of NO. Compound **5** showed moderate inhibition; however, a higher percentage of activity was observed for compounds **6**, **7**, and **10**. Table 6 shows the IC_{50} value for the most active compounds compared with that of aminoguanidine. 6α-Hydroxy-patagonal (**6**) showed an activity comparable with that of the standard; however, a 15% decrease in the viability of macrophages was observed (data shown in Table S4). On the other hand, compounds **7** and **10** showed an IC_{50} lower than that observed for aminoguanidine, with high viability in the RAW 264.7 cells. These results indicate that products **6**, **7**, and **10** have promising anti-inflammatory activity.

Table 6. IC_{50} (μM) values for the inhibition of nitrite production for compounds **7**, **8**, and **11**.

Compound	IC_{50} (μM)
6	26.4 ± 0.4
7	17.3 ± 0.5
10	13.7 ± 2.0
Aminoguanidine	26.2 ± 0.4

The results are expressed as the mean ± S.E.M. of three determinations.

2.3. Taxonomic Considerations

In its original description, *S. guevarae* was classified in section Holwaya Ramamoorthy [9], together with the Mexican species *S. holwayi* Blake, *S. karwinskii* Benth., *S. involucrata* Cav., *S. puberula* Fernald, *S. stolonifera* Benth., and *S. wagneriana* Polak [8]. On the other hand, in 1991, during a taxonomic revision of section Nobiles Epling, *S. adenophora* Fernald, *S. disjuncta* Fernald, and *S. gesneriflora* Lindl & Paxton were transferred to section Holwaya [39]. Although from the taxonomic point of view, *S. guevarae* is closely related to *S. karwinskii*, *S. wagneriana*, *S. involucrata*, and *S. holwayii*, a hierarchical cluster analysis of the diterpenoid content of the members of section Holwaya phytochemically studied thus far, such as *S. adenophora* [40], *S. gesneriflora* [41,42], *S. involucrata* [43], *S. puberula* [44], *S. karwinskii* [45], and *S. wagneriana* [46], including the results obtained in this work from *S. guevarae*, indicated the presence of three groups that can be distinguished (Figure 14). *S. puberula* is, from the chemosystematic point of view, different from the rest of the species in section Holwaya, since *S. puberula* contents only rearranged isosalvipuberulane and salvipuberulane diterpenoids. On the other hand, *S. wagneriana*, *S. karwinskii*, *S. involucrata*, and *S. gesneriflora* constitute a second group with similar diterpenoid constituents. The third group indicates a close similarity between the diterpenoids obtained from *S. adenophora* and *S. guevarae*. Although no phylogenetical analysis has been conducted on *S. guevarae*, the oxidation and substitution pattern of the *neo*-clerodane described in this work support the inclusion of *S. guevarae* in section Holwaya.

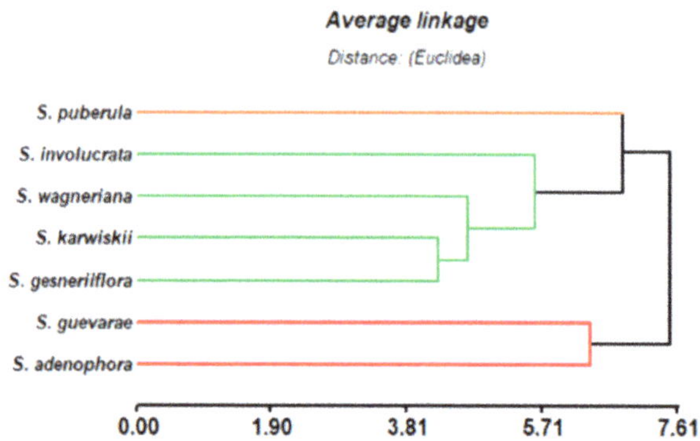

Figure 14. Hierarchical cluster analysis of the *Salvia* species from section *Holwaya* with phytochemicals studies, including *S. guevarae*.

3. Materials and Methods

3.1. General Experimental Procedures

The melting points (uncorrected) were determined on a Fisher Johns apparatus (Fisher Scientific Company, Pittsburgh, PA, USA). Optical rotations were measured on a PerkinElmer 341 polarimeter (PerkinElmer Inc., London, UK). The UV spectra were recorded on a Shimadzu UV 160U spectrophotometer (Shimadzu, Kyoto, Japan). The ECD spectra were measured using a JASCO J-1500 Circular Dichroism Spectrophotometer (JASCO Inc., Easton, MD, USA). The IR spectra were obtained on a Bruker Tensor 27 spectrometer (Bruker Corporation, Billerica, MA, USA); 1D and 2D NMR experiments were performed on a Bruker Advance III HD spectrometer (Bruker Corporation, Billerica, MA, USA) at 700 MHz for ^{1}H and 175 MHz for ^{13}C, a Bruker AVANCE III HD spectrometer (Bruker Corporation, Billerica, MA, USA) at 500 MHz for ^{1}H and 125 MHz for ^{13}C, or a Bruker Avance III (Bruker Corporation, Billerica, MA, USA) at 400 MHz for ^{1}H and 100 MHz for ^{13}C. $CDCl_3$, $(CD_3)_2CO$, and CD_3OD were used as solvents as indicated, and the chemical shifts were attributed to the residual solvents $CHCl_3$ ($\delta_H = 7.26$, $\delta_C = 77.16$), CH_3OH ($\delta_H = 3.31$, $\delta_C = 49$), and $(CH_3)_2CO$ ($\delta_H = 2.05$, $\delta_C = 29.84$). The HR-DART-MS data were obtained on The AccuTOF JMS-T100LC mass spectrometer created by Jeol (Jeol Ltd., Tokyo, Japan) or the HPLC-ESI-QTOF-MS 1260-G6530 model (Agilent Tech. Santa Clara, CA, USA) using a column Zorbax Extend-C18 (Agilent, 50 × 3.0 mm × 3.5 µm), with the mobile phase as follows: A, H_2O with CH_3COOH 0.1% and B, CH_3CN (in a gradient (0–12 min (85% A, 15% B): 100% B), 0.400 mL/min 600.00 bar). The X-ray data were collected on a Bruker APEX II DUO diffractometer (Bruker Corporation, Billerica, MA, USA). Silica gel 230–400 mesh (Macherey-Nagel; Düren, Germany) and Sephadex LH-20 (Pharmacia Biotech AB, Uppsala, Sweden) were used for Column Chromatography (CC). Precoated silica gel TLC plates (Merck, St. Louis, MO, USA) were used for thin layer chromatography (TLC).

3.2. Plant Materials

Salvia guevarae was collected at Xilitla, San Luis Potosi, Mexico, 21°24′34″ N, −99°5′9″ W, and 2100 m altitude, in October 2018. The plant material was identified by Dr. Brenda Y. Bedolla-Garcia and Dr. Sergio Zamudio and deposited in the Herbarium of the Instituto de Ecología, A. C., Centro Regional del Bajío (voucher IEB-266884).

3.3. Extraction and Isolation

The dried and powdered leaves of *S. guevarae* (361 g) were extracted via percolation with CH_2Cl_2 (2 L). The CH_2Cl_2 extract was concentrated at reduced pressures to yield 10.5 g of residue, a portion (9.5 g) of which was subjected to column chromatography (CC, 21 cm in length by 5 cm in internal diameter) on silica gel using a gradient elution with $C_6H_{14}/CH_3COOCH_2CH_3$ (100:0-0:100); $(CH_3)_2CO$ (100%); and finally, CH_3OH as the mobile phase to obtain 80 eluates, 150 mL each, which were combined into 22 major fractions (A−U) after thin-layer chromatography (TLC) evaluation. The acetylation of fraction H (50 mg) and subsequent purification using preparative TLC on silica gel, eluting with $C_6H_{14}/CH_3COOCH_2CH_3$ (80:20) as the mobile phase, gave 3β,28-*O*-diacetyl betulin (13.2 mg) and a mixture of 3β-*O*-acetyl oleanolic acid and 3β-*O*-acetyl betulinic acid (18.9 mg). Oleanolic and ursolic acids were identified as the constituents of fraction I (1296 mg). Fraction M (277 mg) was subjected to CC (35 × 2.5 cm) on silica gel, eluting with $C_6H_{14}/CH_3COOCH_2CH_3$ (40:60) to obtain 25 subfractions, 50 mL each, which were combined into 8 major subfractions (MA−MH) based on a TLC evaluation. Subfraction MC (48 mg) was purified via preparative TLC on silica gel, eluting with $CH_2Cl_2/CH_3COOCH_2CH_3$ (70:30) to give **13** (1.7 mg). Compound **10** (13.7 mg) was obtained as a solid from fraction N, and the mother liquors (369 mg) of this fraction were subjected to CC (20 × 35cm) on silica gel using $C_6H_{14}/(CH_3)_2CO$ (80:20) as the eluent to obtain 14 subfractions (NA−NN) based on a TLC profile. Compound **7** (11 mg) was identified from fraction NC. Compound **10** (116 mg) was crystallized from $C_6H_{14}/CH_3COOCH_2CH_3$ in fraction NJ. Subfraction NK (28.5 mg) was subjected to preparative TLC on silica gel, eluting with $CH_2Cl_2/CH_3COOCH_2CH_3$ (8:2) to give **12** (2 mg). Crystals of compound **1** (711 mg) were obtained from fraction O, and the mother liquor's residue (1079 mg) was subjected to CC on silica gel using $CH_2Cl_2/(CH_3)_2CO$ (90:10) to obtain 18 subfractions (OA−OQ) based on a TLC evaluation. Subfraction OF (156 mg) was subjected to CC (32.5 × 2 cm) on Sephadex LH-20 using CH_3OH as an eluent to obtain four subfractions (OFA−OFD) based on a TLC evaluation. Subfraction OFC (29 mg) was subjected to preparative TLC on silica gel, eluting with $CH_2Cl_2/CH_3COOCH_2CH_3$ (70:30) to give **11** (8 mg). Subfraction OI (55 mg) was purified via TLC on silica gel in the C8 reverse phase (RP-8) using CH_3OH/H_2O (70:30) as the mobile phase to give **2** (30 mg). Compound 3β,20,25-trihydroxylupane (18 mg) was identified as the constituent of fraction ON. Fraction P (398 mg) was subjected to CC (15 × 1.8 cm) on Sephadex LH-20, eluting with methanol to obtain six subfractions (PA−PF) based on a TLC evaluation. Subfraction PC (261 mg) was subjected to CC (12 × 2 cm) on silica gel using $C_6H_{14}/(CH_3)_2CO$ (50:50) to obtain 12 subfractions (PCA−PCL) based on a TLC evaluation. Compound **4** (3 mg) was purified from subfraction PCF via TLC on silica gel, eluting with $C_6H_{14}/CH_3COOCH_2CH_3/CH_3OH/H_2O$ (100:100:8:3.5). Compound **3** (410 mg) was obtained as a powder from fraction Q. Subfraction R (717 mg) was subjected to CC (22 × 2.5 cm) on silica gel using $CH_2Cl_2/(CH_3)_2CO$ (60:40) to obtain 13 subfractions (RA−RM) after TLC evaluation. Subfraction RC (48 mg) was purified via preparative TLC using $C_6H_{14}/C_7H_8/CH_3COOCH_2CH_3$ (30:30:40) as the mobile phase to obtain compound **6** (1.8 mg). Subfraction RD (146 mg) was purified via CC (11 × 1.8 cm) on silica gel using $C_6H_{14}/CH_3COOCH_2CH_3$ (70:30) as the mobile phase to obtain 9 subfractions (RDA−RDI) based on a TLC evaluation. Compound **8** (61.8 mg) was obtained from subfraction RDE. Subfraction RF (100 mg) was purified via CC (11 × 2.5 cm) on silica gel using $C_6H_{14}/CH_3COOCH_2CH_3$ (30:70) as an eluent to obtain 7 subfractions (RFA−RFG) based on a TLC profile. Compound **5** (4 mg) was obtained from subfraction RFD. Subfraction RFE (54 mg) was treated with anhydrous acetone (2 mL) and copper sulfate (120 mg) to obtain a mix of compounds. Compound **9** (2 mg) was obtained after purification via TLC on silica gel, eluting with $CH_2Cl_2/(CH_3)_2CO$ (70:30) as the mobile phase.

The material previously extracted with dichloromethane was subjected to percolation with methanol to obtain 12.8 g of an extract. The methanolic extract was subjected to a liquid–liquid extraction process with a mixture of $(C_6H_{14}:C_6H_6)/(CH_3OH:H_2O)$ (25:25:45:5), and the $CH_3OH:H_2O$ fraction (11.4 g) was fractionated on a Sephadex LH 20 column using methanol as the mobile phase to obtain 7 fractions (A–G). Subfraction C (600 mg) was subjected to flash chromatography (14 × 5 cm) in the C_{18} reverse phase (RP-18), eluting with a mixture of $CH_3CN:H_2O$ (0.1% formic acid) (5:100-100:0) to obtain 20 subfractions (CA-CT) based on an analytical TLC evaluation. Taxifolin-7-*O*-β-glucopyranoside (45 mg) was obtained from subfraction CF. Subfraction CI (35 mg) was purified via TLC on RP-18 using $CH_3COOCH_2CH_3/CH_3OH$ (70:30) to give quercetin-3-*O*-β-xylopyranosyl-(1 → 2)-β-galactopyranoside (12 mg) and caffeic acid (2.5 mg). A mixture of 2*R* and 2*S* eriodictyol-7-*O*-β-glucopyranoside (1.8 mg) was obtained from subfraction CJ. Subfraction CN (20 mg) was subjected to TLC on RP-18 using CH_3OH/H_2O (40:60) as the mobile phase to give naranginin-7-*O*-β-glucopyranoside (6 mg) and rosmarinic acid (10 mg). 3-*O*-Methylrosmarinic acid was identified from subfraction CR.

Guevarain A (1): colorless crystals; mp 136−138 °C; $[\alpha]^{25}_D$ +23.3 (c 0.0045, MeOH); UV (MeOH) λ_{max} (log ε) 207 (3.16) nm; IR (ATR) ν_{max} 3606, 2964, 2932, 2876, 1755, 1654, 1602, 1451, 1349, 1203, 1076, 998 cm^{-1}; ^1H and ^{13}C NMR ($(CD_3)_2CO$): see Table 1; HR-DART-MS *m*/*z* 317.2103 $[M + H - H_2O]^+$; (calcd for $C_{20}H_{29}O_3$, 317.2117).

Guevarain B (2): colorless crystals; mp 112−114 °C; $[\alpha]^{25}_D$ −5.6 (c 0.0006, MeOH); UV (MeOH) λ_{max} (log ε) 214.4 (4.08), 239.8 (4.07), 227.8 (4.01) nm; ECD (*c* 3.01 mM, MeOH) $[\theta]_{257}$ +92349.6, $[\theta]_{278}$ 0, $[\theta]_{325}$ −68602.6; IR (ATR) ν_{max} 3417, 2957, 2930, 2869, 1747, 1644, 1607, 826 cm^{-1}; ^1H and ^{13}C NMR ($CDCl_3$): see Table 1; HR-DART-MS *m*/*z* 333.2063 $[M+H]^+$; (calcd for $C_{20}H_{29}O_4$, 333.2066).

2α,6α-Dihydroxy-patagonol (3): white powder; mp 98−100 °C; $[\alpha]^{25}_D$ +23.1 (c 0.0016, MeOH); UV (MeOH) λ_{max} (log ε) 207.5 (6.45) nm; ECD (*c* 3.14 mM, MeOH) $[\theta]_{213}$ +6266.6, $[\theta]_{229}$ −4287.7, $[\theta]_{255}$ −5936.8, $[\theta]_{321}$ −2968.4; IR (ATR) ν_{max} 3266, 1754, 1649, 1642 cm^{-1}; ^1H and ^{13}C NMR (CD_3OD): see Table 2; HR-DART-MS *m*/*z* 350.2090 $[M-H]^+$; (calcd for $C_{20}H_{30}O_5$, 349.2093).

2-Oxo-patagonol (4): white powder; mp 103−105 °C; $[\alpha]^{25}_D$ −25.6 (c 0.0018, MeOH); UV (MeOH) λ_{max} (log ε) 218.0 (3.65) nm; ECD (*c* 5.41 mM, MeOH) $[\theta]_{215}$ −53430.8, $[\theta]_{244}$ +42876.6, $[\theta]_{322}$ −20448.8; IR (ATR) ν_{max} 3411, 2927, 2872, 1747, 1651, 1050, 773 cm^{-1}; ^1H and ^{13}C NMR ($CDCl_3$): see Table 3; HR-DART-MS *m*/*z* 333.2066 $[M+H]^+$; (calcd for $C_{20}H_{29}O_4$, 333.2066).

6α-Hydroxy-2-oxo-patagonol (5): white powder; mp 92–94 °C; $[\alpha]^{25}_D$ +16 (c 0.001, MeOH); UV (MeOH) λ_{max} (log ε) 241.2 (3.85) nm; ECD (*c* 2.87 mM, MeOH) $[\theta]_{245}$ +40897.7, $[\theta]_{284}$ 0, $[\theta]_{326}$ 21108.5; IR (ATR) ν_{max} 3400, 2956, 2929, 2874, 1741, 1650, 1449, 1266, 1209, 1006, 733 cm^{-1}; ^1H and ^{13}C NMR ($CDCl_3$): see Table 3; HR-DART-MS *m*/*z* 349.2025 $[M+H]^+$; (calcd for $C_{20}H_{29}O_5$, 349.2015).

6α-Hydroxy-2-oxo-patagonal (6): white powder; mp 48−50 °C; $[\alpha]^{25}_D$ −12.7 (c 0.0011, MeOH); UV (MeOH) λ_{max} (log ε) 241.4 (4.08) nm; ECD (*c* 3.17 mM, MeOH) $[\theta]_{251}$ +41557.3, $[\theta]_{295}$ 0, $[\theta]_{338}$ −14512.1; IR (ATR) ν_{max} 3439, 2958, 2931, 2876, 1744, 1676, 1449, 1348, 1261, 1206, 1072, 1048, 832 cm^{-1}; ^1H and ^{13}C NMR ($CDCl_3$): see Table 4; HR-DART-MS *m*/*z* 347.1859 $[M + H]^+$; (calcd for $C_{20}H_{29}O_4$, 347.1859).

2,6-Dioxo-guevarain (1a): Treatment of **1** (50 mg) with pyridinium chlorochromate (20.1 mg) in DCM gave a complex mixture, which was subjected to CC in silica gel using EtOAc as the mobile phase to afford guevarain B (**2**) (14.4 mg) and **1a** (7 mg) as a white powder; mp 148−150 °C; $[\alpha]^{25}_D$ −36 (c 0.003, MeOH); UV (MeOH) λ_{max} (log ε) 241.4 (4.08) nm; IR (ATR) ν_{max} 3416, 1746, 1643, 1607 cm^{-1}; ^{1}H and ^{13}C NMR ($CDCl_3$): see Table 2; HR-DART-MS m/z 331.1898 [M + H]$^+$; (calcd for $C_{20}H_{27}O_4$, 331.1909).

6α-Hydroxy-2-oxo-patagonal (6): Treatment of 3 (24.8 mg) with pyridinium chlorochromate (15.25 mg) gave a complex mixture, which was subjected to CC in silica gel using EtOAc as the mobile phase to afford **5** (2.7 mg) and **6** (7.7 mg) as white powders.

Acetonide 7. Compound 3 (51.4 mg) was dissolved in freshly distilled acetone and treated with anhydrous CuSO4 (35 mg) and stirred for 1 h. A work-up of the reaction afforded 34.4 mg of a compound, identical in all aspects to **7**.

Acetonide 9. The treatment of synthetic diterpenoid **7** (34 mg) was oxidized with 57 mg of PCC in DCM. After stirring at room temperature for 24 h, 26 mg (76%) of a compound identical to acetonide **9** was obtained.

3.4. Electronic Circular Dichroism Calculations

The compounds **2–6** and **10–13** were constructed, and their geometry was optimized using a semiempirical method (PM3), as implemented in Spartan'10. A conformational analysis was performed using the same software and force field. All conformers were filtered and checked for redundancy. Subsequently, the conformers with relativity energies $\leq$ 2.0 or 2.5 Kcal/mol were minimized and optimized with Gaussian 09 using a DFT force field at the B3YLP/DGZVP level of theory for optimization and frequency. The ECD calculations for compounds **2–7** and **12–14** in a MeOH solution were carried out by employing a TD-SCF force field at the B3LYP/6-31G(d) theory level, with the default solvent model. The calculated excitation energy (nm) and rotatory strength (R) in dipole velocity (Rvel) form were simulated into an ECD curve using Equation (1), as implemented in SpecDis software (Version 1.71), where E0k and R0k are the transition energy and rotatory strength of kth electronic transition, respectively, and σ is the exponential half width.

$$\Delta\varepsilon = \frac{1}{2.297 \times 10^{-39}} \times \frac{1}{\sigma\sqrt{\pi}} \sum\nolimits_k E_{0k} R_{0k} exp\left[-\left\{\frac{E - E_{0k}}{\sigma}\right\}^2\right] \quad (1)$$

All calculations were performed on the HP Cluster Platform 3000SL Miztli, a parallel supercomputer with a Linux operating system, containing 25,312 cores and a total of 45,000 GB of RAM.

3.5. Single-Crystal X-Ray Diffraction Analysis of 1 and 10

The relevant details of the crystals, data collection, and structure refinement for compounds **1** and **10** can be found in Table S1. The data for guevarain **A** (**1**) and diterpenoid **10** were collected on a Bruker APEX II CCD Diffractometer at 100 K, using Cu-Ka radiation (k = 1.54178 Å) from an Incoatec ImuS source and Helios optic monochromator. Suitable crystals were coated with hydrocarbon oil, picked up with a nylon loop, and mounted in the cold nitrogen stream of the diffractometer. Frames were collected using ω scans and integrated with SAINT multi-scan absorption correction (SADABS). The structures were solved using direct methods and refined via full-matrix least squares on F2 with SHELXL-2018 [47] using the SHELXLE GUI [48]. The hydrogen atoms of the C–H bonds were placed in idealized positions, the hydrogens of the O–H moiety and the hydrogens of the water molecules were found on a map of residual density, and their position was refined with U_{iso} = aU_{eq} (where a is 1.5 for $-CH_3$ and –OH moieties and 1.2 for others). The molecular graphics were prepared using the POV-RAY and GIMP programs. The crystallographic data for the crystal's structures have been deposited at the Cambridge Crystallographic Data Centre under reference numbers CCDC 2,430,636 and CCDC 2430637 for compounds **1** and **10**, respectively.

The crystal data of **1** were collected from a colorless prism (0.433 × 0.405 × 0.290 mm^3) at 100(2) K: $C_{20}H_{32}O_5$, MW = 352.45, monoclinic, space group $P2_1$, unit cell dimensions a = 8.78990(10) Å, b = 10.45200(10) Å, c = 10.27570(10) Å, α = γ = 90°, β = 90.2546(4)°, V = 944.040(17) $Å^3$, Z = 2, Dc = 1.240 Mg/m^3, F(000) = 384. A total of 33,896 reflections were collected in the range 4.302° < θ < 71.003°, with 3601 independent reflections [R(int) = 0.0304]; completeness to θ_{max} was 99.8%. The structure was solved using direct methods and refined via full-matrix least squares on F^2, with anisotropic temperature factors for non-hydrogen atoms converging at R final indices [I > 2σ(I)], R1 = 0.0266, wR2 = 0.0725; R indices (all data), R1 = 0.0266, wR2 = 0.0725. The absolute Flack, Hooft, and Parsons structure parameters were −0.02(3), −0.02(2), and −0.019(16), respectively, thus indicating that the absolute configuration of compound **1** is that depicted in Figure 3. The configuration of the chiral carbon atoms is 2*R*, 5*R*, 6*S*, 8*R*, 9*S*, and 10*R*.

Crystallographic data for compound **10** were collected from a colorless prism (0.401 × 0.319 × 0.278 mm^3) at 100(2) K, orthorhombic, space group $P2_12_12_1$ (Table S1). A total of 32,163 reflections were collected, and the structure was solved using direct methods. The absolute Flack, Hooft, and Parsons structure parameters were 0.01(5), 0.00(5), and 0.00(3), thus indicating that the absolute configuration of compound **10** is that depicted in Figure 13.

3.6. Chemometric Analysis

A cluster analysis was carried out using a complete chaining method. The data consisted of structural characteristics of 47 diterpenoids reported from the *Salvia* species classified in section *Holwaya*, including *S. guevarae*. The type of diterpenoid scaffolds, the unsaturation index, the oxidation pattern, and the presence of lactones or furan groups in the structure were analyzed. The analysis was carried out using InfoStat software (version 2017, released in 2020).

3.7. Antiproliferative Activity

The crude DCM extracts at 25 ppm and diterpenoids **1–3**, **1a**, **3**, and **5–11** at 25 μM were evaluated in vitro against a panel of six human cancer cell lines: U251 (glioblastoma), PC-3 (prostate cancer), K562 (chronic myelogenous leukemia), HCT-15 (colon cancer), MCF-7 (breast cancer), and SKLU-1 (lung adenocarcinoma). The cell line COS-7 (monkey kidney) was used for the evaluation of the cytotoxicity in a normal cell line. The cell lines were supplied by the National Cancer Institute (USA) and American Type Culture Cells (ATCC). The cytotoxicity was evaluated using the protein-binding dye sulforhodamine B (SRB) in a microculture assay as previously reported by Monks et al. [7,49].

3.8. NO Inhibition in RAW 264.7 Macrophages

RAW 264.7 cells were obtained from the American Type Culture Collection (ATCC TIB-71), and cultured as previously described. Diterpenoids **1–3**, **5–7**, and **9–10** were dissolved in DMSO at 25 μM. The nitrite concentration in the medium was quantified as an indirect indicator of NO production following the Griess reaction and the experimental protocol previously reported [50]. Cell viability was evaluated via the MTT method, according to the protocol described by Mosmann and coworkers [51]. Table S4 shows the results obtained for the inhibition in nitrite production, and Table 6 shows the IC_{50} value for the most active compounds compared with those of aminoguanidine.

4. Conclusions

From the dichloromethane and methanolic extracts of the leaves of the new species *Salvia guevarae*, 13 *neo*-clerodanes diterpenoids (**1–13**) were isolated, of which **1–6** have yet to be described in the literature. The three acetonides **7–9** were artifacts produced via the reaction of diol derivatives with the acetone used in some parts of the separation process. The *neo*-clerodane diterpenoids **10–13** were known diterpenoids previously described from different sources. Six triterpenoids were also isolated and identified: 3β,20,25-trihydroxylupane, oleanolic acid, 3β-*O*-acetyl-oleanolic acid, ursolic acid, 3β-*O*-acetyl-betulinic acid, and 3β,28-*O*-diacetyl-betulin. Additionally, from the methanol extract of *S. guevarae*, several phenolic derivatives were isolated and identified: quercetin-3-*O*-β-xylopyranosyl-(1 → 2)-β-galactopyranoside, taxifolin-7-*O*-β-glucopyranoside, naringenin-7-*O*-β-glucopyranoside, a mixture of 2*R* and 2*S* eriodictyol-7-*O*-β-glucopyranoside, caffeic acid, the methyl ester of rosmarinic acid, and rosmarinic acid. The structure of the isolated compounds was established by spectroscopic means, mainly ^{1}H and ^{13}C NMR, including 1D and 2D homo- and heteronuclear experiments and some chemical reactions. The antiproliferative activity of some diterpenoids was determined via the sulforhodamine B method, where guevarain B (**2**) and 6α-hydroxy patagonol acetonide (**7**) showed moderate activity against the K562 line, with IC_{50} (μM) = 33.0 ± 1.3 and 39.8 ± 1.5, respectively. The NO inhibition in the RAW 264.7 macrophage activity via nitrite formation was also determined for some compounds, where 2-oxo-patagonal (**6**), 6α-hydroxy patagonol acetonide (**7**), and 7α-acetoxy-*ent*-clerodan-3,13-dien-18,19:16,15-diolide (**10**) were proven to be active, with IC_{50} (μM) = 26.4 ± 0.4, 17.3 ± 0.5, and 13.7 ± 2.0, respectively.

The hierarchical cluster analysis of the diterpenoid content of the members of section *Holwaya*, including those obtained in this work, indicated a close phytochemical similarity between *S. adenophora* and *S. guevarae*, thus supporting the classification of the latter in section *Holwaya*.

Supplementary Materials: The following supporting information can be downloaded at https://www.mdpi.com/article/10.3390/molecules30071628/s1, Figures S1–S60: Copies of the 1D and 2D NMR spectra of compounds **1–9**; Figures S61–S63: Comparison between the experimental and calculated ECD for the enantiomers of **11**, **12**, and **13**; Tables S1 and S2: Crystallographic data for compounds **1** and **10**; Table S3: Screening for the antiproliferative activity of the isolated compounds from *Salvia guevarae* (25 μM) and the dichloromethane extract of *S. guevarae* (25 ppm); Table S4: Screening for the inhibition of nitrite (NO) production for compounds **1–3** and **5–10** in the RAW 264.7 macrophages (25 μM); Spectroscopic data of compounds **7–13**.

Author Contributions: Conceptualization, B.E.; methodology, J.P.T.-M., C.B.-B. and B.E.; data curation, J.P.T.-M., D.M.-O., B.Y.B.-G. and S.Z.; validation, J.P.T.-M., C.B.-B., L.Q. and B.E.; formal analysis, J.P.T.-M., T.R.-A. and D.M.-O.; investigation, J.P.T.-M., C.B.-B., L.Q. and B.E.; resources, L.Q. and B.E.; writing—original draft preparation, J.P.T.-M., C.B.-B., D.M.-O., L.Q. and B.E.; writing—review and editing, L.Q., B.E., B.Y.B.-G. and S.Z.; visualization, J.P.T.-M., C.B.-B., B.E., B.Y.B.-G. and D.M.-O.; supervision, C.B.-B., L.Q. and B.E.; project administration, J.P.T.-M., C.B.-B., L.Q. and B.E.; funding acquisition, L.Q. and B.E. All authors have read and agreed to the published version of the manuscript.

Funding: This research received no external funding.

Institutional Review Board Statement: Not applicable.

Informed Consent Statement: Not applicable.

Data Availability Statement: The crystallographic data for compounds **1** and **10** have been deposited at the Cambridge Crystallographic Data Centre under the reference numbers CCDC 2430636 and CCDC 2430637, respectively. Copies of the data can be obtained free of charge via application to the CCDC, 2 Union Road, Cambridge CB2 IEZ, UK. Fax: +44-(0)1223-336033 or email: deposit@ccdc.cam.ac.uk.

Acknowledgments: The authors acknowledge B. Quiroz, E. Huerta, A. Peña, R. A. Romo, C. Garcia, J. Pérez, and E. Tapia for collecting the NMR, UV, IR, and MS data. This study made use of UNAM's NMR lab, LURMN at IQ-UNAM, which was funded under CONACYT-Mexico (project 0224747). J.P.T.-M. is grateful to CONACyT/CONAHCyT for the fellowship provided to pursue graduate studies (CONACyT CVU 968805).

Conflicts of Interest: The authors declare no conflicts of interest.

References

1. Lara-Cabrera, S.I.; de la Luz Perez-Garcia, M.; Maya-Lastra, C.A.; Montero-Castro, J.C.; Godden, G.T.; Cibrian-Jaramillo, A.; Fisher, A.E.; Porter, J.M. Phylogenomics of *Salvia* L. Subgenus *Calosphace* (Lamiaceae). *Front. Plant Sci.* **2021**, *12*, 725900. [CrossRef]
2. Hu, G.X.; Takano, A.; Drew, B.T.; Liu, E.; De Soltis, D.E.; Soltis, P.S.; Peng, H.; Xiang, C.L. Phylogeny and Staminal Evolution of *Salvia* (Lamiaceae, Nepetoideae) in East Asia. *Ann. Bot.* **2018**, *122*, 649–668. [CrossRef] [PubMed]
3. González-Gallegos, J.G.; Bedolla-García, B.Y.; Cornejo-Tenorio, G.; Fernández-Alonso, J.L.; Fragoso-Martínez, I.; García-Peña, M.D.R.; Harley, R.M.; Klitgaard, B.; Martínez-Gordillo, M.J.; Wood, J.R.I.; et al. Richness and Distribution of *Salvia* Subg. *Calosphace (Lamiaceae). Int. J. Plant Sci.* **2020**, *181*, 831–856. [CrossRef]
4. Jenks, A.A.; Kim, S.C. Medicinal Plant Complexes of *Salvia* Subgenus *Calosphace*: An Ethnobotanical Study of New World Sages. *J. Ethnopharmacol.* **2013**, *146*, 214–224. [CrossRef]
5. Li, R.; Morris-Natschke, S.L.; Lee, K.H. Clerodane Diterpenes: Sources, Structures, and Biological Activities. *Nat. Prod. Rep.* **2016**, *33*, 1166–1226. [CrossRef] [PubMed]
6. Bustos-Brito, C.; Nieto-Camacho, A.; Hernandez-Ortega, S.; Rivera-Chávez, J.; Quijano, L.; Esquivel, B. Structural Elucidation of Malonylcommunol and 6β-Hydroxy-Trans-Communic Acid, Two Undescribed Diterpenes from *Salvia cinnabarina.* First Examples of Labdane Diterpenoids from a Mexican *Salvia* Species. *Molecules* **2020**, *25*, 1808. [CrossRef]
7. Bustos-Brito, C.; Torres-Medicis, J.P.; Bedolla-García, B.Y.; Zamudio, S.; Ramírez-Apan, T.O.; Macías-Rubalcava, M.L.; Quijano, L.; Esquivel, B. Structure, Absolute Configuration, Antiproliferative and Phytotoxic Activities of Icetexane and Abietane Diterpenoids from *Salvia carranzae* and Chemotaxonomic Implications. *Molecules* **2024**, *29*, 1226. [CrossRef]
8. Bedolla-García, B.Y.; Zamudio, S. Nueva Especie de *Salvia* (Lamiaceae) del Centro de México. *Phytoneuron* **2017**, *66*, 1–12.
9. Ramamoorthy, T.P. Typifications in *Salvia* (Lamiaceae). *Taxon* **1984**, *33*, 322–324.
10. Adou, E.; Williams, R.B.; Schilling, J.K.; Malone, S.; Meyer, J.; Wisse, J.H.; Frederik, D.; Koese, D.; Werkhoven, M.C.M.; Snipes, C.E.; et al. Cytotoxic Diterpenoids from Two Lianas from the Suriname Rainforest. *Bioorganic Med. Chem.* **2005**, *13*, 6009–6014. [CrossRef]
11. Bruhn, T.; Schaumlöffel, A.; Hemberger, Y.; Bringmann, G. SpecDis: Quantifying the Comparison of Calculated and Experimental Electronic Circular Dichroism Spectra. *Chirality* **2013**, *25*, 243–249. [CrossRef] [PubMed]
12. Esquivel, B.; Hernandez, M.; Cardenas, J.; Ramamoorthy, T.P.; Rodríguez-Hahn, L. Further *ent*-Clerodane Diterpenoids from *Salvia melissodora. Phytochemistry* **1989**, *28*, 566. [CrossRef]
13. Omosa, L.K.; Midiwo, J.O.; Derese, S.; Yenesew, A.; Peter, M.G.; Heydenreich, M. Neo-Clerodane Diterpenoids from the Leaf Exudate of *Dodonaea angustifolia. Phytochem. Lett.* **2010**, *3*, 217–220. [CrossRef]
14. Yürüker, A.; Orjala, J.; Sticher, O.; Rali, T. Triterpenes from *Rhus taitensis. Phytochemistry* **1988**, *48*, 863–866.
15. Ikuta, A.; Itokawa, H. The Triterpenes from *Stauntonia hexaphylla* Callus Tissues and Their Biosynthetic Significance. *J. Nat. Prod.* **1989**, *52*, 37. [CrossRef]
16. Kolak, U.; Topçu, G.; Birteksöz, S.; Ötük, G.; Ulubelen, A. Terpenoids and Steroids from the Roots of *Salvia blepharochlaena. Turk. J. Chem.* **2005**, *29*, 177–186.
17. Migas, P.; Cisowski, W.; Dembinska-Migas, W. Isoprene Derivatives from the Leaves and Callus Cultures of *Vaccinium corymbosum* Var. *Bluecrop. Acta Pol. Pharmacéutica-Drug Res.* **2025**, *62*, 45–51.
18. Sun, I.-C.; Wang, H.-K.; Kashiwada, Y.; Shen, J.-K.; Cosentino, L.M.; Chen, C.-H.; Yang, L.-M.; Lee, K.-H. Anti-AIDS Agents. 34. Synthesis and Structure–Activity Relationships of Betulin Derivatives as Anti-HIV Agents. *J. Med. Chem.* **1998**, *41*, 4648–4657. [CrossRef]
19. Symon, A.V.; Veselova, N.N.; Kaplun, A.P.; Vlasenkova, N.K.; Fedorova, G.A.; Lyutik, A.I.; Gerasimova, G.K.; Shvets, V.I. Synthesis and Antitumor Activity of Cyclopropane Derivatives of Betulinic and Betulonic Acids. *Russ. J. Bioorganic Chem.* **2005**, *31*, 286–291. [CrossRef]
20. Melchior Larsen, L.; Kvist Nielsen, J. Identification of 3-O-[2-O-(β-D-Xylopyranosyl)-β-D-Glactopyranosil] Flavonoids in Horseradish Leaves Acting as Feeding Stimulants for a Flea Beetle. *Phytochemistry* **1982**, *21*, 1029–1033.
21. Hofmann, R.W.; Swinny, E.E.; Bloor, S.J.; Markham, K.R.; Ryan, K.G.; Campbell, B.D.; Jordan, B.R.; Fountain, D.W. Responses of Nine *Trifolium repens* L. Populations to Ultraviolet-B Radiation: Differential Flavonol Glycoside Accumulation and Biomass Production. *Ann. Bot.* **2000**, *86*, 527–537. [CrossRef]

22. Sikorska, M.; Matławska, I. Quercetin and Its Glycosides in the Flowers of *Asclepias syriaca* L. *Acta Pol. Pharm.* **2000**, *57*, 321–324.
23. Olszewska, M.A.; Kwapisz, A. Metabolite Profiling and Antioxidant Activity of *Prunus padus* L. Flowers and Leaves. *Nat. Prod. Res.* **2011**, *25*, 1115–1131. [CrossRef]
24. Iannuzzi, A.M., Giacomelli, C.; De Leo, M.; Pietrobono, D.; Camangi, F.; De Tommasi, N.; Martini, C.; Trincavelli, M.L.; Braca, A. Antioxidant Activity of Compounds Isolated from *Elaeagnus umbellata* Promotes Human Gingival Fibroblast Well-Being. *J. Nat. Prod.* **2020**, *83*, 626–637. [CrossRef] [PubMed]
25. Markham, K.R.; Webby, R.F.; Vilain, C. 7-*O*-Methyl-(2R: 3R)-Dihidroquercetin 5-O-B-D-Glucoside and Other Flavonooids from *Podocarpus nivalis*. *Phytochemistry* **1984**, *23*, 2049–2052. [CrossRef]
26. Yeap Foo, L.; Karchesy, J.J. Polyphenolic Glycosides from Douglas Fir Inner Bark. *Phytochemistry* **1989**, *28*, 1237–1240. [CrossRef]
27. Slimestad, R.; Andersen, Ø.M.; Francis, G.W. Ampelopsin 7-Glucoside and Other Dihydroflavonol 7-Glucosides from Needles of *Picea abies*. *Phytochemistry* **1994**, *35*, 550–552. [CrossRef]
28. Álvarez-Fernández, M.A.; Hornedo-Ortega, R.; Cerezo, A.B.; Troncoso, A.M.; García-Parrilla, M.C. Determination of Nonanthocyanin Phenolic Compounds Using High-Resolution Mass Spectrometry (UHPLC-Orbitrap-MS/MS) and Impact of Storage Conditions in a Beverage Made from Strawberry by Fermentation. *J. Agric. Food Chem.* **2016**, *64*, 1367–1376. [CrossRef]
29. Xu, J.; Yu, Y.; Shi, R.; Xie, G.; Zhu, Y.; Wu, G.; Qin, M. Organ-Specific Metabolic Shifts of Flavonoids in *Scutellaria baicalensis* at Different Growth and Development Stages. *Molecules* **2018**, *23*, 428. [CrossRef]
30. Rayyan, S.; Fossen, T.; Solheim Nateland, H.; Andersen, M. Isolation and Identification of Flavonoids, Including Flavone Rotamers, from the Herbal Drug "Crateagi Folium Cum Flore" (Hawthorn). *Phytochem. Anal.* **2005**, *16*, 334–341. [CrossRef]
31. Pan, J.; Zhang, S.; Yan, L.; Tai, J.; Xiao, Q.; Zou, K.; Zhou, Y.; Wu, J. Separation of Flavanone Enantiomers and Flavanone Glucoside Diastereomers from *Balanophora involucrata* Hook. f. by Capillary Electrophoresis and Reversed-Phase High-Performance Liquid Chromatography on a C_{18} Column. *J. Chromatogr. A* **2008**, *1185*, 117–129. [CrossRef]
32. da Rosa, E.; do Amaral, Q.D.F.; Duarte, J.A.; Limberger, J.T.; Chaves, P.E.E.; Zuravski, L.; de Oliveira, L.F.S.; Machado, M.M. Antigenotoxic, Antimutagenic and Cytoprotective Potential of *Salvia hispanica* L. Seed Extract on Human Leukocytes Exposed to Oxidative Damage. *J. Funct. Foods* **2017**, *38*, 505–509. [CrossRef]
33. Kim, M.H.; Jung, K.; Nam, K.H.; Jang, H.J.; Lee, S.W.; Kim, Y.; Park, C.S.; Lee, T.H.; Park, J.H.; Choi, J.H.; et al. *Salvia* Plebeia R.Br. Inhibits Signal Transduction of IL-6 and Prevents Ovariectomy-Induced Bone Loss by Suppressing Osteoclastogenesis. *Arch. Pharm. Res.* **2016**, *39*, 1671–1681. [CrossRef]
34. Bahadori, M.B.; Asghari, B.; Dinparast, L.; Zengin, G.; Sarikurkcu, C.; Abbas-Mohammadi, M.; Bahadori, S. *Salvia nemorosa* L.: A Novel Source of Bioactive Agents with Functional Connections. *LWT-Food Sci. Technol.* **2017**, *75*, 42–50. [CrossRef]
35. Petersen, M.; Simmonds, M.S.J. Molecules of Interest Rosmarinic Acid. *Phytochemistry* **2003**, *62*, 121–125. [CrossRef] [PubMed]
36. Sharma, Y.; Velamuri, R.; Fagan, J.; Schaefer, J. Full-Spectrum Analysis of Bioactive Compounds in Rosemary (*Rosmarinus officinalis* L.) as Influenced by Different Extraction Methods. *Molecules* **2020**, *25*, 4599. [CrossRef] [PubMed]
37. Forzato, C.; Nitti, P. New Diterpenes with Potential Antitumoral Activity Isolated from Plants in the Years 2017–2022. *Plants* **2022**, *11*, 2240. [CrossRef]
38. Prakash, V. Terpenoids as Source of Anti-Inflamatory Compounds. *Asian J. Pharm. Clin. Res.* **2017**, *10*, 68. [CrossRef]
39. Santos, E.P.; Harley, R.M. Notes on *Salvia* Section *Nobiles* (Lamiaceae) and Two New Species from Brazil. *Kew Bull.* **2004**, *59*, 103–109.
40. Bisio, A.; Schito, A.M.; Ebrahimi, S.N.; Hamburger, M.; Mele, G.; Piatti, G.; Romussi, G.; Dal Piaz, F.; De Tommasi, N. Antibacterial Compounds from *Salvia adenophora* Fernald (Lamiaceae). *Phytochemistry* **2015**, *110*, 120–132. [CrossRef]
41. Jimenez, M.; Moreno, E.D.; Díaz, E. Diterpenos de La *Salvia gensneraefolia* I. Estructuras de La Gensnerofolinas A y B. *Rev. Latinoam. Quim.* **1978**, *10*, 166–171.
42. Esquivel, B.; Flores, E.A. A New *neo*-Clerodane Diterpenoid from *Salvia gensneraeflora* (Labiatae). *Heterocycles* **2001**, *55*, 505–509.
43. Bustos-Brito, C.; Pérez-Juanchi, D.; Rivera-Chávez, J.A.; Hernández-Herrera, A.D.; Bedolla-García, B.Y.; Zamudio, S.; Ramírez-Apan, T.O.; Quijano, L.; Esquivel, B. Clerodane and 5,10-*seco*-Clerodane-Type Diterpenoids from *Salvia involucrata*. *J. Mol. Struct.* **2021**, *1237*, 130367. [CrossRef]
44. Rodriguez-Hahn, L.; Esquivel, B.; Sánchez, A.-A.; Cárdenas, J.; Tovar, O.G.; Soriano-Garcia, M.; Toscano, A. Puberulin and Isopuberulin, Benzonorcaradiene and Benzocycloheptatriene Diterpenoids of Clerodanic Origin from *Salvia puberula*. *J. Org. Chem.* **1988**, *53*, 3933–3936.
45. Esquivel, B.; Calderon, J.S.; Sánchez, L. Neo-Clerodane and Languidulane Diterpenoids from *Salvia sousae* and *S. Karwinskii*. *Phytochemistry* **1997**, *45*, 781–783. [CrossRef]
46. Bisio, A.; De Tommasi, N.; Romussi, G. Diterpenoids from *Salvia wagneriana*. *Planta Med.* **2004**, *70*, 452–457. [CrossRef] [PubMed]
47. Sheldrick, G.M. A Short History of SHELX. *Acta Crystallogr. A* **2008**, *64*, 112–122. [CrossRef] [PubMed]
48. Hübschle, C.B.; Sheldrick, G.M.; Dittrich, B. ShelXle: A Qt Graphical User Interface for SHELXL. *J. Appl. Crystallogr.* **2011**, *44*, 1281–1284. [CrossRef]

49. Monks, A.; Scudiero, D.; Skehan, P.; Shoemaker, R.; Paull, K.; Vistica, D.; Hose, C.; Langley, J.; Cronise, P.; Vaigro-Wolff, A.; et al. Feasibility of a High-Flux Anticancer Drug Screen Using a Diverse Panel of Cultured Human Tumor Cell Lines. *J. Natl. Cancer Inst.* **1991**, *83*, 757–766. [CrossRef]
50. Del-Ángel, M.; Nieto, A.; Ramírez-Apan, T.; Delgado, G. Anti-Inflammatory Effect of Natural and Semi-Synthetic Phthalides. *Eur. J. Pharmacol.* **2015**, *752*, 40–48. [CrossRef]
51. Mosmann, T. Rapid Colorimetric Assay for Cellular Growth and Survival: Application to Proliferation and Cytotoxicity Assays. *J. Lmmunol. Methods* **1983**, *65*, 55–63. [CrossRef] [PubMed]

molecules

MDPI

Review

Harnessing the Power of *Alchemilla*: A Natural Solution for Skin Health and Dermatological Disorders

Sebastian Kanak [1], Barbara Krzemińska [1], Anna Berecka-Rycerz [2], Monika Kopeć [3] and Katarzyna Dos Santos Szewczyk [1,*]

[1] Department of Pharmaceutical Botany, Medical University of Lublin, Chodźki 1, 20-093 Lublin, Poland; sebastian.kanak@umlub.pl (S.K.); barbara.krzem@gmail.com (B.K.)

[2] Department of Medicinal Chemistry, Medical University of Lublin, Jaczewskiego 4, 20-090 Lublin, Poland; anna.berecka-rycerz@umlub.pl

[3] Chair and Department of Obstetrics and Perinatology, Medical University of Lublin, Jaczewskiego 8, 20-090 Lublin, Poland; monika.ruszala@wp.pl

* Correspondence: k.szewczyk@umlub.pl

Abstract: Skin diseases are prevalent and encompass a wide range of disorders with varying clinical manifestations and diverse etiopathogenesis. The response to the necessity of multidirectional treatment is provided by species belonging to the genus *Alchemilla*, which is used in traditional medicine as well as in cosmetic formulations. Responsible for the healing properties of these plants for skin diseases are mainly compounds such as tannins, phenolic acids, flavonoids, and anthocyanins. The aim of the study was to analyze and synthesize the published literature on the *Alchemilla* species in skincare with a timeframe of December 2024. The literature indicates that due to antioxidant, anti-inflammatory, astringent, antimicrobial, elastase activity and tyrosinase inhibitory properties of various *Alchemilla* species, extracts obtained from these plants can be successfully applied in skin rashes, acne, stretch marks, eczema, psoriasis, wrinkles and other dermatological issues. To the best of our knowledge, this is the first review of the cosmetic activities of *Alchemilla* species.

Keywords: *Alchemilla*; Rosaceae; skin disorders; plant extracts; natural agents; anti-aging

1. Introduction

For millennia, medicinal plants and their phytochemicals have been integral to traditional medicine across cultures, including the treatment of skin ailments [1]. Ancient healers in systems from Ayurveda to European folk medicine used herbal preparations for wound care, inflammation, and skin rejuvenation, laying the groundwork for modern phytotherapy [1]. This historical reliance on botanicals is attributed to the presence of bioactive compounds (e.g., polyphenols, tannins, essential oils) that provide therapeutic effects such as antiseptic, anti-inflammatory, and wound-healing actions [1]. These early observations have inspired contemporary research into plant-derived compounds for dermatological uses, with a renewed interest in natural, safer alternatives to synthetic drugs.

In recent years, factors like increasing pollution and consumer demand for "green" skincare have caused a revival in plant-based dermatological products. Botanical extracts offer multidirectional benefits due to the synergism of their constituents, an advantage in managing complex skin disorders that often involve oxidative stress, microbial infection, and inflammation [2]. The genus *Alchemilla* (Rosaceae), commonly known as lady's mantle, is an example of such a plant resource. *Alchemilla* spp. are perennial herbs (about

https://doi.org/10.3390/molecules30081861

795 accepted species worldwide) traditionally used as healing agents for numerous conditions, including dermatological issues [3]. Ethnobotanical records confirm their use for treating wounds and abrasions—for instance, *A. hessii* in Turkey is applied to cuts [4], and *A. monticola* has been used for wounds and burns in Europe [5]. These folkloric uses suggest *Alchemilla* plants possess wound-healing and anti-infective properties.

Alchemilla species are rich in polyphenolic compounds (tannins, flavonoids, phenolic acids, anthocyanins) believed to be responsible for their skin-healing effects [6]. However, a comprehensive evaluation of their dermatological benefits has been lacking. Therefore, the aim of this review is to synthesize current knowledge on the cosmetic and dermatological activities of *Alchemilla* species, including their antioxidant, anti-inflammatory, antimicrobial, anti-aging, and wound-healing properties, and to discuss practical applications and future research directions (Figure 1). To our knowledge, this is the first focused review of *Alchemilla* in skin care and dermatological therapy, highlighting its potential as a multi-functional natural agent.

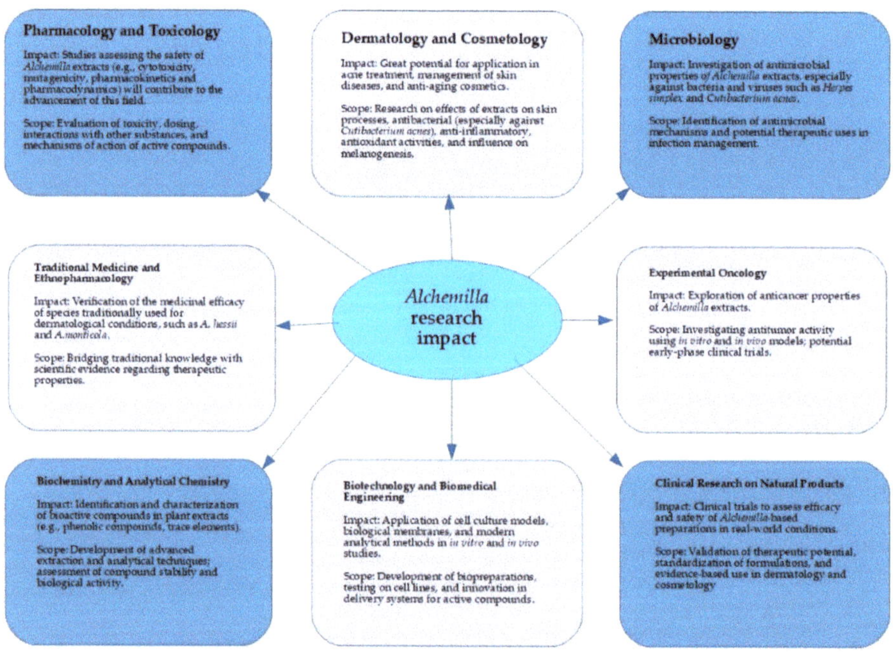

Figure 1. *Alchemilla* research impact.

2. Methodology of Evidence Acquisition

This review analyzed the literature on *Alchemilla* and skin-related applications up to December 2024. Multiple databases were searched (Google Scholar, Scopus, Web of Science, ResearchGate, Medline, SciFinder, ScienceDirect, PubMed) using keywords such as "*Alchemilla* skin", "*Alchemilla* antioxidant", "*Alchemilla* anti-inflammatory", "lady's mantle cosmetic", and related MeSH terms. Inclusion criteria were English-language publications of original studies directly relevant to *Alchemilla* and dermatology. Priority was given to peer-reviewed articles and highly cited papers; however, due to the novelty of this topic, a few conference abstracts (with DOIs) and a patent were included for completeness. Studies where *Alchemilla* was a component of a multi-herb mixture were included if results for *Alchemilla* could be discerned. Exclusion criteria included non-English articles, clearly irrelevant works, duplicate publications, and sources inaccessible online. Using this strategy, we initially identified 230 records. After removing duplicates, 180 unique records remained for screening. Title and abstract screening excluded 100 records that did not meet the inclusion criteria (e.g., unrelated to skin or lacking experimental data). We retrieved 80 full-text articles for detailed assessment, of which 10 were excluded (5 not accessible in full text, 3 non-English, 2 lacking dermatology-related outcomes). In total, 70 publications were included in this review for qualitative synthesis. Figure 2 presents the study selection process in a PRISMA 2020 flowchart, following Page et al. [7] guidelines. The included studies encompass in vitro assays, in vivo animal experiments, and a few clinical or ex vivo investigations, providing a broad evidence base for *Alchemilla*'s dermatological effects. Out of 230 records identified, 70 studies were included in this review after screening and eligibility assessment.

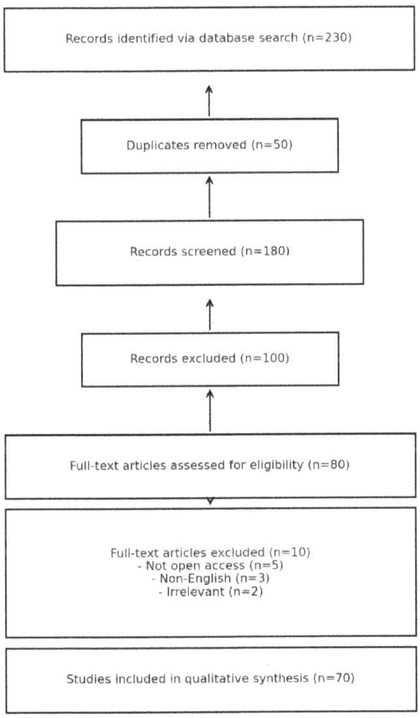

Figure 2. PRISMA flow diagram of the literature search and selection (adapted from [7]). Out of 230 records identified, 70 studies were included in this review after screening and eligibility assessment.

3. Biological Activities of Alchemilla Species Towards Skin

As shown by the gathered evidence, various *Alchemilla* extracts demonstrate a range of beneficial biological activities relevant to skin health (summarized in Table 1 and Figure 3). Key activities include antioxidant effects, anti-inflammatory activity, antimicrobial (antibacterial and antifungal) properties, anti-aging effects (e.g., inhibition of collagenase, elastase, and tyrosinase enzymes), wound-healing promotion, and even anti-tumor effects on skin cancer cells. These activities, discussed below, underlie the traditional uses of *Alchemilla* in treating rashes, acne, eczema, wounds, and other skin ailments. Table 1 organizes the findings by biological activity, summarizing the *Alchemilla* species studied, extract types, experimental models, and main results for each category.

Table 1. Biological activities of *Alchemilla* species are valuable for dermatological diseases and skin care (presented on the basis of original studies published until December 2024).

Biological Activity	*Alchemilla* Species	Part of the Plant	Extraction Used	Study Model	Results	Ref.
antioxidant	*A. acutiloba*	aerial parts and roots	60% methanol extract and its diethyl ether, ethyl acetate and n-butanol fractions	in vitro; DPPH•, ABTS•+, chelating activity	DPPH•—IC_{50} = 51.42–8.83 μg/mL; ABTS•+—IC_{50} = 24.82–1.42 μg/mL; chelating activity—44.12–11.43 μg/mL	[8]
	A. alpina	aerial parts	methanol extract	in vitro; DPPH•	% Inhibition = 45.4–94.4%	[9]
	A. arvensis	leaves	methanol, hexane, acetone, water extracts	in vitro; DPPH•	IC_{50} = 97.72–4.86 μg/mL	[10]
	A. barbatiflora	aerial parts	90% methanol extract and its n-hexane, chloroform and water fractions	in vitro; DPPH•, SOD (superoxide radical scavenging), phosphomolibdenum-reducing antioxidant power (PRAP), ferric-reducing antioxidant power (FRAP)	% Inhibition: DPPH•—18.6–97.17%; SOD—9.80–83.34%. Reducing power: PRAP—0.355–1.516; FRAP—15.76–93.46 mg BHAE/g extract	[11]
	A. ellenbergiana	aerial parts	hexane, ethanol, methanol extracts	in vitro; DPPH•	IC_{50} = 7.1–243.6 μg/mL	[12, 13]
	A. glabra	aerial parts	80% acetone (in 0.2% formic acid) extract	in vitro; ORAC, TRAP, HORAC	ORAC—1337 μmol TE/g; TRAP—1815 μmol TE/g; HORAC—1999 μmol GAE/g	[14]
	A. hybrida		ethanol extract	in vitro; DPPH•	IC_{50} = 0.082 mg/mL	[15]
	A. jumrukczalica	leaves	methanol extract	in vitro; DPPH•	IC_{50} = 12.09 μg/mL	[16]
	A. lithophila	aerial parts	methanol, water and hexane extracts	in vitro; DPPH•, ABTS•+	% Inhibition: DPPH•—10.51–75.38%; ABTS•+—10.56–70.67%	[17]
	A. mollis	leaves	50% ethanol extract	in vitro; DPPH•, ABTS•+, ROS (reactive oxygen species)	DPPH•—IC_{50} = 42.4 μg/mL; ABTS•+—IC_{50} = 7.8 μg/mL; 10 and 100 μg/mL—22.3% and 48.0% decreases in ROS level	[18]
		herb	hexane, ethyl acetate, methanol, 50% methanol, deodorized water extracts	in vitro; DPPH•, ABTS•+	DPPH•—IC_{50} = 0.26–0.15 mg/mL; TEAC—0.90–1.55 mM/L/Trolox	[19]
		aerial parts and roots	80% methanol extract	in vitro; DPPH•	IC_{50} = 39.4 (aerial parts)–114.6 (roots) μg/mL	[20]
		stalks	10–90% ethanol extract	in vitro; DPPH•, ABTS•+, FRAP, CUPRAC	DPPH•—21.50–247.58 mmol TE/dm^3; ABTS•+—27.10–308.44 mmol TE/dm^3; FRAP—67.91–382.78 mmol TE/dm^3; CUPRAC—79.72–363.79 mmol TE/dm^3	[21]
		aerial flowering parts	methanol extract and its ethyl acetate, petroleum, chloroform, water fractions	in vitro; DPPH•	IC_{50} = 9.8–>200 μg/mL	[22]
	A. persica	aerial parts and roots	80% methanol extract	in vitro; DPPH•, TBARS	DPPH•—IC_{50} = 0.055 M (aerial parts), 0.151 M (roots); TBARS—5.9 nmol/mL (aerial parts), 19.08 nmol/mL	[23]

Table 1. *Cont.*

Biological Activity	*Alchemilla* Species	Part of the Plant	Extraction Used	Study Model	Results	Ref.
	A. sericata	aerial parts	95% hexane extract	in vitro; DPPH•	IC_{50} = 185 µg/mL	[24]
	A. vulgaris	herb	aqueous and 70% ethanolic extracts	in vitro; DPPH•	% Inhibition: DPPH•—80.71–87.95%	[25]
		aerial parts and roots	methanol extract	in vitro; DPPH•, ABTS•+, •OH, total antioxidant activity (TAA), metal chelation, reducing capacity, inhibition of lipid peroxidation	DPPH•—IC_{50} = 5.96–11.86 µg/mL; ABTS•+—IC_{50} = 14.80–32.49 µg/mL; •OH—IC_{50} = 13.06–18.44 µg/mL; lipid peroxidation—IC_{50} = 31.91–475.13 µg/mL; TAA—265.62–316.47 mg AA/g of extract; reducing—632.99–607.52 mg Trolox/g of extract	[26]
		aerial parts	80% methanol, 70% ethanol, 70% ethylacetate, water extracts	in vitro; DPPH•, ABTS•+, CUPRAC, FRAP, phosphomolibdenum and metal chelating assays	DPPH•—89.25–502.56 mg TE per g extract; ABTS•+—37.50–174.05 mg TE per g extract; CUPRAC—78.56–283.16 mg TE per g extract; FRAP—3240.09–8745.31 mg AAE per g of extract; Phosphomolibdenum—0.53–2.22 mmol TE per g extract; metal chelating—37.96–42.58 mg EDTAE per g extract	[27]
		aerial parts	50% ethanol extract	in vitro; DPPH•, metal chelating assay	% Inhibition: DPPH•—71.8; metal chelating—84.6%	[28]
		leaves	80% ethanol and water extracts	in vitro; DPPH•	% Inhibition: 131.74%	[29]
		roots	50% ethanol extract	in vitro; ABTS•+, FRAP	ABTS•+—68.21 mmol TE/g DW; FRAP—40.12 mmol of TE/g DW	[30]
	A. xanthochlora	leaves	hexane, chloroform, ethylacetate, methanol, water extracts	in vitro; DPPH•	0.23–2.49 g DPPH/g DE	[31]
anti-inflammatory	*A. acutiloba*	aerial parts and roots	60% methanol extract and its diethyl ether, ethyl acetate and n-butanol fractions	in vitro; COX1, COX2	% Inhibition: COX1—31.27–83.14%; COX2—43.65–90.93	[8]
	A. mollis	aerial parts and roots	80% methanol extract	in vivo; Whittle method	% Inhibition: 5.3–30.6%	[20]
				in vivo; human red blood cell (HRBC) membrane stabilization method	IC_{50} = 1.22–1.24 mg/mL	[32]
	A. persica	aerial parts and roots	80% methanol extract	in vivo; Whittle method	% Inhibition: 3.6–26.6%	[20]
				in vivo; human red blood cell (HRBC) membrane stabilization method	IC_{50} = 1.52–1.82 mg/mL	[32]
	A. vulgaris	aerial parts and roots	methanol extract	in vitro; COX-1 and COX-2	% Inhibition: COX-1—44.1–44.4%; COX-2—40.4–63.6%	[26]

Table 1. *Cont.*

Biological Activity	*Alchemilla* Species	Part of the Plant	Extraction Used	Study Model	Results	Ref.
antibacterial	*A. arvensis*	leaves	methanol, hexane, acetone, water extracts	agar diffusion and micro-broth dilution methods (*Staphylococcus aureus*, *Escherichia coli*, *Pseudomonas aeruginosa*, *Shigella sonnie*)	MIC values 6.3–25.0 mg/mL	[10]
	A. mollis	herb	hexane, ethyl acetate, methanol, 50% methanol, deodorized water extracts	agar dilution method (*S. aureus*, *E. coli*, *P. aeruginosa*, *Enterococcus faecalis*)	MIC values 0.5–7.5 mg/mL MC values 5–10 mg/mL	[19]
		aerial parts and roots	80% methanol extract	microbroth dilution method (*S. aureus*, *E. faecalis*, *B. subtilis*, *E. coli*, *P. aeruginosa*)	MIC values 5–10 mg/mL	[32]
	A. pedata		petroleum ether, chloroform, acetone and methanol extracts	agar well diffusion method (*E. coli*, *P. aeruginosa*, *S. aureus*)	MIC values 12.5–20.16 mg/mL	[33]
	A. persica	aerial parts and roots	80% methanol extract	microbroth dilution method (*S. aureus*, *E. faecalis*, *B. subtilis*, *E. coli*, *P. aeruginosa*)	MIC values 2.5–10.0 mg/mL	[32]
	A. vulgaris	aerial parts	50% ethanol/6% glycerin	agar well diffusion method (*S. epidermis*, *P. acnes*, *P. granulosum*)	inhibitory zone 0–13 mm	[34]
		aerial parts and roots	methanol extract	microdilution method (*Micrococcus lysodeikticus*, *Salmonella typhimurium*, *Bacillus subtilis*, *E. faecalis*, *E. coli*, *Klebsiella pneumoniae*, *P. aeruginosa*, *Bacillus mycoides*, *Azotobacter chroococcum*)	MIC values 0.156–0.625 mg/mL	[26]
antifungal	*A. arvensis*	leaves	methanol, hexane, acetone, water extracts	micro-broth dilution method (*Epidermophyton floccosum*, *Candida albicans*)	MIC values 0.78–12.5 mg/mL	[10]
	A. hybrida		ethanolic extract	microdilution method	MIC values 0.104–1.667 mg/mL	[15]
	A. mollis *A. persica*	aerial parts and roots	80% methanol extract	microbroth dilution method (*Candida albicans*)	MIC values 2.5–10.0 mg/mL	[32]
	A. vulgaris	aerial parts and roots	methanol extract	microdilution method (*Phialophora fastigiata*, *Penicillium canescens*, *Trichoderma viride*, *Trichoderma longibrachiatum*, *Aspergillus brasiliensis*, *A. glaucus*, *Fusarium oxysporum*, *Alternaria alternata*, *Doratomyces stemonitis*, *C. albicans*)	MIC values 2.5–20.0 mg/mL	[26]

Table 1. *Cont.*

Biological Activity	*Alchemilla* Species	Part of the Plant	Extraction Used	Study Model	Results	Ref.
wound-healing	*A. mollis* *A. persica*	aerial parts and roots	80% methanol extract	in vivo; Male Swiss albino mice and Sprague-Dawley rats	tensile strength value 33.3–39.3%; contraction value 43.5–51.4%)	[20]
	A. vulgaris	herb	70% ethanol, water, 80% propylene glycol extracts	in vitro; scratch assay with L929 fibroblasts; in vivo	wound healing potential	[35]
			3% extract in glycerine	in vivo		[36]
			herbal mixture	in vivo; in vitro scratch assay		[37]
anti-aging and skin-lightening (enzyme inhibitory)	*A. vulgaris*	herb	aqueous and 70% ethanolic extracts	in vitro; tyrosinase inhibition	% Inhibition: 71.55%	[25]
		herb	50% methanol extract	in vitro; collagenase inhibition	% Inhibition: 40.0%	[38, 39]
		herb	50% methanol extract	in vitro; elastase inhibition	% Inhibition: 12.0%	[40]
		aerial parts	80% methanol, 70% ethanol, 70% ethylacetate, water extracts	in vitro; tyrosinase inhibition	Inhibition: 73.68–79.84 mg KAE per g extract	[27]
anti-tumor activity (anti-melanoma)	*A. vulgaris*	aerial parts	ethanol extract	in vitro—mouse melanoma cell lines: B16 and B16F10; in vivo—syngeneic mouse melanoma model	significantly reduced tumor growth compared to controls	[41]

Abbreviations: DPPH•—2,2-diphenyl-1-picrylhydrazyl radical scavenging assay; FRAP—ferric reducing antioxidant assay; CUPRAC—cupric-reducing antioxidant capacity; ABTS•+—2,2′-azino-bis-(3-ethyl-benzothiazole-6-sulfonic acid) radical scavenging assay; COX-1/COX-2—cyclooxygenase-1/-2 inhibitory activity; MIC—minimum inhibitory concentration; ORAC—the oxygen radical absorbance capacity; TRAP—total reactive antioxidant potential; HORAC—hydroxyl radical antioxidant capacity assay; KAE—kojic acid; DW—dry weight.

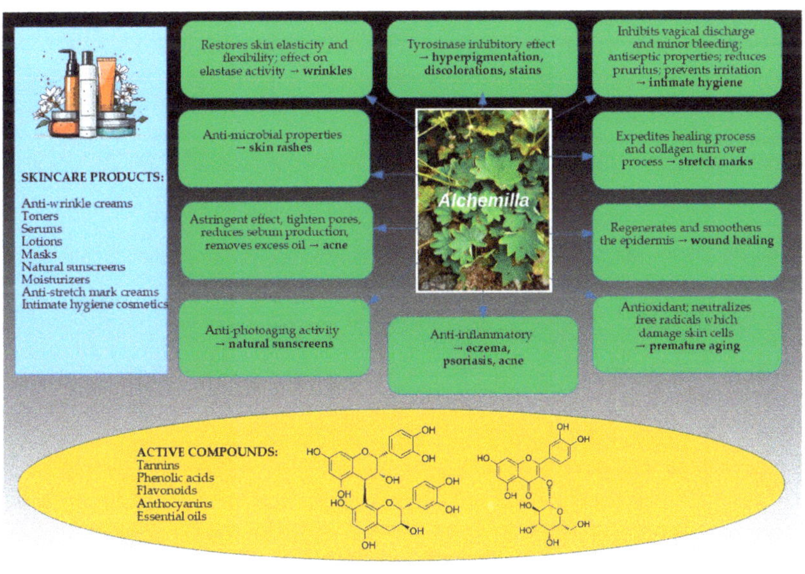

Figure 3. Biological activities towards skin disorders and the applicability of extracts obtained from different *Alchemilla* species in the cosmetic industry.

3.1. Antioxidant Activity

Secondary metabolites such as phenolic compounds of plant origin are a promising tool for preventing skin damage. Increased levels of ROS and oxidative stress lead to the loss of cellular redox homeostasis and, consequently, to damage to proteins, DNA and lipids through various signaling pathways. Reduction of fibroblast functionality contributes to the appearance of clinical features of aging. Normal fibroblast function and increased collagen expression can be restored by treatment with antioxidants such as polyphenols [42]. Oxidative stress contributes to the modification of several biomolecular pathways in cells. Photoaging is connected with MAPKs/AP-1, MMP-1/3/9, p-c-Fos, p-c-Jun pathways, abnormal pigmentation is associated with melanogenic paracrine mediators, tyrosinase and tyrosinase-related protein-1 (TRP-1), while inflammation is generated via p-ERK ½ MAPK, NF-kB, inflammatory cytokines (IL-6, TNFα, IFN-γ) [43]. A study conducted by Garcia-Villegas et al. [44] showed that sometimes, even inconspicuous plant parts, such as cherry stems, may turn out to be a valuable therapeutic raw material for antioxidant activity through cosmetic applications. A comprehensive analysis of the chemical composition using HPLC-ESI-qTOF-MS showed the presence of 146 chemical compounds, including these valuable in the treatment of dermatological disorders, and high values of antioxidant properties in FRAP, TEAC, and ORAC assays. In addition, seemingly well-researched and widely used black tea (the extract obtained through plant small RNA PSRTM technology) has shown excellent anti-aging properties due to its ability to affect the mitochondria, nuclear DNA integrity as well as the extracellular matrix [45]. The above-mentioned examples confirm the necessity to study previously untested species, including so far unexplored *Alchemilla* species.

Among all biological activities, antioxidant properties are most extensively researched in the entire *Alchemilla* genus, and at the same time, this activity is valuable from a cosmetic point of view, which makes this plant material worthy of attention. Interestingly, although antioxidant activity is the most extensively studied property among the genus *Alchemilla*, it turns out that among 795 accepted species, only 12 species have been studied towards this capacity. Methanolic extracts of *A. acutiloba* (and their ethyl acetate and butanol fractions) showed potent free-radical scavenging in DPPH and ABTS assays, quenching ~95% of radicals at 50 μg/mL [8]. The ethyl acetate fraction of aerial parts was especially active (94.8% DPPH scavenging) [8]. Methanol extract of aerial parts of *A. alpina* displayed high DPPH scavenging (45.4% to 94.4% inhibition, depending on concentration) [9], indicating significant antioxidant capacity. Among methanol, hexane, acetone, and water extracts of *A. arvensis* tested, the acetone extract had the strongest DPPH radical scavenging (IC_{50} = 4.9 μg/mL) [10], outperforming other solvents. This suggests moderately polar solvents extract the most active antioxidant compounds. Crude methanolic extract and its fractions (hexane, chloroform, water) from *A. barbatiflora* were evaluated by DPPH, superoxide radical (SOD) scavenging, phosphomolybdenum, and FRAP assays. The methanol extract, and especially its aqueous fraction, showed the highest antioxidant activities [11], highlighting that polyphenols concentrated in polar fractions confer strong antioxidative effects. A leaf hexane extract of *A. ellenbergiana* exhibited very potent DPPH scavenging (IC_{50} = 7.1 μg/mL) [12]. However, ethanol and methanol extracts of this species were less active (IC_{50} = 243 μg/mL) [13], suggesting that specific non-polar constituents (possibly certain flavonoids or other phenolics) in *A. ellenbergiana* contribute to its antioxidant effect. An 80% acetone (in 0.2% formic acid) extract of *A. glabra* demonstrated significant antioxidant capacity in ORAC, TRAP, and HORAC assays [14]. An ethanolic extract of *A. hybrida* also showed strong antioxidant and radical-scavenging effects (DPPH IC_{50} ~ 0.082 mg/mL) [15]. This extract also contained high total phenolics, correlating with its potent activity.

3.2. Anti-Inflammatory Activity

The anti-inflammatory effect of plant extracts is particularly important in the case of chronic inflammatory skin diseases such as psoriasis and atopic dermatitis, in which increased expansion of inflammatory cells and hyperproliferation of keratinocytes are observed. The main focus of active plant extracts is the mTOR (mechanistic target of rapamycin) pathway, which can control the activation and differentiation of keratinocytes. Interestingly, keratinocytes express high levels of glucose transporter (GLUT)1, L-type amino acid transporter (LAT)1, and cationic amino acid transporters (CATs) [46].

Several *Alchemilla* extracts can mitigate inflammation, often assessed via enzyme inhibition or cell-based models.

Butanol and ethyl acetate fractions (50 µg/mL) from *A. acutiloba* showed notable inhibition of pro-inflammatory enzymes cyclooxygenase-1 and -2 (COX-1, COX-2) [8]. In vitro assays indicated COX-2 inhibition up to ~80% by the butanol fraction of aerial parts, comparable to standard anti-inflammatory agents. This suggests *A. acutiloba* contains constituents (likely polyphenols or tannins) that interfere with inflammatory eicosanoid synthesis.

Oral supplementation with *A. mollis* extract in mice has demonstrated anti-inflammatory and anti-photoaging effects. In a UVB-induced skin damage model, dietary *A. mollis* protected against inflammation by downregulating NFATc1 and upregulating Nrf2/ARE pathways, thereby reducing cytokine release and oxidative stress in the skin [18]. This in vivo result aligns with the traditional use of *A. mollis* for soothing skin irritations.

As reported by Oz et al. [20], methanolic extracts of *A. persica* and *A. mollis* in the Whittle method (acetic acid-induced increase in capillary permeability on a group of 10 mice in 0.2 mL/20 g body weight) revealed anti-inflammatory effect at concentration 26.6% at 200 mg/kg dose and 30.6% at 200 mg/kg dose, respectively. Kurtul et al. [32] performed a study using the human red blood cell (HRBC) membrane stabilization method (measuring stabilization capacity against heat-induced hemolysis of HRBC membrane). In this trial, the methanolic extract of *A. mollis* aerial parts revealed the highest anti-inflammatory activity, with IC_{50} = 1.22 mg/mL. For a methanolic extract of *A. persica*, the IC_{50} value for aerial parts extract was 1.52 and in the case of roots, 1.82 mg/mL.

It is worth noting that agrimoniin isolated from *Alchemilla* (e.g., in *A. mollis* extract) has shown anti-inflammatory activity in some studies [47]. Hoffmann et al. [48] demonstrated that agrimoniin possesses significant anti-inflammatory effects, which likely contribute to Alchemilla's activity when present.

3.3. Antibacterial and Antifungal Activity

The rising phenomenon of resistance, as well as unexpected side effects of conventional pharmaceutical drugs, have caused scientists to turn to the plant kingdom as a potential source of new antimicrobial agents. The antibacterial effect of extracts applied to the skin is important because various diseases (such as acne eruptions) result in wounds and associated skin superinfections. According to the latest knowledge, not only the antimicrobial effect but also the interactions of various extracts and other cosmetic ingredients with the network of the skin microbial ecosystem are of significant importance [49].

Alchemilla extracts exhibit broad antimicrobial effects, particularly against Gram-positive skin pathogens, which supports their use in treating infected wounds and acne.

Methanolic, hexane, acetone, and water extracts from *A. arvensis* were tested against bacteria, including *Staphylococcus aureus*, *Escherichia coli*, *Pseudomonas aeruginosa*, and *Shigella sonnei*. All extracts showed antibacterial activity to varying degrees. Notably, S. aureus (a common cause of skin infections) was inhibited by all extracts (inhibition zones 10–20 mm) except a lack of activity against *P. aeruginosa* [10]. MIC values ranged from 6.3 to 25 mg/mL for most bacteria, with *P. aeruginosa* being the least susceptible (no inhibition by some extracts). These results highlight *A. arvensis* potential as a source of topical antibacterial agents, especially for Gram-positive organisms.

Various extracts of *A. mollis* demonstrated significant antibacterial potency. A 50% methanolic extract had MICs of 0.5 mg/mL against *S. aureus*, 2.0 mg/mL against *P. aeruginosa*, and 5.0 mg/mL against *Enterococcus faecalis* [19]. The aqueous and deodorized water extracts showed similar MIC profiles (e.g., 0.5 mg/mL for *S. aureus*). The consistently low MIC for *S. aureus* across extract types indicates *A. mollis* is particularly effective against this bacterium. These findings are promising for developing *A. mollis*-based treatments for staphylococcal skin infections.

Interestingly, although the *Cutibacterium acnes* bacterial strain (formerly called *Propionibacterium acnes*) plays a pivotal role in the etiopathogenesis of *acne vulgaris*, and what is more, the prevalence of acne is very common [50], in the scientific literature, there is only one publication regarding the activity of *Alchemilla* against this strain, i.e., Dzabijeva et al. [34] tested ethanolic extract from *A. vulgaris* against *P. acnes* subsp. acnes MSCL 1521 (ATCC 6919) and *Propionibacterium granulosum* MSCL 1522 (ATCC 25564) using the agar well diffusion method. The obtained diameter of inhibitory zones was 10 mm for *Propionibacterium acnes* and 13 mm for *P. granulosum*. At the same time, in this study, the ethanol extract of *A. vulgaris* turned out to be inactive against *S. epidermidis* [34]. This suggests some efficacy in targeting the anaerobic bacteria involved in acne lesions, which, combined with *Alchemilla*'s anti-inflammatory tannins, could benefit acne treatment. Given the prevalence of acne, further testing of other active species (e.g., *A. mollis*, *A. arvensis*, *A. pedata*) against *C. acnes* is warranted, as they have shown substantial antibacterial effects in general.

As reported by Taddese et al. [33], formulations with 10% of *A. pedata* extract have been assessed for their ability to inhibit *E. coli*, *P. aeruginosa* and *S. aureus* growth. In the case of formulation 1 (extract in Sodium laurylmonosterin cream base), form 2 (in Macrogol cream base), form 3 (in Macrogol blend Ointment base), form 6 (in Polyethylene glycol bases PEG 400:PEG 2000, 1:1) and form 7 (in Polyethylene glycol bases PEG 400:PEG 2000, 1:3) the following MIC values were obtained: *E. coli*: 14.3–16.2 mg/mL, *P. aeruginosa* 14.0–23.5 mg/mL and *S. aureus* 17.5–22.5 mg/mL. At the same time, formulations 4 (extract in simple ointment base) and 5 (white petrolatum) turned out to be inactive. In the study conducted by Boroja et al. [26], *A. vulgaris* extracts showed significant activity against *Enterococcus faecalis*, *Salmonella typhimurium*, *Micrococcus lysodeikticus* and *Bacilus mycoides* with MIC values 0.156–0.625 mg/mL. In summary, only the following *Alchemilla* species have been tested for antibacterial activity: *Alchemilla arvensis*, *A. mollis*, *A. pedata*, *A. persica* and *A. vulgaris*.

Taking into consideration that fungal infections of the skin (including dandruff, oral candidiasis, onychomycosis, and mycosis fungoides of the feet) are very common, the exploration of new substances derived from plants that could support their treatment is an extremely relevant research direction. Moreover, the search for active antifungal substances with a high safety profile has become an important goal of the cosmetics industry. Nevertheless, studies performed so far prove the negligible activity of *Alchemilla* species against *Candida albicans*.

The same *A. arvensis* extracts tested for bacteria were evaluated against fungi such as *C. albicans* and *Epidermophyton floccosum*. The results showed antifungal activity with MICs of 3.7–12.5 mg/mL for *C. albicans* and 0.78–6.3 mg/mL for *E. floccosum* [10]. These ranges suggest that E. floccosum (a dermatophyte causing skin infections) is more susceptible to *A. arvensis* extracts than *Candida*. This antifungal efficacy supports the traditional use of *Alchemilla* for treating rash and eczema, conditions where secondary fungal infections can occur.

An ethanolic extract of *A. hybrida* not only was a strong antioxidant but also exhibited antifungal effects. It inhibited the growth of various fungi with minimum inhibitory concentrations ranging from 0.104 to 1.667 mg/mL and minimum fungicidal concentrations of 0.208 to 2.5 mg/mL [15]. These values (from microdilution assays) indicate a broad-spectrum fungistatic effect, with a complete fungal kill at slightly higher concentrations. The combined antioxidant and antifungal *A. hybrida* profile suggests it could protect the skin by both reducing oxidative stress and directly suppressing fungal pathogens.

A. pedata showed no activity against *C. albicans* in the study conducted by Taddese et al. [33]. Furthermore, *A. mollis* was not active towards this strain in the analysis carried out by Karatoprak et al. [19]. The methanol extract of aerial parts and roots of *A. vulgaris* had no inhibition effect on the growth of *C. albicans* in the survey performed by Boroja et al. [26]. Nonetheless, the same analysis showed the activity of *A. vulgaris* extracts against other fungal strains, namely *Phialophora fastigiata*, *Penicillium canescens*, *Trichoderma viride*, *Trichoderma longibrachiatum*, *Aspergillus brasiliensis*, *Aspergillus glaucus*, *Fusarium oxysporum*, *Alternaria alternata* and *Doratomyces stemonitis* (MIC values ranged from 2.5 to 20 mg/mL). All tested extracts showed weaker antifungal activity than nystatin, which showed activity at concentrations from 0.078 to 5 μg/mL [26].

3.4. Wound Healing Activity

The issue of searching for therapeutic agents with the potential to treat wounds is important, among others, because wounds occur in the course of dermatoses such as acne, eczema or psoriasis. Fibroblasts are relevant in the wound healing process because they proliferate and migrate to the injured area, synthesizing new extracellular matrix. Moreover, keratinocytes re-differentiate and restore the normal epidermal barrier. In the process of wound healing, plant extracts contribute to the suppression of protease activity, which creates a normal environment and restores normal skin functions. Moreover, they enhance angiogenesis quickly by responding to increased macrophage migration and metabolic demand for new tissue [37]. Significant progress in knowledge over the last few years regarding the healing mechanism at the molecular level has allowed scientists to replace experimental animal models with alternative in vitro models. Among such models is an in vitro test based on a monolayer of fibroblasts with artificially formed wounds, which is of great importance. A multidirectional and innovative approach to wound treatment in designing medicinal formulations, taking into account the current understanding of the molecular and cellular basis of tissue healing processes, is of great importance. Different phases of wound healing can be distinguished, namely clot production, re-epithelialization, angiogenesis, and scar deposition. It is well established that keratinocytes, fibroblasts, melanocytes, adipocytes and cutaneous nerves are relevant in this process [51].

A few *Alchemilla* species have been investigated for their ability to accelerate wound closure and skin regeneration, validating their use in folk medicine for wounds.

Tasić-Kostov et al. [35] conducted an extensive study on the effects of *Alchemilla vulgaris* on wound healing processes using in vitro wound healing assay with L929 fibroblasts and in vivo assessment of skin barrier repair potential. The most beneficial effect on fibroblast migration as well as wound healing in vitro was observed for ethanolic extract, which is most likely related to the rich chemical composition of this extract determined by RP-HPLC, i.e., ellagic acid 3.4 mg/g, isoquercetin 4.0 mg/g. What is more, gel with propyleneglycolic extract revealed the most favorable effect on in vitro wound healing and showed the highest value of adhesiveness in TPA—Texture profile analysis (Texture Analyser). In vivo, tests were carried out on 18 volunteers using Corneometer® CM 820 (measurements of stratum corneum hydration on SLS-irritated human skin) and Tewameter® TM 210 (measurements of transepidermal water loss). Gels containing *A. vulgaris* extract revealed significant improvement in the skin hydration level after 3 days of application. Interestingly, after 7 days, stratum corneum hydration was even higher than baseline. These results from Tasić-Kostov et al. demonstrate that *A. vulgaris* facilitates the healing process, likely due to its tannins creating a protective layer and its phytochemicals stimulating tissue repair.

Another study that examined the wound-healing activity of extracts obtained from *A. vulgaris* was conducted by Shrivastava et al. [36]. The effect of *A. vulgaris* on the growth of epithelial cells and myofibroblasts was tested in Chang liver and Madin Darby Bovine Kidney (MDBK) epithelial cell lines and rat aortic myofibroblast cultures. *A. vulgaris* extract at concentration 0.1–1.0% caused a significant increase in cell numbers, namely 21.3% in MDBK, 15.5% in myofibroblast and 10.6% in Chang liver cells. Treatment of rats with the 3% *A. vulgaris* extract resulted in a reduction in the diameter of lesions by 10.0 7% after 2 days and 23.2% after 3 days.

A herbal mixture containing *A. vulgaris* extract (20%), *Mimosa tenuiflora* leaf extract (20%), Glycerol (42%), Honey (10%), and Xanthan Gum (8%) was tested in vivo using a wound model on seven-week-old male BALB/c mice (macroscopic analysis, immunostaining and confocal microscopy) as well as in vitro (scratch assay). The tested plant mixture showed a significant ability to support wound healing [37].

In an in vivo excision and incision wound model on male Swiss albino mice and Sprague-Dawley rats, *A. mollis* methanolic extract showed a remarkable wound healing effect. Treated wounds had ~39% greater tensile strength than controls and significantly faster contraction (51% wound closure) after a set period [20]. Histological analyses confirmed enhanced granulation tissue formation. These results, reported by Oz et al., highlight *A. mollis* as a potent wound healer, validating its traditional use on cuts. The same study found *A. persica* extract improved wound healing, though slightly less than *A. mollis*, with a 33% increase in tensile strength and 43.5% wound contraction [20]. Both *A. mollis* and *A. persica* accelerated healing compared to untreated wounds, suggesting that multiple *Alchemilla* species contain bioactives (likely tannins and flavonoids) that promote collagen deposition and wound closure.

3.5. Anti-Aging and Skin-Lightening (Enzyme Inhibitory) Activity

The skin is the largest organ of the human body (the total surface area is 1.5–2 $m^{2,}$ and the thickness is 1.5–5 mm) and has a complex structure since it consists of three layers: epidermis, dermis (mainly composed of fibroblasts producing collagen) and subcutaneous tissue [42,52]. The Extracellular Matrix (ECM) of the skin is an organized network of insoluble macromolecules that constitute a physical scaffold for cells. It provides unique skin properties, such as elasticity, compressibility and high tensile strength. It consists of polysaccharides, collagen proteins (collagen, elastin—they are responsible for the ECM elasticity), proteoglycans (dermatan sulfate and hyaluronan—they cush-ion cells in the extracellular matrix), hyaluronic acid and water. ECM molecules secreted by fibroblasts and epidermal cells are of great importance [38]. Numerous factors, both external and internal, contribute to the acceleration of the skin aging process. Thus, the following actions should be taken: inhibiting the elastase and collagenase enzymes, decelerating negative changes in fibroblasts, and reducing the amount of free radicals using free radical scavengers.

Skin aging is associated with loss of elasticity, caused by changes in elastin—a protein that forms connective tissue together with collagen and glycosaminoglycans. Miscellaneous factors such as, among others, pregnancy, cellulite, rapid changes in body weight, solar radiation and air pollution affect the connective tissue and contribute to the loss of skin elasticity. Moreover, skin disorders such as psoriasis, contact dermatitis, and atopic dermatitis cause increased elastase activity and degradation of elastin fibers. Enzymes such as elastases (belonging to the chymotrypsin family of proteases) and collagenases are responsible for the breakdown of elastin and collagen. Scientists are still looking for active ingredients that effectively inhibit the elastase and collagenase enzymes with a significant safety profile [2].

Alchemilla extracts have shown the ability to inhibit enzymes that contribute to skin aging and hyperpigmentation, aligning with their use in anti-aging cosmetics. However, only *A. vulgaris* has been tested for its ability to inhibit these enzymes. Some studies indicate that *A. vulgaris* contains compounds that inhibit collagenase, elastase, and tyrosinase—enzymes responsible for collagen breakdown, loss of skin elasticity, and melanin overproduction. As reported by Mandrone et al. [38,39], methanolic extract of *A. vulgaris* at a concentration of 50 µg/mL exhibited collagenase inhibition due to the presence of such compounds as tannins or quercetin-3-*O*-β-glucuronide. The plant complex containing *A. vulgaris*, *Silybum marianum*, *Equisetum arvense*, *Glycine soja*, *Triticum vulgare*, *Medicago sativa* and *Raphanus sativus* in the test of enzymatic inhibition using enzymes porcine pancreatic elastase (PPE) and human leukocyte elastase (HLE), revealed significant inhibition in the order of 41.0% against PPE and 50.0% against HLE [2]. In the same study, in vivo and in vitro tests using the SEM 474 Cutometer (Courage & Khazaka) revealed that applying a cosmetic formulation containing 5% of the plant complex caused a significant increase in skin elasticity [2]. According to Chiocchio et al. [40], methanolic extract of *A. vulgaris* at 50 µg/mL showed 12% elastase inhibitory activity, correlated to the total phenolic and flavonoid content.

Another enzyme involved in the aging process is tyrosinase. Tyrosinase (polyphenol oxidase—PPO) is an enzyme including copper, playing a vital role in two reactions: the conversion of an o-diphenol to the o-quinone as well as the hydroxylation of a monophenol. Furthermore, tyrosinase participates in the biosynthetic pathway of melanin. Thus, it is associated with age-related skin hyperpigmentation. Tyrosinase inhibitors reveal skin-whitening properties [40].

Vlaisavljevic et al. [27] conducted a study assessing the ability of *Alchemilla vulgaris* methanolic, ethanolic, ethylacetate and water extracts to inhibit tyrosinase. The best activity was observed for methanolic, followed by ethanolic, ethylacetate and water extracts (79.84 mg KAE per g for methanolic extract; the enzyme inhibitor effect was evaluated as equivalents of kojic acid—KAE). The compounds that are largely responsible for this effect are apigenin-7-*O*-β-glucoside, luteolin-7-*O*-β-glucoside, quercetin and rutin. Moreover, ethanolic and water extracts of *A. vulgaris* were evaluated spectrophotometrically using l-DOPA as a substrate for their tyrosinase inhibition [25]. Ethanolic extract (3 mg/mL) revealed significant activity (71.55), mainly due to the presence of polyphenols (112.33 GAE µg/mL), proanthocyanidins (130.00 catechine µg/mL) and flavones (497.00 rutin µg/mL). In the discussed publication [25], HPLC analysis showed that the 70% ethanol extract of *A. vulgaris* contains large amounts of ellagic acid (996.6 µg/mL), which, according to Ortiz-Ruiz et al. [53], is a tyrosinase inhibitor and is used in the cosmetic industry as a whitening agent. The complex of Swiss Alpine plant extracts containing *A. vulgaris* significantly reduced the color intensity of dark spots among human volunteers (measured by solar simulator equipment and light meter reading) [54]. On the other hand, *A. vulgaris* methanolic extract showed no tyrosinase inhibitory activity tested at 50 µg/mL in *an* in vitro tyrosinase inhibitory assay [40]. It is worth noting that the only species of the *Alchemilla* genus that has been tested for tyrosinase inhibition is *A. vulgaris*, which provides a large space for further research.

Natural skin aging is associated with changes in peripheral microfibrils. Namely, their number decreases, they become thicker, the surface of these microfibers becomes irregular and granular, and the number of glycosaminoglycans and fibroblasts reduces.

External aging is associated with the presence of amorphous elastin fibers and an increase in cross-links between the fibers. The normal functionality of elastin is prevented due to the increase in the number and changes in glycosaminoglycans, which reduces the functionality of fibroblasts. Fibroblasts create a structural scaffold for tissues, maintain the integrity of connective tissue, release elastic fibers, and, therefore, prevent signs of aging [42].

A study conducted by Borodušķis et al. [55] showed the effect of a complex of seven plant extracts (brand name Cell Repair Bio-Complex CRB), including *A. vulgaris*, on the proliferation of dermal fibroblasts and keratinocytes (using the IncuCyte ZOOM system). Another species of *Alchemilla* showing a beneficial effect on normal human dermal fibroblasts (NHDF) due to AP-1 and Nrf2/ARE signaling pathways is *A. mollis* (ethanolic extract, abundant in gallic acid) [18].

3.6. Protective Effect Against UVB Radiation

UV rays, in addition to their beneficial properties, such as the production of vitamin D in the skin, have many negative consequences related to the condition of the skin. In particular, they significantly accelerate the skin aging process and lead to the development of carcinogenesis, which may result in melanoma. Phytochemicals due to their multidirectional activity reveal a wide range of photoprotective effects, including anti-photoaging, anti-inflammation, and anti-melanogenesis and via activation of nuclear factor erythroid 2-related factor 2 related to the antioxidant response element (Nrf2-ARE) signaling pathway, regulating antioxidant genes (including glutamate cysteine ligase (GCL), glutathione S-transferase (GST), NAD(P)H quinone oxidoreductase-1 (NQO-1), heme oxygenase-1 (HO-1)) [43].

Plants of the genus *Alchemilla* are used in traditional medicine for skin dysfunctions related to excessive exposure to sunlight. Ethnobotanical surveys conducted by Mrabti et al. [56] showed that the powder of leaves obtained from *Alchemilla vulgaris* (local name Gdam sbaa) is used in traditional medicine in the Taza region in Morocco for burns and, therefore, has significant anti-burn activity. Protective effects of ethanolic extract obtained from *Alchemilla mollis* against extrinsic aging caused by UVB radiation were conducted in vitro on UVB-irradiated normal human dermal fibroblasts (NHDF) and hairless mice skin in vivo. The study revealed a significant anti-photoaging effect connected with AP-1 and Nrf2/ARE signaling pathways. Most likely, this effect is related to the presence of significant amounts of gallic acid in the extract [18].

A major direction of research is the search for substances that eliminate melanoma, the main cause of which is overexposure of the skin to the sun's rays. Of course, treatment with plant agents will not replace treatment with traditional chemical drugs, but it can significantly support them due to the multidirectional action of plants. Jelaca et al. [41] carried out a study on the effect of ethanolic extract of *A. vulgaris* against melanoma cells in vitro and in vivo, as well as its effect on tumor microenvironment ex vivo. For this purpose, the following mouse melanoma cell lines were used: B16 and B16F10. Moreover, an in vivo syngeneic mouse melanoma model was employed. The results revealed a dose-dependent decrease of cell viability after 72-h treatment with *A. vulgaris* extract and significantly reduced tumor growth in the B16 melanoma model in vivo [41].

3.7. Moisturizing Properties

Water is a substrate as well as a product of various reactions and a relevant ingredient that plays a significant role in the proper functioning of the skin, especially in the stratum corneum, where it combines with lipids and proteins. In corneocytes, i.e., dead cells of the stratum corneum, proteins adhere tightly to each other. Moreover, they are surrounded by a lipid matrix, which constitutes a specific skin barrier that prevents excessive transepidermal water loss (TEWL). Moreover, The Natural Moisturizing Factor (NMF), which contains free amino acids, pyrrolidone carboxylic acid (PCA), trans urocanic acid (UCA), sugars and lactic acid, is a natural skin protector against dehydration [57].

The study conducted by Załęcki et al. [57] showed that both water consumption as well as physical activity are positively correlated with skin hydration. Topical cosmetic preparations should also be used to maintain skin hydration at a satisfactory level in addition to these types of health-promoting activities. Extracts obtained from *A. vulgaris*, whose moisturizing properties have been scientifically proven, maybe the answer to the need for topical cosmetic application of cosmetic formulations. Other *Alchemilla* species have not yet been tested for their ability to moisturize the epidermis.

Analysis related to the effect of gels with ethanolic, water and propylene glycol extracts obtained from *A. vulgaris* (GAE, GAW, GAP, respectively) on skin hydration levels in vivo revealed that TEWL values measured on SLS-irritated human skin of 18 volunteers by Tewameter® TM 210 were back to normal. Furthermore, SCH (stratum corneum hydration) parameters measured using Corneometer® CM 820 proved action towards skin hydration level after 3 days of application [35].

4. Active Compounds Responsible for Skin Benefits

In *Alchemilla* species with skin-conditioning effects, a variety of compounds have been identified as key factors. These are predominantly polyphenolic compounds, which align with the biological activities observed [6,58]. The chemical profile of *Alchemilla* species is rich and complex, and a full phytochemical inventory is beyond this review's scope; however, notable active compounds include:

- Ellagitannins and gallotannins: These high-molecular-weight polyphenols (e.g., agrimoniin, pedunculagin) are abundant in *Alchemilla* and largely responsible for their astringent, antimicrobial, and antioxidant properties [47]. For instance, agrimoniin (isolated from *A. vulgaris* and *A. mollis*) has demonstrated anti-inflammatory effects by inhibiting NF-κB activation in immune cells [47,48]. Pedunculagin, found in *A. vulgaris* and *A. mollis* leaves, showed significant anti-acne activity; Kim et al. [59] reported that pedunculagin inhibits *Propionibacterium acnes*-induced inflammation and reduces sebum oxidation. These tannins also chelate metals and precipitate proteins, explaining the wound-healing benefit (they can form a protective layer on wounds and contract tissues, aiding clotting and tissue firming).
- Flavonoids: *Alchemilla* species contain various flavonoids (flavonols, flavones) such as quercetin and its glycosides, kaempferol glycosides, and apigenin. Apigenin has been identified in *A. vulgaris* and *A. caucasica* aerial parts [60,61]. This flavonoid is known to protect against UV-induced skin damage, stimulate collagen synthesis, and aid in conditions like psoriasis and vitiligo [62]. A recent comprehensive review by Majma Sanaye et al. [62] highlighted apigenin's dermatological benefits (anti-photoaging, wound healing, anti-cancer). Quercetin-3-*O*-*β*-glucuronide from *A. vulgaris* was shown to be a potent collagenase inhibitor (as mentioned, it can preserve skin elasticity by blocking collagen breakdown) [38,39]. Flavonoids also contribute strongly to *Alchemilla*'s antioxidant activity. Isoquercitrin, juglanin, and other flavonols reported in *Alchemilla* likely synergize to scavenge free radicals and reduce oxidative stress in skin cells.
- Phenolic acids: Gallic acid and ellagic acid are common in *Alchemilla*. Ellagic acid (3.4 mg/g in an ethanolic extract of *A. vulgaris* leaves) was quantified by Tasić-Kostov et al. [35]. Ellagic acid is a known antioxidant and also a tyrosinase inhibitor, contributing to skin-lightening effects. Gallic acid and its derivatives provide antimicrobial action. In an analysis of *A. vulgaris*, gallic acid content correlated with strong DPPH

scavenging [47]. These phenolics, while not unique to *Alchemilla*, bolster their overall efficacy by targeting oxidative and microbial aspects of skin disorders.
- Proanthocyanidins: Oligomeric proanthocyanidins have been detected in some *Alchemilla* species. For example, Mandrone et al. [39] noted procyanidin-type compounds in *A. vulgaris* during their metabolomic identification of active compounds. Proanthocyanidins have anti-enzymatic activity (inhibiting collagenase and elastase) and contribute to vascular health in the skin (strengthening capillaries). Their presence could explain *Alchemilla* extracts' use in anti-redness cosmetics and as firming agents.
- Trace elements: An interesting aspect of *Alchemilla* is its bioaccumulation of certain minerals. *A. velebitica* was found to be a rich source of trace elements like zinc, manganese, and selenium in its leaves and roots [63]. Zinc (18–54 mg/kg in *A. velebitica*) is essential for skin repair and has anti-acne properties when applied topically [63]. The presence of these elements suggests that *Alchemilla* extracts might deliver not only organic compounds but also micronutrients that benefit skin structure and immune defense. However, these findings come from one study of a specific species; it indicates potential, but further analyses of other species are needed.

Notably, many of the above compounds work in concert. For example, *A. vulgaris* extracts contain both ellagitannins and flavonoids; the ellagitannins may provide immediate antibacterial astringency, while flavonoids modulate inflammation and oxidative stress over time. This synergistic complexity is likely why whole-plant extracts often outperform isolated compounds in efficacy—a phenomenon observed in several studies where fractions of *Alchemilla* lost some activity when purified too far [47]. It also underlines the wisdom of traditional medicine using whole extracts or decoctions.

On the other hand, the complexity of *Alchemilla*'s phytochemistry poses challenges: standardizing an extract for consistent bioactivity requires careful control of harvesting (phenolic content can vary with geography and season). Moreover, high-tannin extracts can be irritating if used at excessive concentrations (tannins may cause dryness or rare allergic reactions) [64]. Formulating these extracts in modern delivery systems (nano-formulations, appropriate pH buffers) can improve bioavailability and reduce potential irritation [49]. Studies are starting to explore such approaches—for instance, encapsulating *Alchemilla* extract in lipid nanoparticles to enhance skin penetration of its active compounds [65].

In summary, *Alchemilla*'s skin benefits stem from a diversity of phenolic constituents, with tannins and flavonoids playing the main role. Each compound class tackles a different aspect of skin pathology, making *Alchemilla* extracts inherently multi-functional. Future research that isolates these compounds can further confirm their individual roles (e.g., confirming which specific tannin most strongly inhibits *C. acnes* growth or which flavonoid best stimulates collagen). Importantly, any development of *Alchemilla*-based therapeutics should consider preserving the natural synergy of its compounds to maximize efficacy.

5. Various Cosmetic Formulations and Preparations

Aiming to develop consumer-acceptable products for topical application, in recent years, researchers have attempted to determine which formulations are the most optimal for the effective release of the active factors contained in *Alchemilla* extracts by analyzing such parameters as hardness, consistency or cohesiveness. Due to understanding the mechanisms of skin penetration at the cellular and molecular level, scientists are increasingly examining the impact of advanced technologies, such as nanotechnology, in order to more effectively release and deepen the absorption of active compounds. Inorganic and polymeric nanoparticles (for example, titanium dioxide, zinc oxide or gold nanocarriers) play an important role in this process [65].

A noteworthy example is hydrogels, which are polymeric materials that have the ability to absorb large amounts of water without losing their structure. Both the degree of swelling and the mechanical properties of hydrogels can be changed by selecting the synthesis conditions and monomers so that they respond to external conditions (such as pH temperature) in a desired manner. Hydrogels are employed as vehicles for the modified release of active ingredients [66]. Thermosensitive hydrogels such as poly(N-isopropylacrylamide), p(NIPAM), and poly(Nisopropylacrylamide-co-2-hydroxypropyl methacrylate), p(NIPAM-HPMet) were used for the study conducted by [66]. The ability to release ellagic acid from various hydrogels obtained from the aboveground parts of *A. vulgaris* has been studied using FTIR and scanning electron microscope methods. The experiment indicated that p(NIPAM-HPMet) showed better incorporation and release at 37 °C of ellagic acid (98.87%) and *A. vulgaris* extract (96.45%) compared to p(NIPAM) [66].

As reported in Tasić-Kostov et al. [35], ethanolic, water and propylene glycolic extract obtained from *A. vulgaris* were tested for wound healing and antioxidant properties in combination with gel-based on Carbopol® Ultrez. The most favorable effect on wound healing in vitro was obtained for gel-containing propylene glycolic extract. Values obtained using textural assays demonstrated promising mechanical properties of the gels. Thus, they can be considered vehicles intended for wound treatment with topical application of *A. vulgaris*. It can be concluded that propylene glycol is an effective permeation enhancer in gel formulations and a desirable solvent for the production of herbal extracts.

Another kind of formulation used for topical treatment of *A. vulgaris* extract is an ointment. In the study carried out by Choi et al. [37], the application of ointment, including the herbal mixture on the dorsal skin wounds of mice (wound model on Seven-week-old male BALB/c mice) revealed significant wound healing activity proceeding faster than therapy with fusidic acid [37].

A survey on the effect of using various formulations differing in polarity (such as ointments and creams) on the antibacterial and antifungal activity of *A. pedata* extract was performed by Taddese et al. [33]. Seven formulations (form) were tested, each containing 10% of the extract, namely: form 1: sodium laurylmonosterin cream base; form 2: macrogol cream base; form 3: macrogol blend ointment base; form 4: simple ointment base; form 5: white petrolatum; form 6: polyethylene glycol bases (PEG 400:PEG 2000, 1:1) and form 7: polyethylene glycol bases (PEG 400:PEG 2000, 1:3). The test revealed that releases of the active ingredients from hydrophilic bases were higher and polyethylene glycol-based formulations were more active than formulations prepared with hydrophobic bases. No release has been observed from the simple ointment and white petrolatum (forms 4 and 5). This may be related to the fact that the agar medium is hydrophilic, which results in the adhering of hydrophobic components to the medium for a longer period than they diffuse into the hydrophilic surrounding environment [33].

Another aspect of the application of extracts obtained from the *Alchemilla* genus is the possibility of using them orally to achieve positive health-promoting effects, including activity within the skin tissues. Mansour et al. [67] demonstrated the efficacy of dietary supplementation of *A. vulgaris* powder in the diet of Nile tilapia (*Oreochromis niloticus*) fish in a dose-dependent manner. Oral application of *A. vulgaris* showed antioxidant activity and related increase of antioxidant biomarkers (catalase—CAT, superoxide dismutase—SOD, total antioxidant—TAC, and reduced glutathione—GSH as well as the reduction in myeloperoxidase (MPO) and malondialdehyde (MDA) levels. Nevertheless, further studies on the safety of use in the human body are required.

6. Safety of Application

An essential aspect, not only from the point of view of increasingly conscious consumers but also from the point of view of cosmetics manufacturers, is the assessment of the safety level of products. Accordingly, Boroja et al. [26] performed a biocompatibility analysis of *A. vulgaris* extract using a cell survival assay (immortalized murine BalbC-3 T3 fibroblasts and human normal HaCaT keratinocytes). No significant differences were observed in cell survival between the control group and groups treated with extracts [26]. Moreover, a study performed by Dos Santos Szewczyk et al. [8] employing the MTT assay reported that the butanol fraction of *A. acutiloba* methanolic extract is not cytotoxic towards GMK cells (CC_{50} value was 1000 μg/mL).

7. Comparison with Other Dermatological Medicinal Plants

In our opinion, it is useful to compare *Alchemilla* with other plant species known for treating skin inflammation and disorders to understand the novelty and impact of this genus in the broader context of herbal dermatotherapy. Many medicinal plants have similar phytochemical profiles (rich in polyphenols, tannins, terpenoids, etc.) that provide dermatological benefits such as anti-inflammatory, wound-healing, and antimicrobial effects. Below, we discuss a few notable examples and how *Alchemilla* relates to them:

- *Aloe vera* (L.) Burm.f.: *Aloe vera* gel is a popular natural remedy for skin hydration, wound healing, and mild psoriasis. *Aloe* spp. contain polysaccharides and glycoproteins that soothe irritation and promote tissue repair. Clinical studies have found that topical *Aloe vera* can improve mild to moderate psoriasis plaques, with anti-inflammatory and moisturizing effects [64]. Compared to *Aloe*, *Alchemilla* extracts are more astringent (due to tannins) but similarly anti-inflammatory. Both can reduce skin redness and aid wound closure, though via different mechanisms: *Aloe* mainly provides moisture and growth factors, whereas *Alchemilla* provides antioxidants and antimicrobial tannins. Interestingly, a review of natural psoriasis treatments noted that herbal remedies like *Aloe vera*, *Indigo naturalis*, and *Mahonia aquifolium* have yielded positive outcomes in reducing psoriatic lesions [64]. *Alchemilla* is not yet commonly cited in such contexts, highlighting its under-recognition. Given its properties, *Alchemilla* could complement or enhance treatments like *Aloe*, potentially offering both soothing and antiseptic actions in one.
- *Calendula officinalis* L. (Marigold) and *Matricaria chamomilla* L. (Chamomila): These are classic skin-healing herbs used for anti-inflammatory and soothing purposes in eczema, diaper rash, etc. *Calendula* flowers contain triterpenoids and flavonoids that increase wound healing and reduce dermatitis; *Chamomila* contains bisabolol and chamazulene that calm irritation. Both have established topical uses for skin regeneration. *Alchemilla* shares the wound-healing promotion seen with *Calendula*—for example, *A. mollis* and *A. persica* extracts increased wound tensile strength in animals compared to how *Calendula* ointment accelerates wound closure [20,68,69]. *Chamomila* and *Alchemilla* both have notable antioxidant activity; however, *Alchemilla*'s antimicrobial activity is generally greater, owing to its higher tannin content, while *Chamomila* is milder in that regard. An advantage of *Alchemilla* is its multifaceted action (antioxidant, antimicrobial, and astringent), whereas these other herbs are primarily anti-inflammatory and moisturizing. Thus, *Alchemilla* could potentially replace or complete *Calendula*/*Chamomila* in situations where infection risk is present along with inflammation (such as acne or infected eczema).
- Indigo naturalis: A Traditional Chinese Medicine remedy (Qing Dai) used in psoriasis. Indigo naturalis (derived from *Strobilanthes formosana* S.Moore or related indigo plants) has shown potent anti-psoriatic effects in clinical studies. It reduces inflammation and

excessive keratinocyte proliferation when applied topically (the active compound—indirubin, modulates aryl hydrocarbon receptors in the skin) [64]. *Alchemilla* extracts have not been tested in psoriasis patients yet, but they do mitigate some pathological factors (e.g., oxidative stress). Unlike Indigo naturalis, which can cause a temporary blue staining of skin, *Alchemilla* extracts are tannin-rich and tend to have a brown hue and astringent feel. This difference might affect formulation preferences, but it also indicates that *Alchemilla* could be cosmetically acceptable in products if appropriately prepared.

- *Berberis aquifolium* Pursh (Oregon grape): This plant's root extract is an approved topical remedy for psoriasis, rich in isoquinoline alkaloids (e.g., berberine) that have anti-inflammatory and anti-proliferative effects on keratinocytes. *Berberis* creams have demonstrated significant improvements in psoriatic scaling and inflammation in clinical trials [64]. *Alchemilla* does not contain alkaloids like berberine, but its ellagitannins might achieve some similar anti-inflammatory outcomes via antioxidant pathways. Both *Berberis* and *Alchemilla* have antimicrobial activity that is beneficial for preventing secondary infection in chronic dermatitis. Given *Berberis*' success, *Alchemilla* could be considered a candidate for similar development—especially because it also inhibits tyrosinase (offering an added benefit for managing post-inflammatory hyperpigmentation, where *Berberis* mainly targets inflammation).
- *Withania somnifera* (L.) Dunal (Ashwagandha): This Ayurvedic herb contains withanolides like withaferin A, which have been extensively studied for skin-related pharmacological effects. Withaferin A is a steroidal lactone that exhibits strong anti-inflammatory, anti-proliferative, and antioxidant activities in dermatological disease models [70]. It has shown efficacy against psoriasis and even skin cancers by modulating immune responses and inducing apoptosis in abnormal cells [70]. *Alchemilla* possess some comparable properties—for instance, both *Alchemilla* tannins and withaferin A can reduce inflammatory mediators and oxidative stress. However, *Alchemilla* does not contain a single compound similar to withaferin; instead, it delivers a synergistic mix of polyphenols. Ashwagandha is also a more researched plant (with numerous clinical trials, e.g., in atopic dermatitis), underscoring the need for deeper *Alchemilla* investigations. Nonetheless, the broad-spectrum dermatological effects of *Alchemilla* extracts (antioxidant, antimicrobial, etc.) parallel Ashwagandha's multimodal actions, suggesting that *Alchemilla* could likewise be developed into topical formulations for inflammation-driven skin conditions [70].

In summary, *Alchemilla* stands out as a multi-purpose dermatological herb, much like other known medicinal plants, but it remains less studied and used. Its antioxidant and antimicrobial potency are comparable to or exceeding some well-known skin herbs, and its wound-healing and anti-inflammatory effects complement those of staples like *Aloe* and *Calendula*. The comparison emphasizes that *Alchemilla* has a valuable role to play—it could be considered alongside Ashwagandha for anti-inflammatory uses, or alongside *Berberis* and Indigo naturalis for psoriasis, and as an alternative to *Calendula* in wound and rash remedies. The key novelty of *Alchemilla* is the combination of diverse activities in one genus. Future direct comparative studies (e.g., *Alchemilla* vs. *Calendula* in wound healing efficacy or *Alchemilla* vs. *Berberis* in psoriasis models) would help position this genus in herbal dermatology. Current data already justify integrating *Alchemilla* extracts into modern skin care products, especially given the growing trend of formulating multi-herb complexes for synergistic effects [2]. *Alchemilla*'s inclusion could enhance the impact of such formulations by contributing strong antioxidant and antimicrobial components.

8. Discussion of Key Findings and Practical Implications

Based on the above results and comparisons, several general points emerge regarding how *Alchemilla* extracts can be optimally utilized and what gaps in our knowledge remain:

- Optimal extraction methods: The effectiveness of *Alchemilla* extracts clearly depends on the extraction solvent and method. Generally, hydroalcoholic extracts (e.g., 50–70% ethanol or methanol) and medium-polarity fractions (ethyl acetate, butanol) contain the highest levels of active polyphenols and tend to exhibit the strongest antioxidant and enzyme-inhibiting activities. For instance, partitioning a methanol extract of *A. acutiloba* yielded an ethyl acetate fraction that concentrated most of the antioxidant tannins. In contrast, purely aqueous extracts can be less potent in some assays but still retain significant activity (as seen with *A. mollis* water extracts effective against *S. aureus*). Completely non-polar extracts (hexane) sometimes yield specific actives (like the potent DPPH scavenger in *A. ellenbergiana*), but generally, a mix of water and alcohol is recommended to extract a broad spectrum of actives (tannins, flavonoids, and phenolic acids). Maceration or reflux extraction is commonly used in studies; however, modern techniques like ultrasonic-assisted extraction could improve yield and skin delivery of *Alchemilla* compounds. In practical terms, for topical formulation development, a glycerol- or propylene glycol-containing extract might offer an optimal compromise, harnessing both hydrophilic and lipophilic constituents. The data suggest that no single solvent captures all active compounds, so sequential extraction (graduating from non-polar to polar) might be employed to create a full-spectrum *Alchemilla* extract for maximal efficacy.
- Efficacy of study models: The review encompassed a range of experimental models—from test-tube antioxidant assays to animal wound-healing models—each providing different insights. In vitro assays (DPPH, FRAP, enzymatic inhibition) are useful for screening antioxidant or anti-enzyme potential, but they simplify complex skin physiology. Cell culture models, such as fibroblast scratch assays and keratinocyte inflammation tests, offer more biological relevance by showing how extracts interact with living cells (e.g., promoting cell migration or reducing inflammatory markers). These were effective in demonstrating *Alchemilla* wound-healing stimulation and anti-inflammatory impact on skin cells. The most convincing evidence comes from in vivo models: rodent studies of wound healing illustrated that *Alchemilla* extracts significantly accelerate actual tissue repair and improve the biomechanical strength of healed skin. Such models capture the integrated effect of the extract on inflammation, cell proliferation, and remodeling phases of healing. Similarly, the in vivo melanoma model used for *A. vulgaris* provided crucial evidence that the extract can penetrate a biological system and exert anti-tumor effects. Going forward, ex vivo human skin models (e.g., skin explants) and clinical trials on patients are needed. The existing models have efficiently identified *Alchemilla* extract potential, but human trials will confirm its real-world effectiveness. For example, a small clinical study on an *Alchemilla* cream for acne or eczema would test whether the in vitro antimicrobial and anti-inflammatory effects translate to patient improvement. In summary, the combination of simple and complex models used so far has been effective in characterizing *Alchemilla* activities; the next step is to employ clinical and translational models, which is currently a gap.
- Most potent species and extracts: Among the species studied, certain ones stand out as particularly potent. *A. vulgaris* is the most extensively studied and shows well-rounded efficacy (good antioxidant, antimicrobial, enzyme inhibition, and wound-healing properties), making it a prime candidate for product development. However, *A. vulgaris* is not necessarily the most potent in each category. For example, *A. acutiloba*

and *A. arvensis* exhibited exceptionally high antioxidant power, suggesting these species accumulate certain polyphenols to a higher level. *A. mollis* and *A. persica* exceed in wound-healing assays, indicating their chemical profile is especially suited for tissue repair stimulation. In terms of antimicrobial activity, *A. mollis,* with its low MICs against *S. aureus,* was notably potent, and *A. hybrida* showed strong antifungal activity with low MICs. These findings imply that while any of these *Alchemilla* species can be useful, selecting the right species-extract pair is key for a given application. For an antioxidant-rich serum, *A. acutiloba* or *A. alpina* extracts might provide the strongest effect, whereas, for an acne gel, *A. mollis* (antibacterial) combined with *A. vulgaris* (anti-inflammatory) could be ideal. It is also encouraging that less-common species (e.g., *A. hybrida, A. barbatiflora*) showed potent activities; this diversity means the genus as a whole is a rich resource. Future research could employ bioassay-guided fractionation to specify the most active species and standardize their extracts. Additionally, an interesting note is that some *Alchemilla* species untested so far are used in traditional medicine (like *A. hessii A. monticola*); investigating these could yield even more potent extracts or novel compounds. For now, based on current evidence, *A. vulgaris, A. mollis,* and *A. persica* are good all-around choices (with *A. vulgaris* having the advantage of more safety data historically), while *A. acutiloba* and *A. arvensis* are top performers in antioxidant assays, and *A. hybrida* is notable for antifungal efficacy.

In conclusion of this discussion, *Alchemilla* has demonstrated in vitro and in vivo efficacy that justifies further development, but the translation to clinical use will require addressing the above points: choosing the right extract method for the desired results, confirming efficacy in human models, selecting the most potent species or variety, and ensuring formulations maximize benefits while minimizing any side-effects.

9. Conclusions

In summary, *Alchemilla* (lady's mantle) species exhibit a wide range of beneficial biological activities for skin health, confirming their traditional use in treating dermatological ailments. Key findings of this review highlight that *Alchemilla* extracts are rich in polyphenols with strong antioxidant properties, helping to neutralize free radicals and protect the skin from oxidative stress and aging. They also possess anti-inflammatory and astringent tannins that can soothe irritation, reduce redness, and promote the healing of minor wounds. Various *Alchemilla* extracts showed antimicrobial efficacy, particularly against Gram-positive bacteria implicated in skin infections and acne (e.g., *Staphylococcus aureus* and *Cutibacterium acnes*), as well as activity against certain fungi, which supports their use in preventing or treating infected wounds and rashes. Preliminary studies even indicate anti-tumor potential, with *A. vulgaris* extracts inhibiting melanoma cell growth, though more research is needed in this area.

Practical applications of these findings are already emerging: *Alchemilla* can be incorporated into natural skincare and cosmetic products as an active ingredient for anti-aging (due to its collagenase/elastase inhibitory effects and antioxidants), for acne-care formulations (providing a botanical antibacterial and anti-inflammatory action without the side effects of synthetic agents), and for wound-healing ointments or sprays (to speed up repair and keep wounds clean). The best-studied species, *A. vulgaris,* along with *A. mollis* and *A. persica,* appear particularly promising for such uses. Importantly, this review underlines that among nearly 800 species, just a few have been studied—indicating a rich untapped potential. Future research should focus on exploring these less-studied *Alchemilla* species (e.g., ethnomedicinal plants like *A. hessii* and *A. monticola*), as they may yield new bioactive compounds or even greater efficacy in skin applications.

Continued investigation is also encouraged to fully clarify the mechanisms of action of *Alchemilla* extracts at the molecular level (for example, how exactly they modulate inflammatory pathways or influence skin microbiome balance). Rigorous safety evaluations and clinical trials will be important to translate the in vitro and in vivo findings into approved medical or cosmetic products. This includes confirming that *Alchemilla*'s tyrosinase inhibition is safe for long-term use (ensuring no cytotoxicity to melanocytes) and establishing optimal dosing regimens. Given the current evidence, *Alchemilla* extracts appear to have a favorable safety profile and a low risk of side effects, especially in topical use, but clinical validation will build confidence for consumers and healthcare providers.

In conclusion, *Alchemilla* species represent a versatile and potent natural resource for dermatological therapy and skincare. They combine antioxidant, anti-inflammatory, antimicrobial, and wound-healing activities in one package, a synergy that modern single-target drugs often lack. Using *Alchemilla*-based preparations could reduce reliance on synthetic chemicals (like corticosteroids or antibiotics) in managing certain skin conditions, aligning with the growing demand for gentler, plant-based treatments. To fully realize this potential, future studies should aim to broaden the spectrum of species studied, standardize extract preparations for consistency, and pursue clinical trials in conditions such as acne, eczema, psoriasis, and wound care.

Author Contributions: Conceptualization, K.D.S.S., B.K. and S.K.; methodology, B.K. and S.K.; writing—original draft preparation, B.K., S.K., A.B.-R. and M.K.; writing—review and editing, K.D.S.S., B.K., S.K. and A.B.-R. All authors have read and agreed to the published version of the manuscript.

Funding: This research was funded by the Ministry of Science and Higher Education in Poland DS45 project of the Medical University of Lublin.

Institutional Review Board Statement: Not applicable.

Informed Consent Statement: Not applicable.

Data Availability Statement: No new data were created or analyzed in this study. Data sharing is not applicable to this article.

Conflicts of Interest: The authors declare no conflicts of interest.

References

1. Zhang, X.; You, L.Y.; Zhang, Z.Y.; Jiang, D.X.; Qiu, Y.; Ruan, Y.P.; Mao, Z.J. Integrating pharmacological evaluation and computational identification for deciphering the action mechanism of Yunpi-Huoxue-Sanjie formula alleviates diabetic cardiomyopathy. *Front. Pharmacol.* **2022**, *13*, 957829. [CrossRef] [PubMed]
2. Benaiges, A.; Marcet, P.; Armengol, R.; Betes, C.; Gironés, E. Study of the refirming effect of a plant complex. *Int. J. Cosmet. Sci.* **1998**, *20*, 223–233. [CrossRef] [PubMed]
3. Available online: https://powo.science.kew.org/taxon/urn:lsid:ipni.org:names:30008181-2 (accessed on 15 September 2024).
4. Kaval, I.; Behçet, L.; Cakilcioglu, U. Ethnobotanical study on medicinal plants in Geçitli and its surrounding (Hakkari-Turkey). *J. Ethnopharmacol.* **2014**, *155*, 171–184. [CrossRef] [PubMed]
5. Mladenova, S.G.; Vasileva, L.V.; Savova, M.S.; Marchev, A.S.; Tews, D.; Wabitsch, M.; Ferrante, C.; Orlando, G.; Georgiev, M.I. Anti-adipogenic effect of *Alchemilla monticola* is mediated via PI3K/AKT signaling inhibition in human adipocytes. *Front. Pharmacol.* **2021**, *12*, 707507. [CrossRef]
6. Kanak, S.; Krzemińska, B.; Celiński, R.; Bakalczuk, M.; Dos Santos Szewczyk, K. Phenolic composition and antioxidant activity of *Alchemilla* species. *Plants* **2022**, *11*, 2709. [CrossRef]
7. Page, M.J.; McKenzie, J.E.; Bossuyt, P.M.; Boutron, I.; Hoffmann, T.C.; Mulrow, C.D.; Shamseer, L.; Tetzlaff, J.M.; Moher, D. Updating guidance for reporting systematic reviews: Development of the PRISMA 2020 statement. *J. Clin. Epidemiol.* **2021**, *134*, 103–112. [CrossRef]
8. Dos Santos Szewczyk, K.; Pietrzak, W.; Klimek, K.; Gogacz, M. LC-ESI-MS/MS identification of biologically active phenolics in different extracts of *Alchemilla acutiloba* Opiz. *Molecules* **2022**, *27*, 621. [CrossRef]

9. İnci, Ş.; Eren, A.; Kirbağ, S. Determination of antimicrobial and antioxidant activity of *Alchemilla alpina* L. *Turk. J. Agric. Food Sci. Technol.* **2021**, *9*, 2260–2264. [CrossRef]
10. Ali, H.; Alkowni, R.; Jaradat, N.; Masri, M. Evaluation of phytochemical and pharmacological activities of *Taraxacum syriacum* and *Alchemilla arvensis*. *Jordan. J. Pharm. Sci.* **2021**, *14*, 457–472.
11. Renda, G.; Özel, A.; Barut, B.; Korkmaz, B.; Šoral, M.; Kandemir, Ü.; Liptaj, T. Bioassay guided isolation of active compounds from *Alchemilla barbatiflora* Juz. *Rec. Nat. Prod.* **2018**, *12*, 76–85. [CrossRef]
12. Acet, T.; Özcan, K. Determination of antioxidant and antimicrobial properties of lady's mantle (*Alchemilla ellenbergiana*) extracts. *Gümüşhane Üniversitesi Fen. Bilim. Enstitüsü Derg.* **2018**, *8*, 113–121. [CrossRef]
13. Uçar Sözmen, E.; Eruygur, N.; Akpolat, A.; Çetin, M.D.; Durukan, H.; Demirba, A.; Karaköy, T. Sivas Ili Do gal Florasından Toplanan Sarı Kantaron (*Hypericum scabrum* L.) ve Aslan Pençesi (*Alchemilla mollis* (Buser) Rothm) Bitkilerinin Bazı Kalite Kriterlerinin Belirlenmesi. *J. Inst. Sci. Tech.* **2020**, *10*, 1410–1418.
14. Denev, P.; Kratchanova, M.; Ciz, M.; Lojek, A.; Vasicek, O.; Blazheva, D.; Nedelcheva, P.; Vojtek, L.; Hyrsl, P. Antioxidant, antimicrobial and neutrophil-modulating activities of herb extracts. *Acta Biochim. Pol.* **2014**, *61*, 359–367. [CrossRef]
15. Unkovic, N.; Ćoćić, D.; Džamić, A.; Savković, Z.; Živković, L.; Ljaljević Grbić, M. Fungal contamination of make-up products and assessment of *Alchemilla hybrida* L. extracts as potential cosmetic ingredients. In *FEMS Conference on Microbiology, Electronic Abstract Book*; University of Belgrade: Belgrade, Serbia, 2022; p. 824.
16. Nikolova, M.; Dincheva, I.; Vitkova, A.; Badjakov, I. Phenolic acids and free radical scavenging activity of Bulgarian endemic—*Alchemilla jumrukczalica* Pawl. *Planta Med.* **2011**, *77*, 802–804. [CrossRef]
17. Güzel, A. Assessment of antioxidant, acetylcholinesterase, paraoxonase inhibition activities and phenolic content of *Alchemilla lithophila*. *Pak. J. Pharm. Sci.* **2024**, *37*, 25–32. [PubMed]
18. Hwang, E.; Ngo, H.T.T.; Seo, S.A.; Park, B.; Zhang, M.; Yi, T.H. Protective effect of dietary *Alchemilla mollis* on UVB-irradiated premature skin aging through regulation of transcription factor NFATc1 and Nrf2/ARE pathways. *Phytomedicine* **2018**, *39*, 125–136. [CrossRef] [PubMed]
19. Karatoprak, G.Ş.; İlgün, S.; Koşar, M. Antiradical, antimicrobial and cytotoxic activity evaluations of *Alchemilla mollis* (Buser) Rothm. *Int. J. Herb. Med.* **2018**, *6*, 33–38.
20. Oz, B.E.; Ilhan, M.; Özbilgin, S.; Akkol, E.K.; Acıkara, O.B.; Saltan, G.; Keles, H.; Süntar, I. Effects of *Alchemilla mollis* and *Alchemilla persica* on the wound healing process. *Bangladesh J. Pharmacol.* **2016**, *11*, 577–584. [CrossRef]
21. Nedyalkov, P.; Kaneva, M.; Mihaylova, D.; Kostov, G.; Kemilev, S. Influence of the ethanol concentration on the antioxidant capacity and polyphenol content of *Alchemilla mollis* extracts. *Comptes Rendus L'Academie Bulg. Sci.* **2015**, *68*, 1491–1502.
22. Trendafilova, A.; Todorova, M.; Nikolova, M.; Gavrilova, A.; Vitkova, A. Flavonoid constituents and free radical scavenging activity of *Alchemilla mollis*. *Nat. Prod. Commun.* **2011**, *6*, 1851–1854. [CrossRef]
23. Ergene, B.; Bahadir Acikara, Ö.; Bakar, F.; Saltan, G.; Nebioğlu, S. Antioxidant activity and phytochemical analysis of *Alchemilla persica* Rothm. *Ank. Univ. Eczac. Fak. Derg.* **2010**, *39*, 145–154. [CrossRef]
24. Shafaghat, A. Chemical constituents, antioxidant and antibacterial activities of the hexane extract of *Alchemilla sericata* Reichenb. *J. Food Biochem.* **2019**, *43*, 9–14. [CrossRef]
25. Neagu, E.; Paun, G.; Albu, C.; Radu, G.L. Assessment of acetylcholinesterase and tyrosinase inhibitory and antioxidant activity of *Alchemilla vulgaris* and *Filipendula ulmaria* extracts. *J. Taiwan. Inst. Chem. Eng.* **2015**, *52*, 26. [CrossRef]
26. Boroja, T.; Mihailović, V.; Katanić, J.; Pan, S.P.; Nikles, S.; Imbimbo, P.; Monti, D.M.; Stanković, N.; Stanković, M.S.; Bauer, R. The biological activities of roots and aerial parts of *Alchemilla vulgaris* L. *S. Afr. J. Bot.* **2018**, *116*, 175–184. [CrossRef]
27. Vlaisavljević, S.; Jelača, S.; Zengin, G.; Mimica-Dukić, N.; Berežni, S.; Miljić, M.; Stevanović, Z.D. *Alchemilla vulgaris* agg. (Lady's mantle) from central Balkan: Antioxidant, anticancer and enzyme inhibition properties. *RSC Adv.* **2019**, *9*, 37474–37483. [CrossRef]
28. Oktyabrsky, O.; Vysochina, G.; Muzyka, N.; Samoilova, Z.; Kukushkina, T.; Smirnova, G. Assessment of anti-oxidant activity of plant extracts using microbial test systems. *J. Appl. Microbiol.* **2009**, *106*, 1175–1183. [CrossRef] [PubMed]
29. El-Hadidy, E.M.; Refat, O.G.; Halaby, M.S.; Elmetwaly, E.M.; Omar, A.A. Effect of Lion's Foot (*Alchemilla vulgaris*) on liver and renal functions in rats induced by CCl4. *Food Nutr. Sci.* **2018**, *9*, 46–62. [CrossRef]
30. Hamid, K. *Alchemilla vulgaris* and *Filipendula ulmaria* extracts as potential natural preservatives in beef patties. *Malays. J. Anal. Sci.* **2017**, *21*, 986–995. [CrossRef]
31. Ondrejovič, M.; Ondrigová, Z.; Kubincová, J. Isolation of antioxidants from *Alchemilla xanthochlora*. *Nov. Biotechnol. Chim.* **2009**, *9*, 313–318. [CrossRef]
32. Kurtul, E.; Eryilmaz, M.; Sarialtin, S.Y.; Tekin, M.; Acikara, Ö.B.; Çoban, T. Bioactivities of *Alchemilla mollis*, *Alchemilla persica* and their active constituents. *Braz. J. Pharm. Sci.* **2022**, *58*, e18373. [CrossRef]
33. Taddese, S.; Asres, K.; Gebre-Mariam, T. Formulation of topical antimicrobials containing the extracts of *Alchemilla pedata* and *Maesa lanceolata*. *Ethiop. Pharm. J.* **2009**, *21*, 13–24.

34. Dzabijeva, D.; Boroduske, A.; Ramata-Stunda, A.; Mazarova, N.; Nikolajeva, V.; Boroduskis, M.; Nakurte, I. Anti-bacterial activity and online HPLC-DPPH based antiradical kinetics of medicinal plant extracts of high relevance for cosmetics production. *Key Eng. Mater.* **2018**, *762*, 8–13. [CrossRef]
35. Tasić-Kostov, M.; Arsić, I.; Pavlović, D.; Stojanović, S.; Najman, S.; Naumović, S.; Tadić, V. Towards a modern approach to traditional use: In vitro and in vivo evaluation of *Alchemilla vulgaris* L. gel wound healing potential. *J. Ethnopharmacol.* **2019**, *238*, 16. [CrossRef] [PubMed]
36. Shrivastava, R.; John, G.W. Treatment of aphthous stomatitis with topical *Alchemilla vulgaris* in glycerine. *Clin. Drug Investig.* **2006**, *26*, 567–573. [CrossRef] [PubMed]
37. Choi, J.; Park, Y.G.; Yun, M.S.; Seol, J.W. Effect of herbal mixture composed of *Alchemilla vulgaris* and *Mimosa* on wound healing process. *Biomed. Pharmacother.* **2018**, *106*, 326–332. [CrossRef]
38. Mandrone, M. Medicinal Plants from Ancient Tradition as a Source for Matrix Proteases Inhibitors. Study of Correlation Between Biological Activity and Phytochemical Profile. Ph.D. Thesis, University of Bologna, Bologna, Italy, 2016; pp. 1–57.
39. Mandrone, M.; Coqueiro, A.; Poli, F.; Antognoni, F.; Choi, Y.H. Identification of a collagenase-inhibiting flavonoid from *Alchemilla vulgaris* using NMR-based metabolomics. *Planta Med.* **2018**, *84*, 941–946. [CrossRef]
40. Chiocchio, I.; Mandrone, M.; Sanna, C.; Maxia, A.; Tacchini, M.; Poli, F. Screening of a hundred plant extracts as tyrosinase and elastase inhibitors, two enzymatic targets of cosmetic interest. *Ind. Crops Prod.* **2018**, *122*, 498–505. [CrossRef]
41. Jelača, S.; Drača, D.; Stevanović, Z.D.; Jovanović, I.; Pavlović, S.; Gajović, N.; Mijatović, S.; Arsenijević, N.; Maksimović Ivanić, D. Multiple effects of *Alchemilla vulgaris* L. extract on melanoma cells and tumor microenvironment. *Eur. J. Immunol.* **2021**, *51*, 352. [CrossRef]
42. Merecz-Sadowska, A.; Sitarek, P.; Kucharska, E.; Kowalczyk, T.; Zajdel, K.; Cegliński, T.; Zajdel, R. Antioxidant properties of plant-derived phenolic compounds and their effect on skin fibroblast cells. *Antioxidants* **2021**, *10*, 726. [CrossRef]
43. Chaiprasongsuk, A.; Panich, U. Role of phytochemicals in skin photoprotection via regulation of Nrf2. *Front. Pharmacol.* **2022**, *13*, 823881. [CrossRef]
44. García-Villegas, A.; Fernández-Ochoa, Á.; Alañón, M.E.; Rojas-García, A.; Arráez-Román, D.; Cádiz-Gurrea, M.D.L.L.; Segura-Carretero, A. Bioactive compounds and potential health benefits through cosmetic applications of Cherry stem extract. *Int. J. Mol. Sci.* **2024**, *25*, 3723. [CrossRef] [PubMed]
45. Moreau, M.; Naiken, T.; Bru, G.; Marteau, C.; Canaple, L.; Gourguillon, L.; Leblanc, E.; Oger, E.; Le Mestr, A.; Mantelin, J.; et al. The impact of PSR^{TM} (plant small RNA technology), tea extract, and its principal components on mitochondrial function and antioxidant properties in skin cells. *Cosmetics* **2023**, *10*, 172. [CrossRef]
46. Cibrian, D.; de la Fuente, H.; Sánchez-Madrid, F. Metabolic pathways that control skin homeostasis and inflammation. *Trends Mol. Med.* **2020**, *26*, 975–986. [CrossRef]
47. Duckstein, S.M.; Lotter, E.M.; Meyer, U.; Lindequist, U.; Stintzing, F.C. Phenolic constituents from *Alchemilla vulgaris* L. and *Alchemilla mollis* (Buser) rothm. at different dates of harvest. *Z. Naturforsch. Sect. C J. Biosci.* **2012**, *67C*, 529–540. [CrossRef]
48. Hoffmann, J.; Casetti, F.; Bullerkotte, U.; Haarhaus, B.; Vagedes, J.; Schempp, C.M.; Wölfle, U. Anti-inflammatory effects of agrimoniin-enriched fractions of *Potentilla erecta*. *Molecules* **2016**, *21*, 792. [CrossRef]
49. Melnyk, N.; Vlasova, I.; Skowrońska, W.; Bazylko, A.; Piwowarski, J.P.; Granica, S. Current knowledge on interactions of plant materials traditionally used in skin diseases in Poland and Ukraine with human skin microbiota. *Int. J. Mol. Sci.* **2022**, *23*, 9644. [CrossRef] [PubMed]
50. Dreno, B.; Dekio, I.; Baldwin, H.; Demessant, A.L.; Dagnelie, M.A.; Khammari, A.; Corvec, S. Acne microbiome: From phyla to phylotypes. *J. Eur. Acad. Dermatol. Venereol.* **2024**, *38*, 657–664. [CrossRef] [PubMed]
51. Peña, O.A.; Martin, P. Cellular and molecular mechanisms of skin wound healing. *Nat. Rev. Mol. Cell Biol.* **2024**, *25*, 599–616. [CrossRef] [PubMed]
52. Costa, E.F.; Magalhães, W.V.; Di Stasi, L.C. Recent advances in herbal-derived products with skin anti-aging properties and cosmetic applications. *Molecules* **2022**, *27*, 7518. [CrossRef]
53. Ortiz-Ruiz, C.V.; Berna, J.; Tudela, J.; Varon, R.; Garcia-Canovas, F. Action of ellagic acid on the melanin biosynthesis pathway. *J. Dermatol. Sci.* **2016**, *82*, 115–122. [CrossRef]
54. Gupta, S.K. Boosting Tyrosinase Inhibiting Activity of Skin Whitening and Sunscreen Compositions. U.S. Patent 2004/0092606A1,, 26 August 2004.
55. Boroduškis, M.; Kaktiņa, E.; Blāķe, I.; Nakurte, I.; Dzabijeva, D. Chemical characterization and *in vitro* evaluation of birch sap and a complex of plant extracts for potential use in cosmetic anti-ageing products. *Environ. Exp. Biol.* **2017**, *15*, 29–36. [CrossRef]
56. Mrabti, H.N.; Doudach, L.; Mekkaoui, M.; Khalil, Z.; Harraqui, K.; Fozia, F.; Naceiri Mrabti, N.; El-Shazly, M.; Alotaibi, A.; Ullah, R.; et al. Profile of medicinal plants traditionally used for the treatment of skin burns. *Evid. Based Complement. Altern. Med.* **2022**, *2022*, 3436665. [CrossRef]
57. Załęcki, P.; Rogowska, K.; Wąs, P.; Łuczak, K.; Wysocka, M.; Nowicka, D. Impact of lifestyle on differences in skin hydration of selected body areas in young women. *Cosmetics* **2024**, *11*, 13. [CrossRef]

58. Jakimiuk, K.; Tomczyk, M. A review of the traditional uses, phytochemistry, pharmacology, and clinical evidence for the use of the genus *Alchemilla* (Rosaceae). *J. Ethnopharmacol.* **2024**, *320*, 117439. [CrossRef]
59. Kim, M.; Yin, J.; Hwang, I.H.; Park, D.H.; Lee, E.K.; Kim, M.J.; Lee, M.W. Anti-acne vulgaris effects of pedunculagin from the leaves of *Quercus mongolica* by anti-inflammatory activity and 5α-reductase inhibition. *Molecules* **2020**, *25*, 2154. [CrossRef] [PubMed]
60. Jurić, T.; Katanić Stanković, J.S.; Rosić, G.; Selaković, D.; Joksimović, J.; Mišić, D.; Stanković, V.; Mihailović, V. Protective effects of *Alchemilla vulgaris* L. extracts against cisplatin-induced toxicological alterations in rats. *South. Afr. J. Bot.* **2020**, *128*, 141–151. [CrossRef]
61. Karaoglan, E.S.; Bayir, Y.; Albayrak, A.; Toktay, E.; Ozgen, U.; Kazaz, C.; Kahramanlar, A.; Cadirci, E. Isolation of major compounds and gastroprotective activity of *Alchemilla caucasica* on indomethacin induced gastric ulcers in rats. *Eurasian J. Med.* **2020**, *52*, 249–253. [CrossRef]
62. Majma Sanaye, P.; Mojaveri, M.R.; Ahmadian, R.; Sabet Jahromi, M.; Bahramsoltani, R. Apigenin and its dermatological applications: A comprehensive review. *Phytochemistry* **2022**, *203*, 113390. [CrossRef]
63. Juranović Cindrić, I.; Zeiner, M.; Požgaj, M.; Šilić, T.; Stingeder, G. Elemental characterisation of the medical plant *Alchemilla velebitica*. *J. Trace Elem. Med. Biol.* **2015**, *31*, 274–278. [CrossRef]
64. Radu, A.; Tit, D.M.; Endres, L.M.; Radu, A.F.; Vesa, C.M.; Bungau, S.G. Naturally derived bioactive compounds as precision modulators of immune and inflammatory mechanisms in psoriatic conditions. *Inflammopharmacology* **2025**, *33*, 527–549. [CrossRef]
65. Achagar, R.; Ait-Touchente, Z.; El Ati, R.; Boujdi, K.; Thoume, A.; Abdou, A.; Touzani, R. A Comprehensive review of essential oil–nanotechnology synergy for advanced dermocosmetic delivery. *Cosmetics* **2024**, *11*, 48. [CrossRef]
66. Ilić-Stojanović, S.; Nikolić, V.; Kundaković, T.; Savić, I.; Savić-Gajić, I.; Jocić, E.; Nikolić, L. Thermosensitive hydrogels for modified release of ellagic acid obtained from *Alchemilla vulgaris* L. extract. *Int. J. Polym. Mater. Polym. Biomater.* **2018**, *67*, 553–563. [CrossRef]
67. Mansour, A.T.; Mahboub, H.H.; Elshopakey, G.E.; Aziz, E.K.; Alhajji, A.H.M.; Rayan, G.; Ghazzawy, H.S.; El-Houseiny, W. Physiological performance, antioxidant and immune status, columnaris resistance, and growth of *Nile tilapia* that received *Alchemilla vulgaris*—supplemented diets. *Antioxidants* **2022**, *11*, 1494. [CrossRef]
68. Givol, O.; Kornhaber, R.; Visentin, D.; Cleary, M.; Haik, J.; Harats, M. A systematic review of *Calendula officinalis* extract for wound healing. *Wound Repair. Regen.* **2019**, *27*, 548–561. [CrossRef] [PubMed]
69. Ferreira, E.B.; Vasques, C.I.; Jesus, C.A.C.; Reis, P.E.D. Topical effects of *Chamomilla recutita* in skin damage: A literature review. *Pharmacologyonline* **2015**, *3*, 123–130.
70. Bungau, S.; Vesa, C.M.; Abid, A.; Behl, T.; Tit, D.M.; Purza, A.L.; Pasca, B.; Todan, L.M.; Endres, L. Withaferin A—A promising phytochemical compound with multiple results in dermatological diseases. *Molecules* **2021**, *26*, 2407. [CrossRef]

molecules

Review

Sacha Inchi (*Plukenetia volubilis*): Potential Bioactivity, Extraction Methods, and Microencapsulation Techniques

Sarah Gustia Redjeki [1], Alfa Fildzah Hulwana [1], Rizqa Nurul Aulia [2], Ira Maya [2], Anis Yohana Chaerunisaa [3] and Sriwidodo Sriwidodo [3,*]

1 Undergraduate Program in Pharmacy, Faculty of Pharmacy, Universitas Padjadjaran, Sumedang 45363, Indonesia; sarah21006@mail.unpad.ac.id (S.G.R.); alfa21001@mail.unpad.ac.id (A.F.H.)
2 Master Program in Pharmacy, Faculty of Pharmacy, Universitas Padjadjaran, Sumedang 45363, Indonesia; rizqa16001@mail.unpad.ac.id (R.N.A.); ira16001@mail.unpad.ac.id (I.M.)
3 Department of Pharmaceutics and Pharmaceutical Technology, Faculty of Pharmacy, Universitas Padjadjaran, Sumedang 45363, Indonesia; anis.yohana.chaerunisaa@unpad.ac.id
* Correspondence: sriwidodo@unpad.ac.id

Abstract: Sacha inchi (*Plukenetia volubilis* L.), an oilseed native to the Peruvian rainforest, has garnered attention for its valuable components and its potential applications in the food, pharmaceutical, and nutraceutical industries. Sacha inchi oil is rich in fatty acids, particularly omega-3, omega-6, and omega-9, along with antioxidants such as tocopherols, which collectively contribute to cardiovascular health, antioxidant, anti-inflammatory, antiproliferative, and neuroprotective effects. The susceptibility of the oil to oxidation poses significant challenges for both storage and processing, making it essential to employ microencapsulation technologies to preserve its integrity and extend shelf life. This paper aims to provide a review of the therapeutic potential, extraction methods, and microencapsulation strategies for enhancing the oil's stability and bioavailability. Optimizing both extraction processes and encapsulation strategies would enhance the oil's stability and bioavailability, enabling it to be more effectively utilized in functional foods and therapeutic applications across the nutraceutical and pharmaceutical fields.

Keywords: sacha inchi oil; oil recovery; alternative medicine; oxidative stability; microcapsule technologies

1. Introduction

Sacha inchi (*Plukenetia volubilis* Linneo), a plant native to the Peruvian rainforest, is part of the Euphorbiaceae family. It is also known as Inca peanut, wild peanut, or mountain peanut. The name "sacha inchi" comes from the Quechua language which means "wild peanut". This is because it was originally eaten as a nut by the Chanka and Mochica-Chimú tribes before the Inca. Characterized by its star-shaped capsules, sacha inchi fruit grows to a size of 3 to 5 cm. As it ripens, the fruit undergoes a color transformation from green to a blackish-brown shade. Each capsule contains edible seeds, which are dark brown and oval in shape [1,2]. Sacha inchi cultivation requires a warm climate, with temperatures ranging from 10 to 36 °C, annual rainfall of 850–1000 mm, and well-drained acidic soils, such as sandy or clay loams, at altitudes of 200–1500 m under high light exposure, primarily in moist-to-wet lowland forest environments [3–5]. The flowering of sacha inchi occurs within 3–5 months after planting, while the fruiting process is observed around 8–9 months after the initial planting [6]. Sacha inchi is a climbing plant with diverse applications, requiring a single planting while allowing for multiple harvests per year over a productive period of 15–20 years [4]. This plant is now grown in many places, including Asia (Thailand, China, Vietnam, Indonesia) and Central and South America. It is not only a good source of nutrition but also contributes to economic development [7–9]. Sacha inchi is renowned for its abundance of unsaturated fatty acids, particularly in its seed oil [10].

Sacha inchi oil (SIO) has promising applications in the food, pharmaceutical, and nutraceutical industries due to its valuable components. It is primarily composed of polyunsaturated fatty acids, comprising approximately 85–93% of its total fatty acid content [11]. Linolenic acid (omega-3) and linoleic acid (omega-6) are the predominant fatty acids present within this composition. These essential fatty acids are necessary for human health and can only be acquired through dietary intake. Additionally, oleic acid (omega-9) has been identified as a notable constituent of SIO. Omega-3, omega-6, and omega-9 are present in SIO in proportions of approximately 48%, 33.5%, and 9%, respectively [4]. It is noteworthy that the specific fatty acid composition of sacha inchi seeds can exhibit variation depending on factors such as cultivar, cultivation conditions, and the processing methods employed [2,12,13]. In general, the composition of oilseeds is shaped by the interplay between genetic and environmental factors. Environmental factors, such as temperature, water availability, and the length of the cultivation period, play a crucial role in influencing the composition of fatty acids in seed oil [14,15]. Processing methods, such as pre-extraction roasting, and extraction conditions play a significant role in determining the composition of oils. Research has demonstrated that different extraction techniques yield differences in fatty acid profiles [2].

In addition to having anti-inflammatory, antioxidant, and blood lipid-lowering properties, SIO also has potential as an anti-aging agent. A study by Musquera et al. (2012) [16] tested the anti-aging effects of SIO on cosmetic formulas. In this study, 30 women with signs of skin aging used cosmetic products containing SIO for four weeks. The results showed significant improvements in skin firmness, elasticity, and smoothness after regular use. These findings were supported by clinical and instrumental evaluations conducted using a skin elasticity meter.

Despite its various benefits, SIO contains unsaturated fatty acids, especially omega-3 acids, which have a high susceptibility to oxidation, so SIO was developed into a microencapsulated preparation. This microencapsulation of SIO will inhibit or delay the deterioration of unsaturated fatty acids from environmental factors, such as light, air, or moisture [17]. The unsaturated fatty acid content of oxidized SIO can also give rise to an unpleasant odor and taste. This leads to low acceptability for direct oral consumption. With microencapsulation technology, the unpleasant taste and odor of SIO can be well covered and can be accepted by the public for oral consumption [18].

The microencapsulation process involves enclosing small particles or droplets within a coating or embedding them in a matrix, either homogeneous or heterogeneous, to produce small capsules with advantageous properties. Through this technique, the encapsulated ingredients are fully surrounded by a coating material, thereby enhancing desirable characteristics or eliminating undesirable ones from the original substance [19]. Microencapsulation serves as a strategy to maintain the quality and enhance the physicochemical stability of components that are vulnerable to thermal or photodegradation, such as omega-3 fatty acid [20].

This study focuses on the biological activity, extraction and microencapsulation of SIO, three studies that have been individually researched but rarely explored together. By bridging these fields, this study aims to propose a comprehensive method for improving the efficiency and application of this natural resource.

2. Biological Activity and Recommended Dosing of Sacha Inchi Oil (SIO)

Sacha inchi, or *Plukenetia volubilis*, is a plant native to the Amazon region that is known for its abundance of essential fatty acids, especially omega-3, omega-6, and omega-9, as well as many antioxidants. SIO contains a diverse array of bioactive compounds that play a significant role in enhancing its nutritional value and therapeutic applications [3]. Essential fatty acids dominate the composition of SIO, with α-Linolenic and linoleic acid together contributing up to 82% to its content. Other bioactive components, such as tocopherols, carotenoids, polyphenols, and phytosterols, have also been identified in this oil [12,21–24].

Omega-3 and omega-6 fatty acids play a crucial role in reducing cardiovascular disease risk by lowering LDL cholesterol (omega-6) and triglycerides (omega-3), enhancing vascular health, and managing inflammation. They also contribute to brain development, cognitive health, and offer therapeutic benefits for conditions involving chronic inflammation, oxidative stress, and neurological disorders [12,25]. Omega-9 fatty acids, especially oleic acid, exhibit significant health-promoting properties that aid in wound healing and decrease eye inflammation by regulating inflammatory pathways. They also show potential anti-cancer properties, particularly in breast cancer, by limiting tumor cell growth and migration, though their efficacy varies across cancer types and require further research [26].

Tocopherols support cellular homeostasis, mitigate inflammation through antioxidant activity, and regulate signaling pathways, enzymatic functions, and gene expression [27]. Carotenoids contribute to reducing oxidative stress and minimizing the likelihood of developing chronic diseases, including cardiovascular, neurological, and metabolic disorders, as well as specific cancers [28]. Phytosterols demonstrate a range of health benefits such as lowering cholesterol levels and providing anticancer, anti-inflammatory, and immunomodulatory properties [29]. Similarly, phenolic compounds reduce cancer risk, enhance insulin sensitivity, reduce inflammation, and prevent liver-related and infectious diseases [30]. Table 1 presents the fatty acid content and bioactive compounds in SIO.

Due to its exceptional nutritional content, SIO has many pharmacological activities that are good for human health. Recent studies have shown that this oil has treatment potential for a variety of conditions, including cardiovascular health, anti-inflammatory, antioxidant, antiproliferative, and neuroprotection [7,31]. Table 2 is a summary of the therapeutic applications of SIO.

One of the pharmacological properties of SIO is that it benefits the heart and blood vessels. Clinical studies have shown that SIO contains Omega-3, specifically α-linolenic acid (ALA), which lowers LDL cholesterol and triglyceride levels in the blood [32]. ALA is metabolized in the body into eicosapentaenoic acid (EPA), which is further converted into docosahexaenoic acid (DHA). These omega-3 fatty acids, EPA and DHA, are also recommended for cardiovascular health [33,34]. To determine the levels of fatty acid exposure, especially ALA, after a single administration of SIO, Gonzales et al. analyzed the plasma fatty acid levels in participants who consumed SIO versus sunflower oil. The study involved 18 healthy participants (9 males and 9 females, aged 20–55) consuming 10 or 15 mL of cold-pressed SIO. ALA peaked 4 h after intake, with plasma levels significantly higher in women (2.84 ± 0.36) than in men (0.94 ± 0.57). DHA levels were also elevated in both groups. This effect was not detected in those consuming sunflower oil [34]. In another study, they also found that the consumption of SIO has demonstrated efficacy in preventing dyslipidemia in healthy individuals. It was found that after 16 weeks of consuming 10 or 15 mL of SIO, participants experienced a significant decrease in total cholesterol and LDL cholesterol, along with an increase in HDL cholesterol [35].

In the study by Li et al., the activity of lipid dysmetabolism improvement was measured in obese rats. The findings show that 0.5–1.5 mL/kg SIO consumption for 8 weeks reduces gut microbiota dysbiosis and improves lipid metabolism in rats fed a high-fat diet

(HFD). This process decreases de novo lipogenesis and promotes the β-oxidation of fatty acids, thereby correcting the imbalances in triglyceride (TG), glycerophospholipid, and sphingolipid metabolism. These improvements contribute to a reduction in low-grade inflammation, liver fat accumulation, and hyperlipidemia in mice on a high-fat diet [36]. The randomized controlled trial (RCT) study by Garmendia et al. on hypercholesterolemia patients also reported significant reductions in TC, LDL, non-HDL cholesterol, TGs, VLDL, and non-esterified fatty acids (NEFA). Simultaneously, HDL cholesterol levels rose significantly, achieving a 30% increase from baseline [37].

Table 1. Composition of fatty acids and bioactive compounds in SIO.

Component	Composition	Reference
Fatty acids		
(Palmitic) $C_{16:0}$	3.95 ± 0.21%	[21]
(Palmitoleic) $C_{16:1}$	0.06 ± 0.01%	
(Margaric) $C_{17:0}$	0.09 ± 0.01%	
(Heptadecenoic) $C_{17:1}$	0.05 ± 0.01%	
(Stearic) $C_{18:0}$	3.05 ± 0.15%	
(Oleic) $C_{18:1}$	9.90 ± 0.35%	
(Linoleic) $C_{18:2}$	34.42 ± 0.58%	
(α-Linolenic) C18:3	47.88 ± 0.44%	
(Arachidic) $C_{20:0}$	0.32 ± 0.15%	
(Gadoleic) $C_{20:1}$	0.28 ± 0.15%	
Tocopherols		
γ-tocopherol	1142 ± 4 mg/kg	[22]
δ-tocopherol	715 ± 6.7 mg/kg	
Total tocopherol	1856 mg/kg	
Total carotenoids	1.0 ± 0.0 mg/kg	
Phytosterols		
Campesterol	10.47%	[23]
Stigmasterol	20.27%	
β-Sitosterol	54.44%	
Polyphenols		
Secoiridoids	40.96%	[24]
Flavonoids	14.40%	
Lignans	19.69%	
Isocoumarin	10.56%	
Phenyl alcohols	14.39%	

In addition to their well-documented benefits for cardiovascular health, polyunsaturated fatty acids (PUFAs) have been associated with neuroprotective properties [38,39]. Herrera-Calderon et al., therefore, examined the anticonvulsant activity of SIO against pentylenetetrazole (PTZ)-induced seizures. The experimental design consisted of five groups. Group I (control) received PTZ (80 mg/kg, s.c.), while Group II was given PTZ and diazepam (1 mg/kg, s.c.). Groups III, IV, and V were treated with PTZ along with single oral doses of SIO at 250, 500, and 1000 mg/kg, respectively. The oil was administered 30 min prior to PTZ-induced seizure induction. The study concluded that SIO demonstrated significant anticonvulsant effects at the highest tested doses, with effects closely resembling those of diazepam. The underlying mechanism is likely associated with its ability to reduce free radicals and enhance GABA levels in the brain [40].

SIO also has strong anti-inflammatory properties. The production of inflammatory mediators such as prostaglandins and leukotrienes can be reduced by the polyunsaturated fatty acids contained in this oil. Chronic inflammatory diseases such as arthritis and asthma can be treated with this anti-inflammatory effect. Eicosapentaenoic acid (EPA, ω-3) competes with arachidonic acid (ω-6) for cyclooxygenase and lipoxygenase enzymes, reducing the production of prostaglandin E2 (PGE2), thromboxane A2 (TXA2), and leukotriene B4 (LTB4), which are involved in platelet aggregation, vasoconstriction, inflammation, and leukocyte adhesion [7].

Alayón et al. (2019) conducted a study to investigate the effects of adding SIO on postprandial inflammation and lipid profile due to high-fat intake. Two kinds of breakfasts were given to 20 metabolically healthy (MH) and 22 metabolically unhealthy (MU). The first breakfast was termed high saturated breakfast (HFM), and the second breakfast was HFM+S, which included an additional 15 mL of commercial SIO. The results showed that the addition of SIO induced a reduced postprandial serum total cholesterol (TC) and IL-6 in both groups and completely returned it to baseline in the MH group. However, it showed no significant effect on HDL-C and TG. This result may be due to the limited period of SIO consumption. SIO intake also resulted in a notable decrease in serum IL-6, especially within the MH group. In the MU group, SIO consumption reduced the increase in LPS and weakened the relationship between LPS and TG. This may suggest a potential inhibitory role of PUFAs in limiting LPS entry into circulation [41]. In another study, they also found that SIO consumption improved insulin sensitivity in the group with less favorable metabolic profiles and heightened glycemic responses to fat intake. Furthermore, increased expression of Sirtuin 1 (SIRT-1) was noted in individuals with higher initial triglyceride levels and glycemic responses. SIRT-1 expression in peripheral blood mononuclear cells (PBMC) was linked to enhanced postprandial insulin sensitivity [42].

Ambulay et al. reported in their study that the administration of 2.5 mL of SIO emulsion with different concentrations of ω-3 (0.5 g/day and 0.25 g/day) led to reduced levels of LDL-C, TC, and TG, while simultaneously increasing HDL-C levels. A reduction in malondialdehyde (MDA) and advanced oxidation protein products (AOPPs), along with an increase in catalase activity, was observed, indicating antioxidant effects. Additionally, SIO emulsion reduced inflammation in obese rats, as indicated by the decreased levels of pro-inflammatory cytokines IL-6 and TNF-α [43]. Another study conducted by Suthiphasil et al. demonstrated the anti-inflammatory and antibacterial activities of SIO. The combination of 6 mL of SIO after breakfast, accompanied by a 250 mg erythromycin tablet before meals, four times a day for 8 weeks long, was significant for reducing acne severity and total acne count [44].

SIO also contains tocopherols, phenols, and carotenoids, providing antioxidant properties that aid in preventing oxidation [3,45]. The total tocopherol content in *P. volubilis* L. for the shell and seeds exceeds that of other oilseed crops, such as rye. Recognized as natural antioxidants, tocopherols prevent lipid oxidation by stabilizing hydroperoxyl and free radicals. Besides enhancing oil stability, they are crucial for human health, associated with delayed aging, lower cardiovascular disease risk, and cancer regression in cell cultures [3,46].

As of now, there is limited information regarding the association between sacha inchi or its derivatives and the prevention of neoplasia or tumors [7]. Despite this, Schiessel et al. produced noteworthy findings regarding the effects of a sacha inchi fatty acid supplement, which primarily consists of ALA, in the context of antineoplastic control. This was demonstrated by a reduction in tumor mass and Walker 256 cell proliferation by up to 2.3-fold and 3-fold, respectively, in a murine model of breast cancer. These findings align with data obtained for a fish oil diet and are accompanied by decreases of 65%, 62,5%, and 50% in plasma concentrations of TNF-α, IL-6, and triacylglycerides [47]. Centurion-Rodriguez et al. assessed the potential protective effects of SIO on colon cancer (CC) induced with 1,2-dimethylhydrazine (DMH) in Holtzman rats. The study was conducted by randomly assigning the rats into four groups: a positive control group receiving DMH (C1), a negative control group treated with SIO at 150 μL/kg/day (C2), and two experimental groups treated with both DMH and SIO at 150 μL/kg/day (E1) or 300 μL/kg/day (E2). DMH was administered for 8 weeks, with the total duration of induction lasting 22 weeks. The preventive effect was assessed by comparing the proportion of rats without lesions in the DMH-exposed groups. In this study, a 12.5% higher proportion of rats in the E1 group were protected from tumor induction, showing no injury, compared to the control group. Despite this, no statistically significant differences were observed, preventing a definitive link between SIO consumption and the prevention of neoplastic lesion formation [48].

Table 2. SIO therapeutic Applications.

Activity	SI Preparation	Dose	Experimental Models	Results	Reference
Antidyslipidemic	SIO suspension	5 or 10 mL for 4 months	Hypercholesterolemia patients aged 35–75	Significantly reduced the concentrations of TC, LDL, non-HDL cholesterol, triglycerides, VLDL, and NEFA. In contrast, HDL cholesterol levels rose significantly, reaching 30% above the initial measurement.	[37]
Antidyslipidemic	SIO	10 or 15 mL	18 healthy volunteers (9 males and 9 females) aged 20–55 years	Significant increase in plasma ALA 4 h after intake, (2.84 ± 0.36) mg/mL in women and (0.94 ± 0.57) mg/mL in men. As well as increase in DHA, (2.60 ± 0.84) mg/mL in women and (1.00 ± 0.38) mg/mL in men.	[34]
Antidyslipidemic	SIO	10 or 15 mL for 16 weeks	Non-vegetarian men and women aged 25–55 years, BMI ranging from 20 to 35 kg/m^2, no history of hyperlipidemia or conditions that could influence lipid metabolism, not taking fatty acid, lipid, antioxidant supplements or medications; 18 healthy volunteers (9 males and 9 females) aged 20–55 years	At month-4, serum HDL-C increased, serum TC and LDL-C decreased, and arterial blood pressures reduced	[35]

Table 2. *Cont.*

Activity	SI Preparation	Dose	Experimental Models	Results	Reference
Antiproliferative and antitumoral	SIO	1 g/kg for 4 weeks	Walker 256 tumor-bearing rats	Reduced tumor mass and proliferation of Walker 256 tumor cells ex vivo, increased lipoperoxidation in the tumor tissues, and reduced plasma levels of glycemia, triglycerides, and inflammatory cytokines	[47]
Antidyslipidemic and antioxidant	SIO	10% of the whole diet for 21 days	Male Wistar rats	Reduced ω-6/ω-3 LCPUFAs from (9.24 ± 0.6) to (0.29 ± 0.03) g per 100 g of fatty acid methyl esters (FAME), and reduced expression and activity of Δ-5 and Δ-6 desaturases	[49]
Antiproliferative	SIO	150 and 300 µL/kg/day	Holtzman male albino rats	Cancerous lesions were present in two samples from group C_1 (exposed to only DMH), one sample from group E_1 (exposed to DMH with SIO 150 µL/kg/day), and two samples from group E_2 (exposed to DMH with SIO 300 µL/kg/day). Group C_2 (exposed to SIO 150 µL/kg/day) showed no intestinal lesions. The proportions of specimens without injury were 75% for group C_1, 87.5% for group E_1, and 75% for group E_2, with no significant differences observed.	[48]
Antibacterial and anti-inflammation	SIO	6 mL for 8 weeks	32 volunteers with acne global severity 1–4	The combination of SIO extraction and oral erythromycin significantly reduced acne severity and total acne lesions	[44]

Table 2. *Cont.*

Activity	SI Preparation	Dose	Experimental Models	Results	Reference
Antidyslipidemic and antihyper-glycemic	SIO	15 mL	42 men aged 29–64, non-smokers, engaged in little physical activity	Increased insulin sensitivity, reduced postprandial hyperglycemia, and increased expression of SIRT-1 were noted in individuals with higher initial triglyceride levels and glycemic responses	[42]
Antidyslipidemic and anti-inflammation	SIO	15 mL	20 metabolically healthy (MH) and 22 metabolically unhealthy (MU) individuals given a high-fat meal	Reduced postprandial TC and IL-6 in both groups and the reverse in the MH group, no effect on HDL-C and TAG, and reduced LPS along with a suppression of the correlation between LPS and TAG in the MU group.	[41]
Antidyslipidemic	SIO	0.5–1.5 mL/kg for 8 weeks	High-fat diet (HFD)-fed rats	Reduced TC, TG, and LDL-C restored gut microbiota balance and enhanced bile acid profiles.	[36]
Neuroprotective	SIO	250, 500, 1000 mg/kg	Male Balb/C albino mice	The administration of SIO at its highest tested dose of 1000 mg/kg in the experimental group yielded better outcomes against PTZ-induced seizures, including decreased severity, reduced frequency, and shorter duration.	[40]
Antidyslipidemic, antioxidant and anti-inflammation	SIO emulsion	2.5 mL with different ω-3 contents (0.5 g/day and 0.25 g/day) for 8 weeks	Obese rats	Reduced LDL-C, TC, and TGs and increased HDL-C. Reduced MDA and AOPP and increased catalase activity. Reduced levels of IL-6 and TNF-α.	[43]
Anti-inflammation	SIO	2 × 530 mg softgel	Non-vegetarian adults aged 30 or older, with a BMI ranging from >20 to <35 kg/m^2	Reduced the Systolic Blood Pressure (SBP) of the participants.	[50]

Table 2. *Cont.*

Activity	SI Preparation	Dose	Experimental Models	Results	Reference
Anti-aging	SIO	Applied twice daily on the face and forearm area, with gentle massage until fully absorbed.	Thirty women aged between 26 and 65 years old with a certain degree of photo-aging were selected.	A 28-day treatment with TM001, TM003 and TM004 creams improved the condition of the volunteers' facial skin. According to clinical evaluation, the creams improved the brightness and smoothness of the volunteers' facial skin, while instrumental evaluation showed an increase in skin firmness and elasticity.	[16]
Anti-aging	SIO	30 and 15 mg/mL	Normal human fibroblasts (NHFs)	Sacha inchi was proven to be a promising plant for nutraceutical products, being rich in α-linolenic and linoleic acids, fatty acids that have health benefits.	[51]
Moiturizing	SIO	Applied on the left or right lower leg of the subjects for 14 days followed by application discontinuation for 2 days.	Skin tissues from surgery to remove excess skin from females in the age range of 50–65 years old were collected using 6 mm, full-thickness punch biopsies.	The oil was mild to the skin and had a beneficial effect on dry skin. Its moisturizing effect was comparable to that of olive oil.	[52]

Its important fatty acid content, especially omega-3, omega-6, and omega-9, which have antidyslipidemic and anti-inflammatory functions, makes SIO very popular. SIO contains alpha-linolenic acid (ALA), which functions as an antidyslipidemic, lowering blood levels of triglycerides and LDL cholesterol while also increasing HDL cholesterol levels. Both of these actions benefit heart health [34,35]. The ability of unsaturated fatty acids to stop the production of inflammatory mediators such as prostaglandins and leukotrienes is the reason for the anti-inflammatory properties of this oil [7]. The natural antioxidant content in SIO enhances this anti-inflammatory effect. This content protects body tissues from oxidative damage and oxidative stress, which aggravate inflammation [53].

As it is known that SIO is rich in omega-3, omega-6, and omega-9 fatty acids, SIO offers an optimal fatty acid profile for heart and brain health, making it suitable as a base for various food preparations. The distinctive texture and flavor of SIO make it suitable for use as a substitute for regular cooking oil, or as an addition to salad dressings and stir fry dishes, just like olive oil. SIO products have been sold widely and one that has been circulating in the Indonesian market is Svarga, from the collaboration between Quilla and the Faculty of Pharmacy, Padjadjaran University. However, people still rarely hear about this product and the great benefits of SIO. Therefore, more promotion is needed to increase interest in SIO products.

SIO is also still difficult to commercialize, not only as a food ingredient but also in other applications such as microencapsulation or even in cosmetics and pharmaceuticals. Some of the barriers to commercialization of SIO products include the following:

- Production Cost: The high production cost of SIO is due to the need for specialized equipment and advanced technology for the extraction and microencapsulation processes, as well as fluctuations in raw material prices.
- Production Limitations: The limited supply of sacha inchi seeds from certain regions and lack of large-scale production infrastructure are major constraints in meeting global market demand.
- Consumer Awareness: The lack of consumer awareness of the unique benefits of SIO over other vegetable oils, such as olive oil, necessitates more intensive promotional and educational efforts.
- Health and Safety Issues: The potential allergenicity and anti-nutritional compounds in SIO require special attention in the processing process to ensure product safety.
- Market Competition: Intense competition in the edible oil market, with the dominance of products such as olive oil and coconut oil, makes the penetration of SIO a challenge.

3. Extraction of Sacha Inchi Oil

The quality and bioactivity of SIO are determined by both upstream and downstream phases of production. In the upstream phase, the cultivation of sacha inchi plants is influenced by environmental and agricultural factors such as soil conditions, weather, and farming practices, all of which affect seed composition and oil yield [5,14]. Post-harvest operations, including drying and storage, also play a pivotal role in preventing oxidative deterioration and ensuring raw material quality [54,55].

Following these initial steps, downstream processes focus on the extraction and refinement of oil. A range of techniques have been explored for the extraction of natural oils, with variable yields depending on the specific method utilized [56]. Common techniques for extracting oil from plant seeds include traditional methods such as mechanical pressing, cold pressing, Soxhlet extraction, and shaking extraction (SE), as well as eco-friendly approaches like ultrasound-assisted extraction (UAE), microwave-assisted extraction (MAE), subcritical extraction (SubE), and supercritical fluid extraction [57]. SIO can be obtained from the sacha inchi seeds through several extraction techniques, such as cold pressing, conventional solvent extraction with polar and non-polar solvents, and enzymatic extraction [13]. The choice of extraction method has a significant impact on both the yield and the composition of bioactive compounds in SIO. Due to the oil's rich content of valuable compounds and its numerous health benefits, many studies have concentrated on enhancing oil yield by exploring various extraction techniques [56,58]. Understanding the optimal extraction techniques is crucial for maximizing the benefits of SIO in industrial applications. A comparative analysis of the SIO yield produced by different extraction techniques is shown in Table 3.

The conventional production of SIO comprises a sequence of steps, beginning with the selection of sacha inchi seeds, followed by dehulling, cleaning, pressing, filtration, and final bottling. Dehulling is an advisable step in the processing of oilseeds [59,60]. A study by Gutiérrez et al. revealed that the oil extraction yield from whole sacha inchi seeds was substantially lower than that from dehulled seeds, likely due to the low lipid content of the seed shell, which accounts for approximately 35% of the total seed weight [61].

Among the different extraction methods, mechanical extraction stands out for its ease of setup, low investment and operational costs, lack of toxic solvents, and its effectiveness in achieving high oil yields [58,62]. Mechanical oil extraction employs either hydraulic presses or motor-driven screw presses [63]. The process involves placing the seeds between barriers, where compression reduces the space around the seeds, forcing the oil to be released [64,65]. Cold press extraction is a mechanical technique that is more energy-efficient than many other oil extraction methods and is environmentally sustainable. It is widely utilized for extracting oil from various sources, particularly oilseeds, and is considered eco-friendly as it does not involve the use of solvents. Furthermore, cold pressing avoids the use of heat or chemical processes to maintain the seeds' nutritional value [66,67]. However, pressing methods have a relatively low extraction efficiency, leaving a significant amount of oil in the press cake, which is subsequently extracted using solvents like hexane [68].

Garcia et al. employed the cold pressing method using a filter press with 75 rpm and 240 Watt of power. The dehulled seeds were individually fed into the press, with an approximate interval of 5 s between each seed, then filtered before storage. The duration of the pressing and filtering process is approximately one hour, during which 120 mL of oil is directly obtained [67]. Gutiérrez et al. employed a similar method, where dehulled and whole sacha inchi seeds (1 kg each) were placed in separate filtration sleeves and pressed twice at 200 bar using a 15.24 cm diameter piston cylinder press. The pressing temperature remained below 30 °C throughout the process. The extraction yield from dehulled seeds was significantly higher (40.15 ± 2.50% w/w) than that from whole seeds (27.20 ± 1.90% w/w) [61].

To compare oil yield between different roasting temperatures, Cisneros et al. conducted a study by employing the pressing method to extract SIO. The kernels were roasted using a commercial gas-fired roaster, with each batch being approximately 4.5 kg. Three roasting conditions were tested: lightly roasted (75–81 °C for 9 min), medium roasted (83–86 °C for 10 min), and highly roasted (99–102 °C for 10 min). After roasting, the kernels were cooled using the roaster's integrated fan. The unroasted sample and the three roasted variants were pressed with a temperature of 100–110 °C. The yield of non-clarified oil exhibited a progressive increase with higher roasting temperatures, achieving weights of approximately 42%, 49%, and 65% for lightly, medium, and highly roasted samples, respectively [55].

One of the approaches used in cold-pressed oil production is extraction via mechanical screw presses. Screw pressing offers several advantages, such as yielding high-quality oil with bioactive compounds, the potential use of the residual cake, and lower initial investment and operational expenses [69]. Muangrat et al. conducted research to assess the effects of operational parameters, including drying temperature (60, 75, 90 °C) and press head temperature (60, 75, 90 °C), on SIO extraction by utilizing a single screw press machine. The combined conditions of a feeding rate of 1.5 kg/h, a drying temperature of 90 °C, and a press head temperature of 90 °C resulted in a maximum extraction yield of 40.63% of SIO [62]. Mai et al. also employed screw pressing to obtain SIO. The extraction conditions were not directly reported, but the procedure yielded 47.5% oil [45]. This result is not significantly different from the oil yield achieved through screw pressing, as documented by Muangrat et al.

Hydraulic pressing is another mechanical extraction method that provides oil yields comparable to screw press extraction and higher quality oil than solvent extraction. However, it produces a lower oil yield than solvent extraction [58,70]. In hydraulic presses, pressure is generated by hydraulic equipment, which utilizes higher pressure than screw presses and can be operated either manually or with power [65]. A study by Chasquibol et al. reported the use of hydraulic pressing of *P. huayllabambana* L. seeds to obtain SIO. The procedure was conducted by applying pressure to the seeds using a piston driven by a hydraulic system, assisted by a 1-horsepower (HP) motor. Compared to *P. volubilis*, which is the most commonly used cultivar for oil extraction and commercialization, *P. huayllabambana* is nearly twice as large and heavy, yielding an oil content of 30.3 to 41.25% after pressing and filtration of the shelled seeds [71].

Kong et al. reported a study to determine the impact of pressure and pressing time on SIO yields [58]. A hydraulic cold-press extraction of the dehulled seeds was carried out at a fixed temperature of 25 ± 1 °C, with pressures ranging from 30 to 50 MPa and pressing times varying from 10 to 30 min. The study revealed that both pressure and pressing time significantly affected the yields of SIO, with the optimal oil recovery of 86.31% achieved at 50 MPa over 30 min. The oil yield obtained in this study was similar to the findings of Muangrat et al. regarding screw press extraction and Chasquibol et al. concerning hydraulic pressing [58]. Hidalgo et al. also implemented mechanical extraction through the use of extrusion. The extraction, carried out at room temperature with 1000 g of sacha inchi seeds, produced 26.92% oil. This yield was considered low, likely due to the absence of elevated temperatures during extraction [72].

Another method for extracting vegetable oils near room temperature is supercritical fluid extraction (SFE), often referred to as supercritical carbon dioxide extraction. SFE extracts substances from a matrix using supercritical fluids. A substance is classified as a supercritical fluid when it is held at pressures and temperatures beyond its critical points. These fluids exhibit molecular permeability and viscosity similar to gases, allowing for easy flow. Additionally, their low surface tension enhances mass transfer by increasing the contact area between phases during separation processes [73,74]. The use of low-to-moderate temperatures helps prevent unwanted reactions and product degradation. A primary advantage of this method is its suitability for extracting heat-sensitive compounds without the use of toxic solvents [13,64]. However, SFE could be considered too costly due to its high investment costs [75]. Additionally, SFE requires the careful optimization of various process parameters, such as temperature, pressure, flow rate, and solvent type, to achieve optimal extraction yields and product quality. This optimization process can be both time-consuming and resource-intensive [76]. Subtle changes in temperature and pressure can significantly impact the extraction yield and selectivity. Therefore, the precise control of these parameters is essential to maintain consistent product quality [77].

In their study, Zanqui et al. selected n-propane as the solvent for SFE due to its faster performance compared to CO_2, attributed to its higher lipid solubility. The solvent n-propane was pressurized using a syringe pump, with temperature regulated by a thermostatic bath set at 10 °C. A flow of 1 mL/min was maintained for 1 h, regulated by an expansion valve at 80 °C. Temperature and pressure variations were also applied. The combination of a temperature of 60 °C and a pressure of 12 MPa resulted in the highest oil yield of 29.7 ± 0.5% [53].

Triana-Maldonado et al. (2017) also obtained SIO through SFE, employing CO_2 as solvent. The extraction process involved a 200 g sample placed in a 1 L tank, operated at a temperature of 60 °C, with pressures between 400 and 500 bar, a CO_2 flow rate varying from 40 to 80 g/min, and an extraction time between 120 and 180 min. The optimal oil extraction yield of 23.48 g of oil/100 g of samples was attained at a temperature of 60 °C, a pressure of 500 bar, a CO_2 flow rate of 40 g/min, and an extraction duration of 180 min [78].

A similar approach was employed by Jitpinit et al. The extraction of SIO was carried out in a 100 mL extraction vessel. CO_2 from an external cylinder was pressurized and liquefied using a high-pressure pump and a coolant bath attached to the pump head. The CO_2 was then heated in a CO_2 heater to reach supercritical conditions before entering the vessel, where 70 g of ground seed kernels was loaded. To evaluate the impact of temperature and pressure on the extraction of SIO using supercritical CO_2, the process was carried out at temperatures of 40, 50, and 60 °C, and pressures of 300 and 400 bar. The CO_2 flow rate remained constant at 1.5 L/min, with extraction continuing for up to 6 h. A maximum oil yield of 38.1% was achieved during supercritical CO_2 extraction conducted at 400 bar and 60 °C, and optimum extraction time of 3 h [13].

Another extraction method that might be preferred is the solvent extraction method due to its cost-effectiveness and ease of use. This method relies on the solvent's capacity to dissolve and extract oils from seeds. Thus, the solvent must effectively solubilize the oil to ensure efficient extraction. The primary drawbacks of solvent extraction are associated with the use of organic solvents, which can contribute to environmental pollution and pose health risks [79]. Moreover, residual solvent can negatively impact the quality, safety, and flavor of the final product. However, the complete elimination of solvent from the extracted oil can be difficult to achieve [80]. The solvent extraction process comprises three primary stages: cleaning and conditioning of the oilseeds, the extraction of oil, and the separation of the miscella [64]. Bueno-Borges et al. reported a study that utilized solvent extraction to obtain SIO. Around 5 g of ground seeds was placed in stoppered Erlenmeyer flasks and extracted with 30 mL of n-hexane under agitation for 4 h at room temperature. The mixture was then filtered and concentrated via a rotary evaporator at 30 °C, yielding around 1.9 g of oil [81]. Cordero-Clavijo et al. adopted a similar approach, which is extracting SIO by the solvent extraction method. In summary, SI seeds were ground and mixed with n-hexane at a 1:2 weight-to-volume ratio in amber glass bottles. The solution was incubated at 150 rpm and 30 °C for one hour. After a 30 min settling period, the supernatant (n-hexane and SIO) was filtered using Büchner funnels with Whatman No. 1 filter paper. The n-hexane was then removed from the SIO through rotary evaporation under vacuum at 50 °C, resulting in 97.22 ± 0.12% of oil [82].

The use of aqueous enzymatic extraction as an eco-friendly oil extraction method has become increasingly popular. Enzymes hydrolyze cell wall components, promoting the release of oil which can be effortlessly separated from the water phase, thereby making purification easier [83–85]. Nevertheless, aqueous enzymatic extraction has certain drawbacks, such as extended processing times, the potential for hydrolysis and oxidation of compounds, relatively high costs associated with enzymes or enzyme preparations, and the need for rapid processing of the unstable aqueous phase [86]. A study reported by Nguyen et al. demonstrated the extraction of SIO with aqueous enzymatic extraction. For this process, 2 g of seed powder was incubated with 1% (w/w) of various enzymes (chamzyme FP, flavourzyme, protamex, bromelain, papain, cellulase A, or a 1:1 blend of papain and cellulase A) in 10 mL of water at 40 °C for 4 h with stirring (6000 rpm). The mixtures were then centrifuged at 4000× g for 30 min, and the oil was collected, dried with anhydrous sodium sulfate, and heated at 105 °C for 3 h. Papain showed the highest efficacy for oil extraction, yielding 24.67% oil, outperforming the other enzymes tested [85].

Table 3. Different extraction methods for SIO.

Source	Extraction Method	Extraction Solvent	Extraction Conditions	Yield	Reference
P. huayllabambana seeds	Hydraulic cold pressing	-	Hydraulic piston with a 1 HP motor	30.3–41.25% of oil quantity	[71]
P. volubilis seeds	Pressing	-	Press temperature of 100–110 °C	65% of oil quantity	[55]
P. volubilis seeds	Supercritical fluid extraction (SFE)	n-propane	Temperature of 60 °C, pressure of 12 MPa, n-propane flow duration of 60 min, and extraction duration of 1 h	29.7 ± 0.5% of oil quantity	[53]

Table 3. *Cont.*

Source	Extraction Method	Extraction Solvent	Extraction Conditions	Yield	Reference
P. volubilis seeds	Supercritical fluid extraction (SFE)	Carbon dioxide	Temperature of 60 °C, pressure of 500 bar, CO_2 flow rate of 40 g/min, and extraction duration of 180 min	23.48 g/100 g of samples	[78]
P. volubilis seeds	Screw pressing	-	Feeding rate of 1.5 kg/h, drying temperature of 90 °C, and press head temperature of 90 °C	40.63% of oil quantity	[62]
P. volubilis seeds	Solvent extraction	n-hexane	Temperature of 25 °C, extraction duration for 4 h and solvent volume of 30 mL	1.9 g of oil	[81]
P. volubilis seeds	Extrusion method	-	Temperature of 25 °C	26.92% of oil quantity	[72]
P. volubilis seeds	Cold pressing	-	Filter press with 75 rpm and 240 W of power	17.46% (120 mL) of oil quantity	[67]
P. volubilis seeds	Cold pressing	-	Piston cylinder press with pressure of 200 bar and temperature kept below 30 °C	40.15 ± 2.50% of oil quantity	[61]
P. volubilis seeds	Screw pressing	-	-	47.5% of oil quantity	[45]
P. volubilis seeds	Aqueous enzymatic extraction	Water	Mixture of seed powder with 1% *w*/*w* enzyme, 10 mL of solvent, temperature of 40 °C, extraction duration of 4 h, and stirring speed of 600 rpm	24.67% of oil quantity	[85]
P. volubilis seeds	Supercritical fluid extraction (SFE)	Carbon dioxide	Temperature of 60 °C, pressure of 400 bar, extraction duration of 3 h, and CO_2 flow rate of 1.5 L/min	38.1% of oil quantity	[13]
P. volubilis seeds	Cold pressing	-	-	200 mL of oil	[14]
P. volubilis seeds	Hydraulic cold pressing	-	Temperature of 25 ± 1 °C, pressure of 50 MPa, extraction duration of 30 min	86.31% of oil quantity	[58]
P. volubilis seeds	Cold pressing	-	-	50% (1000 mL) of oil quantity	[87]
P. volubilis seeds	Solvent extraction	n-hexane	1 to 2 ratio of solids to solvent, stirring speed of 150 rpm, temperature of 30 °C, and extraction duration of 1 h	97.22 ± 0.12% of oil quantity	[82]
P. volubilis seeds	Supercritical fluid extraction (SFE)	CO_2 and aqueous ethanol as cosolvent	Pressure of 400 bar, temperature of 60 °C, CO_2 flow rate 10 g/min, extraction duration of 1 h	99.07 ± 0.03% of oil quantity	

Based on the table above, it can be presumed that supercritical CO_2 extraction is a promising alternative for extracting SIO from P. volubilis seeds. This method enables the extraction of heat-sensitive compounds without the use of toxic solvents with faster extraction processes, excellent selectivity (resulting in high-quality extracts), and enhanced extraction yields. Furthermore, this method avoids the use of harmful solvents, preventing the formation of toxic byproducts and ensuring that the final food product is free from chemical residues [88,89].

4. Microencapsulation of Sacha Inchi Oil

Following extraction, microencapsulation techniques are utilized to augment the stability and bioavailability of SIO. These encapsulation methods safeguard the oil from oxidative degradation and enable its integration into diverse delivery systems [90]. Recent trends in the food sector show a significant increase in consumer preference for products categorized as healthy and natural [91]. This reflects people's growing awareness of the importance of a nutritious and sustainable diet for long-term health. In response to this change in consumer behavior, research into new methods for incorporating nutritional supplements and bioactive compounds into people's daily diets is gaining momentum. This research aims to create innovations in food formulations that not only fulfill nutritional needs but also enhance overall health benefits, thereby assisting consumers in achieving a healthier and more balanced lifestyle.

Essential oils, antioxidants, polyphenols, minerals, vitamins, and other bioactive compounds are examples of a wide variety of bioactive compounds with very diverse chemical properties. Beyond the basic nutrients commonly found in foods, these compounds have great potential to provide significant health benefits. They have anti-inflammatory activity that can help reduce chronic inflammation, anti-diabetic activity that can help regulate blood glucose levels, anti-cancer activity that can help fight cancer cell growth, anti-viral activity that can fight viral infections, and anti-tumor activity that can help treat malignant tumors [92]. However, these bioactive compounds must be protected to maintain their biological properties during storage and further incorporation into food formulations as they are susceptible to external stimuli such as light, oxygen, and temperature.

As is known, microencapsulation is an excellent technology to modify preparations containing bioactive compounds, especially fatty acid content. Microencapsulation is also one option to improve the bioavailability and stability of SIO, which is rich in omega-3 and omega-6 fatty acids that have many health benefits, such as improving heart health, reducing inflammation, and supporting brain function. However, the high content of unsaturated fatty acids makes this oil highly susceptible to oxidation, which in turn can reduce its quality, stability, and health benefits. Microencapsulation is therefore an excellent way to protect SIO from oxidation due to exposure to oxygen, heat, and light. It also increases its shelf life and stability. Microencapsulation encapsulates the oil with a protective coating such as maltodextrin or gum arabic. This preserves the bioactive properties of the oil during storage and allows the body to control its release when consumed [18]. Studies show that this method effectively reduces the peroxide value and TBARS (thiobarbituric acid reactivated substance) which are key indicators of lipid oxidation. In addition, this method removes the unpleasant taste and odor from the oil, making it easier to consume orally [20]. The process involves encasing the oil in a protective coating, which results in microcapsules that protect the vulnerable parts against heat, light, and oxygen. When used in food, medicine, or cosmetics, this method improves delivery and maintains the functional properties of the oil during storage [93].

One of the most commonly used microencapsulation techniques for oils, including SIO, is spray drying. In this method, an oil-in-water emulsion is created by mixing the oil with a wall material such as a protein, carbohydrate, or gum, such as maltodextrin, whey protein, or gum arabic. The emulsion is then atomized into fine droplets and dried quickly using hot air, resulting in microcapsules with a stable matrix. Spray drying has been shown to effectively improve the stability of SIO, reduce oxidation and extend shelf life, while maintaining the beneficial fatty acid profile [17].

Emulsions are highly susceptible to the negative impact of external stimuli, this can lead to fatty acid oxidation and during storage, thus limiting their application in the food industry [94]. Thus, the microencapsulation of emulsions via the spray-drying method has emerged as a promising strategy to extend product shelf life [95]. However, researchers have optimized the use of stabilizers and wall materials in this formulation, improving the stability of the emulsion during the spray drying process. This is because the stabilizers in the interfacial layer of the emulsion can be disrupted during the spray-drying process, leading to unstable emulsions and demulsification under high temperatures [32].

Spray-dried microencapsulation methods generally use protective materials such as maltodextrin, gum arabic, and OSA starch to protect the SIO emulsion. The spray-drying process using the B-290 apparatus involves the optimization of parameters such as inlet and outlet temperatures and flow rate. Temperature variation allows customization of the process for different types of samples. Inlet temperatures of 140–150 °C and outlet temperatures of 70–90 °C are used for the rapid evaporation of water and maintaining the stability of sensitive samples [90,96]. The flow rate of the feed solution and air significantly affects the atomization and drying process, thus having a direct impact on the size and particle size distribution of the final product [17,97].

Coacervation is a microencapsulation technique that involves forming a thin film around oil droplets using biopolymers such as gelatin or alginate. This method is preferred over spray drying for several reasons:

- High encapsulation efficiency: almost all oils can be encapsulated well.
- Better protection: heat-sensitive materials such as SIO are better protected.
- More uniform particle size: the resulting capsules tend to be larger and more uniform.
- Controlled release: the content in the capsule can be released slowly [98–100].

However, coacervation also has a more complex process. Ingredients such as tannic acid, pectin, and ovalbumin are often used as additional coacervation agents. Calcium chloride ($CaCl_2$) plays an important role as a cross-linker to form a stable microcapsule structure [101–103].

Freeze drying is a microencapsulation technique that freezes the material first before removing the water directly, resulting in stable microcapsules. This method is particularly suitable for sensitive ingredients such as probiotics as it preserves their original physical and nutritional properties. In addition, the use of binders such as maltodextrin can increase the strength and protection of the microcapsules [18,104].

Each microencapsulation method has unique challenges. Spray drying can cause nutrient degradation in SIO due to high temperature-induced oxidation, as well as producing less uniform particles due to the high viscosity of the oil. Freeze drying requires a large capital investment for equipment and energy, as well as a long process time, making it less economically efficient. Coacervation has high process complexity due to sensitivity to various variables, and often results in lower encapsulation efficiency for oils with physicochemical properties such as sacha inchi.

In the food industry, spray drying, as it is known, is the most common method for drying microcapsules; freeze-drying is also frequently used. However, the two different types of drying are used to process the product. Each method results in variations in microstructure and particle size because it is performed at different temperatures and times. Freeze drying, on the other hand, is ideal for drying thermosensitive compounds because it is processed continuously at low temperatures. In the study by Suwannasang et al. in 2022, the authors used zein as a wall material for microencapsulation [105].

The oxidative stability of SIO was improved after being modified in the form of microencapsulation by various methods such as spray drying, freeze drying, and coacervation. Specifically, these microcapsules exhibit lower moisture content, water activity, hygroscopicity, and shorter sol time. Thus, a longer shelf life stored under controlled conditions with lower oxidation levels of the oil is expected. This was confirmed by the NMR results conducted by the researcher. Studies have shown that microencapsulation significantly improves the oxidative stability of SIO as shown in Table 4. Studies using encapsulation techniques such as spray drying and coacervation reported decreased peroxide and TBARS (thiobarbituric acid reactive substances) values, indicators of lipid oxidation, compared to non-encapsulated oils. This demonstrates the efficacy of this method in protecting the polyunsaturated fatty acids of SIO, thus making it more suitable for various applications that require long-term stability.

Table 4. Different microencapsulation methods for SIO.

Microencapsulation Method	Coating Materials	Microencapsulation Conditions	Oxidative Stability	Reference
Coacervation	Ovalbumin and sodium alginate	OVA and SIO solutions were mixed in an oil-in-water (O/W) emulsion, then homogenized with AL solution. The emulsion was set at pH 3.8, cooled to 10 °C for complex coacervation, and centrifuged. The microcapsules formed were cross-linked with $CaCl_2$ solution, then dried using lyophilization after freezing at −40 °C.	This method improved the thermal resistance of the isolated bio-polymers (OVA and AL). This was confirmed by DSC and encapsulation by complex coacervation. The oxidative state of SIO was not affected by this method (as confirmed by 1H NMR).	[98]
Freeze-dried	Ovalbumin, XG, and PEC	Emulsions were prepared with varying concentrations of Ova, XG, or Pec, homogenized with UltraTurrax at 18,000 rpm, sonicated for 12 min, and freeze-dried to form microencapsulated products.	Freeze-drying and emulsion systems protect the omega-3 s without damaging the contents, as evidenced by NMR analysis for 180 min. Omega-3 is protected in SIO-Ova-Pec and SIO-Ova-XG microcapsules.	[20]
Spray-dried	Maltodextrin and Sodium caseinate	Microencapsulation was carried out by the spray-drying method using a Mini Spray B-290 at an inlet temperature of 150–170 °C and outlet temperature of 120–130 °C, with a 90% suction rate and 10% pumping rate; then, the microcapsules were stored in a dryer for further characterization.	In particular, these microcapsules exhibit lower moisture levels, water activity, and hygroscopicity, and shorter sol time. Thus, a longer shelf life stored under controlled conditions with lower oil oxidation levels is expected.	[90]
Spray-dried	Gum arabic	A solution with GA and distilled water containing camu camu and mango peel extracts was mixed with SIO (18% total solids) and homogenized. The emulsion was dried using a spray dryer at 140 °C and 70 °C with a flow rate of 55 mL/min, and the dried powder was stored in airtight bags at −5 °C for analysis.	Oxidative stabilization of microcapsules: natural (188–198 °C) vs. commercial (174 °C) antioxidants for inchi sacha oil.	[17]

Table 4. *Cont.*

Microencapsulation Method	Coating Materials	Microencapsulation Conditions	Oxidative Stability	Reference
Coacervation	Ovalbumin, PEC, and tannic acid	The microencapsulation process was carried out through these main steps: O/W primary emulsion with SIO and OVA-TA, followed by complex coacervation with PEC solution at pH 3.5, slow cooling, centrifugation, and drying by lyophilization.	There were no oxidatively decayed SIO products seen during the microencapsulation procedure.	[106]
Spray-dried	Gum arabic and maltodextrin	The microencapsulation method was performed by mixing gum arabic, maltodextrin, and whey protein isolate as encapsulation materials together with SIPHO oil, then homogenized at 9000 rpm for 10 min. After that, the emulsion was dried using a spray dryer, and the resulting powder was stored for further analysis at 5 °C.	Better oxidative stability and shelf life than microcapsules with BHT at 200 ppm.	[107]
Freeze-dried	Zein and maltodextrin	The emulsion was prepared through the liquid–liquid dispersion process, zein stock solution was prepared by dissolving zein in aqueous ethanol, and surfactant stock solution was prepared with Tween 80 and lecithin in pH adjusted deionized water. The mixture of surfactant solution, zein solution, and SO was homogenized at low temperature; then, ethanol was evaporated before the samples were frozen and dried to produce FDSOM powders.	The oxidative stability of microencapsulated SO in freeze-dried powders is anticipated to last longer than 15 days because yogurt is kept in a refrigerator.	[18]
Spray-dried	OSA starch and maltodextrin	Microencapsulation was carried out by preparing emulsions of hydrated starch MD and OSA, then mixing with SO and homogenizing. The emulsion was dried using a spray dryer at 150 °C (inlet) and 90 °C (outlet), with a feed rate of 0.8 L/h and an air flow of 35 L/min.	The oxidative stability of microencapsulated SO in spray-dried powders is anticipated to last longer than 15 days because yogurt is kept in a refrigerator.	[18]
Spray-dried	Gum arabic	Microcapsules were prepared from a mixture of phenolic camu camu and/or mango peel extracts with gum arabic and sacha inchi *P. huayllabambana* oil. Emulsions were made using distilled water containing camu camu and mango peel extracts. The drying process was carried out with inlet and outlet air temperatures of 140 °C and 70 °C, respectively, and an optimal flow rate of 55 mL/min.	The microcapsulated antioxidants camu-camu peel and mango peel proved to be better at protecting against oxidation than the synthetic antioxidant BHT.	[108]

Table 4. *Cont.*

Microencapsulation Method	Coating Materials	Microencapsulation Conditions	Oxidative Stability	Reference
Spray-dried	Gum arabic, maltodextrin, whey protein isolate, Hi-cap, Capsul Tapioca starch	Coating material solutions were prepared with MD, Capsul TA, Hi-cap, AG, and WPI according to specifications. Emulsions were made with a homogenizer at low temperature before being dried using a spray dryer at 150–80 °C with a certain flow rate. The resultant dried powder was stored at low temperature for subsequent analysis.	The encapsulation process transformed the oil with a loss of 6.2% of the 3-Ln major fatty acids. SIHO with ternary coating materials (AG + MD + WPI) resulted in a 3% loss, while SIVO with Capsul TA as wall material only 0.2–0.9 mgg 1 oil for TG-P. The largest losses were tocopherols (30–15% for SIHO and surface, 28–24% for SIVO).	[21]
Spray-dried	Gum arabic and maltodextrin	AG and MD were used as encapsulating agents according to the previous method. CP was dispersed in ultrapure water at 80 °C with a concentration of 0.6% for 3 h. Antioxidant extracts GOE and ACHPE were added to the formulation. The total solids were adjusted to 30%. SIO was added at a concentration of 33.33% of the total solids. A homogeneous emulsion was obtained with a Silverson homogenizer. Spray drying was performed at 140–70 °C and a flow rate of 55 mL/min.	Formulation 3 (CP + SIOPH + GOE (200 ppm) + GA) with orujo grape extract had the longest shelf life (4908 ± 184 h). Formulation 5 (PC + SIOPH + ACHPE (200 ppm) + GA) (4740 ± 59 h) with aji charapita pepper extract was also stable.	[109]
Spray-dried	Gum arabic	Feed solution was prepared from AG-Inu and distilled water, and stirred for 12 h. SIO and polysorbate 80 were added, homogenized, and dried into microparticles.	-	[110]
Spray-dried	Lycopodium clavatum spores (average diameter of 25 μm)	SIO was dissolved in ethanol (9% v/v, 2 mL) and stirred for 5 min. Microcapsules (150 mg) were resuspended in SIO solution and rotated for 5 min at 1000 rpm. The SIO/spore ratios were 0.25:1.00, 0.50:1.00, 0.75:1.00, and 1.00:1.00 with codenames SIO@spore-0.25, SIO@spore-0.50, SIO@spore-0.75, and SIO@spore-1.00, respectively. The original spores were processed similarly. The mixture was shaken horizontally at 250 rpm for 24 h; then, the microcapsule spores (SIO@spore) were dried and stored at 4 °C before use.	The encapsulated microcapsule spore maintained its same form after 336 h of UV exposure, exhibiting little damage or distortion, indicating that UV radiation had a limited influence on its shell structure.	[111]

Table 4. *Cont.*

Microencapsulation Method	Coating Materials	Microencapsulation Conditions	Oxidative Stability	Reference
Spray-dried	Gum arabic and maltodextrin	The spray drying process was carried out using a laboratory-scale Büchi B-290 spray dryer with a 0.7 mm diameter nozzle, an air flow rate of 31.5 m^3/h, and an air pressure of 50 mbar. The microcapsules were collected at −15 °C.	The use of WPC slows down the oxidation of SIO lipids in microencapsulation, indicating better oxidative stability.	[112]

Based on Table 4, it is found that the spray-drying method is better used for the microencapsulation of SIO. The spray-drying process is an excellent choice for processing SIO microencapsulation due to its high efficiency, relatively low operating costs, and ability to produce highly stable microencapsulations. In this method, SIO emulsion containing coating materials such as maltodextrin and gum arabic is sprayed in the form of fine droplets into hot air, resulting in encapsulated dry microparticles. The main advantage of spray drying over other methods such as freeze drying and coacervation is its ability to produce microencapsulations in a short time with longer shelf life and sufficient protection against oxidation of unsaturated fatty acids [17]. In addition, spray drying is easy to implement on an industrial scale and can effectively preserve the nutritional properties of oils without requiring excessive temperatures, making it suitable for food and pharmaceutical applications [105].

Research has also shown that the microencapsulation of SIO using spray drying exhibits lower peroxide levels and better oxidative stability than other methods [18].

Microencapsulation of SIO has great potential but has not been optimally utilized. Some of its potential uses include the following:

- Pharmaceutical industry: the combination of omega-3 fatty acids in SIO with other bioactive compounds can increase drug effectiveness and facilitate body absorption.
- Food industry: microencapsulated SIO can be used to create innovative functional food products, such as chocolate or chewing gum with customized fatty acid profiles.
- Cosmetics industry: Microencapsulated SIO can be an active ingredient in skincare products, especially for anti-aging products. Its combination with natural antioxidants can enhance the effectiveness of the product.

In essence, microencapsulation of SIO opens up great opportunities for the development of innovative products in various industries, ranging from pharmaceuticals to cosmetics.

5. Conclusions, Limitations, and Future Perspectives

SIO exhibits considerable potential for implementation in the food, pharmaceutical, and nutraceutical fields due to its composition of essential fatty acids, particularly omega-3 fatty acids, and bioactive compounds. Numerous studies have demonstrated SIO, in various preparations, shows therapeutic potential for a range of health conditions, including benefits for cardiovascular health, antioxidant effects, anti-inflammatory properties, antiproliferative, and neuroprotective activity. This implies that SIO could be an important element in dietary regimens intended to enhance overall health and target specific medical issues. A notable limitation of this review is the insufficient number of large-scale clinical trials focusing on SIO, with the current evidence predominantly based on preclinical and small-scale clinical studies. Although these findings provide foundational knowledge, they may not be entirely representative of broader population groups, emphasizing the importance of conducting large-scale randomized trials. Moreover, sacha inchi research tends to emphasize certain cultivars or locales, with plant composition variations driven by genetic and environmental factors posing challenges to the universal applicability of the findings.

While the health benefits of SIO are promising and research gaps remain, it is imperative to also focus on resolving the practical issues related to its industrial utilization. The stability of SIO is a significant concern throughout the processes of extraction, handling, and storage. Thus, various studies have been conducted to optimize extraction parameters to enhance the efficacy of SIO in industrial applications. Additionally, the development of advanced microencapsulation techniques has been actively explored in order to enhance its stability and bioavailability. Further research should prioritize clinical trials aimed at validating the health benefits of SIO, and exploring its synergistic interactions with other nutraceuticals may also uncover additional therapeutic advantages.

Author Contributions: Conceptualization, A.F.H., S.G.R. and R.N.A.; methodology, A.F.H. and S.G.R.; data curation, A.F.H. and S.G.R.; writing—original draft preparation, S.G.R. and A.F.H.; writing—review and editing, R.N.A., I.M., S.G.R. and A.F.H.; supervision, S.S. and A.Y.C. All authors have read and agreed to the published version of the manuscript.

Funding: This research received no external funding.

Institutional Review Board Statement: Not applicable.

Informed Consent Statement: Not applicable.

Data Availability Statement: All data are contained within the article.

Acknowledgments: The authors thank Universitas Padjadjaran and PT Habbatussauda International.

Conflicts of Interest: The authors declare no conflicts of interest.

References

1. Fu, Q.; Niu, L.; Zhang, Q.; Pan, B.-Z.; He, H.; Xu, Z.-F. Benzyladenine treatment promotes floral feminization and fruiting in a promising oilseed crop *Plukenetia volubilis*. *Ind. Crops Prod.* **2014**, *59*, 295–298. [CrossRef]
2. Wang, S.; Zhu, F.; Kakuda, Y. Sacha inchi (*Plukenetia volubilis* L.): Nutritional composition, biological activity, and uses. *Food Chem.* **2018**, *265*, 316–328. [CrossRef] [PubMed]
3. Mhd Rodzi, N.A.R.; Lee, L.K. Sacha Inchi (*Plukenetia volubilis* L.): Recent insight on phytochemistry, pharmacology, organoleptic, safety and toxicity perspectives. *Heliyon* **2022**, *8*, e10572. [CrossRef]
4. Van, Q.V.; Thi, N.Y.P.; Thi, T.N.; Van, M.N.; Le Van, T.; Thi, B.H.N. Variation in Growth and Yield of Sacha Inchi (*Plukenetia Volubilis* L.) Under Different Ecological Regions in Vietnam. *J. Ecol. Eng.* **2022**, *23*, 161–168. [CrossRef]
5. Kodahl, N.; Sørensen, M. Sacha Inchi (*Plukenetia volubilis* L.) Is an Underutilized Crop with a Great Potential. *Agronomy* **2021**, *11*, 1066. [CrossRef]
6. Kodahl, N. Sacha inchi (*Plukenetia volubilis* L.)—From lost crop of the Incas to part of the solution to global challenges? *Planta* **2020**, *251*, 80. [CrossRef]
7. Sierra, D.M.C.; Rave, L.J.G.; Soto, J.A. Biological Activity of Sacha Inchi (*Plukenetia volubilis* Linneo) and Potential Uses in Human Health: A Review. *Food Technol. Biotechnol.* **2021**, *59*, 253–266. [CrossRef]
8. Medina-Mendoza, M.; Rodriguez-Pérez, R.J.; Rojas-Ocampo, E.; Torrejón-Valqui, L.; Fernández-Jeri, A.B.; Idrogo-Vásquez, G.; Cayo-Colca, I.S.; Castro-Alayo, E.M. Rheological, bioactive properties and sensory preferences of dark chocolates with partial incorporation of Sacha Inchi (*Plukenetia volubilis* L.) oil. *Heliyon* **2021**, *7*, e06154. [CrossRef]
9. Silva, N.C.; Rivera, R.A.; Gómez-Coca, R.B.; Moreda, W.; Pérez-Camino, M.C. Characterization and Preservation of the Bioactive Compounds of Sacha Inchi (*Plukenetia volubilis* and *P. huayllabambana*) Oils. In *Native Crops in Latin America*; Repo-Carrasco-Valencia, R., Tomás, M.C., Eds.; CRC Press: Boca Raton, FL, USA, 2022; pp. 185–208. [CrossRef]
10. Yanti, S.; Agrawal, D.C.; Saputri, D.S.; Lin, H.-Y.; Chien, W.-J. Nutritional Comparison of Sacha Inchi (*Plukenetia volubilis*) Residue with Edible Seeds and Nuts in Taiwan: A Chromatographic and Spectroscopic Study. *Int. J. Food Sci.* **2022**, *2022*, 9825551. [CrossRef]

11. Niu, L.; Li, J.; Chen, M.-S.; Xu, Z.-F. Determination of oil contents in Sacha inchi (*Plukenetia volubilis*) seeds at different developmental stages by two methods: Soxhlet extraction and time-domain nuclear magnetic resonance. *Ind. Crops Prod.* **2014**, *56*, 187–190. [CrossRef]
12. Chirinos, R.; Zuloeta, G.; Pedreschi, R.; Mignolet, E.; Larondelle, Y.; Campos, D. Sacha inchi (*Plukenetia volubilis*): A seed source of polyunsaturated fatty acids, tocopherols, phytosterols, phenolic compounds and antioxidant capacity. *Food Chem.* **2013**, *141*, 1732–1739. [CrossRef]
13. Jitpinit, S.; Siraworakun, C.; Sookklay, Y.; Nuithitikul, K. Enhancement of omega-3 content in sacha inchi seed oil extracted with supercritical carbon dioxide in semi-continuous process. *Heliyon* **2022**, *8*, e08780. [CrossRef] [PubMed]
14. Supriyanto, S.; Imran, Z.; Ardiansyah, R.; Auliyai, B.; Pratama, A.; Kadha, F. The Effect of Cultivation Conditions on Sacha Inchi (*Plukenetia volubilis* L.) Seed Production and Oil Quality (Omega 3, 6, 9). *Agronomy* **2022**, *12*, 636. [CrossRef]
15. Bocianowski, J.; Liersch, A.; Nowosad, K. Genotype by environment interaction for alkenyl glucosinolates content in winter oilseed rape (*Brassica napus* L.) using additive main effects and multiplicative interaction model. *Curr. Plant Biol.* **2020**, *21*, 100137. [CrossRef]
16. Mosquera, T.; Noriega, P.; Tapia, W.; Nowosad, K. Evaluación de la eficacia cosmética de cremas elaboradas con aceites extraídos de especies vegetales Amazónicas: Mauritia Flexuosa (Morete), *Plukenetia volubilis* (Sacha Inchi) y *Oenocarpus Bataua* (Ungurahua). *Granja* **2012**, *16*, 14. [CrossRef]
17. Alarcón, R.; Gonzales, B.; Sotelo, A.; Gallardo, G.; Pérez-Camino, M.D.C.; Chasquibol, N. Microencapsulation of Sacha Inchi (Plukenetia huayllabambana) Oil by Spray Drying with Camu Camu (Myrciaria dubia (H.B.K.) Mc Vaugh) and Mango (Mangifera indica) Skins. In Proceedings of the 2nd International Conference of Ia ValSe-Food Network, Lisbon, Portugal, 21–22 October 2019; MDPI: Basel, Switzerland, 2020; p. 11. [CrossRef]
18. Suwannasang, S.; Zhong, Q.; Thumthanaruk, B.; Vatanyoopaisarn, S.; Uttapap, D.; Puttanlek, C.; Rungsardthong, V. Physicochemical properties of yogurt fortified with microencapsulated Sacha Inchi oil. *LWT* **2022**, *161*, 113375. [CrossRef]
19. Pittia, P.; Gharsallaoui, A. Conventional product formation. In *Food Waste Recovery*; Elsevier: Amsterdam, The Netherlands, 2015; pp. 173–193. [CrossRef]
20. Vicente, J.; de Souza Cezarino, T.; Pereira, L.J.B.; da Rocha, E.P.; Sá, G.R.; Gamallo, O.D.; de Carvalho, M.G.; Garcia-Rojas, E.E. Microencapsulation of sacha inchi oil using emulsion-based delivery systems. *Food Res. Int.* **2017**, *99*, 612–622. [CrossRef]
21. Chasquibol, N.A.; Gallardo, G.; Gómez-Coca, R.B.; Trujillo, D.; Moreda, W.; Pérez-Camino, M.C. Glyceridic and Unsaponifiable Components of Microencapsulated Sacha Inchi (*Plukenetia huayllabambana* L. and *Plukenetia volubilis* L.) Edible Oils. *Foods* **2019**, *8*, 671. [CrossRef] [PubMed]
22. Valencia, A.; Muñoz, A.M.; Ramos-Escudero, M.; Chavez, K.C.; Carotenoid, F.R.-E. Carotenoid, Tocopherol, and Volatile Aroma Compounds in Eight Sacha Inchi Seed (*Plukenetia volubilis* L.) Oil Accessions. *Jpn. J. Oleo Sci.* **2024**, *73*, 665–674. [CrossRef]
23. Ramos-Escudero, F.; Muñoz, A.M.; Escudero, M.R.; Viñas-Ospino, A.; Morales, M.T.; Asuero, A.G. Characterization of commercial Sacha inchi oil according to its composition: Tocopherols, fatty acids, sterols, triterpene and aliphatic alcohols. *J. Food Sci. Technol.* **2019**, *56*, 4503–4515. [CrossRef]
24. Ramos-Escudero, F.; Morales, M.T.; Escudero, M.R.; Muñoz, A.M.; Chavez, K.C.; Asuero, A.G. Assessment of phenolic and volatile compounds of commercial Sacha inchi oils and sensory evaluation. *Food Res. Int.* **2021**, *140*, 110022. [CrossRef] [PubMed]
25. Djuricic, I.; Calder, P.C. Beneficial Outcomes of Omega-6 and Omega-3 Polyunsaturated Fatty Acids on Human Health: An Update for 2021. *Nutrients* **2021**, *13*, 2421. [CrossRef]
26. Farag, M.A.; Gad, M.Z. Omega-9 fatty acids: Potential roles in inflammation and cancer management. *J. Genet. Eng. Biotechnol.* **2022**, *20*, 48. [CrossRef] [PubMed]
27. Szewczyk, K.; Chojnacka, A.; Górnicka, M. Tocopherols and Tocotrienols—Bioactive Dietary Compounds; What Is Certain, What Is Doubt? *Int. J. Mol. Sci.* **2021**, *22*, 6222. [CrossRef] [PubMed]
28. Crupi, P.; Faienza, M.F.; Naeem, M.Y.; Corbo, F.; Clodoveo, M.L.; Muraglia, M. Overview of the Potential Beneficial Effects of Carotenoids on Consumer Health and Well-Being. *Antioxidants* **2023**, *12*, 1069. [CrossRef] [PubMed]
29. Shen, M.; Yuan, L.; Zhang, J.; Wang, X.; Zhang, M.; Li, H.; Jing, Y.; Zeng, F.; Xie, J. Phytosterols: Physiological Functions and Potential Application. *Foods* **2024**, *13*, 1754. [CrossRef]
30. Rasouli, H.; Farzaei, M.H.; Khodarahmi, R. Polyphenols and their benefits: A review. *Int. J. Food Prop.* **2017**, *20*, 1700–1741. [CrossRef]
31. Chirinos, R.; Necochea, O.; Pedreschi, R.; Campos, D. Sacha inchi (*Plukenetia volubilis* L.) shell: An alternative source of phenolic compounds and antioxidants. *Int. J. Food Sci. Technol.* **2016**, *51*, 986–993. [CrossRef]
32. Liua, Q.; Xu, Y.K.; Zhang, P.; Na, Z.; Tang, T.; Shi, Y.X. Chemical composition and oxidative evolution of Sacha Inchi (*Plukentia volubilis* L.) oil from Xishuangbanna (China). *Grasas Aceites* **2014**, *65*, e012. [CrossRef]
33. Takic, M.; Pokimica, B.; Petrovic-Oggiano, G.; Popovic, T. Effects of Dietary α-Linolenic Acid Treatment and the Efficiency of Its Conversion to Eicosapentaenoic and Docosahexaenoic Acids in Obesity and Related Diseases. *Molecules* **2022**, *27*, 4471. [CrossRef] [PubMed]

34. Gonzales, G.F.; Gonzales, C.; Villegas, L. Exposure of fatty acids after a single oral administration of sacha inchi (*Plukenetia volubilis* L.) and sunflower oil in human adult subjects. *Toxicol. Mech. Methods* **2014**, *24*, 60–69. [CrossRef] [PubMed]
35. Gonzales, G.F.; Gonzales, C. A randomized, double-blind placebo-controlled study on acceptability, safety and efficacy of oral administration of sacha inchi oil (*Plukenetia volubilis* L.) in adult human subjects. *Food Chem. Toxicol.* **2014**, *65*, 168–176. [CrossRef] [PubMed]
36. Li, P.; Huang, J.; Xiao, N.; Cai, X.; Yang, Y.; Deng, J.; Zhang, L.-H.; Du, B. Sacha inchi oil alleviates gut microbiota dysbiosis and improves hepatic lipid dysmetabolism in high-fat diet-fed rats. *Food Funct.* **2020**, *11*, 5827–5841. [CrossRef]
37. Garmendia, F.; Pando, R.; Ronceros, G. Effect of sacha inchi oil (*Plukenetia volúbilis* L.) on the lipid profile of patients with hyperlipoproteinemia. *Rev. Peru. Med. Exp. Salud Publica* **2011**, *28*, 628–632.
38. Bjornevik, K.; Cortese, M.; Furtado, J.D.; Paganoni, S.; Schwarzschild, M.A.; Cudkowicz, M.E.; Ascherio, A. Association of Polyunsaturated Fatty Acids and Clinical Progression in Patients with ALS. *Neurology* **2023**, *101*, E690–E698. [CrossRef] [PubMed]
39. Taha, Y.; Burnham, W.M.; Auvin, S. Polyunsaturated fatty acids and epilepsy. *Epilepsia* **2010**, *51*, 1348–1358. [CrossRef] [PubMed]
40. Herrera-Calderon, O.; Yuli-Posadas, R.A.; Tinco-Jayo, J.A.; Enciso-Roca, E.; Franco-Quino, C.; Chumpitaz-Cerrate, V.; Figueroa-Salvador, L. Neuroprotective Effect of Sacha Inchi Oil (*Plukenetia volubilis* L.) in an Experimental Model of Epilepsy. *Pharmacogn. J.* **2019**, *11*, 1591–1596. [CrossRef]
41. Alayón, N.; Ávila, J.G.O.; Echeverri Jiménez, I. Metabolic status is related to the effects of adding of sacha inchi (*Plukenetia volubilis* L.) oil on postprandial inflammation and lipid profile: Randomized, crossover clinical trial. *J. Food Biochem.* **2019**, *43*, e12703. [CrossRef]
42. Alayón, N.; Avila, J.G.O.; Echeverri Jiménez, I. Carbohydrate metabolism and gene expression of sirtuin 1 in healthy subjects after Sacha inchi oil supplementation: A randomized trial. *Food Funct.* **2018**, *9*, 1570–1577. [CrossRef] [PubMed]
43. Ambulay, J.P.; Rojas, P.A.; Timoteo, O.S.; Barreto, T.V.; Colarossi, A. Effect of the emulsion of Sacha Inchi (*Plukenetia huayabambana*) oil on oxidative stress and inflammation in rats induced to obesity. *J. Funct. Foods* **2020**, *64*, 103631. [CrossRef]
44. Suthiphasil, P.; Rintha, J.; Nararatwanchai, T.; Sittiprapaporn, P. Comparative study of oral administration of Sacha Inchi oil extraction with erythromycin versus oral erythromycin on the treatment of Acne Vulgaris. In Proceedings of the 2018 International Conference on Digital Arts, Media and Technology (ICDAMT), Phayao, Thailand, 25–28 February 2018; IEEE: New York, NY, USA; pp. 309–312. [CrossRef]
45. Mai, H.C.; Nguyen, D.C.; Nhan, N.P.T.; Bach, L.G. Physico-Chemical Properties of Sacha Inchi (*Plukenetia volubilis* L.) Seed Oil from Vietnam. *Asian J. Chem.* **2020**, *32*, 335–338. [CrossRef]
46. Aguirrezábal, L.; Martre, P.; Pereyra-Irujo, G.; Echarte, M.M.; Izquierdo, N. Improving grain quality: Ecophysiological and modeling tools to develop management and breeding strategies. In *Crop Physiology*; Elsevier: Amsterdam, The Netherlands, 2015; pp. 423–465. [CrossRef]
47. Schiessel, D.L.; Yamazaki, R.K.; Kryczyk, M.; Coelho, I.; Yamaguchi, A.A.; Pequito, D.C.T.; Brito, G.A.P.; Borghetti, G.; Fernandes, L.C. α-Linolenic Fatty Acid Supplementation Decreases Tumor Growth and Cachexia Parameters in Walker 256 Tumor-Bearing Rats. *Nutr. Cancer* **2015**, *67*, 839–846. [CrossRef] [PubMed]
48. Centurión-Rodríguez, A.; Huamán-Saavedra, J.J.; Requena-Fuentes, V.R. Effect of Sacha Inchi oil (*Plukenetia volubilis* L.) on 1,2-dimethylhydrazine-induced colon carcinogenesis in Holtzman rats. *Rev. Gastroenterol.* **2017**, *37*, 129–136.
49. Rincón-Cervera, M.; Valenzuela, R.; Hernandez-Rodas, M.C.; Barrera, C.; Espinosa, A.; Marambio, M.; Valenzuela, A. Vegetable oils rich in alpha linolenic acid increment hepatic n-3 LCPUFA, modulating the fatty acid metabolism and antioxidant response in rats. *Prostaglandins Leukot. Essent. Fatty Acids* **2016**, *111*, 25–35. [CrossRef]
50. En, Y.; Udin, N.A.B.; Vanoh, D.A.; Leng, S.K. Effect of Sacha Inchi Oil on Human Blood Pressure and Lipid Profile: A Preliminary Study in Malaysia. *J. Gizi Dan Pangan* **2024**, *19*, 61–68. [CrossRef]
51. Lourith, N.; Kanlayavattanakul, M.; Chaikul, P. Sacha Inchi: The Promising Source of Functional Oil for Anti-Aging Product. *J. Oleo Sci.* **2024**, *73*, 429–435. [CrossRef] [PubMed]
52. Soimee, W.; Nakyai, W.; Charoensit, P.; Grandmottet, F.; Worasakwutiphong, S.; Phimnuan, P.; Viyoch, J. Evaluation of moisturizing and irritation potential of sacha inchi oil. *J. Cosmet. Dermatol.* **2020**, *19*, 915–924. [CrossRef] [PubMed]
53. Zanqui, A.B.; da Silva, C.M.; de Morais, D.R.; Santos, J.M.; Ribeiro, S.A.O.; Eberlin, M.N.; Cardozo-Filho, L.; Visentainer, J.V.; Gomes, S.T.M.; Matsushita, M. Sacha inchi (*Plukenetia volubilis* L.) oil composition varies with changes in temperature and pressure in subcritical extraction with n-propane. *Ind. Crops Prod.* **2016**, *87*, 64–70. [CrossRef]
54. Chan, Y.-J.; Chiu, C.-S.; Li, P.-H.; Lu, W.-C. Evaluation of different roasting condition on yield, physico-chemical characteristics, and antioxidant activity of cold-pressed sacha inchi (*Plukenetia volubilis*) oil. *LWT* **2024**, *203*, 116343. [CrossRef]
55. Cisneros, F.H.; Paredes, D.; Arana, A.; Composition, L.C.-Z.C. Oxidative Stability and Antioxidant Capacity of Oil Extracted from Roasted Seeds of Sacha-Inchi (*Plukenetia volubilis* L.). *J. Agric. Food Chem.* **2014**, *62*, 5191–5197. [CrossRef] [PubMed]
56. Norhazlindah, M.F.; A Jahurul, M.H.; Norliza, M.; Shihabul, A.; Islam, S.; Nyam, K.L.; Zaidul, I.S.M. Techniques for extraction, characterization, and application of oil from sacha inchi (*Plukenetia volubilis* L.) seed: A review. *J. Food Meas. Charact.* **2023**, *17*, 904–915. [CrossRef]

57. Liu, N.; Ren, G.; Faiza, M.; Li, D.; Cui, J.; Zhang, K.; Yao, X.; Zhao, M. Comparison of conventional and green extraction methods on oil yield, physicochemical properties, and lipid compositions of pomegranate seed oil. *J. Food Compos. Anal.* **2022**, *114*, 104747. [CrossRef]
58. Kong, S.; Keang, T.; Bunthan, M.; Say, M.; Nat, Y.; Tan, C.P.; Tan, R. Hydraulic Cold-Pressed Extraction of Sacha Inchi Seeds: Oil Yield and Its Physicochemical Properties. *ChemEngineering* **2023**, *7*, 69. [CrossRef]
59. Matthäus, B. Oil Technology. In *Technological Innovations in Major World Oil Crops*; Springer: New York, NY, USA, 2012; Volume 2, pp. 23–92. [CrossRef]
60. Rękas, A.; Siger, A.; Wroniak, M.; Ścibisz, I.; Derewiaka, D.; Anders, A. Dehulling and microwave pretreatment effects on the physicochemical composition and antioxidant capacity of virgin rapeseed oil. *J. Food Sci. Technol.* **2017**, *54*, 627–638. [CrossRef] [PubMed]
61. Gutiérrez, L.; Sanchez-Reinoso, Z.; Quiñones-Segura, Y. Effects of Dehulling Sacha Inchi (*Plukenetia volubilis* L.) Seeds on the Physicochemical and Sensory Properties of Oils Extracted by Means of Cold Pressing. *J. Am. Oil Chem. Soc.* **2019**, *96*, 1187–1195. [CrossRef]
62. Muangrat, R.; Veeraphong, P.; Chantee, N. Screw press extraction of Sacha inchi seeds: Oil yield and its chemical composition and antioxidant properties. *J. Food Process Preserv.* **2018**, *42*, e13635. [CrossRef]
63. Bhuiya, M.M.K.; Rasul, M.G.; Khan, M.M.K.; Ashwath, N.; Azad, A.K.; Mofijur, M. Optimisation of Oil Extraction Process from Australian Native Beauty Leaf Seed (*Calophyllum inophyllum*). *Energy Procedia* **2015**, *75*, 56–61. [CrossRef]
64. Nde, D.B.; Foncha, A.C. Optimization Methods for the Extraction of Vegetable Oils: A Review. *Processes* **2020**, *8*, 209. [CrossRef]
65. Sheikh, S.M.; Kazi, Z.S. Technologies for Oil Extraction: A Review. *Int. J. Environ. Agric. Biotechnol.* **2016**, *1*, 106–110.
66. Çakaloğlu, B.; Özyurt, V.H.; Ötleş, S. Cold press in oil extraction. A review. *Ukr. Food J.* **2018**, *7*, 640–654. [CrossRef]
67. García, M.; Samaniego, A.; Coyachamín, F.; Vallejo, S.; Caluña, E. Obtaining Vegetable Oil from Sacha-Inchi (*Plukenetia volubilis*) by the Cold Pressing Method for Industrial Processing. *Int. J. Curr. Res. Acad. Rev.* **2019**, *7*, 11–15. [CrossRef]
68. Bhuiya, M.M.K.; Rasul, M.; Khan, M.; Ashwath, N.; Mofijur, M. Comparison of oil extraction between screw press and solvent (n-hexane) extraction technique from beauty leaf (*Calophyllum inophyllum* L.) feedstock. *Ind. Crops Prod.* **2020**, *144*, 112024. [CrossRef]
69. Mašán, V.; Vaštík, L.; Burg, P.; Sotolář, R.; Macák, M. The evaluation of extraction of some nut oils using screw pressing. *Potravin. Slovak. J. Food Sci.* **2020**, *14*, 847–853. [CrossRef] [PubMed]
70. Wang, S.; Wang, J.; Dong, G.; Chen, X.; Wang, S.; Lei, F.; Su, X.; Bai, Q. Effect of Different Extraction Methods on Quality Characteristics of Rapeseed and Flaxseed Oils. *J. Food Qual.* **2022**, *2022*, 8296212. [CrossRef]
71. Chasquibol, N.A.; del Aguila, C.; Yácono, J.C.; Guinda, A.; Moreda, W.; Gómez-Coca, R.B.; Pérez-Camino, M.C. Characterization of Glyceridic and Unsaponifiable Compounds of Sacha Inchi (*Plukenetia huayllabambana* L.) Oils. *J. Agric. Food Chem.* **2014**, *62*, 10162–10169. [CrossRef] [PubMed]
72. Valdiviezo, C.J.; Hidalgo, L.E.R.; Bermeo, S.M.B. Caracterización del aceite de la semilla de Sacha Inchi (*Plukenetia volubilis*) del cantón San Vicente, Manabí, Ecuador, obtenida mediante procesos no térmicos de extrusión. *Granja* **2019**, *30*, 77–87. [CrossRef]
73. Kataoka, H. Pharmaceutical Analysis Sample Preparation. In *Reference Module in Chemistry, Molecular Sciences and Chemical Engineering*; Elsevier: Amsterdam, The Netherlands, 2018. [CrossRef]
74. Moghimi, M.; Honarvar, M.; Ghavami, M. Betalain Extraction from Beetroot Using Supercritical Carbon Dioxide and Microwave Pretreatment by Response Surface Method (RSM). *Iran. J. Chem. Chem. Eng.* **2023**, *42*, 925–938.
75. Hassim, N.; Markom, M.; Rosli, M.I.; Harun, S. Scale-up approach for supercritical fluid extraction with ethanol–water modified carbon dioxide on *Phyllanthus niruri* for safe enriched herbal extracts. *Sci. Rep.* **2021**, *11*, 15818. [CrossRef]
76. Sharif, K.; Rahman, M.; Azmir, J.; Mohamed, A.; Jahurul, M.; Sahena, F.; Zaidul, I. Experimental design of supercritical fluid extraction—A review. *J. Food Eng.* **2014**, *124*, 105–116. [CrossRef]
77. Capuzzo, A.; Maffei, M.E.; Occhipinti, A. Supercritical Fluid Extraction of Plant Flavors and Fragrances. *Molecules* **2013**, *18*, 7194–7238. [CrossRef]
78. Triana-Maldonado, D.M.; Torijano-Gutiérrez, S.A.; Giraldo-Estrada, C. Supercritical CO_2; extraction of oil and omega-3 concentrate from Sacha inchi (*Plukenetia volubilis* L.) from Antioquia, Colombia. *Grasas Aceites* **2017**, *68*, 172. [CrossRef]
79. Costa, R.; Dugo, P.; Mondello, L. Sampling and Sample Preparation Techniques for the Determination of the Volatile Components of Milk and Dairy Products. In *Comprehensive Sampling and Sample Preparation*; Elsevier: Amsterdam, The Netherlands, 2012; pp. 43–59. [CrossRef]
80. Kua, Y.L.; Gan, S.; Ng, H.K. Non-evaporative method to remove high boiling point solvent (ethyl lactate) from palm oil extract at atmospheric conditions. *Int. Food Res. J.* **2018**, *25*, 97–103.
81. Bueno-Borges, L.B.; Sartim, M.A.; Gil, C.C.; Sampaio, S.V.; Rodrigues, P.H.V.; Regitano-d'Arce, M.A.B. Sacha inchi seeds from sub-tropical cultivation: Effects of roasting on antinutrients, antioxidant capacity and oxidative stability. *J. Food Sci. Technol.* **2018**, *55*, 4159–4166. [CrossRef] [PubMed]

82. Cordero-Clavijo, L.M.; Mejía-Valdez, D.; Antunes-Ricardo, M.; Lazo-Vélez, M.A.; Guajardo-Flores, D. Evaluating sacha inchi (*Plukenetia volubilis*) oil stability and physicochemical properties: A comparison between conventional extraction and supercritical fluids. *Food Chem.* **2025**, *463*, 141132. [CrossRef] [PubMed]
83. Liu, Z.; Gui, M.; Xu, T.; Zhang, L.; Kong, L.; Qin, L.; Zou, Z. Efficient aqueous enzymatic-ultrasonication extraction of oil from *Sapindus mukorossi* seed kernels. *Ind. Crops Prod.* **2019**, *134*, 124–133. [CrossRef]
84. Liu, Q.; Li, P.; Chen, J.; Li, C.; Jiang, L.; Luo, M.; Sun, A. Optimization of Aqueous Enzymatic Extraction of Castor (*Ricinus communis*) Seeds Oil Using Response Surface Methodology. *J. Biobased Mater. Bioenergy* **2019**, *13*, 114–122. [CrossRef]
85. Nguyen, H.C.; Vuong, D.P.; Nguyen, N.T.T.; Nguyen, N.P.; Su, C.-H.; Wang, F.-M.; Juan, H.-Y. Aqueous enzymatic extraction of polyunsaturated fatty acid–rich sacha inchi (*Plukenetia volubilis* L.) seed oil: An eco-friendly approach. *LWT* **2020**, *133*, 109992. [CrossRef]
86. Konopka, I.; Roszkowska, B.; Czaplicki, S.; Tańska, M. Optimization of Pumpkin Oil Recovery by Using Aqueous Enzymatic Extraction and Comparison of the Quality of the Obtained Oil with the Quality of Cold-Pressed Oil. *Food Technol. Biotechnol.* **2016**, *54*, 413–420. [CrossRef]
87. Maya, I.; Winardi, D.O.; Amalia, E.; Mita, S.R.; Kusumawulan, C.K.; Putriana, N.A.; Sriwidodo, S. Physicochemical Characteristics, Fatty Acid Profile, and In Vitro Antioxidant Activity Evaluation of Sacha Inchi Seed Oil from Indonesia. *Cosmetics* **2023**, *10*, 171. [CrossRef]
88. Sieber, R.; Eyer, H. LIPIDS | Cholesterol Removal from Dairy Products. In *Encyclopedia of Dairy Sciences*; Elsevier: Amsterdam, The Netherlands, 2002; pp. 1611–1617. [CrossRef]
89. Lai, W.T.; Khong, N.M.; Lim, S.S.; Hee, Y.Y.; Sim, B.I.; Lau, K.Y.; Lai, O.M. A review: Modified agricultural by-products for the development and fortification of food products and nutraceuticals. *Trends Food Sci. Technol.* **2017**, *59*, 148–160. [CrossRef]
90. Rodríguez-Cortina, A.; Hernández-Carrión, M. Microcapsules of Sacha Inchi seed oil (*Plukenetia volubilis* L.) obtained by spray drying as a potential ingredient to formulate functional foods. *Food Res. Int.* **2023**, *170*, 113014. [CrossRef]
91. Sun, Y.; Zhong, M.; Liao, Y.; Kang, M.; Qi, B.; Li, Y. Pickering emulsions stabilized by reassembled oleosome protein nanoparticles for co-encapsulating hydrophobic nutrients. *Food Hydrocoll.* **2022**, *138*, 108445. [CrossRef]
92. Sarkar, T.; Salauddin, M.; Roy, A.; Sharma, N.; Sharma, A.; Yadav, S.; Jha, V.; Rebezov, M.; Khayrullin, M.; Thiruvengadam, M.; et al. Minor tropical fruits as a potential source of bioactive and functional foods. *Crit. Rev. Food Sci. Nutr.* **2023**, *63*, 6491–6535. [CrossRef] [PubMed]
93. Chang, C.; Nickerson, M.T. Nickerson. Encapsulation of omega 3-6-9 fatty acids-rich oils using protein-based emulsions with spray drying. *J. Food Sci. Technol.* **2018**, *55*, 2850–2861. [CrossRef] [PubMed]
94. Rahman, S.N.R.; Agarwal, N.; Goswami, A.; Sree, A.; Jala, A.; Venuganti, A.; Deka, A.; Borkar, R.M.; Singh, V.; Das, D.; et al. Studies on spray dried topical ophthalmic emulsions containing cyclosporin A (0.05% *w*/*w*): Systematic optimization, in vitro preclinical toxicity and in vivo assessments. *Drug Deliv. Transl. Res.* **2023**, *13*, 1654–1674. [CrossRef]
95. Zhang, L.; Zhou, C.; Xing, S.; Chen, Y.; Su, W.; Wang, H.; Tan, M. Sea bass protein-polyphenol complex stabilized high internal phase of algal oil Pickering emulsions to stabilize astaxanthin for 3D food printing. *Food Chem.* **2023**, *417*, 135824. [CrossRef]
96. Yunilawati, R.; Yemirta, Y.; Cahyaningtyas, A.A.; Aviandharie, S.A.; Hidayati, N.; Rahmi, D. Optimasi Proses Spray Drying Pada Enkapsulasi Antosianin Ubi Ungu. *J. Kim. Dan Kemasan* **2018**, *40*, 17. [CrossRef]
97. Meng, W.; Sun, H.; Mu, T.; Garcia-Vaquero, M. Future trends in the field of Pickering emulsions: Stabilizers, spray-dried microencapsulation and rehydration for food applications. *Trends Food Sci. Technol.* **2024**, *150*, 104610. [CrossRef]
98. da Silva Soares, B.; Siqueira, R.P.; de Carvalho, M.G.; Vicente, J.; Garcia-Rojas, E.E. Microencapsulation of sacha inchi oil (*Plukenetia volubilis* L.) using complex coacervation: Formation and structural characterization. *Food Chem.* **2019**, *298*, 125045. [CrossRef] [PubMed]
99. Yan, Z.; Xue, Y. Algorithms to Calculate Exact Inclusion Probabilities for a Non-Rejective Approximate ps Sampling Design. *Rev. Colomb. Estad.* **2014**, *37*, 127. [CrossRef]
100. Santos, M.B.; da Costa, A.R.; Garcia-Rojas, E.E. Heteroprotein complex coacervates of ovalbumin and lysozyme: Formation and thermodynamic characterization. *Int. J. Biol. Macromol.* **2018**, *106*, 1323–1329. [CrossRef]
101. Xiong, W.; Ren, C.; Tian, M.; Yang, X.; Li, J.; Li, B. Complex coacervation of ovalbumin-carboxymethylcellulose assessed by isothermal titration calorimeter and rheology: Effect of ionic strength and charge density of polysaccharide. *Food Hydrocoll.* **2017**, *73*, 41–50. [CrossRef]
102. Amiruddin, M.; Rijal, A.S.; Hariyadi, D.M. Effect of $CaCl_2$ Crosslinker Concentration on The Characteristics, Release and Stability of Ciprofloxacin HCl-Alginate-Carrageenan Microspheres. *J. Farm. Dan Ilmu Kefarmasian Indones.* **2023**, *10*, 312–323. [CrossRef]
103. Sponton, E.; Perez, A.A.; Santiago, L.G. Protein-polysaccharide associative phase separation applied to obtain a linoleic acid dried ingredient. *Food Hydrocoll.* **2017**, *71*, 158–167. [CrossRef]
104. Zahara, A.; Ulfa, S.M.; Safitri, A. Comparative Analysis of Different Natural Polymers as Coating Agents for Freeze-Dried Microencapsulation of *Cosmos caudatus* Kunth Compounds. *Sci. World J.* **2024**, *2024*, 6833341. [CrossRef]

105. Zhang, H.; Zhu, L.; Shao, Y.; Wang, L.; He, J.; He, Y. Microencapsulation of Monascus red pigments by emulsification/internal gelation with freeze/spray-drying: Process optimization, morphological characteristics, and stability. *LWT* **2023**, *173*, 114227. [CrossRef]
106. da Silva Soares, B.; de Carvalho, C.W.P.; Garcia-Rojas, E.E. Microencapsulation of Sacha Inchi Oil by Complex Coacervates using Ovalbumin-Tannic Acid and Pectin as Wall Materials. *Food Bioproc. Technol.* **2021**, *14*, 817–830. [CrossRef]
107. Chasquibol, N.; Gonzales, B.F.; Alarcón, R.; Sotelo, A.; Gallardo, G.; García, B.; Pérez-Camino, M.D.C. Co-Microencapsulation of Sacha Inchi (*Plukenetia huayllabambana*) Oil with Natural Antioxidants Extracts. *Foods* **2023**, *12*, 2126. [CrossRef]
108. Chasquibol, N.; Alarcón, R.; Gonzales, B.F.; Sotelo, A.; Landoni, L.; Gallardo, G.; García, B.; Pérez-Camino, M.C. Design of Functional Powdered Beverages Containing Co-Microcapsules of Sacha Inchi *P. huayllabambana* Oil and Antioxidant Extracts of Camu Camu and Mango Skins. *Antioxidants* **2022**, *11*, 1420. [CrossRef] [PubMed]
109. Chasquibol, N.; Sotelo, A.; Tapia, M.; Alarcón, R.; Goycoolea, F.; Perez-Camino, M.D.C. Perez-Camino. Co-Microencapsulation of Cushuro (*Nostoc sphaericum*) Polysaccharide with Sacha Inchi Oil (*Plukenetia huayllabambana*) and Natural Antioxidant Extracts. *Antioxidants* **2024**, *13*, 680. [CrossRef]
110. Rengifo, E.; Rios-Mera, J.D.; Huamaní, P.; Vela-Paredes, R.; Vásquez, J.; Saldaña, E.; Siche, R.; Tello, F. Fish Burgers Fortified with Microencapsulated Sacha Inchi Oil: Effects on Technological and Sensory Properties. *Foods* **2024**, *13*, 1004. [CrossRef]
111. Khann, B.; Polpanich, D.; Opaprakasit, P.; Wongngam, Y.; Thananukul, K.; Kaewsaneha, C. Fabrication of Sacha Inchi Oil-Loaded Microcapsules Employing Natural-Templated *Lycopodium clavatum* Spores and Their Pressure-Stimuli Release Behavior. *ACS Omega* **2023**, *8*, 20937–20948. [CrossRef] [PubMed]
112. Landoni, L.; Alarcon, R.; Vilca, L.; Chasquibol, N.; Pérez-Camino, M.C.; Gallardo, G. Physicochemical characterization and oxidative stability of microencapsulated edible sacha inchi seed oil by spray drying. *Grasas Aceites* **2020**, *71*, 387. [CrossRef]

molecules

MDPI

Review

Advancing the Potential of *Polyscias fruticosa* as a Source of Bioactive Compounds: Biotechnological and Pharmacological Perspectives

Anita A. Śliwińska [1,*] and Karolina Tomiczak [2]

1 Department of Pharmaceutical Biology and Medicinal Plant Biotechnology, Faculty of Pharmacy, Medical University of Warsaw, 1 Banacha St., 02-097 Warsaw, Poland

2 Plant Breeding and Acclimatization Institute—National Research Institute, Radzików, 05-870 Błonie, Poland; k.tomiczak@ihar.edu.pl

* Correspondence: anita.sliwinska@wum.edu.pl

Abstract

Polyscias fruticosa (L.) Harms, a Southeast Asian medicinal plant of the Araliaceae family, has gained increasing attention due to its rich phytochemical profile and potential pharmacological applications. This review provides an up-to-date synthesis of biotechnological strategies and chemical investigations related to this species. In vitro propagation methods, including somatic embryogenesis, adventitious root, and cell suspension cultures, are discussed with emphasis on elicitation and bioreactor systems to enhance the production of secondary metabolites. Phytochemical analyses using gas chromatography–mass spectrometry (GC-MS), high-performance liquid chromatography (HPLC), and nuclear magnetic resonance (NMR) have identified over 120 metabolites, including triterpenoid saponins, polyphenols, sterols, volatile terpenoids, polyacetylenes, and fatty acids. Several compounds, such as tocopherols, conjugated linoleic acids, and alismol, were identified for the first time in the genus. These constituents exhibit antioxidant, anti-inflammatory, antimicrobial, antidiabetic, anticancer, and neuroprotective activities, with selected saponins (e.g., chikusetsusaponin IVa, *Polyscias fruticosa* saponin [PFS], zingibroside R1) showing confirmed molecular mechanisms of action. The combination of biotechnological tools with phytochemical and pharmacological evaluation supports *P. fruticosa* as a promising candidate for further functional, therapeutic, and nutraceutical development. This review also identifies knowledge gaps related to compound characterization and mechanistic studies, suggesting future directions for interdisciplinary research.

Keywords: *Polyscias fruticosa*; in vitro propagation; triterpenoid saponins; flavonoids; pharmacological potential; biotechnological applications; phytoremediation

1. Introduction

Polyscias fruticosa (L.) Harms, commonly referred to as Ming aralia or "Vietnamese ginseng", is an important medicinal plant of the Araliaceae family, native to Southeast Asia and widely cultivated across tropical and subtropical regions [1,2]. It has a longstanding role in traditional medicine systems in Vietnam, the Philippines, and Indonesia, where it is used to treat a broad spectrum of conditions, including fatigue, asthma, metabolic disorders, inflammation, and neurodegenerative diseases [2–4]. These ethnomedical applications are consistent with the plant's chemically diverse profile. Recent pharmacological findings also indicate similarities to *Panax ginseng*, particularly with regard to adaptogenic and immunomodulatory properties.

Phytochemical investigations have identified a wide array of bioactive constituents in *P. fruticosa*, including triterpenoid saponins, flavonoids and phenolic acids, sterols, essential oils, polyacetylenes, and fatty acids [3,5–11]. These structurally diverse compounds have been associated with a broad spectrum of biological activities, such as anti-inflammatory, antioxidant, antidiabetic, antimicrobial, antiasthmatic, antitussive, anti-osteoclastogenic, and neuroprotective effects [10–21]. Due to their structural and functional similarity to ginsenosides, these saponins have garnered increasing interest as potential functional analogs to those found in *Panax* species, supporting their use in both pharmaceutical and nutraceutical applications [16]. However, the broader utilization of *P. fruticosa* is hindered by slow vegetative growth, seasonal variation, and low natural yields of pharmacologically active metabolites [22]. To overcome these limitations, several in vitro culture techniques have been employed, including micropropagation, somatic embryogenesis, callus and suspension cultures, and adventitious root formation [22–25]. These biotechnological strategies not only enable sustainable biomass production but also enhance the yield of targeted secondary metabolites. For instance, elicitation with compounds such as jasmonic acid and chitosan has been shown to significantly increase flavonoid and saponin accumulation in vitro [26,27], offering a platform for the metabolic enhancement of high-value phytochemicals.

Despite significant research progress, no comprehensive review has yet addressed the multifaceted properties of *Polyscias fruticosa* as a medicinal plant. Therefore, the aim of this critical review is to integrate current knowledge on the following: (i) biotechnological methods enhancing biomass and secondary metabolite production; (ii) phytochemical diversity, with particular emphasis on compound classification and structural characteristics; and (iii) pharmacological activities supported by mechanistic evidence. In addition, this review provides the authors' perspective on research gaps, the biosynthetic plausibility of identified compounds, and directions for future studies. By presenting *P. fruticosa* as a plant species with high research potential in the fields of biotechnology and pharmacology, this work aims to highlight its relevance for further investigations into natural products and plant-derived therapeutic strategies.

2. Materials and Methods

The literature for this review was collected through a comprehensive search of scientific databases including PubMed, Scopus, Web of Science, and Google Scholar. Keywords such as "*Polyscias fruticosa*," "bioactive compounds," "in vitro culture," "pharmacological activity," and "biotechnology" were used. Studies published in English between 2000 and 2024 were prioritized; however, earlier foundational works and historically significant publications were also included when relevant, particularly those providing essential methodological background or pioneering data.

The selection criteria encompassed relevance to the topic, experimental rigor, and contribution to understanding the biotechnological and pharmacological potential of *Polyscias fruticosa*. Priority was given to peer-reviewed original research articles, reviews, and phytochemical studies reporting detailed extraction methods, compound identification (e.g., by GC-MS, HPLC, NMR), and bioactivity assessments.

Duplicate reports and publications lacking primary data or methodological transparency were excluded. Data were organized thematically and interpreted critically to identify key findings, research gaps, and emerging perspectives in the field.

3. Morphology, Systematics, Distribution, and Ethnobotanical Relevance of *Polyscias fruticosa* (L.) Harms

Polyscias fruticosa is a perennial, glabrous shrub or undershrub in the Araliaceae family, characterized by a woody, sparsely to moderately branched stem and a distinctive crown of finely dissected, compound leaves. The species is widely cultivated in tropical and subtropical regions of Asia, the Pacific Islands, Africa, and the Caribbean, primarily for its ornamental and medicinal properties. It typically grows to a height of 1.5 to 4 m, depending on environmental conditions and cultivation practices [1,2].

Leaves are alternate, bipinnate to tripinnate and imparipinnate, with long petioles (7–16 cm) and total dimensions reaching up to 29 × 25 cm. Each leaf comprises 7 to 15 pinnae, with pinnules bearing two–three pairs per pinna. The leaflets are narrowly lanceolate to elliptical (0.3–3 cm wide, 4.5–5 cm long), cuneate at the base, long-acuminate at the apex, and irregularly dentate to laciniate along the margins. Leaf coloration ranges from deep green in shade-grown specimens to yellowish hues or variegated forms in sun-exposed or horticultural varieties (Figure 1) [28]. The intricate leaf morphology and variable coloring enhance its visual distinctiveness and ornamental appeal [1,2].

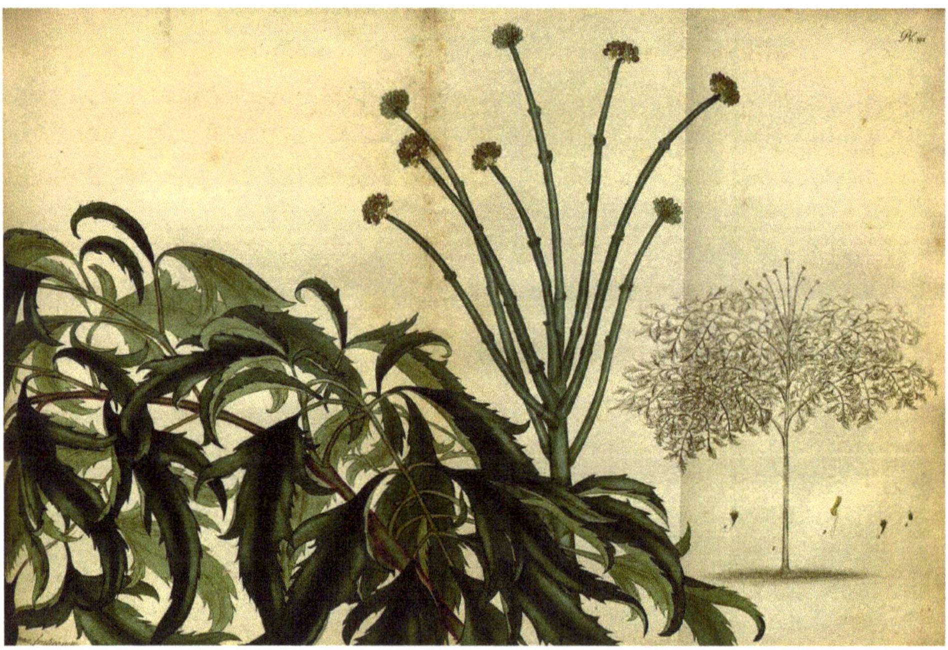

Figure 1. Botanical illustration of *Polyscias fruticosa* (L.) Harms (as *Panax fruticosus* L.), family Araliaceae, from *The Botanist's Repository*, Vol. 9 (1809), Plate 595, drawn by H.C. Andrews. The image depicts the compound, serrated leaves, thick inflorescence-bearing stems, and the overall growth habit of the plant. Source: Missouri Botanical Garden, St. Louis, MO, USA. Public domain. Available online at http://www.plantillustrations.org/illustration.php?id_illustration=111562 (accessed on 30 April 2025) [28].

The inflorescences are terminal or axillary panicles (10–30 cm) composed of numerous umbellate cymes (12–20 per inflorescence). Flowers are actinomorphic, hermaphroditic, or functionally male, with articulated pedicels, a ring-like gamosepalous calyx, five deciduous ovate petals (2–4 mm), and five stamens with beige filaments and ovate yellow to white anthers. The inferior ovary comprises two–three carpels with initially fused styles that may separate or twist during fruit maturation (Figure 2) [29]. The fruit is a laterally compressed drupe (3–4 mm in diameter), dark purple to black at maturity, containing two flattened pyrenes and a seed with smooth endosperm [1,2].

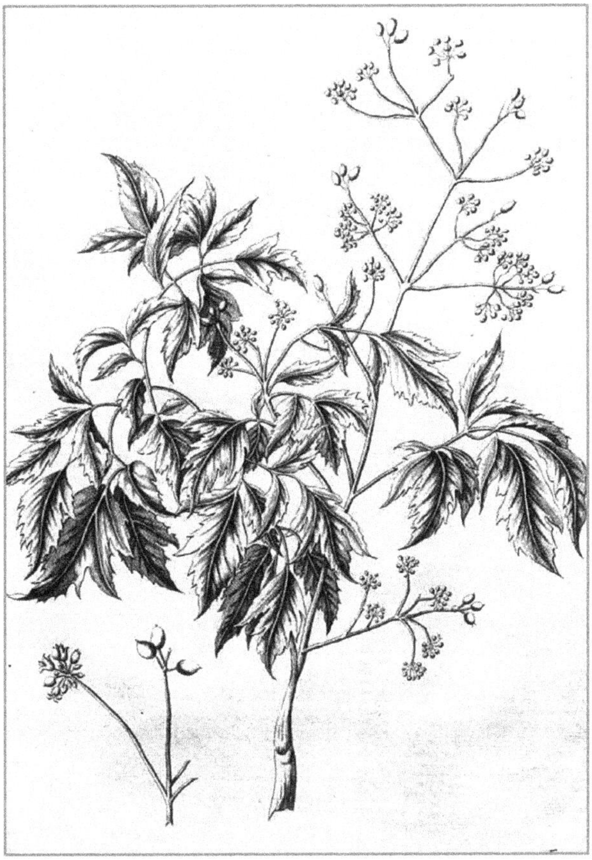

Figure 2. *Polyscias fruticosa* (L.) Harms (synonym: *Panax fruticosus* L.). Historical botanical illustration by Georgius Everhardus Rumphius (Rumpf), from *Herbarium Amboinense*, Vol. 4, Tab. XXXIII, p. 78 (1743). Image obtained from the website of the Missouri Botanical Garden, St. Louis, MO, USA. Public domain. Available online at http://www.plantillustrations.org/illustration.php?id_illustration=121516 (accessed on 13 June 2025) [29].

The species belongs to the genus *Polyscias*, originally described by J.R. and G. Forster in 1775. Historically heterogeneous, the genus was redefined by Lowry and Plunkett [3], who integrated six previously separate genera (*Arthrophyllum*, *Gastonia*, *Reynoldsia*, *Cuphocarpus*, *Tetraplasandra*, and *Munroidendron*) based on molecular phylogenetic data. As a result, the recircumscribed genus now includes approximately 159 accepted species, systematically organized into ten subgenera. *P. fruticosa* is classified within *Polyscias* sensu stricto, a lineage characterized by articulated pedicels, sheathing petiole bases, and a distinct foliar fragrance upon drying [3].

The native range of *P. fruticosa* includes Southeast Asia and western Oceania, from where it has spread through human-mediated cultivation. It is now distributed in Vietnam, Laos, Cambodia, the Philippines, Indonesia, Papua New Guinea, India, China, and many Pacific and Caribbean islands, including Cuba, Puerto Rico, and the Virgin Islands [2]. In

Cuba, the plant has been cultivated since at least the late 19th century and is commonly used in urban landscaping as a hedge or potted ornamental. It prefers well-drained, fertile soils and thrives under full sun or partial shade, although its growth is generally slow and benefits from periodic pruning and organic amendments.

Genetic and morphological studies conducted in Vietnam revealed high phenotypic plasticity and significant intraspecific variation within *P. fruticosa*. Using leaf morphology and internal transcribed spacer (ITS) rDNA sequencing, over 20 morphotypes were differentiated among 23 accessions, including several subspecies and potential hybrids. These findings support the hypothesis of regional domestication and extensive cultivar development driven by traditional medicinal use and esthetic selection [30].

According to Plants of the World Online (POWO) [31], *P. fruticosa* has 18 accepted synonyms, reflecting historical taxonomic revisions. Notable examples include *Panax fruticosus* L., *Nothopanax fruticosus* (L.) Miq., *Aralia fruticosa* (L.) L.H. Bailey, and *Tieghemopanax fruticosus* (L.) R.Vig. The name *Polyscias* is derived from the Greek "poly" (many) and "skia" (shade), referring to the plant's dense, spreading foliage [2].

From an ethnopharmacological standpoint, *P. fruticosa* is a widely used medicinal species. In Vietnam, it is traditionally known as "đinh lăng" and used as a tonic, adaptogen, and treatment for inflammation, respiratory disorders, and fatigue [9]. In Indonesian jamu medicine, it features in postpartum and gynecological formulations. Ethnobotanical records from the Philippines and Oceania describe its use as an antipyretic, analgesic, and diuretic, applied as decoctions or topical poultices [9]. The widespread use of *P. fruticosa* in traditional medicine aligns with its confirmed phytochemical richness, including oleanane-type triterpenoid saponins (e.g., polysciosides A–K), chikusetsusaponin IVa, flavonoids, polyacetylenes, and sterols [3–11]. Pharmacological studies have confirmed its antioxidant, anti-inflammatory, antidiabetic, immunomodulatory, and antimicrobial effects [12–17].

Overall, *P. fruticosa* represents a phytochemically and ethnomedically important species. Its morphological plasticity, wide geographic distribution, and medicinal versatility make it a promising subject for integrative research spanning taxonomy, molecular phylogenetics, and evidence-based phytotherapy.

4. Micropropagation Strategies for *Polyscias fruticosa*

4.1. Historical Background of In Vitro Studies on *Polyscias fruticosa*

The development of in vitro culture systems for *Polyscias fruticosa* has played a critical role in advancing plant biotechnology, particularly with respect to secondary metabolite production in the Araliaceae family. Foundational studies were conducted at the K.A. Timiryazev Institute of Plant Physiology (IPPRAS, Moscow, Russia) in the mid-to-late 20th century, laying the groundwork for successful cultivation of this species under controlled conditions. Led by Professor Raisa G. Butenko, the IPPRAS team pioneered the induction of stable cell lines in medicinal plants, including *Panax ginseng*, *Catharanthus roseus*, and *Dioscorea deltoidea*, providing both methodological and conceptual frameworks for subsequent research on lesser-known taxa such as *P. fruticosa* [32].

The first callus and suspension cultures of *P. fruticosa* were initiated using leaf explants from greenhouse-grown donor plants, stabilized aseptically, and incorporated into the All-Russian Collection of Plant Cell Cultures—one of the largest repositories of medicinal plant cell lines in Eastern Europe. Suspension cultures demonstrated stable biosynthesis of triterpenoid saponins, including polysciosides and their derivatives, with concentrations ranging from 0.5 to 3.0% dry weight. This capacity supports the pharmacological potential of *P. fruticosa* as an adaptogen and immunomodulator and reinforces its viability as a phytopharmaceutical alternative to *Panax* species [32].

The scale-up of cultures was achieved in 20 L and 75 L bubble-type bioreactors operated in semi-continuous regimes, ensuring reproducible biomass accumulation and maintaining metabolite productivity. Notably, two compounds—*Polyscias fruticosa* saponin (PFS) and ladyginoside A—were identified and quantified at concentrations of 0.91 $mg \cdot g^{-1}$ DW and 0.77 $mg \cdot g^{-1}$ DW, respectively, surpassing yields obtained in flask cultures [17]. The resulting biomass was utilized for phytopharmaceutical development, including the commercial adaptogen Vitagmal©, produced by SMC 'Biopharmtox', St. Petersburg, Russia, and introduced in Russia in the 1990s—one of the earliest examples of a semi-industrial product based on plant cell cultures [32,33].

To preserve biosynthetic competence and genetic stability, selected cell lines were cryopreserved in liquid nitrogen at −196 °C. Post-thaw recovery confirmed the retention of both metabolic competence and regenerative capacity, validating the IPPRAS cryobank as an effective model for preserving elite *P. fruticosa* genotypes [33].

Currently, *P. fruticosa* is one of the few Araliaceae species with comprehensively documented in vitro protocols, including callogenesis, suspension culture, bioreactor cultivation, and cryopreservation. These developments provide a robust platform for further studies in micropropagation, metabolite enhancement, and sustainable biomass production [17,33].

4.2. Biotechnological Strategies for In Vitro Culture of *Polyscias fruticosa*

In vitro culture techniques are fundamental tools in the biotechnological propagation, conservation, and phytochemical exploitation of medicinal plants. They enable year-round controlled biomass production, independent of environmental fluctuations, and are widely used in pharmaceutical and cosmetic applications [34]. Tissue culture enables the rapid, clonal propagation of selected genotypes and allows for the stabilization and enhancement of secondary metabolite production through elicitation and genetic transformation strategies [35]. Such methodologies are particularly relevant for slow-growing species, those with limited natural distribution, or taxa threatened by overharvesting, offering a sustainable and scalable alternative to conventional cultivation practices [34,36].

Polyscias fruticosa, a pharmacologically promising member of the Araliaceae family, has gained attention due to its rich content of bioactive secondary metabolites, particularly triterpenoid saponins. However, the traditional cultivation of this species is constrained by low biomass yield, poor seed germination rates, and an extended vegetative period, significantly limiting its applicability in industrial phytopharmaceutical production [17,22].

In vitro propagation systems represent a viable solution to these constraints, providing rapid, reproducible, and environmentally independent means of generating uniform plant material. These systems also facilitate metabolic studies and the targeted enhancement of pharmacologically relevant compounds through the use of biotic and abiotic elicitors. The present study reviews and compares the efficacy of the main regenerative strategies for *P. fruticose*—namely, somatic embryogenesis, adventitious root culture, and suspension culture—with particular emphasis on their applicability in phytochemical and pharmacognostic research.

4.2.1. In Vitro Regeneration of *Polyscias fruticosa*: Embryogenesis and Shoot Apices

Somatic embryogenesis remains a widely adopted method for clonal propagation in plant biotechnology [37,38]. Within the Araliaceae family, this technique has been successfully applied to species such as *Panax ginseng*, *Eleutherococcus senticosus*, and *Aralia elata* [35–38]. The process involves the differentiation of somatic cells into embryogenic structures that mimic the developmental stages of zygotic embryos—globular, heart-shaped, torpedo, and cotyledonary. The embryogenic transition can proceed directly from explants or indirectly through a callus phase, offering high regeneration efficiency and facilitating adaptation to bioreactor-based systems [39,40].

Meristem-based micropropagation utilizes shoot apices or axillary buds as explants and exploits the high mitotic activity and low differentiation status of meristematic tissues [41]. This approach allows for the rapid proliferation of genetically stable and pathogen-free plantlets, minimizing somaclonal variation and chimerism. It is particularly advantageous when maintaining clonal fidelity is essential for phytopharmaceutical applications.

Both somatic embryogenesis and meristematic propagation have proven effective for *P. fruticosa*, enabling the generation of uniform, high-quality explants for downstream metabolic and biotechnological applications [42].

Tram et al. [43] established an efficient protocol for somatic embryogenesis of *P. fruticosa* using leaf explants from two-year-old ex vitro plants. Callus induction was achieved on MS [44] medium with 0.3 mg·L^{-1} 2,4-D, 2.0 mg·L^{-1} BAP, and 7 mL/L coconut water. Subculturing onto MS medium with 0.5 mg·L^{-1} BAP and 100 mL/L CW resulted in a high embryogenesis rate (75.5%). Embryos developed into shoots on MS medium with 0.1 mg·L^{-1} kinetin and 150 mL/L CW, producing on average 6.3 shoots per explant.

These results indicate that the combination of BAP and CW is highly effective in promoting embryogenesis and shoot conversion, confirming the morphogenic potential of coconut-derived additives.

Phuong et al. [24] established embryogenic suspension cultures from leaf-derived calli in liquid MS medium with 2,4-D or NAA (0.5–2.0 mg·L^{-1}), achieving the highest biomass (5.7 g/flask) and somatic embryo yield (489/flask) at 1.5 mg·L^{-1} NAA. The occurrence of rhizogenic cells suggests a robust regeneration pathway combining embryogenesis and rooting.

Sakr et al. [23] developed a shoot-apex-based protocol for juvenile plants using B5 [45] medium enriched with BAP and kinetin, reaching up to 6.7 shoots per explant. Rooting on MS medium with 1.0 mg·L^{-1} NAA produced 6.42 cm long roots, with over 80% acclimatization success.

These protocols highlight the species' high regenerative plasticity and suggest that adjusting cytokinin/auxin ratios is key to optimizing micropropagation. This regenerative responsiveness underscores the biotechnological potential of *P. fruticosa*, enabling its application in efficient biomass propagation, metabolic profiling, and long-term conservation strategies.

A simplified micropropagation protocol was introduced by Pandya et al. [22], using MS medium supplemented only with kinetin (0.5 mg·L^{-1}). Shoot emergence occurred within 20 d, and the complete regeneration cycle—including elongation, rooting, and hardening—was achieved in 60 d. This method, by eliminating auxins and reducing hormonal inputs, shortened the production time compared to conventional 80 d systems and offers a cost-effective alternative for large-scale propagation. Its minimalistic design highlights the intrinsic morphogenetic potential of *P. fruticosa*, even under reduced hormonal stimulation.

Collectively, somatic embryogenesis and meristem-based propagation strategies offer robust platforms for the rapid and standardized production of *P. fruticosa* plantlets. These plantlets can be used for callus induction, genetic transformation, elicitor studies, and secondary metabolite production. Meanwhile, meristematic approaches remain critical for maintaining genetic fidelity, eliminating pathogens, and ensuring consistency in phytopharmaceutical applications.

In the authors' view, these complementary strategies fulfill both research and industrial objectives: while embryogenic systems are suited for scalable production and bioreactor implementation, meristem culture offers quality assurance for pharmaceutical-grade propagation. The integration of both approaches is essential for ensuring efficient, reproducible, and sustainable exploitation of *P. fruticosa* in modern biotechnology.

4.2.2. Adventitious Root Cultures of *Polyscias fruticosa*: Induction, Optimization, and Saponin Production

The induction of callus and regeneration of adventitious roots constitute essential in vitro techniques for obtaining root-derived organs capable of synthesizing secondary metabolites of pharmacological relevance, especially when full-plant regeneration is not necessary [46–49]. Callus, as an undifferentiated tissue, can be hormonally directed towards root morphogenesis using specific auxins, such as 2,4-dichlorophenoxyacetic acid (2,4-D), indole-3-acetic acid (IAA), indole-3-butyric acid (IBA), or α-naphthaleneacetic acid (NAA), either individually or in combination with cytokinins [50–52].

Root cultures offer the opportunity to apply elicitation strategies that enhance secondary metabolite biosynthesis via biochemically induced stress responses. Elicitors such as jasmonic acid (JA), yeast extract (YE), or mannitol activate cellular defense mechanisms and stimulate the accumulation of bioactive compounds, providing a promising approach for the optimized production of high-value phytochemicals [50,53–55].

In the case of *P. fruticosa*, this approach is particularly relevant, as roots are the primary site of biosynthesis and storage of triterpenoid saponins a class of compounds known for their anti-inflammatory, cytotoxic, and antihyperglycemic properties [56,57]. However, their natural concentration is relatively low, and the plant's cultivation cycle spans three to five years, rendering conventional harvesting economically inefficient [22,58,59].

In the study by Lộc et al. [60], adventitious roots were induced from leaf explants of three-year-old greenhouse-grown *P. fruticosa* plants. The explants were cultured on MS medium supplemented with 2,4-D at concentrations ranging from 0 to 4.0 mg·L^{-1}. The highest callus induction rate (100%) was observed at 2.0 mg·L^{-1} 2,4-D. After four weeks, the resulting calli were transferred to MS medium containing 1.0 mg·L^{-1} IBA and 0.1 mg·L^{-1} NAA, which promoted robust root formation. The induction and development of roots followed a two-step protocol involving auxin-specific stimulation for morphogenic differentiation. Qualitative analysis confirmed the presence of saponins in the in vitro-derived roots, with a dry weight content of 1.67%, corresponding to 83.5% of the concentration found in field-grown roots (1.99%). The identification of saponins was conducted using phytochemical tests and gravimetric analysis.

Subsequently, Le et al. [12] evaluated the effects of three elicitors—JA, YE, and mannitol—on secondary metabolite production in *P. fruticosa* adventitious root cultures. Roots obtained through NAA-induced rhizogenesis (2.0 mg·L^{-1}) were transferred to media supplemented with varying concentrations of elicitors: JA (0.5, 1.0, and 2.5 mM), YE (100, 300, and 500 mg·L^{-1}), and mannitol (50, 100, and 150 mM). The highest total saponin content (167.19 ± 3.29 mg·L^{-1} extract, expressed as aescin equivalents) was recorded in cultures treated with 2.5 mM JA, representing more than a threefold increase compared to the control (54.08 mg·L^{-1}) and surpassing the levels found in wild-type roots (137.37 mg·L^{-1}). Saponins were extracted using ethanol-based solvent systems and quantified spectrophotometrically via vanillin–sulfuric acid assay.

These results demonstrate that elicitation of *P. fruticosa* root cultures significantly enhances the biosynthesis of triterpenoid saponins, offering an efficient and reproducible system for the scaled production of pharmacologically valuable compounds.

This approach ensures metabolic stability of the root system in vitro, reduces production time, and may serve as an ecologically and economically viable alternative to field cultivation.

4.2.3. Cell Suspension Cultures of *Polyscias fruticosa*: Optimization, Bioreactor Scaling, and Production of Bioactive Triterpenoids

Plant cell suspension cultures offer a controlled and scalable system for the production of high-value secondary metabolites. Typically initiated from friable callus derived from explants, these cultures are maintained in agitated liquid MS-based media under regulated temperature and photoperiod conditions. Agitation and aeration ensure uniform cell proliferation and support metabolite biosynthesis, independent of environmental fluctuations [61]. This approach has been validated in numerous medicinal plants, including *Taxus* spp., *Panax* spp., and *Catharanthus roseus*, for the production of taxanes, ginsenosides, and alkaloids, respectively [62,63]. Suspension cultures provide high reproducibility and process standardization, while allowing the synthesis of both native and novel compounds via metabolic reprogramming [63].

Nevertheless, these systems face certain limitations, such as genetic instability, low metabolite yields, and microbial contamination. Optimization strategies—such as the selection of productive cell lines, modulation of plant growth regulators, elicitor treatments, and bioreactor scaling—have been employed to overcome these challenges. Within the Araliaceae family, *Polyscias fruticosa* has emerged as a promising candidate for cell suspension culture due to its ability to biosynthesize bioactive triterpenoid saponins [62,63].

In an early study, Kim et al. [25] established a suspension culture from 30 d-old stem-derived callus. Cultures were maintained in MS medium with 30 g·L^{-1} sucrose, 1.0 mg·L^{-1} BAP, and 0.5 mg·L^{-1} 2,4-D under a 12 h/12 h light/dark cycle at 25 ± 2 °C and 120 rpm. After 16 days, dry biomass reached 0.43 g per flask (a 3.7-fold increase), and oleanolic acid accumulated to 25.4 mg·L^{-1}, nearly five times higher than in in vitro leaves (5.2 mg/g DW) [25]. Further experiments by the same group [26] revealed that sucrose (30 g·L^{-1}) outperformed other carbon sources in biomass promotion, while elicitors like yeast extract and silver nitrate induced a shift towards secondary metabolism at the expense of biomass. This suggests that a trade-off exists between growth and metabolite accumulation, which must be optimized depending on the intended application. In comparative studies, the application of malonyl ginsenosides (M-GS) as elicitors in two cell lines—6a (*P. fruticosa*) and VDK (*P. filicifolia*)—revealed contrasting responses [27]. The 6a line showed a 79.7% increase in polyscioside E and a 70.7% rise in ladyginoside A, despite a ~45% reduction in biomass. In contrast, the VDK line exhibited lower biomass, but a 63.3% increase in only polyscioside A, highlighting cell-line-specific responses.

Scalability was demonstrated by Titova et al. [17], who used a 20 L bubble-type bioreactor operated semi-continuously. Peak biomass reached 6.8 g·L^{-1} DW, with productivity of 0.32 g·L^{-1}·d^{-1}and over 70% cell viability. Saponin content significantly increased: PFS (3-O-[β-D-glucopyranosyl-(1→4)-β-D-glucuronopyranosyl] oleanolic acid 28-O-β-D-glucopyranosyl ester) reached 0.91 mg·L^{-1} DW (82% higher than in flask cultures), while ladyginoside A reached 0.77 mg·L^{-1} DW (3.5-fold increase). The extracts exhibited antimicrobial activity (MIC = 250–2000 µg·mL^{-1}) against *Staphylococcus aureus*, MRSA, *Pseudomonas aeruginosa*, and *Escherichia coli*, outperforming leaf-derived extracts (MIC = 4000 µg·mL^{-1}). Antioxidant activity was also confirmed via DPPH and TEAC assays, indicating the retention of pharmacologically active compounds under in vitro conditions [17].

The suspension culture system of *P. fruticosa* provides a biotechnologically robust platform for triterpenoid saponin production, with documented scalability and responsiveness to elicitation. The observed trade-off between growth and metabolite synthesis, alongside cell-line-specific metabolic behavior, underlines the need for tailored optimization. Bioreactor systems, when properly configured, enhance both productivity and phytochemical enrichment, positioning *P. fruticosa* as a viable candidate for pharmaceutical-scale bioproduction.

4.3. In Vitro Propagation and Phytoremediation Potential of Polyscias fruticosa

Beyond its pharmacological significance, *P. fruticosa* exhibits notable potential for phytoremediation, particularly in the detoxification of heavy metals from contaminated environments. A comparative study by Pandya et al. [64] demonstrated that plants regenerated through in vitro methods accumulate significantly higher levels of lead (Pb) and cadmium (Cd) than conventionally propagated (in vivo) specimens.

In this study, in vitro-derived plants were obtained via a shoot apex micropropagation protocol using apical meristems cultured on Murashige and Skoog (MS) medium supplemented solely with 0.5 mg·L^{-1} kinetin, without the addition of auxins. This simplified, hormone-restricted protocol enabled the generation of genetically uniform and physiologically vigorous plantlets. Following in vitro rooting and successful acclimatization, the plants were transplanted to Pb- and Cd-contaminated soils to assess phytoremediation capacity.

At the highest tested soil concentration of Pb (800 mg·kg^{-1}), in vitro-propagated plants accumulated 1420 mg·kg^{-1} in roots and 979 in leaves, compared to 1331 and 667, respectively, in in vivo-grown controls. Similarly, for Cd, in vitro-derived plants exhibited greater accumulation (89.09 in roots and 33.33 in leaves) than in vivo plants (80.81 and 23.13, respectively).

These results suggest that the superior phytoremediation performance of in vitro-regenerated plants may be due to their increased uniformity, higher metabolic rates, and greater physiological adaptability under stress conditions. Moreover, tissue-culture-derived lines may be selectively enriched or genetically engineered to further improve metal tolerance and detoxification efficiency.

Given the global urgency of remediating heavy-metal-polluted soils and the scalable nature of micropropagation systems, *P. fruticosa* represents a viable candidate for eco-friendly biotechnological applications. Its potential applicability in post-industrial soil recovery, urban ecological restoration, and as part of phytoprotective green infrastructure highlights the need for further investigation.

4.4. Author's Perspective and Future Directions

The accumulated data confirm that *Polyscias fruticosa* exhibits remarkable morphogenetic plasticity across diverse in vitro systems, including somatic embryogenesis, shoot apex-based micropropagation, adventitious root cultures, and cell suspension cultures. This developmental versatility enables both rapid clonal propagation and targeted biosynthesis of pharmacologically active secondary metabolites, particularly triterpenoid saponins [12,17,22,24–27].

Among these strategies, somatic embryogenesis and meristem-based protocols ensure the highest genetic stability, making them ideal for transformation, virus elimination, and germplasm conservation. In contrast, adventitious root and suspension cultures offer rapidly proliferating undifferentiated biomass suitable for elicitor-driven secondary metabolism and phytopharmaceutical production [17,23–25].

Comparative elicitation studies highlight the complementary potential of these systems. Adventitious root cultures treated with 2.5 mM jasmonic acid (JA) achieved the highest saponin content (167.19 mg·L^{-1}), exceeding that of both untreated and wild-type roots. Meanwhile, suspension cultures maintained in 20 L bioreactors demonstrated superior biomass accumulation (6.8 g·L^{-1} DW) and elevated yields of individual saponins, such as PFS (0.91 mg·g^{-1} DW) and ladyginoside A (0.77 mg·g^{-1} DW), outperforming conventional flask cultures [12,17]. These findings suggest that adventitious roots respond more strongly to elicitation, while suspension cultures are better suited for upscaling and process optimization under bioreactor conditions.

Despite these promising outcomes, key knowledge gaps remain. The molecular mechanisms underlying saponin biosynthesis, hormonal signaling, and elicitor-induced responses in *P. fruticosa* have yet to be elucidated. To date, no transcriptomic, metabolomic, or proteomic analyses have been conducted for any in vitro culture type of this species. Furthermore, there is a lack of direct comparative analyses of metabolite profiles between adventitious roots and suspension cultures using harmonized extraction procedures and chromatographic parameters. Additionally, the long-term genetic and metabolic stability of in vitro-derived lines, particularly under elicitor treatment or bioreactor conditions, requires further assessment.

Future research should prioritize the following directions:

- The integration of transcriptomic, metabolomic, and proteomic analyses to unravel biosynthetic regulatory networks;
- The optimization of culture parameters using metabolic modeling, combinatorial elicitation, and environmental stimuli (e.g., light, temperature);
- Comparative profiling of triterpenoid production across culture types and elicitation regimes;
- The evaluation of genetic and biochemical stability under long-term and large-scale in vitro propagation.

For industrial translation, both adventitious root and suspension cultures should be scaled up in air-lift or stirred-tank bioreactors, coupled with life-cycle assessment (LCA) and techno-economic analysis. This would facilitate the standardized, sustainable production of targeted saponins with validated pharmacological properties, potentially reducing dependence on wild or field-grown biomass.

From an applied perspective, *P. fruticosa* also emerges as a promising candidate for phytoremediation. In vitro-regenerated plants demonstrated enhanced accumulation of heavy metals such as lead and cadmium, underscoring their dual function as both phytopharmaceutical and environmental bioresources [65]. Ultimately, integrating micropropagation with metabolic engineering and stress conditioning may unlock the full biotechnological value of this underutilized Araliaceae species.

5. Chemical Composition and Structural Diversity of Bioactive Compounds in *Polyscias fruticosa*

5.1. Triterpenoid Saponins

Triterpenoid saponins are a class of glycosidic secondary metabolites derived from pentacyclic triterpenes such as oleanolic acid and are widely distributed across the Araliaceae family. These compounds exhibit a broad spectrum of pharmacological activities, including anti-inflammatory, antidiabetic, immunomodulatory, cytotoxic, and neuroprotective effects, which are largely attributed to their amphipathic structures that enable interactions with cellular membranes, enzymes, and signaling pathways [65–68]. Their relevance in drug discovery has gained particular attention due to their potential application as natural therapeutics or adjuvants in the treatment of metabolic, inflammatory, and oncological disorders [65]. In *P. fruticosa*, triterpenoid saponins constitute the dominant class of bioactive constituents, and their structural diversity provides a valuable basis for both pharmacological evaluation and biotechnological exploitation. Importantly, selected saponins have demonstrated immunostimulatory or antimicrobial properties, reinforcing their therapeutic value.

5.1.1. Contextual Account of Triterpenoid Saponin Discovery in *Polyscias fruticosa*

The presence of triterpenoid saponins in *P. fruticosa* was first reported in the mid-1990s, marking a key milestone in the phytochemical exploration of this species (Table 1). In 1995, Chaboud and colleagues isolated a saponin from the leaves of *P. fruticosa*, identified as 3-O-[β-D-galactopyranosyl-(1→2)-β-D-glucuronopyranosyl] oleanolic acid [69]. This compound was characterized as a monodesmosidic saponin, featuring a disaccharide chain at the C-3 position of the oleanolic acid aglycone and lacking substitution at the C-28 position. Its structure confirmed the occurrence of oleanane-type saponins, which are typical for members of the Araliaceae family. The predominance of oleanane-type structures among the saponins isolated from *P. fruticosa* confirms its chemotaxonomic affiliation with other medicinally relevant Araliaceae species such as *Panax* and *Aralia*. The presence of shared compounds (e.g., chikusetsusaponin IVa) further supports this classification.

Table 1. Summary of triterpenoid glycosides isolated from roots, leaves, and in vitro cultures of *P. fruticosa*.

No.	Trivial Name	Systematic Name	Molecular Formula	Molecular Weight [g/mol]	Plant Source	Identification Method	Ref.
1	-	3-O-[β-D-galactopyranosyl-(1→2)-β-D-glucuronopyranosyl] oleanolic acid	$C_{42}H_{66}O_{14}$	794.44	Leaves	FAB, MS (negative)	[69]
2	-	3-O-[α-L-rhamnopyranosyl-(1→4)-β-D-glucuronopyranosyl]28-O-β-D-glucopyranosyl oleanolic acid	$C_{48}H_{76}O_{19}$	940	Leaves (yellow variety)	FAB, MS (negative)	[5]
3	Polyscioside A	3-O-(β-D-glucopyranosyl-(1→2)-β-D-glucopyranosyl-(1→4)-β-D-glucuronopyranosyl) oleanolic acid	$C_{48}H_{76}O_{19}$	956.49	Leaves, roots	HR FAB-MS (negative), NMR	[3]
4	Polyscioside B	3-O-[α-L-arabinopyranosyl-(1→4)-β-D-glucopyranosyl-(1→2)-β-D-glucuronopyranosyl] oleanolic acid	$C_{47}H_{74}O_{18}$	926.47	Roots	HR FAB-MS (negative), NMR	[3]
5	Polyscioside C	3-O-[β-D-galactopyranosyl-(1→2)-β-D-glucopyranosyl-(1→3)-β-D-glucuronopyranosyl] oleanolic acid	$C_{48}H_{76}O_{19}$	956.49	Roots	HR-FAB-MS (negative), NMR	[3]
6	Polyscioside D	3-O-[β-D-glucopyranosyl-(1→2)-[β-D-glucopyranosyl-(1→4)]-β-D-glucuronopyranosyl]- oleanolic acid 28-O-β-D-glucopyranosyl ester	$C_{54}H_{86}O_{24}$	1118.54	Leaves, roots	HR FAB-MS (negative), NMR	[3]
7	Polyscioside E	3-O-[α-L-arabinopyranosyl-(1→4)-[β-D-glucopyranosyl-(1→2)]-β-D-glucuronopyranosyl]oleanolic acid 28-O-β-D-glucopyranosyl ester	$C_{53}H_{84}O_{23}$	1088.53	Roots	HR FAB-MS (negative), NMR	[3]
8	Polyscioside F	3-O-[β-D-galactopyranosyl-(1→2)-[β-D-glucopyranosyl-(1→3)]-β-D-glucuronopyranosyl] oleanolic acid 28-O-β-D-glucopyranosyl ester	$C_{54}H_{86}O_{24}$	1118.54	Leaves	HR FAB-MS (negative), NMR	[3]
9	Polyscioside G	3-O-[β-D-glucopyranosyl-(1→4)-β-D-glucuronopyranosyl]oleanolic acid 28-O-α-L-rhamnopyranosyl-(1→3)-β-D-glucopyranosyl ester	$C_{54}H_{86}O_{23}$	1102.55	Leaves	HR FAB-MS (negative), NMR	[3]
10	Polyscioside H	3-O-[β-D-glucopyranosyl-(1→4)-β-D-glucopyranosyl-(1→2)-β-D-glucuronopyranosyl] oleanolic acid 28-O-α-L-rhamnopyranosyl-(1→3)-β-D-glucopyranosyl ester	$C_{60}H_{96}O_{28}$	1264.65	Leaves	HR FAB-MS (negative), NMR	[3]

Table 1. *Cont.*

No.	Trivial Name	Systematic Name	Molecular Formula	Molecular Weight [g/mol]	Plant Source	Identification Method	Ref.
11	Ladyginoside A (calendulaglycoside E)	3-*O*-[*β*-D-glucopyranosyl (1-4)-*β*-D-glucuronopyranosyl] oleanolic acid	$C_{42}H_{66}O_{14}$	794.44	Leaves, cell suspension culture	UPLC-ESI-MS	[3]
12	Zingibroside R1	3-*O*-[*β*-D-glucopyranosyl (1-2)-*β*-D-glucuronopyranosyl] oleanolic acid	$C_{42}H_{66}O_{14}$	794.44	Leaves	NMR, MS	[3]
13	Saponin PFS	3-O-[*β*-D-glucopyranosyl-(1→4)-*β*-D-glucuronopyranosyl] oleanolic acid 28-O-*β*-D-glucopyranosyl ester	$C_{48}H_{76}O_{19}$	956.49	Leaves, root, cell suspension culture	HR-ESI-MS (negative)	[3,57]
14	-	oleanolic acid-28-O-*β*-D-glucopyranosyl-D-glucopyranosyl-rhamnopyranoside		926	Leaves, roots	ESI-MS, NMR	[6]
15	-	3-O-*α*-L-arabinopyranosyl-oleanolic acid-28-O-*β*-D-glucopyranosyl-D-glucopyranosyl-rhamnopyranoside		1058	Leaves, roots	ESI-MS, NMR	[6]
16	Polyscioside I	3-O-[*β*-D-glucopyranosyl-(1→2)-[*β*-D-glucopyranosyl-(1→4)]-*β*-D-glucuronopyranosyl] oleanolic acid 28-O-*β*-D-glucopyranosyl-(1→2)-*β*-D-galactopyranosyl ester	$C_{60}H_{97}O_{29}$	1280.61	Leaves	HR ESI-MS, NMR	[14]
17	Polyscioside J	3-O-[*β*-D-glucopyranosyl-(1→4)]-β-D-(6-O-methyl)glucuronopyranosyl] oleanolic acid 28-O-*β*-D-glucopyranosyl ester	$C_{49}H_{78}O_{19}$	970.50	Leaves	HR ESI-MS (negative)	[7]
18	Polyscioside K	3-O-[*β*-D-glucopyranosyl-(1→4), β-D-glucopyranosyl-(1→2)]-*β*-D-(6-O-methyl)glucuronopyranosyl] oleanolic acid	$C_{49}H_{78}O_{19}$	970.50	Leaves	HR-ESI-MS (negative)	[7]
19	Chikusetsusaponin IVa	3-*O*-[*β*-D-glucuronopyranosyl] oleanolic acid 28-*O*-*β*-D-glucopyranosyl ester	$C_{42}H_{66}O_{14}$	794.44	Leaves	NMR, MS	[7]

HR FAB-MS—high-resolution fast atom bombardment mass spectrometry; NMR—nuclear magnetic resonance.

In 1996, Proliac et al. [5] reported the isolation of another oleanane-type saponin from the yellow-leaved variant of *P. fruticosa*, structurally identified as 3-O-[α-L-rhamnopyranosyl-(1→4)-β-D-glucuronopyranosyl]-28-O-β-D-glucopyranosyl oleanolic acid. Unlike the compound described by Chaboud et al. [69], this saponin exhibited a bisdesmosidic structure, with glycosidic substitutions at both the C-3 and C-28 positions of the aglycone, a feature commonly observed in Araliaceae saponins.

A major advancement occurred in 1998, when Vo Duy Huan and colleagues conducted a comprehensive phytochemical analysis of *P. fruticosa* leaf and root extracts, resulting in the isolation of eleven triterpenoid saponins [3]. Eight of these were novel compounds, designated polysciosides A–H. All were based on oleanolic acid aglycones and exhibited bisdesmosidic structures with varying sugar compositions and glycosidic linkages. Several of these novel saponins were subsequently reported to exhibit cytotoxicity against tumor cell lines or antioxidant potential. The structural variation among polysciosides A–H, particularly the nature and position of sugar moieties, is likely to influence membrane interaction and bioactivity, although systematic structure–activity relationship (SAR) studies are still lacking.

The remaining three compounds had previously been reported: ladyginoside A from *Ladyginia bucharica* [70], zingibroside R1 from *Panax zingiberensis* [3], and a compound later referred to as PFS (*Polyscias fruticosa* saponin), originally isolated from *Swartzia simplex* and identified as 3-O-[β-D-glucopyranosyl-(1→4)-β-D-glucuronopyranosyl] oleanolic acid 28-O-β-D-glucopyranosyl ester [71].

In 2003, Divakar and co-workers [6] isolated two additional novel saponins: oleanolic acid-28-O-β-D-glucopyranosyl-D-glucopyranosyl-rhamnopyranoside and 3-O-α-L-arabinopyranosyl-oleanolic acid-28-O-β-D-glucopyranosyl-D-glucopyranosyl-rhamnopyranoside. Although the linkages between sugar moieties were not fully elucidated, both compounds demonstrated significant immunostimulatory activity. They enhanced the phagocytic activity of leukocytes against *Candida albicans* in vitro and stimulated carbon clearance in mice. Importantly, neither compound exhibited toxicity in brine shrimp lethality assays (LC_{50} > 800 $\mu g \cdot mL^{-1}$) or in acute oral toxicity tests in Swiss albino mice at doses up to 1.5 g kg^{-1} body weight. These findings suggest that the immunomodulatory effects of certain saponins from *P. fruticosa* may be mediated through enhanced phagocytic responses and macrophage activation, although mechanistic studies at the molecular level remain to be conducted.

Since 2010, research has focused on expanding the inventory of triterpenoid saponins in *P. fruticosa*, aided by advances in chromatographic and spectroscopic techniques such as high-performance liquid chromatography (HPLC), gel filtration, high-resolution mass spectrometry (HR-MS), and multidimensional NMR spectroscopy. These modern approaches have improved structure elucidation and supported pharmacokinetic evaluations. However, no pharmacokinetic or bioavailability studies have yet been reported for individual *P. fruticosa* saponins in vivo, which limits their translational potential.

In 2016, Tran et al. [14] isolated three bisdesmosidic saponins from *P. fruticosa* leaves, including a novel compound designated as polyscioside I, which displayed the characteristic Araliaceae glycosylation pattern at both the C-3 and C-28 positions.

Further discoveries by Do et al. in 2020 [7] led to the isolation of four saponins from the leaves, two of which were newly identified and named polyscioside J and polyscioside K. Notably, this study also confirmed—for the first time—the presence of chikusetsusaponin IVa in *P. fruticosa*, a compound previously reported in *Panax ginseng*, thereby reinforcing the chemotaxonomic relationship between *P. fruticosa* and other medicinally important genera of the Araliaceae family [8].

To date, at least 19 triterpenoid saponins have been isolated and structurally characterized from *P. fruticosa*. This group includes both unique compounds and saponins shared with other Araliaceae species, providing a robust foundation for future pharmacological and biotechnological investigations. However, the biosynthetic pathways responsible for this diversity remain poorly characterized, and the correlation between specific structures and bioactivities has yet to be systematically explored. Further studies integrating metabolomics and enzymatic profiling are warranted to clarify these relationships.

Despite the growing inventory of saponins in *P. fruticosa*, their pharmacological relevance remains underexplored in preclinical models. Most reports are limited to in vitro assays, and few compounds have been tested for toxicity, bioavailability, or efficacy in animal systems. A systematic evaluation of their immunomodulatory and cytotoxic properties, particularly for bisdesmosidic saponins, could identify promising therapeutic leads. Furthermore, understanding how glycosylation patterns influence biological activity may guide future efforts in semi-synthetic modification and metabolic engineering.

5.1.2. Extraction Strategies for Triterpenoid Saponins

Given the therapeutic relevance of triterpenoid saponins, considerable efforts have been made to develop efficient extraction methods for *P. fruticosa* plant material. Aqueous ethanol-based protocols remain standard, but recent innovations offer greater selectivity and sustainability.

Among these, ultrasound-assisted extraction (UAE) has demonstrated notable efficacy. Khoang et al. [58] applied UAE in combination with response surface methodology (RSM) to optimize the recovery of saponins from *P. fruticosa* roots. Under optimal conditions, i.e., 60 °C, 60% ethanol, 65 min, and 180 W ultrasonic power, the total saponin yield reached 14.5% of the dry root mass, and the extract contained approximately 41 $mg \cdot g^{-1}$ of saponins. The extract showed cytotoxicity against A549, HepG2, PC-3, and HeLa cell lines.

In a complementary study, Chuyen et al. [72] evaluated the influence of extraction parameters on both saponin recovery and antioxidant activity. Extraction with 40% ethanol at 50 °C for 90 min, using a solvent-to-solid ratio of 40:1, resulted in high yields of saponins and co-extracted phenolic compounds. The obtained extracts demonstrated enhanced antioxidant capacity, suggesting saponin–polyphenol synergy.

Such optimization supports both pharmacological efficacy and product standardization.

5.1.3. Pharmacological Potential of *Polyscias fruticosa* Saponins

Numerous pharmacological studies have validated the traditional uses of *P. fruticosa* and demonstrated the broad spectrum of biological activities exerted by its triterpenoid saponins [4,6,7,14,16,17]. One of the most extensively studied compounds is PFS, identified as 3-O-[β-D-glucopyranosyl-(1→4)-β-D-glucuronopyranosyl] oleanolic acid 28-O-β-D-glucopyranosyl ester (**13**). This saponin exhibited significant inhibitory activity against key carbohydrate-hydrolyzing enzymes: porcine pancreatic α-amylase (IC_{50} = 27.1 $\mu g \cdot mL^{-1}$, ~21.2 μM) and yeast α-glucosidase (IC_{50} = 440.5 $\mu g \cdot mL^{-1}$, ~344 μM) [4,57]. In vivo, oral administration of PFS at a dose of 100 $mg \cdot kg^{-1}$ significantly reduced postprandial blood glucose levels in mice subjected to an oral sucrose tolerance test, resulting in decreases of 16.6% at 30 min and 27.9% at 60 min, along with a reduced area under the curve ($AUC_{0–120}$ min) compared to controls [57]. These results confirm its potential in metabolic disorder management.

Another triterpenoid saponin identified in *P. fruticosa* is chikusetsusaponin IVa (**19**) [7], a compound with well-documented pharmacological activity. It possesses anti-inflammatory properties by suppressing the nuclear factor kappa B (NF-κB) signaling pathway and inhibiting activation of the NOD-like receptor protein 3 (NLRP3) inflammasome, leading to reduced expression of pro-inflammatory mediators such as TNF-α, IL-6, COX-2, and iNOS [73–76]. Under oxidative stress conditions, it enhances endogenous antioxidant defenses by upregulating superoxide dismutase (SOD), glutathione (GSH), and catalase (CAT), thereby mitigating cellular oxidative damage [74,75]. It also exerts significant antihyperglycemic effects by activating AMP-activated protein kinase (AMPK), which promotes glucose uptake and fatty acid oxidation via increased GLUT4 translocation and CPT-1 activation in insulin-resistant skeletal muscle cells [75,76]. In metabolic dysfunction models induced by high-fat diets, chikusetsusaponin IVa improves insulin sensitivity, regulates lipid profiles, and modulates macrophage polarization in adipose tissue [73,75].

Moreover, chikusetsusaponin IVa exhibits anticancer activity by inducing cell cycle arrest and apoptosis, suppressing metastasis-related pathways such as Wnt/β-catenin and IL-6/STAT3, and inhibiting matrix metalloproteinases (MMP-2 and MMP-9) [75]. It also demonstrates neuroprotective and cardioprotective effects through activation of SIRT1 and ERK1/2 pathways, reduction in ROS, and maintenance of mitochondrial function [75]. Its confirmed occurrence in *P. fruticosa* highlights its relevance and warrants further mechanistic research.

In addition to individual saponins, saponin-rich extracts from *P. fruticosa* have exhibited notable pharmacological effects. Despite this, polysciosides J (**17**) and K (**18**) alone showed low cytotoxicity, whereas saponin-enriched extracts were active against cancer cells, likely due to synergy with polyphenols [7]. These results support the potential therapeutic advantage of standardized phytocomplexes and encourage further in vivo and mechanistic studies.

Extracts derived from *P. fruticosa* suspension cell cultures grown in bubble-type bioreactors, containing triterpenoid saponins such as PFS and ladyginoside A (**11**), demonstrated potent antibacterial activity. In vitro assays revealed inhibitory effects against *Escherichia coli*, *Staphylococcus aureus*, and *Candida albicans*, with minimum inhibitory concentrations (MICs) of 250, 500, and 500 $\mu g \cdot mL^{-1}$, respectively [17]. The MIC for *E. coli* was markedly lower than that of extracts from greenhouse-grown leaves (MIC = 4000 $\mu g \cdot mL^{-1}$), suggesting enhanced antimicrobial potential of in vitro-derived biomass. The presence of saponins supports their contribution to antimicrobial activity.

Zingibroside R1 (**12**) is another confirmed oleanane-type saponin in *P. fruticosa*. In a *Caenorhabditis elegans* model, it demonstrated antioxidant and anti-aging properties by reducing intracellular ROS levels, enhancing locomotion, increasing resistance to oxidative and thermal stress, and extending lifespan [77]. In vitro, it inhibited glucose uptake in tumor cells and showed cytotoxicity against MT-4 human T-lymphocytes and Ehrlich ascites tumor cells ($IC_{50} \approx 91$ μM) [78]. Antiviral activity against HIV-1 was also reported at subtoxic concentrations, with greater efficacy than glycyrrhizin [78]. In silico analyses using PASS software (version 2019) predicted high probabilities for antioxidant (Pa = 0.829), free radical scavenging (Pa = 0.411), and antihypoxic activity (Pa = 0.378), while PharmaExpert software was used to analyze possible synergistic or additive effects of these phytoconstituents [78]. Further predictions suggest neuroprotection via various mechanisms, including lipid peroxidation inhibition and NGF agonism [79]. These multifaceted effects justify further pharmaceutical investigation of Zingibroside R1.

From a pharmacotechnical perspective, the chemical stability of triterpenoid saponins is a crucial factor affecting extract quality. Le et al. [80] demonstrated that storage temperature significantly influences the integrity of ethanol extracts from *P. fruticosa* leaves. After 30 d, samples stored at 5 °C retained over 90% of their initial saponin content, whereas those stored at 30 °C and 60 °C exhibited reductions of 29.65 and 57.82%, respectively. These losses were accompanied by proportional declines in antioxidant activity, confirming that elevated storage temperatures accelerate saponin degradation and diminish biological efficacy. Therefore, cold storage is essential to maintain extract quality and efficacy.

5.1.4. Proposed Biosynthetic Pathway of Triterpenoid Saponins (TSBP) in *Polyscias fruticosa*

Based on the available literature and comparative analyses, a complete triterpenoid saponin biosynthetic pathway (TSBP) is proposed here for the first time in *P. fruticosa* (Figure 3). This reconstruction integrates structural and biochemical data from closely related Araliaceae species, such as *Aralia elata* [81], *Aralia spinosa* [82], and *Panax ginseng* [83].

In *P. fruticosa*, the TSBP proceeds via the canonical cytosolic mevalonate (MVA) pathway, yielding isopentenyl diphosphate (IPP) and dimethylallyl diphosphate (DMAPP) as key isoprenoid precursors. Their condensation forms farnesyl pyrophosphate (FPP), which dimerizes to squalene. Oxidation by squalene epoxidase generates 2,3-oxidosqualene, which is cyclized by β-amyrin synthase into β-amyrin, the oleanane-type triterpenoid core predominant in this species [84]. This reaction is catalyzed by oxidosqualene cyclases (OSCs), which determine the aglycone skeleton; in *P. fruticosa*, β-amyrin predominates, whereas dammarane- and ursane-type skeletons dominate in *Panax* and *Centella*, respectively [84].

Further oxidation at the C-28 position, likely catalyzed by cytochrome P450 monooxygenases from the CYP716 subfamily, converts β-amyrin to oleanolic acid (OA), the principal sapogenin in *P. fruticosa* [83]. This step mirrors CYP716A12 and CYP716A94 catalysis in *Medicago* and *Kalopanax*, and may involve CYP716A52v2-like or CYP716A75-like enzymes [83].

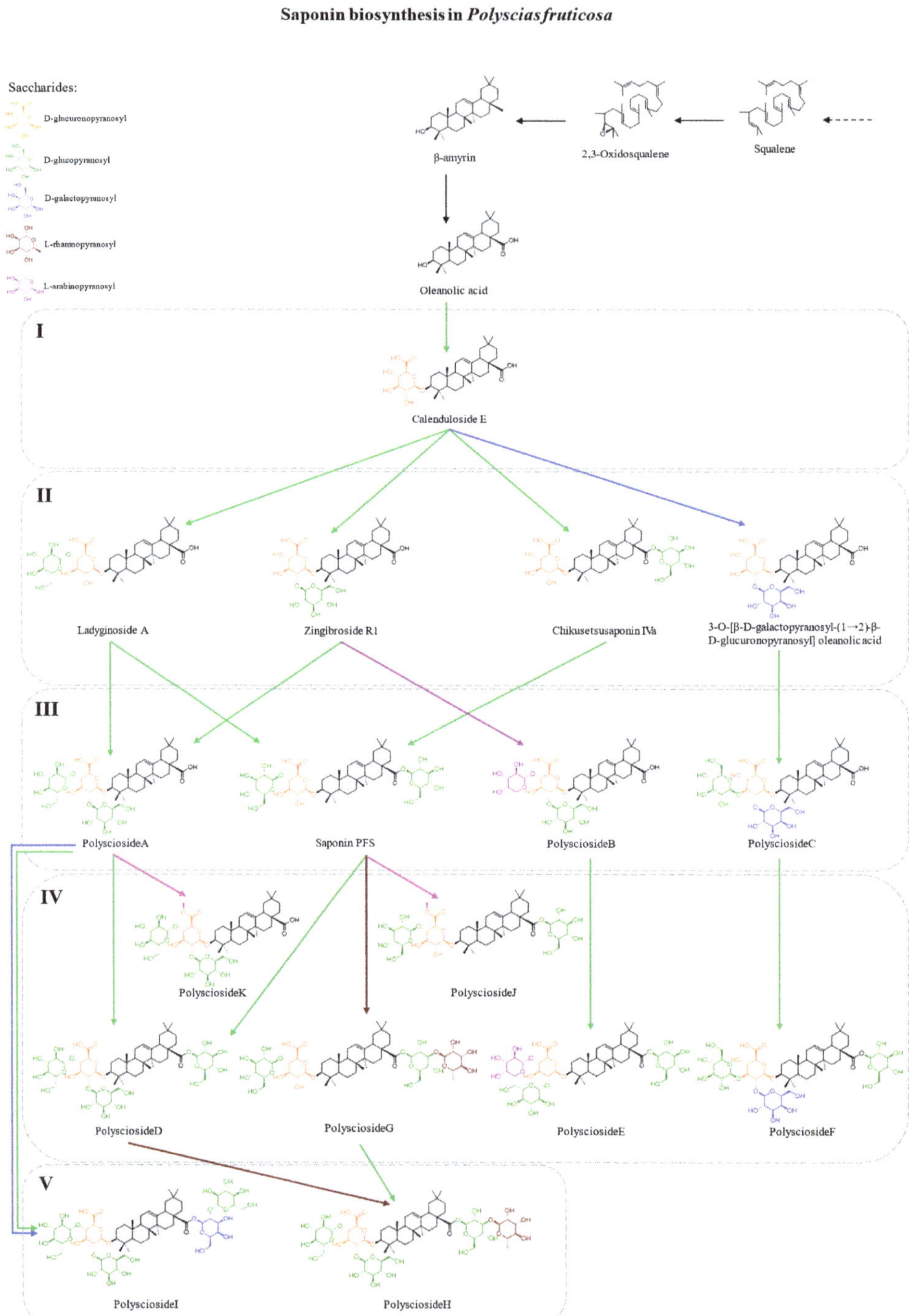

Figure 3. Proposed biosynthetic pathway of triterpenoid saponins in *Polyscias fruticosa*.

Subsequent glycosylation steps are catalyzed by UDP-dependent glycosyltransferases (UGTs), incorporating saccharides such as pentoses (L-arabinopyranosyl, Ara), deoxyhexoses (L-rhamnopyranosyl, Rha), hexoses (D-glucopyranosyl, Glc; D-galactopyranosyl, Gal), and uronic acids (D-glucuronopyranosyl, GluA). Sugar chains are typically attached at the C-3 hydroxyl and C-28 carboxyl groups. UGTs implicated in these reactions may include members of the UGT73, UGT74, and UGT94 subfamilies, as demonstrated in other Araliaceae. Initial glucosylation at C-3 is often followed by sugar branching at O-2, O-3, or O-4 of the glycosidic residues [83,84].

The proposed TSBP comprises five sequential stages of glycosylation and methylation, culminating in the structurally diverse array of saponins found in *P. fruticosa*. The first committed intermediate is presumed to be calenduloside E, formed by glycosylation of OA at C-3 with GluA. Although not yet isolated from *P. fruticosa*, this compound is likely a transient precursor rapidly converted to more complex saponins [85].

Glycosylation with Glc or Gal yields zingibroside R1 and ladyginoside A through substitutions at O-2 and O-4 of GluA, respectively. Alternatively, glycosylation at C-3 with Glc leads to chikusetsusaponin IVa, whereas conjugation of Gal to Calenduloside E produces 3-O-[β-D-galactopyranosyl-(1→2)-β-D-glucuronopyranosyl] oleanolic acid (Figure 3).

Additional sugar modifications diversify the saponin pool. For example, polyscioside A likely arises from Glc attachment to the sugar chains of zingibroside R1 or ladyginoside A. Polyscioside B is proposed to originate from zingibroside R1 via Ara substitution at O-4 of GluA, while polyscioside C may form through Glc addition at O-3 of the Gal–GluA chain. PFS (3-O-[β-D-glucopyranosyl-(1→4)-β-D-glucuronopyranosyl] oleanolic acid 28-O-β-D-glucopyranosyl ester) can be generated via esterification of C-28 in ladyginoside A or glycosylation of the same site in chikusetsusaponin IVa (Figure 3).

In addition to classical O-glycosylation, the TSBP in *P. fruticosa* appears to involve O-methylation of sugar moieties. At least six additional saponins arise from such modifications. Polyscioside D may result from Glc esterification of polyscioside A or from Glc attachment to the sugar chain of PFS. Polyscioside E is generated by Glc esterification at C-28 of polyscioside B, while polyscioside F forms analogously from polyscioside C. Polyscioside G likely results from Rha addition to the C-28 sugar chain of PFS. Furthermore, O-methylation of the GluA carboxyl in PFS or polyscioside A may yield polyscriosides J and K, respectively.

Terminal steps in the pathway may involve the formation of polyscioside H and I. Polyscioside H could arise from Glc addition to polyscioside G or Rha conjugation to polyscioside D. Polyscioside I is proposed to form via the addition of a disaccharide unit (Gal–Glc) at the C-28 position of polyscioside A. A putative intermediate, 3-O-[β-D-glucopyranosyl-(1→2)-[β-D-glucopyranosyl-(1→4)]-β-D-glucuronopyranosyl] oleanolic acid 28-O-β-D-galactopyranosyl ester, is hypothesized to precede polyscioside I formation, although it has not yet been isolated from *P. fruticosa*.

Overall, the proposed TSBP in *P. fruticosa* suggests that its triterpenoid saponins are biosynthesized via both linear and convergent pathways. Some compounds, such as polyscioside E, are likely formed through a strictly linear progression (OA → calenduloside E → zingibroside R1 → polyscioside B → polyscioside E), whereas others, like polyscioside H, may derive from alternative branches. This model integrates structural, biochemical, and comparative insights, providing a robust framework for future experimental validation of saponin biosynthesis in *P. fruticosa* and supporting pathway engineering and synthetic biology applications. From the authors' perspective, this model provides a biosynthetically coherent explanation of saponin diversity in *P. fruticosa*, integrating structural, enzymatic, and comparative data. It offers a foundation for future experimental validation and supports applications in metabolic engineering and synthetic biology.

5.1.5. Concluding Remarks on Triterpenoid Saponins

Triterpenoid saponins constitute the principal class of bioactive metabolites in *P. fruticosa*, characterized by considerable structural diversity and a wide spectrum of pharmacological activities. To date, 19 saponins have been isolated and structurally characterized from this species, including both unique glycosides and compounds common to other Araliaceae taxa. Experimental studies have demonstrated their anti-inflammatory, antidiabetic, cytotoxic, antioxidant, and neuroprotective properties in various in vitro and in vivo models [8,14,16,17,20,56,57].

Efficient extraction techniques, particularly ultrasound-assisted extraction (UAE), have been developed to maximize saponin yield and preserve bioactivity. Moreover, the observed synergism between saponins and co-extracted phytochemicals enhances the therapeutic value of standardized saponin-rich extracts. Based on comparative phytochemical and biochemical data, a complete triterpenoid saponin biosynthetic pathway (TSBP) has been proposed for the first time in *P. fruticosa*, encompassing the mevalonate pathway, β-amyrin cyclization, oxidation to oleanolic acid, and subsequent glycosylation and methylation reactions.

From the authors' perspective, the integration of structural, pharmacological, and biosynthetic insights offers a robust and coherent foundation for future studies focused on metabolic engineering, quality control of herbal preparations, and the exploration of *P. fruticosa* saponins as candidates for pharmaceutical and biotechnological applications.

5.2. Phenolic Constituents of Polyscias fruticosa: Chemotaxonomic Significance and Pharmacological Perspectives

5.2.1. Flavonoids and Phenolic Acids in *Polyscias fruticosa*

To date, only one comprehensive review on phenolic compounds in the genus *Polyscias* has been published, authored by Ashmawy et al. [4]. Identified compounds include quercetin-3-O-glucoside (*P. fulva*), luteolin (*P. nodosa*), lichexanthone (*P. fulva*), tamaraxetin 3,7-di-O-α-L-rhamnopyranoside (*P. balfouriana*, *P. guilfoylei*), and various other phenolic derivatives. The 2020 review by Ashmawy et al. [4] did not include phenolic compounds from *P. fruticosa*, as these constituents were only confirmed in subsequent studies published between 2021 and 2023. This section provides, for the first time, a comprehensive summary and discussion of 20 phenolic compounds, encompassing both simple phenolics (e.g., 2,6-dimethoxyphenol) and more complex lignin-derived eugenol-type structures (e.g., sinapyl alcohol, 1′-hydroxyeugenol, 1,2-bis(4-hydroxy-3-methoxyphenyl)ethylene) (Table 2).

Table 2. Phenolic compounds identified in *Polyscias fruticosa*: structural characteristics, plant sources, and extraction methods.

No.	Compound Name	Compound Class	Molecular Formula	Exact Mass	Plant Source	Extraction Method	Ref.
20	Kaempferol-3-rhamnoside/afzelin/kaempferol-3-O-alpha-L-rhamnoside	Flavonoids	$C_{21}H_{20}O_{10}$	432.10	Leaves	EtOH (95%), maceration 72 h, 25 °C, EtOAc/n-hexane fraction	[8]
21	Quercetin-3-rhamnoside/quercitrin/quercetin 3-L-rhamnoside	Flavonoids	$C_{21}H_{20}O_{11}$	448.10	Leaves	EtOH (95%), maceration 72 h, 25 °C, EtOAc/n-hexane fraction	[8]
22	Esculetin/aesculetin	Phenolic compounds	$C_9H_6O_4$	286.24	Leaves	EtOH (95%), maceration 72 h, 25 °C, EtOAc/n-hexane fraction	[8]

Table 2. *Cont.*

No.	Compound Name	Compound Class	Molecular Formula	Exact Mass	Plant Source	Extraction Method	Ref.
23	Liquiritigenin/ 7-hydroxy-2-(4-hydroxy-phenyl)-chroman-4-one	Flavanones	$C_{15}H_{12}O_4$	256.07	Leaves	EtOH (95%), maceration 72 h, 25 °C, EtOAc/n-hexane fraction	[8]
24	(*E*)-3,4-dihydroxycinnamic Acid/ caffeic acid	Phenolic acids	$C_9H_8O_4$	180.04	Leaves	EtOH (95%), maceration 72 h, 25 °C, EtOAc/n-hexane fraction	[8]
25	4-hydroxycinnamaldehyde	Phenolic compounds	$C_9H_8O_2$	148.05	Leaves	EtOH (95%), maceration 72 h, 25 °C, EtOAc/n-hexane fraction	[8]
26	(*E*)-isoferulaldehyde/ 3-hydroxy-4-methoxycinnamaldehyde	Phenolic compounds	$C_{10}H_{10}O_3$	178.06	Leaves	EtOH (95%), maceration 72 h, 25 °C, EtOAc/n-hexane fraction	[8]
27	Protocatechuic acid/ 3,4-dihydroxybenzoic acid	Phenolic acids	$C_7H_6O_4$	154.02	Roots	EtOH 95%, maceration at RT Et_2O fraction	[21]
28	Politoic acid/ (E)-2-(4-((E)-2-carboxyvinyl)-2-methoxyphenoxy)-3-(4-hydroxyphenyl)acrylic acid	Phenolic acids	$C_{18}H_{16}O_7$	344.32	Roots	EtOH 95%, maceration at RT, Et_2O fraction	[21]
29	8-O-4-dehydrodiferulic acid	Phenolic acids	$C_{20}H_{18}O_8$	386.35	Roots	EtOH 95%, maceration at RT, Et_2O fraction	[21]
30	8-O-4/8-O-4-dehydrotriferulic acid	Phenolic acids	$C_{30}H_{26}O_{12}$	578.52	Roots	EtOH 95%, maceration at RT, Et_2O fraction	[21]
31	1′-hydroxyeugenol/ 4-(1-hydroxy-allyl)-2-methoxy-phenol	Polyphenols	$C_{10}H_{12}O_3$	180.07	Leaves	UAE EtOH (95%), n-hexane/DCM (PFLD) 1 h, 30 °C	[10]
32	2,6-dimethoxy-4-vinylphenol/ 4-ethenyl-2,6-dimethoxyphenol	Polyphenols	$C_{10}H_{12}O_3$	180.07	Leaves	UAE EtOH (95%), n-hexane/DCM (PFLD) 1 h, 30 °C	[10]
33	2,6-dimethoxyphenol/ syringol/ pyrogallol 1,3-dimethyl ether	Polyphenols	$C_8H_{10}O_3$	154.06	Leaves	UAE EtOH (95%), n-hexane/DCM (PFLD) 1 h, 30 °C)	[10]
34	4-vinylphenol/ 4-hydroxystyrene/	Polyphenols	C_8H_8O	120.05	Leaves	UAE EtOH (95%), n-hexane/DCM (PFLD) 1 h, 30 °C	[10]

Table 2. *Cont.*

No.	Compound Name	Compound Class	Molecular Formula	Exact Mass	Plant Source	Extraction Method	Ref.
35	vanillin/ 4-hydroxy-3-methoxybenzaldehyde/ vanillaldehyde	Polyphenols	$C_8H_8O_3$	152.04	Leaves	UAE EtOH (95%), n-hexane/DCM (PFLD) 1 h, 30 °C	[10]
36	2-methoxy-4-vinylphenol/ 4-vinylguaiacol/ p-vinylguaiacol	Polyphenols	$C_9H_{10}O_2$	150.06	Leaves	UAE EtOH (95%), n-hexane/DCM (PFLD) 1 h, 30 °C	[10]
37	4-allyl-2,6-dimethoxyphenol/ methoxyeugenol/ 4-allylsyringol	Polyphenols	$C_{11}H_{14}O_3$	194.09	Leaves	UAE EtOH (95%), n-hexane/DCM (PFLD) 1 h, 30 °C	[10]
38	1,2-bis(4-hydroxy-3-methoxyphenyl)ethylene	Polyphenols	$C_{16}H_{16}O_4$	272.10	Leaves	UAE EtOH (95%), n-hexane/DCM (PFLD) 1 h, 30 °C	[10]
39	Sinapyl alcohol/ 4-(3-hydroxyprop-1-en-1-yl)-2,6-dimethoxyphenol	Phenylpropanoid (lignin precursor)	$C_{11}H_{14}O_4$	210.08	Leaves	UAE EtOH (95%), n-hexane/DCM (PFLD) 1 h, 30 °C	[10]

EtOH (95%)—95% ethanol extraction, Et_2O—diethyl ether fraction (liquid–liquid partitioning with diethyl ether), DCM (PFLD)—dichloromethane fraction (*Polyscias fruticosa* leaf dichloromethane fraction), EEPF (EtOAc fraction)—ethyl acetate fraction of ethanol extract from *P. fruticosa* roots; UAE, n-hexane—ultrasound-assisted extraction using n-hexane at 30 °C for 1 h [10]; maceration, EtOH (95%), 72 h, 25 °C—ethanol maceration at room temperature [8].

Rarison et al. [10] identified nine phenolic compounds in the dichloromethane fraction (PFLD) of *P. fruticosa* leaf extract. After extraction with 95% ethanol and partitioning with n-hexane and dichloromethane, GC-MS analysis revealed several low-polarity phenolics, including 2-methoxy-4-vinylphenol (**36**), 2,6-dimethoxy-4-vinylphenol (**32**), sinapyl alcohol (**39**), 4-allyl-2,6-dimethoxyphenol (**37**), 1′-hydroxyeugenol (31), 2,6-dimethoxyphenol (**33**), and the dimeric 1,2-bis(4-hydroxy-3-methoxyphenyl)ethylene (**38**). Two additional compounds, 4-vinylphenol (**34**) and vanillin (**35**), were also detected; however, their identification remains tentative. These two structures are commonly recognized as potential thermal artifacts or lignin degradation products and are known to occur as contaminants in GC-MS profiles. In the absence of orthogonal validation (e.g., LC–MS or NMR), their biosynthetic origin in *P. fruticosa* remains speculative and should be interpreted with caution. Therefore, their inclusion in the phenolic profile of this species should be treated with caution. These findings suggest that the lipophilic leaf fraction of *P. fruticosa* may represent an underexplored source of structurally unusual phenolic compounds with potential antioxidant and anti-inflammatory activities, warranting further investigation (Table 2).

Selvaraj et al. [21] identified phenolic compounds in the ethyl acetate fraction derived from a 75% ethanol extract of *P. fruticosa* roots (EEPF). Chromatographic purification yielded four phenolic compounds, including one novel and three previously known structures. The newly discovered compound, named politoic acid (**28**), was characterized by HRESI-MS and 1D/2D NMR (^{1}H, ^{13}C, HSQC, HMBC) as (E)-2-(4-((E)-2-carboxyvinyl)-2-methoxyphenoxy)-3-(4-hydroxyphenyl)acrylic acid—a unique lignin-derived dimer not previously reported in any *Polyscias* species, thereby extending the chemotaxonomic spectrum of this genus.

Additionally, two oligomers were isolated: 8-O-4-dehydrodiferulic acid (**29**) and 8-O-4/8-O-4-dehydrotriferulic acid (**30**), representing a ferulic acid dimer and trimer, respectively, both with known antioxidant and neuroprotective effects. These compounds were identified for the first time in *P. fruticosa* and the *Polyscias* genus overall, substantially expanding its known phenolic repertoire [21].

The same fraction also contained protocatechuic acid (PCA) (**27**), a well-known plant-derived phenolic acid with potent antioxidant activity [86]. Although structurally familiar, this compound had not previously been reported in *P. fruticosa*, making its identification a notable contribution to the species' phytochemistry and potentially linking it to the documented pharmacological properties of other Araliaceae taxa. PCA acts through ROS scavenging, metal chelation, and inhibition of lipid peroxidation. Furthermore, it exhibits antidiabetic properties by inhibiting α-amylase and α-glucosidase, thereby reducing postprandial hyperglycemia. Notably, it inhibited α-glucosidase with an IC_{50} of 1.76 μM [86,87]. PCA has also shown anticancer activity by suppressing proliferation, inducing apoptosis, and modulating signaling pathways (NF-κB, PI3K/AKT, MAPK), and exerts chemopreventive effects by normalizing redox balance and cellular metabolism [88].

Do et al. [8] conducted a detailed phytochemical study of *P. fruticosa* leaves extracted with 95% ethanol, followed by partitioning with diethyl ether, ethyl acetate, and n-butanol. From the diethyl ether fraction (26 g), obtained from 859 g of dried leaves, nine phenolic compounds were isolated using silica gel and Sephadex LH-20 chromatography.

Among them were two flavonol glycosides, kaempferol-3-O-rhamnoside (**20**) and quercetin-3-O-rhamnoside (**21**), along with one flavanone (liquiritigenin) (**23**), one coumarin (esculetin) (**22**), and one phenolic acid (caffeic acid) (**24**). Additionally, two cinnamic aldehyde derivatives, 4-hydroxycinnamaldehyde (**25**) and (E)-isoferulaldehyde (**26**), were identified. Despite their structural simplicity, these compounds contribute to the overall phenolic content due to their hydroxylated aromatic systems, which suggests that these compounds may play a relevant role in the antioxidant profile of *P. fruticosa*. (Table 2).

Structural elucidation was confirmed by ^{1}H and ^{13}C NMR and HRESI-MS, supported by a comparison of the available literature. Interestingly, two triterpenoids, 6,15α-epoxy-1β,4β-dihydroxyeudesmane and olean-12-ene-3β,15α-diol, were also isolated for the first time in the *Polyscias* genus. The aldehydic and acidic phenolics identified in this fraction were previously unreported in *P. fruticosa*.

Altogether, these findings significantly expand the known phenolic profile of *P. fruticosa*, particularly regarding its lipophilic constituents. The discovery of novel dimers and oligomers, as well as rare cinnamic derivatives and eugenol-related compounds, underscores the species' chemical diversity and potential pharmacological relevance. However, further validation using non-volatile analysis methods (e.g., LC-MS, NMR) is recommended, especially for structurally labile or thermally sensitive molecules.

5.2.2. Extraction and Analysis of Phenolic Compound Fractions

In recent years, research on phenolic compounds in *P. fruticosa* has increasingly focused on optimizing extraction protocols and conducting comprehensive phytochemical analyses of plant fractions. Studies have particularly emphasized the role of extraction variables in determining the qualitative and quantitative profile of phenolic metabolites. Particular attention has been paid to evaluating the efficacy of solvents with different polarities, applying assisted extraction techniques, and assessing the influence of physicochemical parameters, including extraction time, temperature, and plant-to-solvent ratio.

Nguyen et al. [89] systematically examined the impact of ethanol concentration (50–90%) on the extraction efficiency of *P. fruticosa* roots.

Using 90% ethanol at 30 °C for 3 h (1:20 ratio), the authors achieved the highest total phenolic and flavonoid contents (96.09 mg GAE·g^{-1} and 58.30 mg QE·g^{-1}, respectively), which positively correlated with antioxidant activity (DPPH, ABTS). Building upon these findings, Quoc et al. [59] implemented ultrasound-assisted extraction (UAE), which significantly enhanced TPC and TFC compared to maceration. Under 80% ethanol, 40 °C, and 30 min treatment (300 W), UAE resulted in higher TPC/TFC values and improved antioxidant readouts (DPPH, ABTS, FRAP). These results suggest that UAE provides a more efficient and reproducible alternative for extracting antioxidant phenolics from this species.

Notably, the use of low-polarity solvents such as dichloromethane [10] and diethyl ether [9] enabled the detection of lipophilic compounds, including sinapyl alcohol, eugenol-type dimers, vinylphenols, and ferulic acid oligomers. However, some of these—particularly 4-vinylphenol and vanillin—may represent degradation products or analytical artifacts, rather than genuine biosynthetic metabolites. Therefore, we caution against overinterpretation of these GC-MS-derived compounds without orthogonal structural confirmation (e.g., NMR, LC-MS).

Moreover, in vitro culture experiments conducted by Le et al. [12] demonstrated that elicitation with jasmonic acid, mannitol, and yeast extract significantly enhanced both phenolic biosynthesis and the activity of antioxidant enzymes, such as peroxidase (POD) and catalase (CAT). Although promising, the reproducibility and scalability of such elicitor-driven enhancements require further validation, especially under industrially relevant conditions.

In summary, the phytochemical study of phenolics in *P. fruticosa* benefits from well-designed extraction strategies, especially UAE and solvent polarity gradients. These approaches facilitate the recovery of structurally diverse phenolics. Nonetheless, further chemical verification is required to confirm the natural occurrence of several low-polarity compounds before attributing pharmacological activity or biosynthetic significance.

5.2.3. Pharmacological Significance of Selected Phenolic Compounds Identified in *Polyscias fruticosa*

Phenolic compounds are key contributors to the biological activity of medicinal plants, exhibiting a wide range of pharmacological effects, including antioxidant, anti-inflammatory, antimicrobial, and neuroprotective properties [90]. In *P. fruticosa*, accumulating evidence suggests that these metabolites—comprising both ubiquitous constituents (e.g., quercetin, caffeic acid) and unique lignin-derived derivatives—play a substantial role in the therapeutic effects traditionally associated with this species [4,17,21].

In this section, only selected phenolic compounds with either confirmed structural identity or significant biological activity have been discussed in detail. This selective approach reflects the authors' intention to emphasize pharmacologically relevant metabolites while avoiding speculative interpretation of tentative or potentially artifactual identifications.

In vitro studies have confirmed strong antioxidant activity in ethanol extracts from *P. fruticosa* roots and leaves, which correlates positively with their phenolic content. Nguyen et al. [89] reported that root extracts exhibited potent radical-scavenging activity against DPPH (IC_{50} = 96.14 $\mu g \cdot mL^{-1}$) and ABTS (IC_{50} = 38.76 $\mu g \cdot mL^{-1}$), with total phenolic content (TPC) and total flavonoid content (TFC) being strongly associated with antioxidant potential. Similar results were obtained for leaf extracts by Ly et al. [20], which showed pronounced free radical scavenging activity and inhibition of lipid peroxidation in TBARS assays.

Phenolic compounds isolated from lipophilic fractions, including 1′-hydroxyeugenol (**31**), sinapyl alcohol (**39**), and the dimeric 1,2-bis(4-hydroxy-3-methoxyphenyl)ethylene (**38**), exhibited significant anti-inflammatory activity through inhibition of nitric oxide (NO) production in LPS-stimulated RAW 264.7 macrophages [17]. These findings suggest that lipophilic phenolics may modulate key inflammatory signaling pathways. Its chemical structure, featuring both methoxy and hydroxyl groups on the aromatic ring, confers high antioxidant capacity and facilitates redox regulation [91].

Le Roy et al. [91] showed that sinapyl alcohol is stored in plants as glucosides, which can be mobilized in response to environmental stimuli, providing protection against pathogens and UV radiation.

Further evidence supports the anti-inflammatory and antinociceptive properties of sinapyl alcohol in vivo. Oral administration significantly reduced edema and pain in formalin- and carrageenan-induced inflammation models, highlighting its therapeutic potential in inflammatory and pain-related disorders [92]. Additionally, sinapyl alcohol exhibits moderate antimicrobial activity and regulates lignin biosynthesis by modulating cell wall differentiation, which may underlie its cytotoxic and neuroprotective potential [93].

Ferulic acid derivatives isolated from *P. fruticosa* roots, including 8-O-4-dehydrodiferulic acid (**29**) and 8-O-4/8-O-4-dehydrotriferulic acid (**30**), demonstrated neuroprotective effects in oxidative stress models. Selvaraj et al. [21] attributed these effects to their antioxidant capacity and modulation of apoptotic and intracellular signaling pathways in neuronal cells.

Elicitation with jasmonic acid and other stressors enhanced phenolic biosynthesis and antioxidant potential in in vitro cultures of *P. fruticosa* [12]. This observation suggests that elicitation strategies could be further optimized to boost pharmacologically valuable phenolic content in vitro.

Quercetin derivatives may also contribute to the antimicrobial activity of *P. fruticosa*. A review by Mawea et al. [94] highlighted the antibacterial efficacy of quercetin and quercitrin in other plant models, supporting the ethnomedicinal use of *P. fruticosa* for treating infections and inflammatory skin conditions.

Among the most pharmacologically significant polyphenols in *P. fruticosa* is kaempferol-3-O-α-L-rhamnoside (afzelin) (**20**), isolated from the diethyl ether fraction of leaf extracts [8]. Afzelin exhibits antioxidant, cytoprotective, anti-inflammatory, and anticancer properties [95–99]. In lung cancer models, afzelin induced immunogenic cell death (ICD) by downregulating NAD(P)H: quinone oxidoreductase 2 (NQO2), triggering ER stress, and promoting DAMP release (ATP, HMGB1, calreticulin), thereby stimulating antitumor immune responses [96]. In murine models, afzelin suppressed Ehrlich ascites carcinoma (EAC) proliferation by ~71% at 50 $mg \cdot kg^{-1}$ with minimal toxicity [97]. It also enhanced SPF values in sunscreen formulations and exhibited mild anti-adipogenic activity in 3T3-L1 cells, broadening its potential applications in cosmetics and metabolic health [95,99].

Quercitrin (quercetin-3-O-α-L-rhamnoside) (**21**), another flavonol glycoside identified in the same fraction [8], is known for its antioxidant, anti-inflammatory, and cytoprotective properties. In osteoarthritis models, quercitrin inhibited NF-κB signaling and suppressed matrix metalloproteinases and pro-inflammatory cytokines [100]. In myocardial infarction models, it improved cardiac function by promoting M2 macrophage polarization and enhancing mitochondrial respiration [101]. Quercitrin also improved gut microbiota composition and reduced serum cholesterol in zebrafish models, confirming its multifaceted health benefits [102,103].

Esculetin (6,7-dihydroxycoumarin) (**22**), a coumarin derivative identified for the first time in *P. fruticosa* [8], exhibits anticancer, lipid-lowering, and metabolic regulatory activities [104–107]. In hepatocellular carcinoma models, it induced ferroptosis by inhibiting the Nrf2–xCT/GPx4 axis and impairing glycolysis through GPI inhibition [104–107]. Additionally, it promoted HDL formation via CD36 upregulation in adipose macrophages and reduced fat accumulation in *C. elegans* via insulin/IGF-1 and AMPK signaling pathways [105,106].

Caffeic acid (**24**), a hydroxycinnamic acid detected in *P. fruticosa* for the first time [8], exhibits robust antioxidant and anti-inflammatory properties. It scavenges reactive radicals, chelates metal ions, and inhibits pro-inflammatory cytokines via NF-κB and MAPK suppression [108–110]. It also exerts anticancer effects, particularly against HCC, by suppressing STAT3 signaling and promoting apoptosis [108].

The identification of such well-known bioactives in *P. fruticosa* contributes to the chemotaxonomic characterization of the species and its alignment with other pharmacologically rich Araliaceae taxa.

4-hydroxycinnamaldehyde (**25**), identified by Do et al. [8], demonstrated antiproliferative and pro-apoptotic effects via Wnt/β-catenin and BAG3/HSF1 pathway inhibition [111,112]. It also suppresses NF-κB activity via ERK modulation, supporting its anti-inflammatory potential [113].

Finally, (E)-isoferulaldehyde (**26**), an aldehydic derivative of ferulic acid, was shown to inhibit NO production in LPS-stimulated macrophages (IC_{50} = 19.0 mg·dm^{-3}), and exhibits antimicrobial and cytotoxic effects [114,115]. Its presence in *P. fruticosa* supports its chemotaxonomic classification among phenylpropanoid-rich species and may explain some of its neuroprotective and immunomodulatory effects.

Taken together, this critical analysis of selected phenolic compounds in *P. fruticosa* highlights their diverse pharmacological profiles and supports the ethnomedical relevance of the species. Further integrative studies are needed to confirm their bioactivity in vivo and to validate the most promising compounds as lead candidates for therapeutic development.

5.3. *Sterols and Steroidal Derivatives Identified in Polyscias fruticosa*

Sterols are fundamental components of plant cell membranes, contributing to membrane fluidity, permeability, and receptor-mediated signaling. In medicinal plants, phytosterols are valued for their roles in modulating inflammation, oxidative stress, and lipid metabolism [116,117].

In *P. fruticosa*, recent phytochemical investigations have confirmed the presence of sterols and steroidal derivatives, enhancing the known chemical diversity of the species (Table 3). Rarison et al. [10] identified two sterols, stigmasterol (**40**) and (3β,5α)-stigmasta-7,16-dien-3-ol (**41**), in both the n-hexane (PFLH) and dichloromethane (PFLD) leaf extracts. The identification of these sterols in both moderately and strongly non-polar fractions confirms their high lipophilicity and supports their accumulation in membrane-rich tissues.

Table 3. Sterols and steroidal derivatives identified in *Polyscias fruticosa*: molecular characteristics, extraction conditions, and analytical methods.

No.	Compound Name	Type	Molecular Formula	Plant Source	Extraction Method	Identification Method	Ref.
40	Stigmasterol	Phytosterol	$C_{29}H_{48}O$	leaves	UAE EtOH (95%), n-hexane/DCM (PFLD) 1 h, 30 °C	GC-MS	[4,10]
41	(3β,5α)-Stigmasta-7,16-dien-3-ol	Sterol derivative	$C_{29}H_{48}O$	leaves	UAE EtOH (95%), n-hexane/DCM (PFLD) 1 h, 30 °C	GC-MS	[10]
42	22-dehydro-24-isopropylcholesterol	Atypical sterol	$C_{30}H_{48}O$	roots	Petroleum ether/diethyl ether (1:1)	X-ray crystallography	[118]

DCM extraction—dichloromethane extraction, EtOH (95%)—extraction using 95% ethanol; petroleum ether/diethyl ether (1:1)—extraction with a mixture of petroleum ether and diethyl ether (1:1, *v/v*); GC-MS—gas chromatography–mass spectrometry, X-ray crystallography—X-ray diffraction-based structural analysis. Identification of compounds 40 and 41 by GC-MS was based on comparison with the NIST spectral library and published reference data [10]. Chromatographic parameters: Rxi-5MS column (30 m × 0.25 mm i.d., 0.25 μm), helium carrier gas (1.12 mL/min), 1 μL injection (split ratio 1:20), injector temperature 280 °C, oven temperature 50–280 °C (10 °C/min), EI mode (70 eV), scan range *m/z* 50–600.

Additionally, Nguyen et al. [118] isolated an unusual sterol, 22-dehydro-24-isopropylcholesterol (**42**), from petroleum ether–diethyl ether (1:1, *v/v*) root extracts (Table 3). This sterol, previously described mainly in marine taxa, constitutes a rare occurrence in terrestrial flora, suggesting that *P. fruticosa* may possess biosynthetic traits not yet fully characterized within Araliaceae.

Earlier reviews by Ashmawy et al. [4] documented the presence of β-sitosterol and 3-O-β-D-glucopyranosyl-sitosterol in other *Polyscias* species, such as *P. fulva*, *P. nodosa*, and *P. guilfoyeli* [4,119,120]. However, their presence in *P. fruticosa* was not confirmed until the reports by Rarison et al. [10] and Nguyen et al. [118]. The confirmation of these sterols in *P. fruticosa* aligns with previous reports in congeneric species and reinforces its position within a phytochemically rich lineage. From a chemotaxonomic perspective, the diversity of sterols in *P. fruticosa* supports its classification among phytosterol-producing Araliaceae and provides a foundation for comparative biosynthetic studies.

From the authors' perspective, the current state of research on sterols in *Polyscias fruticosa* remains limited, particularly in comparison to the extensive studies on triterpenoid saponins and polyphenols. Although several phytosterols have been identified, including rare or unusual compounds such as 22-dehydro-24-isopropylcholesterol (**42**), their biosynthetic origins, tissue-specific distribution, and regulatory mechanisms have not been elucidated. Moreover, the lack of in vivo studies hinders a comprehensive understanding of their pharmacological roles, including potential synergistic effects with other lipophilic metabolites. Further investigations should aim to characterize the sterol biosynthetic pathway, assess the bioavailability of individual compounds, and explore their therapeutic relevance through integrative pharmacological models. Such studies would clarify the contribution of sterols to the traditional and modern medicinal use of *P. fruticosa* and enhance the rationale for their inclusion in phytopharmaceutical formulations.

Biological Properties of Sterols and Steroidal Derivatives in *Polyscias fruticosa*

Polyscias fruticosa contains a diverse array of sterolic constituents with distinct structural features and pharmacological implications. Among them, stigmasterol, detected in both n-hexane and dichloromethane extracts, is the most thoroughly studied [4]. Stigmasterol (**40**) is known for its anti-inflammatory, antioxidant, antidiabetic, and anticancer effects [118–120]. Its anti-inflammatory activity involves suppression of cyclooxygenase-2 (COX-2) and inducible nitric oxide synthase (iNOS), inhibition of NF-κB translocation, and downregulation of pro-inflammatory cytokines including TNF-α, IL-1β, and IL-6.

The antioxidant effects result from both direct ROS scavenging and induction of endogenous antioxidant enzymes such as catalase, superoxide dismutase (SOD), and glutathione peroxidase (GPx).

Anticancer effects are mediated through modulation oncogenic signaling via inhibition of Akt/mTOR and JAK/STAT pathways and downregulation of anti-apoptotic proteins such as Bcl-2 and Bcl-xL [119,120].

(3β,5α)-Stigmasta-7,16-dien-3-ol (**41**), a less commonly reported Δ^7-sterol with double bonds at C-7 and C-16, was also identified in *P. fruticosa* [10]. Although direct pharmacological data on this compound are limited, structurally similar Δ^7-sterols have demonstrated membrane-stabilizing, antifungal, and cytostatic properties [116]. Their rigid steroidal structure is thought to support membrane integrity under oxidative and osmotic stress. The co-occurrence of this sterol with stigmasterol in lipophilic extracts may imply cooperative effect in modulating membrane fluidity and lipid raft-associated signaling.

Of particular interest is 22-dehydro-24-isopropylcholesterol (**42**), an atypical marine-type sterol isolated from the roots of *P. fruticosa* [118]. This sterol, characterized by a double bond at C-22 and an isopropyl group at C-24, is rarely found in terrestrial plants. In marine systems, related sterols have demonstrated cytotoxic, antimicrobial, and immunomodulatory effects, while its biological activity in *P. fruticosa* has not been investigated, its structural similarity to marine sterols suggests potential bioactivity, including membrane disruption, apoptosis induction in cancer cells, and inhibition of microbial enzymes. Its presence in *P. fruticosa* suggests a unique biosynthetic route and warrants further study as a potentially bioactive and taxonomically significant metabolite.

Altogether, the sterolic profile of *P. fruticosa*—comprising stigmasterol, (3β,5α)-stigmasta-7,16-dien-3-ol, and 22-dehydro-24-isopropylcholesterol—underscores its biochemical complexity and value as a source of bioactive natural products. These compounds likely contribute synergistically to the modulation of inflammation, oxidative stress, and cellular homeostasis.

From the authors' perspective, their diversity highlights the need for in-depth studies on biosynthesis, subcellular distribution, and functional activity. Their structural features also make them promising lead scaffolds for further drug development [10].

5.4. *Essential Oils and Volatile Constituents Identified in Polyscias fruticosa*

Studies on the essential oils of *P. fruticosa* have revealed a complex composition of terpenoid constituents, with marked variation depending on the extraction method employed. Comparative analysis of n-hexane and dichloromethane extracts has demonstrated distinct chemical profiles, with specific classes of terpenoids predominating in each fraction (Table 4) [10].

Table 4. Volatile and lipophilic constituents of *Polyscias fruticosa* identified by GC-MS and other analytical methods.

No.	Compound Name	Class of Compounds	Molecular Formula	Plant Source	Identification Method	Ref.
43	Limonene	Monoterpene	$C_{10}H_{16}$	Leaves	GC-MS	[9]
44	(Z)-Hex-3-en-1-yl acetate	Monoterpene	$C_8H_{14}O_2$	Leaves	GC-MS	[9]
45	1-hexanol	Monoterpene	$C_6H_{14}O$	Leaves	GC-MS	[9]
46	(Z)-Hex-3-en-l-ol	Monoterpenoid	$C_6H_{12}O$	Leaves	GC-MS	[9]
47	3-bornanone oxime	Oxygenated Monoterpenes	$C_{10}H_{17}NO$	Leaves	GC-MS	[10]
48	Actinidiolide	Norisoprenoid lactone	$C_{11}H_{16}O_2$	Leaves	GC-MS	[10]
49	Loliolide	Norisoprenoid lactone	$C_{11}H_{16}O_3$	Leaves	GC-MS	[10]
50	®-1-(7,7-dimethyl-1,3,4,5,6,7-hexahydroisobenzofuran-1α-yl)-2-propanol	Monoterpenoid derivative (furan)	$C_{13}H_{22}O_2$	Leaves	GC-MS	[10]
51	(E)-γ-bisabolene	Sesquiterpene	$C_{15}H_{24}$	Leaves	GC-MS	[9]
52	α-bergamotene	Sesquiterpene	$C_{15}H_{24}$	Leaves	GC-MS	[9,10]
53	α-cubebene	Sesquiterpene	$C_{15}H_{24}$	Leaves	GC-MS	[9]
54	α-ylangene	Sesquiterpene	$C_{15}H_{24}$	Leaves	GC-MS	[9,10]
55	Germacrene D	Sesquiterpene	$C_{15}H_{24}$	Leaves	GC-MS	[9,10]
56	Germacrene B	Sesquiterpene	$C_{15}H_{24}$	Leaves	GC-MS	[9]
57	β-caryphyllene	Sesquiterpene	$C_{15}H_{24}$	Leaves	GC-MS	[9]
58	β-elemene	Sesquiterpene	$C_{15}H_{24}$	Leaves	GC-MS	[9]
59	δ-elemene	Sesquiterpene	$C_{15}H_{24}$	Leaves	GC-MS	[9]
60	γ-elemene	Sesquiterpene	$C_{15}H_{24}$	Leaves	GC-MS	[9]

Table 4. *Cont.*

No.	Compound Name	Class of Compounds	Molecular Formula	Plant Source	Identification Method	Ref.
61	α-copaene	Sesquiterpene	$C_{15}H_{24}$	Leaves	GC-MS	[9,10]
62	Aromadedrene	Sesquiterpene	$C_{15}H_{24}$	Leaves	GC-MS	[9,10]
63	α-humulene	Sesquiterpene	$C_{15}H_{24}$	Leaves	GC-MS	[9]
64	δ-cadinene	Sesquiterpene	$C_{15}H_{24}$	Leaves	GC-MS	[9]
65	α-ylangene	Sesquiterpene	$C_{15}H_{24}$	Leaves	GC-MS	[9,10]
66	α-copaene	Sesquiterpene	$C_{15}H_{24}$	Leaves	GC-MS	[9,10]
67	β-bourbonene	Sesquiterpene	$C_{15}H_{24}$	Leaves	GC-MS	[9]
68	β-cubebene	Sesquiterpene	$C_{15}H_{24}$	Leaves	GC-MS	[9]
69	β-gurjunene	Sesquiterpene	$C_{15}H_{24}$	Leaves	GC-MS	[9,10]
70	Calacorene	Sesquiterpene	$C_{15}H_{24}$	Leaves	GC-MS	[9]
71	γ-cadinene	Sesquiterpene	$C_{15}H_{24}$	Leaves	GC-MS	[10]
72	Caryophyllene oxide	Oxygenated sesquiterpene	$C_{15}H_{24}O$	Leaves	GC-MS	[10]
73	Calamenene	Oxygenated sesquiterpene	$C_{15}H_{22}O$	Leaves	GC-MS	[9]
74	Alismol	Oxygenated sesquiterpene	$C_{15}H_{26}O$	Leaves	GC-MS	[10]
75	Opposita-4(15),7(11)-dien-1β-ol	Oxygenated sesquiterpene	$C_{15}H_{24}O$	Leaves	GC-MS	[10]
76	Alloisolongifolene alcohol	Oxygenated sesquiterpene	$C_{15}H_{24}O$	Leaves	GC-MS	[10]
77	(4S,5R)-5-hydroxycaryophyll-8(13)-ene-4,12-epoxide	Oxygenated sesquiterpene	$C_{15}H_{24}O_2$	Leaves	GC-MS	[10]
78	Alismoxide	Oxygenated sesquiterpene	$C_{15}H_{24}O_2$	Leaves	GC-MS	[10]
79	β-Oplopenone	Oxygenated sesquiterpene	$C_{15}H_{22}O$	Leaves	GC-MS	[10]
80	Neoclovene oxide	Oxygenated sesquiterpene	$C_{15}H_{22}O$	Leaves	GC-MS	[10]
81	(−)-isolongifolol methyl ether	Oxygenated sesquiterpene (ether)	$C_{16}H_{28}O$	Leaves	GC-MS	[10]
82	Ledol	Oxygenated sesquiterpene	$C_{15}H_{22}O$	Leaves	GC-MS	[10]
83	Caryophyllenol II	Oxygenated sesquiterpene	$C_{15}H_{24}O$	Leaves	GC-MS	[10]
84	6,10,14-trimethylpentadecan-2-one	Aliphatic ketone	$C_{18}H_{36}O$	Leaves	GC-MS	[10]
85	Neophytadiene	Diterpenoid hydrocarbon	$C_{20}H_{38}$	Leaves	GC-MS	[10]
86	Phytol	Diterpenoid alcohol	$C_{20}H_{40}O$	Leaves	GC-MS	[10]
87	(Z)-1,3-Phytadiene	acyclic diterpene	$C_{20}H_{38}$	Leaves	GC-MS	[10]

GS-MS—gas chromatography–mass spectrometry. All volatile and lipophilic compounds listed in Table 4 were identified using GC-MS. For the majority of samples, analyses were performed on an Rxi-5MS capillary column (30 m × 0.25 mm i.d., 0.25 μm film thickness) with helium as carrier gas (1.12 mL/min), injector temperature 280 °C, injection volume 1 μL (split 1:20), and oven program from 50 °C (3 min hold) to 280 °C (10 min hold) at 10 °C/min. Mass spectra were recorded in EI mode at 70 eV (scan range m/z 50–600). Earlier GC-MS identifications (e.g., Brophy et al. [9]) did not report full chromatographic parameters. Biological activity data are discussed in Sections 5.4 and 5.5. Only compounds with documented or presumed pharmacological significance are addressed in the discussion.

The n-hexane extract, obtained by maceration, was notably enriched in hydrocarbon sesquiterpenes, including β-caryophyllene (**57**), germacrene D (**55**), α-humulene (**64**), and α-ylangene (**66**). These lipophilic compounds occurred in high concentrations and are known for their anti-inflammatory properties and potential modulatory effects on the endocannabinoid system.

In contrast, the dichloromethane extract was characterized by a higher content of oxygenated sesquiterpenes, notably spathulenol, caryophyllene oxide (**73**), and globulol, which have been associated with antioxidant, cytotoxic, and topical anti-inflammatory activities. This fraction also contained structurally distinct terpenoids such as ledol (**83**) and (4S,5R)-5-hydroxycarvophyll-8(13)-ene-4,12-epoxide (**78**), compounds of interest for their potential roles in redox modulation [10].

Comparative profiling of both fractions revealed that the n-hexane fraction is dominated by hydrocarbon sesquiterpenes with pronounced lipophilicity and potential activity at CB2 receptors and pro-inflammatory signaling pathways, whereas the dichloromethane extract was richer in oxygenated sesquiterpenes with stronger antioxidant and antiproliferative potential [10]. These observations suggest that the pharmacological effects of *P. fruticosa* extracts may be selectively enhanced through targeted extraction strategies, emphasizing the need for receptor-level studies to validate their mechanisms of action.

These compositional differences reflect solvent polarity and selectivity: n-hexane preferentially extracts nonpolar hydrocarbon terpenoids, while dichloromethane, with moderate polarity, facilitates the extraction of more functionally diverse and oxygenated constituents. Such differentiation is crucial, as the lipophilic and oxygenated fractions are likely to elicit distinct biological responses depending on their structural features. These findings underscore the critical importance of extraction methodology in shaping the chemical and pharmacological profiles of *P. fruticosa* preparations.

From the authors' perspective, the presence of sesquiterpenes with documented affinity for CB2 and TRPV1 receptors, such as β-caryophyllene and caryophyllene oxide, lends strong support to the ethnomedicinal use of *P. fruticosa* in inflammatory and pain-related conditions. Although preliminary in vitro and in silico studies are promising [10], we emphasize the need for in vivo validation, pharmacokinetic characterization, and mechanistic analyses to substantiate these bioactivities. In particular, sesquiterpenes with lipophilic properties and receptor-binding potential represent attractive candidates for development into topical or transdermal formulations, aligning with the traditional modes of administration.

The foundational study by Brophy et al. [9] provided one of the first comprehensive GC-MS analyses of essential oils distilled from *P. fruticosa* leaves collected in Fiji and Thailand. Hydrodistillation of the leaf material yielded approximately 24 sesquiterpenes, among which β-elemene (**60**), α-bergamotene (**52**), germacrene D (**55**), and (E)-γ-bisabolene (**51**) were predominant. Other constituents included α-humulene (**64**), β-caryophyllene (**57**), and aromadendrene (**63**), as well as trace amounts of monoterpenes (e.g., limonene) (**43**) and low-molecular-weight alcohols such as 1-hexanol (**45**) and (Z)-hex-3-en-1-ol (**46**) (Table 4) [9].

Importantly, Brophy et al. [9] observed considerable qualitative and quantitative variation in oil composition depending on geographical origin. For example, oxygenated sesquiterpenes accounted for ~20% in the Bangkok I sample, were nearly absent in the Bangkok II sample, and reached intermediate levels (~7%) in the Fiji sample. These differences may be attributed to environmental and genetic factors, as well as to chemical transformations such as isomerization or oxidation induced by light or heat during distillation. The detection of sesquiterpene isomers, including β-bourbonene (**68**) and δ-cadinene (**65**), may reflect such degradation processes. In light of these concerns, we support the future application of orthogonal techniques such as NMR or GC×GC to confirm compound identity and eliminate possible artifacts.

Whereas Brophy et al. [9] focused on hydrodistilled essential oils, Rarison et al. [10] extended the analysis to include solvent-extracted fractions, thereby broadening the understanding of the chemical variability and potential pharmacological significance of *P. fruticosa* terpenoids. The combination of hydrodistillation and solvent extraction techniques allows for a more complete characterization of both volatile and semi-volatile constituents with differing biological potential.

From the authors' perspective, the sesquiterpene-rich essential oil profile of *P. fruticosa* demonstrates high pharmacological potential, especially for compounds such as β-caryophyllene, caryophyllene oxide, and germacrene D. Due to their lipophilicity and documented bioactivities, these metabolites warrant further investigation as candidates for topical or transdermal therapies. Standardization efforts should also account for chemical variability linked to environmental and genetic factors. To ensure compound authenticity and uncover novel activities, advanced analytical methods such as NMR or GC×GC are recommended.

5.5. *Pharmacologically Relevant Rare Terpenoids and Norisoprenoids Identified in Polyscias fruticosa*

Polyscias fruticosa is recognized for its complex phytochemical profile, which includes numerous structurally unique compounds with potential pharmacological applications. In addition to the commonly reported sesquiterpenes and monoterpenes, advanced gas chromatography–mass spectrometry (GC-MS) analyses have revealed the presence of several rare and structurally distinctive terpenoids and norisoprenoids in *P. fruticosa*.

Although many of these constituents occur in low abundance, their structural uniqueness and bioactivities—also documented in other species—suggest potential relevance in pharmacological or ecological contexts.

However, the possibility that some volatile constituents may result from analytical artifacts or thermal degradation during GC-MS analysis should be taken into account. Therefore, conclusions based solely on GC-MS data require confirmation by complementary analytical techniques such as NMR or LC-MS to ensure structural accuracy. Despite their minor abundance, these metabolites may contribute substantially to the plant's biological activity and adaptive responses to environmental stressors.

Among these newly identified compounds is loliolide (**49**), a norisoprenoid lactone known for its potent antioxidant, anti-inflammatory, and anti-aging properties. While loliolide is commonly found in marine algae [121] and was recently confirmed in *Camellia ptilosperma* leaves [122], its detection in *P. fruticosa* is uncommon. This suggests possible chemotypic variability or previously unrecognized biosynthetic pathways within the Araliaceae family. Loliolide efficiently scavenges reactive oxygen species (DPPH, H_2O_2), protects cells against oxidative damage, and exerts cytoprotective effects in both in vitro and in vivo models (including Vero cells and zebrafish embryos) [123]. It also acts as a natural herbivore resistance inducer, functioning independently of the jasmonic acid pathway [124], and enhances dermal papilla cell activity via AKT/β-catenin signaling [125]. Recent studies further highlight its neuroprotective properties against glutamate-induced excitotoxicity, mediated through the MAPK/Nrf2 pathway and improved mitochondrial function [126]. These diverse effects render loliolide a promising multipotent molecule that may contribute to both the ecological and pharmacological profile of *P. fruticosa*.

Actinidiolide (**48**), another norisoprenoid lactone detected in *P. fruticosa*, is a degradation product of carotenoids and shares structural features with loliolide. While its specific activity has not yet been confirmed in *P. fruticosa*, studies in other species suggest its involvement in cytoprotective and antioxidant pathways. Its presence further supports the relevance of norisoprenoids in the chemotaxonomic and ecological profile of the species [10].

Alismol (**75**), an oxygenated sesquiterpene originally isolated from *Alisma orientale* and later reported in *Vladimiria souliei* [127], has also been identified in *P. fruticosa*. This compound displays notable anti-inflammatory activity via activation of the Nrf2 pathway and inhibition of pro-inflammatory mediators, including TNF-α, IL-1β, IL-6, and COX-2 expression [128,129]. In LPS-stimulated microglial cells, alismol suppresses nitric oxide (NO) and prostaglandin E_2 (PGE_2) production by inhibiting NF-κB signaling while sparing MAPK pathways [127]. Additionally, it exhibits neuroprotective effects by mitigating microglia-mediated neuronal cytotoxicity and alleviating lung injury in LPS-induced inflammatory models [128,129].

α-bergamotene (**52**), a hydrocarbon sesquiterpene detected in the essential oil of *P. fruticosa*, has been reported in other plant species such as *Guarea cedrata* and *Schisandra perulata* [130,131]. It demonstrates a moderate antioxidant capacity and exhibits antibacterial and antifungal activities against *Escherichia coli*, *Salmonella typhimurium*, and *Candida albicans*, thereby contributing to the antimicrobial potential of *P. fruticosa* extracts [132,133].

Another notable component is α-gurjunene (**70**), a hydrocarbon sesquiterpene identified in the n-hexane fraction of *P. fruticosa* leaf extracts. The presence of α-gurjunene significantly enhances both the pharmacological and aromatic profiles of the essential oil. Studies in other species, such as *Araucaria columnaris* [134] and *Globba schomburgkii* [135], have shown that α-gurjunene exhibits strong antibacterial and antifungal properties, supporting its relevance in plant defense mechanisms.

It is noteworthy that α-gurjunene, together with other sesquiterpenes such as β-caryophyllene (**57**) and caryophyllene oxide (**73**), may act synergistically to enhance the antioxidant and antimicrobial properties of *P. fruticosa* extracts. Their abundance in lipophilic fractions (n-hexane and dichloromethane) suggests their potential applicability in phytotherapeutic formulations and nutraceutical development [134,135].

Of particular interest is 6,10,14-trimethylpentadecan-2-one (**79**), a C18 isoprenoid ketone derived from the oxidative degradation of phytol (**87**). This compound may result from abiotic breakdown of (E)-phytenal or from the hydrolysis of photochemically generated phytyl-chain derivatives of chlorophyll [136]. Its detection in *P. fruticosa* indicates possible environmental influences on the plant's metabolome and highlights how endogenous metabolism can interact with ecological conditions. However, as this compound can be a photodegradation product, its presence should be interpreted with caution in the context of GC-MS-based metabolite profiling.

In summary, these rare terpenoids and norisoprenoids highlight the importance of comprehensive chemical profiling in *P. fruticose*. Among them, loliolide (**76**) stands out for its multifunctional activities, including antioxidant and anti-inflammatory effects [123,137], induction of herbivore resistance [124], stimulation of dermal papilla cell activity [125], and neuroprotective effects [126]. Similarly, alismol (**71**), α-bergamotene (**48**), α-gurjunene (**66**), and 6,10,14-trimethylpentadecan-2-one (**79**) contribute to the plant's potential therapeutic spectrum, particularly its anti-inflammatory, antioxidant, antimicrobial, and ecological defense properties. Future studies should aim to confirm the occurrence of these compounds using orthogonal analytical tools and to evaluate their synergistic interactions with major bioactive constituents of *P. fruticosa*.

5.6. First Identification and Biological Role of Tocopherols in Polyscias fruticosa

According to the comprehensive phytochemical review by Ashmawy et al. [4], there had been no previous evidence confirming the presence of tocopherols (vitamin E and its derivatives) (Table 5) in any species of the genus *Polyscias*. The authors cataloged a wide range of phytochemical constituents, such as triterpenoid saponins, terpenoids, and sterols, but tocopherols were notably absent. This observation supports the novelty and taxonomic importance of recent findings by Rarison et al. [10], who reported, for the first time, the occurrence of tocopherols in *P. fruticosa*, specifically within the n-hexane fraction of leaf extracts. This finding represents a notable expansion of the known metabolomic diversity of the species and underscores the importance of including lipophilic fractions in phytochemical screening.

Table 5. Tocopherols identified in *Polyscias fruticosa* leaf extracts by GC-MS.

No.	Compound Name	Class of Compound	Molecular Formula	Plant Source	Identification Method	Ref.
88	δ-tocopherol	Tocol (Vitamin E)	$C_{27}H_{46}O_2$	Leaves	GC-MS	[10]
89	β-tocopherol	Tocol (Vitamin E)	$C_{28}H_{48}O_2$	Leaves	GC-MS	[10]
90	DL-α-tocopherol	Tocol (Vitamin E)	$C_{29}H_{50}O_2$	Leaves	GC-MS	[10]
91	α-tocopherol	Tocol (Vitamin E)	$C_{29}H_{50}O_2$	Leaves	GC-MS	[10]

GC-MS—gas chromatography–mass spectrometry. Compounds were identified using the following conditions: Rxi-5MS capillary column (30 m × 0.25 mm i.d., 0.25 μm film), helium as carrier gas (1.12 mL/min), injector at 280 °C, split 1:20, injection volume 1 μL. Oven program: 50–280 °C at 10 °C/min (3 min initial, 10 min final hold). EI at 70 eV, scan range m/z 50–600 [10]. The biological functions of tocopherols are discussed in Section 5.6.

Tocopherols, particularly α-tocopherol, are well-established lipid-soluble antioxidants in both plant and animal systems [138]. Their principal function has traditionally been attributed to the scavenging of reactive oxygen species (ROS) and the protection of membrane lipids from peroxidation. However, emerging evidence indicates that α-tocopherol also exerts biological functions independent of its antioxidant properties. These include modulation of gene expression, regulation of intracellular signaling cascades, and involvement in lipid metabolism [138,139]. From a phytopharmacological perspective, such pleiotropic effects may enhance the adaptogenic potential of *P. fruticosa* and partially explain its traditional use in managing oxidative stress and inflammation.

The detection of tocopherols in *P. fruticosa* may also reflect their physiological role in stabilizing membrane structures and influencing lipid raft composition (Table 5). Tocopherols are known to interact with phospholipids and sterols in the lipid bilayer, potentially affecting membrane fluidity and signal transduction under stress conditions [138]. This membrane-level modulation may act synergistically with sterols previously identified in *P. fruticosa*, suggesting coordinated functions of lipophilic compounds in the plant's response to abiotic stress. Furthermore, metabolites of tocopherols, including carboxychromanols and CEHCs (2-(β-carboxyethyl)-6-hydroxychromans), have demonstrated a range of bioactivities, such as anti-inflammatory, antiproliferative, and cytoprotective effects in mammalian systems [139]. Although these metabolites have not yet been reported in *P. fruticosa*, their biosynthetic plausibility invites targeted metabolomic studies.

In our opinion, the functional role of tocopherols in *P. fruticosa* warrants further investigation not only due to their pharmacological relevance, but also their potential contribution to stress resilience and chemotaxonomic distinction within Araliaceae.

This first report of tocopherols in the *Polyscias* genus emphasizes the importance of detailed phytochemical investigation and invites further study into their functional roles in plant physiology and therapeutic potential. Future research should focus on quantification, localization, and possible synergistic interactions of tocopherols with other lipophilic constituents in *P. fruticosa*, such as sesquiterpenes, diterpenes, and triterpenoids. Such investigations may shed light on the integrative defense mechanisms of the plant and support its potential for phytopharmacological and nutraceutical applications.

5.7. *Bioactive Polyacetylenes in Polyscias fruticosa: Phytochemical Identification and Pharmacological Relevance*

Polyacetylenes are a class of unsaturated aliphatic compounds characterized by the presence of one or more carbon–carbon triple bonds. In *P. fruticosa*, these metabolites constitute a pharmacologically significant group of secondary metabolites, exhibiting a broad range of biological activities, including anti-inflammatory, cytotoxic, antimicrobial, and immunomodulatory effects (Table 6) [11,132,133,140].

Table 6. Polyacetylenes identified in *Polyscias fruticosa*, including compound class, plant source, and analytical methods.

No.	Compound Name	Class of Compounds	Molecular Formula	Plant Source	Identification Method	Ref.
92	Falcarinol (panaxynol)	C17 polyacetylene; monoacetylene alcohol	$C_{17}H_{24}O$	Roots, leaves	GC-MS, NMR	[4,10,11]
93	Heptadeca-1,8-diene-4,6-diyne-3-ol-10-one	C17 polyacetylene; diacetylene diol	$C_{17}H_{22}O_2$	Roots, leaves	GC-MS, NMR	[4,11]
94	Heptadeca-1,8-diene-4,6-diyne-3,10-diol/ (seselidiol)	C17 polyacetylene; diacetylene alcohol-ketone	$C_{17}H_{24}O_2$	Roots, leaves	GC-MS, NMR	[4,11]
95	Hexadeca-5,7,9,11-tetrayne-1,16-diol	C17 polyacetylene; polyacetylene diol	$C_{16}H_{18}O_2$	Leaves	GC-MS	[10]

GC-MS—gas chromatography–mass spectrometry. NMR—nuclear magnetic resonance. All compounds were identified based on GC-MS analysis and comparison with literature data [4,10,11]. Their biological activities are discussed in detail in Section 5.7.

The presence of polyacetylenes in *P. fruticosa* was initially suggested by earlier studies referenced by Do et al. [7], which reported their occurrence in the roots and associated them with the plant's traditional use in treating inflammatory conditions. Subsequent phytochemical investigations confirmed the presence of four principal polyacetylenes, namely falcarinol (**92**) (also known as panaxynol), falcarindiol, heptadeca-1,8-diene-4,6-diyne-3,10-diol (**93**), and heptadeca-1,8-diene-4,6-diyne-3-ol-10-one (**94**), in both root and leaf tissues. Rarison et al. [10] further expanded the understanding of polyacetylene distribution in *P. fruticosa* by identifying falcarinol (**92**) and hexadeca-5,7,9,11-tetrayne-1,16-diol (**95**) in different solvent fractions of the leaf extract. Falcarinol was predominantly present in the n-hexane fraction (PFLH), consistent with its high lipophilicity, while hexadeca-5,7,9,11-tetrayne-1,16-diol was selectively detected in the dichloromethane fraction (PFLD) at a concentration of $0.94 \pm 0.01\%$. These findings indicate solvent-dependent extraction efficiency and suggest differential tissue distribution and solubility of polyacetylenes within the species. Such solvent-specific activity supports the importance of fractionation strategies in metabolite profiling and bioactivity correlation.

Falcarinol (**92**), a monoacetylene alcohol, has been extensively studied for its pharmacological potential. It exhibits strong anti-inflammatory activity by downregulating inducible nitric oxide synthase (iNOS) and cyclooxygenase-2 (COX-2), suppressing nuclear factor-κB (NF-κB) activation, and reducing the secretion of pro-inflammatory cytokines such as TNF-α and IL-6 [141]. In vitro cytotoxicity has also been reported across diverse cancer cell lines, primarily through oxidative stress and apoptosis-related pathways. However, despite promising preclinical outcomes, its translation to clinical models remains unexplored.

The antimicrobial activity of falcarinol has also been well documented. Lutomski et al. [11] reported its activity against Gram-positive bacteria (*Staphylococcus aureus, Streptococcus pyogenes*) and fungal strains (*Candida albicans, Microsporum gypseum*), suggesting its relevance in the treatment of infections. Additionally, Rarison et al. [10] demonstrated that falcarinol modulates immune responses by downregulating costimulatory molecules on antigen-presenting cells and suppressing T-cell proliferation in inflammatory environments, supporting its immunomodulatory role.

Mechanistic studies by Alfurayhi et al. [140] have further elucidated the multi-targeted pharmacological profile of falcarinol-type polyacetylenes. These compounds were shown to inhibit iNOS and COX-2 expression, suppress pro-inflammatory cytokine production, activate the Nrf2-mediated antioxidant defense system, and modulate key signaling pathways such as PI3K/Akt and MAPK. This pleiotropic mode of action may underlie their efficacy in both inflammatory and tumorigenic settings.

Neuroprotective effects—though preliminary—have been linked to calcium channel inhibition and mitochondrial preservation under oxidative stress [132]. However, further studies are needed to establish their pharmacodynamic profile and therapeutic index.

Polyacetylenes, especially falcarinol, emerge as promising multifunctional agents in *P. fruticosa*, with reported anti-inflammatory, cytotoxic, antimicrobial, immunomodulatory, and neuroprotective activities. However, compared to triterpenoid saponins or polyphenols, this class remains underexplored. Future studies should prioritize their biosynthetic origins, stability under extraction conditions, and potential synergistic interactions with other lipophilic compounds. Bridging phytochemical data with pharmacodynamic endpoints will be essential to assess their translational potential in phytomedicine.

5.8. Fatty Acids in Polyscias fruticosa and Their Pharmacological Significance

Phytochemical investigations of *P. fruticosa* have revealed a diverse composition of fatty acids (FAs), identified by gas chromatography–mass spectrometry (GC-MS) in both the n-hexane (PFLH) and dichloromethane (PFLD) leaf extract fractions [10]. A total of 14 distinct fatty acid-related compounds were identified across both fractions, with 13 compounds detected in the PFLH and 8 in the PFLD. This fraction-dependent distribution reflects the solvent-selective extraction efficiency, where the nonpolar solvent (*n*-hexane) favors the recovery of saturated and unsaturated lipids with low polarity, while dichloromethane, exhibiting intermediate polarity, enables the extraction of moderately polar constituents (Table 7) [10]. Compounds were identified by comparing the resulting spectra with NIST and Wiley libraries [10]. In our view, the differential presence of fatty acids in PFLH and PFLD extracts underscores the influence of solvent polarity on the lipidomic profile of *P. fruticosa*, which may have implications for bioavailability and formulation strategies in phytopharmaceutical development.

Table 7. Fatty acid derivatives identified in *Polyscias fruticosa* by GC-MS and their classification.

No.	Compound Name	Type	Molecular Formula	Molecular Weight (g/mol)	Plant Source	Identification Method	Ref.
96	9,11-octadecadienoic acid	CLA isomer	$C_{18}H_{32}O_2$	280.24	Leaves	GC-MS	[10]
97	10-trans,12-cis-linoleic acid	CLA isomer	$C_{18}H_{32}O_2$	280.24	Leaves	GC-MS	[10]
98	2-linoleoylglycerol	Monoacylglycerol (MAG)	$C_{21}H_{38}O_4$	354.27	Leaves	GC-MS	[10]
99	Linoleic acid	Polyunsaturated fatty acid (PUFA)	$C_{18}H_{32}O_2$	280.24	Leaves	GC-MS	[10]
100	Linolenic acid	Polyunsaturated fatty acid (PUFA)	$C_{18}H_{30}O_2$	278.22	Leaves	GC-MS	[10]

Table 7. *Cont.*

No.	Compound Name	Type	Molecular Formula	Molecular Weight (g/mol)	Plant Source	Identification Method	Ref.
101	Lionoelaidic acid	Polyunsaturated fatty acid (PUFA)	$C_{18}H_{30}O_2$		Leaves	GC-MS	[10]
102	Palmitic acid	Saturated fatty acid (SFA)	$C_{16}H_{32}O_2$	256.24	Leaves	GC-MS	[10]
103	Stearic acid	Saturated fatty acid (SFA)	$C_{18}H_{36}O_2$	284.27	Leaves	GC-MS	[10]
104	Methyl linoleate	Fatty acid methyl ester (FAME)	$C_{19}H_{34}O_2$	294.25	Leaves	GC-MS	[10]
105	Ethyl palmitate	Fatty acid ethyl ester (FAEE)	$C_{18}H_{36}O_2$	284.27	Leaves	GC-MS	[10]
106	Myristic acid	Saturated fatty acid (SFA)	$C_{14}H_{28}O_2$	228.20	Leaves	GC-MS	[10]
107	Octanoic acid	Fatty acid ester	$C_8H_{16}O_2$	144.12	Leaves	GC-MS	[10]
108	2-palmitoylglycerol	Monoacylglycerol (MAG)	$C_{19}H_{38}O_4$	330.28	Leaves	GC-MS	[10]
109	Diisobutyl adipate	Aliphatic diester of a dicarboxylic acid	$C_{14}H_{26}O_4$	298.51	Leaves	GC-MS	[10]

GC-MS—gas chromatography–mass spectrometry. All fatty acids and related compounds were identified using GC-MS under the same analytical conditions previously described (see footnote to Table 4). The biological activities of selected compounds are discussed in Section 5.8.

In the hexane fraction, saturated FAs such as palmitic acid (**102**, 10.72%) and stearic acid (**103**, 2.28%) were among the most abundant, alongside unsaturated FAs including linolenic acid (**100**, 7.73%), linoleic acid (**99**), and 10-trans,12-cis-linoleic acid (**97**, 8.15%). A particularly notable compound, 9,11-octadecadienoic acid (**96**), a rare positional isomer of linoleic acid, was exclusively identified in the PFLH at 0.24% [10]. Its presence in *P. fruticosa*, not previously reported in the Araliaceae family, may hold chemotaxonomic relevance and suggests that this species biosynthesizes unique lipid mediators with potential therapeutic value [142]. This observation underscores the importance of minor lipid constituents in the pharmacological profiling of medicinal plants.

By contrast, the PFLD displayed a simplified FA profile with lower relative abundances of linolenic acid (2.56%), 10-trans,12-cis-linoleic acid (2.85%), and palmitic acid (5.04%) [10]. However, it contained monoacylglycerol derivatives, including 2-linoleoylglycerol (**98**) and 2-palmitoylglycerol (**108**), possibly resulting from partial hydrolysis or esterification processes. These compounds may participate in lipid signaling pathways and warrant further investigation regarding their metabolic roles. The observed differences between PFLH and PFLD reinforce the critical influence of extraction polarity on the fatty acid composition and reflect the physicochemical diversity of these metabolites in planta.

Among the unsaturated fatty acids, conjugated linoleic acid (CLA)—especially the 10-trans,12-cis isomer—stands out due to its multifaceted pharmacological effects. Recent studies have demonstrated its ability to modulate lipid and glucose homeostasis through activation of PPARγ and PPARδ pathways, upregulation of β-oxidation enzymes such as CPT1A, and increased expression of stearoyl-CoA desaturase (SCD) [143]. Additionally, CLA reduces intracellular triglyceride accumulation and influences fatty acid-binding proteins (FABP1, FABP6), while enhancing short-chain fatty acid (SCFA) production via modulation of the gut microbiome, contributing to improved systemic metabolic function. Special attention should be directed to 9,11-octadecadienoic acid (**96**) due to its dual antioxidant and anti-inflammatory activity. Mechanistic studies have shown that this isomer suppresses COX-2 expression, reduces pro-inflammatory cytokines such as IL-6 and TNF-α, and activates PPARγ-dependent lipid-regulating pathways [144]. It also upregulates the Nrf2/HO-1 antioxidant defense axis and enhances glutathione reductase activity, offering cellular protection against oxidative stress [145]. Related conjugated dienes, such as 13-KODE ((9Z,11E)-13-oxooctadeca-9,11-dienoic acid), exert similar anti-inflammatory effects via inhibition of NF-κB/MAPK signaling and activation of Nrf2 [146].

In our view, the identification of rare fatty acids such as 9,11-octadecadienoic acid positions *P. fruticosa* as a potential source of specialized lipid mediators beyond nutritional relevance. These metabolites may contribute to the anti-inflammatory and metabolic regulatory effects traditionally attributed to this species. However, the lack of in vivo validation, bioavailability data, and mechanistic studies remains a major gap in current research. Future investigations should prioritize the pharmacokinetics, metabolic stability, and synergistic interactions of these fatty acids—particularly in comparison with other Araliaceae taxa—to substantiate their potential for phytotherapeutic or nutraceutical applications.

5.9. *Newly Identified Volatile and Lipophilic Constituents in Polyscias fruticosa*

Recent phytochemical investigations of *P. fruticosa* leaf extracts have led to the identification of several volatile and lipophilic metabolites previously unreported within the *Polyscias* genus [4]. These compounds were characterized by gas chromatography–mass spectrometry (GC-MS) in two solvent-derived fractions: n-hexane (PFLH) and dichloromethane (PFLD) [10]. In total, five newly identified constituents were detected, with the majority either exclusively present or more abundant in the PFLD fraction, highlighting the influence of solvent polarity on metabolite recovery (Table 8).

Table 8. Newly identified volatile and lipophilic constituents of *Polyscias fruticosa* detected by GC-MS.

No.	Compound Name	Type	Molecular Formula	Molecular Weight (g/mol)	Plant Source	Identification Method	Ref.
110	3-hydroxy-4,5-dimethylfuran-2(5H)-one	Furanone-type lactone (oxygenated heterocycle)	$C_6H_8O_3$	128.05	Leaves	GC-MS	[10]
111	Octanal	Aliphatic aldehyde	$C_8H_{16}O$	128.12	Leaves	GC-MS	[10]
112	Hexadecanal	Long-chain saturated aliphatic aldehyde	$C_{16}H_{32}O$	240.25	Leaves	GC-MS	[10]
113	3-methylene-7,11-dimethyl-1-dodecene	Branched unsaturated hydrocarbon	$C_{15}H_{28}$	208.22	Leaves	GC-MS	[10]
114	Linoleyl alcohol	Long-chain unsaturated fatty alcohol	$C_{18}H_{34}O_2$	266.26	Leaves	GC-MS	[10]

GC-MS—gas chromatography–mass spectrometry. Compounds (**110–114**) were identified using GC-MS under the same analytical conditions previously described (see footnote to Table 4). Their biological activities are discussed in Section 5.9.

The presence of unique volatile and lipophilic compounds in PFLD highlights the underexplored chemical space of *P. fruticosa*, especially with regard to less polar but pharmacologically active constituents that may escape detection in aqueous or ethanol-based extracts.

Among these, 3-hydroxy-4,5-dimethylfuran-2(5H)-one (**110**), a furanone-type lactone, stands out due to its known antioxidant and antimicrobial activities. Detected in the PFLD at 0.95 $\pm$ 0.03%, this semi-volatile compound may contribute significantly to the pharmacological properties of *P. fruticosa* extracts. Although this compound has been reported in other medicinal plants, its occurrence in *P. fruticosa* may reflect species-specific stress-related biosynthetic pathways that deserve further study.

Additionally, four aliphatic hydrocarbon-related compounds were identified: octanal (**111**), hexadecanal (**112**), 3-methylene-7,11-dimethyl-1-dodecene (**113**), and linoleyl alcohol (**114**) (Table 8). Octanal, a short-chain aldehyde with a citrus aroma, exhibits potent antibacterial and cytotoxic effects, with IC_{50} values below 20 $\mu g \cdot mL^{-1}$ against selected cancer cell lines [147,148]. Hexadecanal (palmitaldehyde), a saturated long-chain aldehyde, is a known lipid peroxidation byproduct and sphingolipid metabolism intermediate, linked to oxidative stress mechanisms and inflammatory responses relevant to vascular health [148,149].

3-methylene-7,11-dimethyl-1-dodecene (**113**), an unsaturated hydrocarbon likely of terpenoid origin, may act as a semiochemical involved in plant–environment interactions, particularly in defense signaling. In turn, linoleyl alcohol (**114**), a long-chain unsaturated fatty alcohol, plays a role in the structural organization of plant cuticular waxes and membranes. In other botanical systems, it has demonstrated cytoprotective and membrane-stabilizing properties, supporting its potential bioactivity in *P. fruticosa* [149].

The identification of 3-methylene-7,11-dimethyl-1-dodecene and linoleyl alcohol, although not confirmed by isolation or reference standards, suggests that *P. fruticosa* synthesizes functionally diverse lipophilic compounds that may participate in both structural and signaling functions.

The predominance of these compounds in the PFLD fraction emphasizes the efficiency of medium-polarity solvents in isolating structurally diverse lipophilic metabolites. Their absence in previous reports such as that by Ashmawy et al. [4] may reflect either differences in extraction and detection methods or genuine chemotaxonomic distinctiveness. Caution is warranted before assuming novelty, and targeted confirmation using authentic standards and tandem MS is recommended.

Moreover, given the documented biological activities of structurally analogous compounds—particularly octanal and hexadecanal—these newly identified metabolites warrant further pharmacological investigation to evaluate their contributions to the therapeutic potential of *P. fruticosa* extracts.

The lack of functional assays for these lipophilic constituents remains a critical limitation. Future studies should integrate isolation-guided bioassays and metabolomic comparisons across Araliaceae species to validate their relevance in inflammation, oxidative stress, and membrane-associated signaling.

5.10. *Newly Identified Structurally Diverse Compounds in Polyscias fruticosa*

Comprehensive GC-MS analysis of *P. fruticosa* leaf extracts, as performed by Rarison et al. [10], led to the identification of several structurally diverse metabolites that appear to be previously unreported in this species or in the *Polyscias* genus as a whole, based on comparison with the phytochemical inventory by Ashmawy et al. [4]. These constituents, tentatively grouped as "other compounds" due to their chemical heterogeneity, were detected in either the dichloromethane (PFLD) or hexane (PFLH) fractions (Table 9), indicating that untargeted metabolomic profiling can uncover minor, but structurally significant, constituents. Notably, 4,3′-difluoro-4′-methoxybiphenyl was detected exclusively in the PFLH fraction, indicating that nonpolar solvents facilitate the isolation of halogenated aromatic compounds from lipophilic matrices.

Among the identified metabolites, malic acid (**117**) and 4-ethoxy-4-oxobutanoic (**115**) acid are low-molecular-weight carboxylic acids of potential metabolic and antioxidant relevance. Malic acid, a central intermediate of the tricarboxylic acid (TCA) cycle, may serve as a marker of active primary metabolism and intracellular pH regulation. In contrast, the presence of levoglucosan (**118**), a 1,6-anhydrosugar associated with the pyrolytic degradation of lignocellulosic biomass, could reflect oxidative stress responses or senescence-related remodeling of plant cell walls. However, it should be noted that levoglucosan is also a known thermal degradation product, and its detection in GC-MS analysis may represent an analytical artifact rather than a true endogenous metabolite. This highlights a key limitation of GC-MS-based profiling and warrants further validation using non-thermal extraction and detection methods. A particularly noteworthy finding is the detection of 2,3-dihydrothiophene (**116**), a sulfur-containing heterocycle rarely observed in higher plants. Its ecological roles may include allelopathic interactions or microbial defense. Also of significant interest is indole-3-carboxaldehyde (**120**), a tryptophan-derived indolic aldehyde with demonstrated antibacterial and anti-inflammatory activities. This compound is a known natural agonist of the aryl hydrocarbon receptor (AhR), a transcriptional regulator involved in mucosal immunity and epithelial barrier function [141,150]. Recent studies have shown that enteric formulations of indole-3-carboxaldehyde alleviate colitis and modulate host–microbiota interactions through AhR-dependent mechanisms [151]. Furthermore, hydrazone derivatives of this molecule exhibit marked antimicrobial activity against *Staphylococcus aureus* and *Candida albicans*, underscoring its potential as a bioactive lead structure [141]. Its occurrence in *P. fruticosa* suggests a broader distribution of AhR-active indoles within Araliaceae and highlights the need to investigate immunomodulatory effects of this species beyond the currently described anti-inflammatory activity.

Table 9. Structurally diverse metabolites newly identified in *Polyscias fruticosa* detected by GC-MS analysis.

No.	Compound Name	Type	Molecular Formula	Molecular Weight (g/mol)	Plant Source	Identification Method	Ref.
115	4-ethoxy-4-oxobutanoic acid	Carboxylic acid derivative (β-ketoester-type compound)	$C_6H_{10}O_4$	146.06	Leaves	GC-MS	[10]
116	2,3-dihydrothiophene	Sulfur-containing heterocyclic compound	C_4H_6S	86.02	Leaves	GC-MS	[10]
117	Malic acid	Dicarboxylic acid (α-hydroxy acid)	$C_4H_6O_5$	134.02	Leaves	GC-MS	[10]
118	Levoglucosan	Carbohydrate derivative (1,6-anhydro sugar)	$C_6H_{10}O_5$	162.05	Leaves	GC-MS	[10]
119	4,3′-difluoro-4′-methoxybiphenyl	Halogenated aromatic hydrocarbon (fluoroalkylated biphenyl)	$C_{13}H_{10}F_2O$	220.07	Leaves	GC-MS	[10]
120	Indole-3-carboxaldehyde	Indole derivative (aromatic heterocyclic aldehyde)	C_9H_7NO	145.05	Leaves	GC-MS	[10]
121	4,6,6-trimethyl-2-(3-methylbuta-1,3-dienyl)-3-oxatricyclo[5.1.0.0(2,4)]octane	Oxygenated polycyclic hydrocarbon (tricyclic ether–terpenoid-like compound)	$C_{15}H_{22}O$	218.16	Leaves	GC-MS	[10]

GC-MS—gas chromatography–mass spectrometry. Compounds (**115–121**) were identified using GC-MS under the same analytical conditions previously described (see footnote to Table 4). Their biological activities are discussed in Section 5.10.

The identification of 4,3′-difluoro-4′-methoxybiphenyl (**119**), a halogenated biphenyl derivative, is also of interest. This compound has demonstrated moderate antibacterial activity in vitro [152]. While fluorinated aromatics are often associated with anthropogenic origins or environmental contamination, their presence in *P. fruticosa* may reflect either an unrecognized endogenous biosynthetic route or biotransformation capability inherent to the plant. Alternatively, these compounds might arise from environmental uptake or microbial symbiosis, emphasizing the importance of discriminating endogenous metabolites from external contaminants.

Lastly, 4,6,6-Trimethyl-2-(3-methylbuta-1,3-dienyl)-3-oxatricyclo[5.1.0.0(2,4)]octane (**121**), a polycyclic oxygenated hydrocarbon, further exemplifies the chemical complexity of *P. fruticosa*. Its structural features suggest a potential terpenoid origin and may contribute to the plant's pharmacological or ecological interactions. However, its precise biosynthetic origin remains unclear and deserves further structural elucidation and biosynthetic pathway analysis.

From a critical perspective, the identification of these structurally diverse and often uncommon compounds raises several key points. First, their detection underscores the importance of fractionated extraction and non-targeted GC-MS profiling in revealing low-abundance phytochemicals. Second, the bioactivity of several identified molecules—or their close analogs—supports the hypothesis that *P. fruticosa* harbors unexplored pharmacologically relevant chemistry. Third, some constituents, such as levoglucosan or fluorinated aromatics, may be artifacts or of exogenous origin, highlighting the need for rigorous methodological controls and confirmatory studies.

Collectively, these newly identified compounds broaden the phytochemical landscape of *P. fruticosa*, reinforce its chemotaxonomic uniqueness within Araliaceae, and suggest its potential as a source of bioactive and structurally novel natural products. Future investigations should focus on confirming the endogenous origin of these metabolites, elucidating their biosynthetic pathways, and evaluating their pharmacological relevance through isolation and bioassay-guided studies.

5.11. Critical Review and Future Directions in the Phytochemical Research of Polyscias fruticosa

The phytochemical investigation of *Polyscias fruticosa* has significantly advanced in recent years, shifting from descriptive cataloging to more mechanistically driven exploration of bioactive constituents. The current review integrates both historical and newly identified compounds, highlighting the species' remarkable chemical diversity and its relevance to ethnopharmacology and drug discovery.

A critical finding is the first confirmed occurrence of tocopherols within the *Polyscias* genus, as reported by Rarison et al. [10]. This compound group was absent from earlier comprehensive reviews, including Ashmawy et al. [4]. This observation demonstrates the added value of revisiting known species with optimized solvent systems and modern GC-MS workflows. Tocopherols, known for their antioxidant and anti-inflammatory roles, suggest that *P. fruticosa* may contribute to redox balance not only through polyphenols and saponins, but also via lipophilic antioxidants. Nonetheless, their relative abundance in extracts is low, and their physiological relevance remains speculative without targeted quantification and in vivo confirmation.

Similarly, the identification of rare fatty acid isomers, notably 9,11-octadecadienoic acid and CLA-type compounds (e.g., 10-trans,12-cis-linoleic acid), adds a new dimension to the pharmacological potential of this plant. These lipids show activity via PPARγ and Nrf2 pathways, suggesting implications for metabolic and inflammatory disorders [142–146]. However, most of these findings are derived from mechanistic in vitro studies using non-purified fractions, which limits their direct pharmacological interpretation. Additional studies on bioavailability, metabolic stability, and formulation strategies are needed to assess their translational potential.

The discovery of previously undetected norisoprenoids, terpenoids, sulfur-containing heterocycles, and halogenated aromatics—such as indole-3-carboxaldehyde and 4,3′-difluoro-4′-methoxybiphenyl—expands the chemotaxonomic boundaries of the genus. These compounds, some with established biological relevance in other systems, such as AhR-mediated immunomodulation and antibacterial activity, provide leads for future drug discovery pipelines [10]. Their presence in *P. fruticosa*, particularly in lipophilic fractions, may support the species' distinct biosynthetic repertoire within Araliaceae and merits comparative chemotaxonomic studies with *Panax* and *Aralia* species. Nevertheless, their low abundance and analytical sensitivity challenge isolation and characterization efforts, requiring the development of efficient enrichment protocols and high-resolution analytical tools.

Although numerous studies have cataloged the presence of triterpenoid saponins and flavonoids [3,4,7,8,17], their biosynthetic pathways in *P. fruticosa* remain largely uncharacterized. Comparative transcriptomic and metabolomic studies, especially in relation to *Panax* and *Aralia* species, could help clarify the evolution and regulation of secondary metabolite biosynthesis in *Polyscias* [30]. In our view, such studies would enable functional annotation of biosynthetic gene clusters and support metabolic engineering or biotechnological production strategies.

From a methodological perspective, the application of GC-MS has proven essential in revealing volatile and lipophilic components. Nevertheless, this technique has limitations in detecting thermolabile or highly polar molecules. For instance, compounds such as levoglucosan may represent pyrolytic artifacts rather than true endogenous metabolites. Future research would benefit from integrating LC-MS/MS, NMR-based metabolomics, and spatial metabolite mapping (e.g., MALDI imaging) to provide a more comprehensive profile. Moreover, method validation using authentic standards and isotopically labeled compounds is needed to confirm the endogenous nature of low-abundance features.

In conclusion, *P. fruticosa* should be considered a chemically rich and pharmacologically versatile species. Its documented pharmacological effects—including anti-inflammatory, antidiabetic, antioxidant, and cytoprotective activities—can now be linked to a broader spectrum of structurally diverse metabolites.

The underutilization of its potential is primarily due to the limited integration of biosynthetic, pharmacokinetic, and clinical investigations. A systematic research agenda focusing on bioactivity-guided isolation, in vivo efficacy, and molecular mechanisms will be instrumental in unlocking its full therapeutic potential.

We also emphasize the need for chemotaxonomic and phylogenetic studies to better position *P. fruticosa* within the metabolic diversity of Araliaceae and to identify unique metabolite signatures that may guide drug discovery and standardization efforts.

6. Pharmacological Properties of *Polyscias fruticosa*: An Overview of Current Evidence

Polyscias fruticosa has been extensively used in traditional medicine across Southeast Asia for the management of inflammatory disorders, respiratory diseases, metabolic dysfunctions, and stress-related conditions. The pharmacological interest in this species stems not only from its diverse ethnomedicinal applications and the growing body of experimental evidence supporting its therapeutic potential. Notably, in vitro and in vivo studies have demonstrated anti-inflammatory, antiasthmatic, antidiabetic, antioxidant, antimicrobial, and neuroprotective activities [4,10,15–17,20,21].

A comprehensive characterization of the phytochemical constituents of *P. fruticosa*—including triterpenoid saponins, flavonoids, sterols, polyacetylenes, phenolic acids, and various volatile and lipophilic compounds—has been provided in Section 5: Chemical Composition and Structural Diversity of Bioactive Compounds in *Polyscias fruticosa*. Accordingly, the present section focuses exclusively on summarizing the current pharmacological findings and elucidating the underlying mechanisms of action where available.

This section aims to synthesize current experimental findings related to the biological activities of *P. fruticosa*, with particular emphasis on pharmacodynamic mechanisms and disease-relevant applications.

Although the current body of pharmacological evidence is promising, it remains fragmented and largely limited to preclinical studies. In our opinion, a critical gap persists in the form of well-designed in vivo studies and clinical trials that would validate the therapeutic relevance of *P. fruticosa*. Furthermore, few studies have directly linked specific compounds to distinct bioactivities using bioassay-guided isolation or mechanistic validation. Addressing these limitations will require interdisciplinary approaches combining phytochemistry, pharmacology, and systems biology to elucidate compound–target interactions and therapeutic pathways.

6.1. Bronchial Asthma—Clinical Background and Treatment Challenges

Bronchial asthma is a chronic inflammatory disorder of the airways characterized by variable clinical symptoms and reversible airflow limitation. It affects both children and adults, with global prevalence steadily rising. According to the World Health Organization, more than 300 million people are affected worldwide, with projections exceeding 400 million by 2025 [153].

The pathophysiology of asthma is complex, involving genetic predispositions, environmental exposures, and dysregulated immune responses. A hallmark feature is eosinophilic inflammation leading to hyperresponsiveness, obstruction, and structural airway remodeling. T-helper type 2 (Th2) lymphocytes play a central role by secreting IL-4, IL-5, and IL-13, which promote IgE production, eosinophil recruitment, and mediator release from mast cells [154].

Chronic inflammation also induces basement membrane thickening, smooth muscle hypertrophy, and mucus hypersecretion.

Pharmacologic management of asthma typically involves inhaled corticosteroids (ICS), β2-adrenergic agonists, leukotriene receptor antagonists, anticholinergic agents, and targeted biologic therapies such as monoclonal antibodies against IL-5, IL-4Rα, and IgE. However, many patients continue to experience exacerbations, and long-term drug use may cause adverse effects that reduce adherence and efficacy [153].

These limitations have fueled interest in complementary plant-based therapies with anti-inflammatory, antioxidant, and immunomodulatory potential. Among these is *P. fruticosa*, a member of the Araliaceae family that is traditionally used in the treatment of inflammatory conditions, respiratory ailments, and as a general tonic [4,155]. Recent studies suggest that *P. fruticosa* extracts can modulate airway inflammation, oxidative stress, bronchial tone, and mucus secretion, supporting its potential as a phytotherapeutic agent in asthma [10,56].

6.1.1. Antiasthmatic Potential of *Polyscias fruticosa*: Pharmacological and Mechanistic Insights

The ovalbumin (OVA)-induced asthma model is a widely accepted preclinical approach for evaluating immunopathological features and therapeutic responses in allergic asthma. It reproduces hallmark features of human asthma, such as eosinophilic airway inflammation, bronchial hyperresponsiveness, increased IgE levels, and a Th2-skewed cytokine profile.

In a study by Koffuor et al. [56], guinea pigs were sensitized and challenged with OVA and subsequently treated orally with an ethanolic leaf extract of *P. fruticosa* (PFE) at doses of 100, 250, and 500 mg·kg^{-1} for 21 consecutive days. Therapeutic efficacy was assessed via BALF eosinophil counts, serum CRP, ESR, and histopathological analysis of lung tissue.

Administration of PFE at (500 mg·kg^{-1}) resulted in a 56.3% reduction in eosinophils, a 43% decrease in CRP, and notable histological improvements. The treated animals showed reduced peribronchial infiltration and preserved bronchial epithelium. These effects were comparable to those of prednisolone (2 mg·kg^{-1}), underscoring the extract's anti-inflammatory potency.

Although cytokine levels were not directly measured, the results suggest Th2 suppression-possibly via reduced IL-4, IL-5, and IL-13 activity. Furthermore, hematological assessments and histological analysis of major organs revealed no signs of systemic toxicity, indicating the safety of prolonged PFE administration.

These findings confirm the antiasthmatic potential of *P. fruticosa*, particularly in reducing airway inflammation and systemic inflammatory markers, without inducing toxicity, supporting its development as a phytotherapeutic for allergic asthma [56]. These results confirm the antiasthmatic activity of *P. fruticosa* in vivo; however, the lack of cytokine data limits mechanistic understanding. Further studies should clarify immunomodulatory pathways and identify active constituents.

6.1.2. Mucolytic and Antitussive Activity

Effective control of mucus hypersecretion and cough is critical in the management of symptomatic asthma, particularly in mucus-dominant phenotypes. In a study conducted by Koffuor et al. [18], two complementary animal models were employed to assess the mucolytic and antitussive effects of *P. fruticosa*: (1) ammonium chloride (NH_4Cl)-induced bronchial secretion in ICR mice and (2) citric-acid-induced cough in guinea pigs. An aqueous root extract of *P. fruticosa* (PFE) was administered orally at doses of 100, 200, and 400 mg·kg^{-1} body weight.

In the NH_4Cl-induced mucus model, semi-quantitative evaluation using phenol red dye revealed a significant reduction in bronchial secretion. PFE at 400 mg·kg^{-1} reduced mucus volume by 49.7% versus control, with efficacy comparable to bromhexine, a reference mucolytic agent. The dose-dependent nature of this response indicates a consistent pharmacodynamic effect of the extract.

In the citric-acid-induced cough model, PFE significantly reduced the number of cough episodes by 67% and prolonged the latency to first cough by 82%, compared to the vehicle-treated group. These results indicate both suppression of chemically induced cough and possible modulation of airway sensory responsiveness. The antitussive effect was comparable to that of dihydrocodeine, a centrally acting reference drug.

Biochemical safety assessments, including serum levels of alanine aminotransferase (ALT), aspartate aminotransferase (AST), creatinine, and urea, showed no significant deviations from normal values, confirming the absence of systemic toxicity following subacute oral administration of PFE at doses up to 400 mg·kg^{-1}.

Triterpenoid saponins and glycosides may underlie the mucolytic effect, potentially by promoting mucociliary clearance and epithelial hydration. Although the precise mechanism of the antitussive action remains unclear, the observed effects suggest peripheral modulation of the cough reflex, possibly through desensitization of vagal afferents or through the regulation of TRPV1 and TRPA1 ion channels, both of which are involved in mediating airway sensory signaling [18].

In our opinion, these findings support the therapeutic relevance of *Polyscias fruticosa* in managing airway symptoms such as mucus hypersecretion and cough. Nonetheless, further studies are needed to elucidate its underlying mechanisms and confirm the observed effects in clinical settings.

6.1.3. Bronchodilatory and Antihistaminic Effects

The ability to induce bronchial smooth muscle relaxation and counteract the effects of bronchoconstrictors such as histamine and acetylcholine is central to the pharmacological management of asthma. In a study by Koffuor et al. [15], the bronchodilatory effects of *P. fruticosa* extract (PFE) was evaluated in guinea pigs subjected to bronchospasm induced by inhalation of histamine (5.8×10^{-2} mg·mL^{-1}) and acetylcholine (2.0×10^{-2} mg·mL^{-1}). Following provocation, animals received oral doses of PFE at 100, 250, and 500 mg·kg^{-1}, and responses were compared to those of reference drugs: mepyramine (an H_1 receptor antagonist) and atropine (a muscarinic M_3 receptor antagonist).

PFE significantly prolonged the time to onset of pre-convulsive dyspnea (PCD) in a dose-dependent manner, with increases ranging from 70% to 110%. It also reduced recovery time by 44–63% compared to control, confirming effective bronchodilation. These bronchodilatory effects were corroborated by in vitro experiments using isolated guinea pig ileum, in which PFE attenuated contractile responses to exogenously applied histamine and acetylcholine, indicating potential antagonism at H_1 and M_3 receptors [15].

These effects may be mediated by flavonoids, sesquiterpenes, and alkaloids that modulate G protein-coupled receptors regulating airway tone. Additionally, PFE may stabilize mast cells, reducing the release of bronchoconstrictors such as histamine, prostaglandins, and leukotrienes.

No adverse effects were reported at oral doses up to 500 mg·kg^{-1}, supporting the safety profile of the extract under subacute exposure conditions [15,18].

Collectively, the data support the bronchodilatory and antihistaminic potential of *P. fruticosa*, highlighting its relevance as a safe phytotherapeutic option for obstructive airway conditions including asthma and COPD.

In our opinion, these findings highlight the potential of *P. fruticosa* as a dual-acting bronchodilator and antihistaminic agent. However, further mechanistic studies and clinical validation are warranted to confirm its role in airway pharmacotherapy.

6.1.4. Molecular Mechanisms: Anti-Inflammatory and Antioxidant Pathways

Contemporary pharmacological research emphasizes the need to elucidate molecular mechanisms in order to identify therapeutic targets of plant-derived compounds. In this regard, Rarison et al. [10] employed an integrative approach combining network pharmacology, molecular docking, and in vitro assays using LPS-stimulated RAW 264.7 macrophages to evaluate the bioactivity of lipophilic extracts from *P. fruticosa*. The extract, tested at concentrations of 12.5, 25, and 50 μg·mL^{-1}, significantly inhibited nitric oxide (NO) production without inducing cytotoxicity, as confirmed by MTT assay. These effects were consistent with in silico predictions, indicating interactions with inflammation-related targets such as NF-κB, MAPK1, and PTGS2. A total of 71 phytoconstituents were identified in the extract, including sesquiterpenes (e.g., α-humulene), phytosterols (e.g., β-sitosterol), flavonoids, and phenolic acids. Molecular docking revealed strong binding to proteins involved in inflammatory and oxidative stress pathways, such as PTGS2 (COX-2), KEAP1, NFKB1, PRKCD, and TLR4. These findings suggest a dual modulatory potential—both anti-inflammatory and antioxidant.

In vitro assays further demonstrated that the extract significantly reduced the expression of pro-inflammatory cytokines TNF-α, IL-1β, and IL-6 in LPS-activated RAW 264.7 cells. ELISA confirmed cytokine suppression, while RT-qPCR and Western blotting showed downregulation at both mRNA and protein levels.

Importantly, the extract also upregulated the expression of antioxidant enzymes, including heme oxygenase-1 (HO-1) and catalase, which are under transcriptional control of the nuclear factor erythroid 2-related factor 2 (Nrf2). This indicates concurrent activation of the Nrf2-ARE pathway and inhibition of the TLR4-NF-κB inflammatory axis, contributing to a broad-spectrum protective mechanism [10].

Given the interplay between oxidative damage and chronic inflammation in asthma pathogenesis, the multimodal activity of *P. fruticosa* is of particular therapeutic interest.

By simultaneously suppressing pro-inflammatory signaling and enhancing cytoprotective defenses, *P. fruticosa* may aid both symptom management and long-term disease control in asthma, where oxidative stress and inflammation are synergistic contributors.

In our opinion, the ability of *P. fruticosa* extracts to simultaneously modulate key inflammatory and antioxidant pathways provides a strong rationale for further mechanistic and translational studies. Future work should focus on compound-specific activity and in vivo confirmation to validate therapeutic relevance.

6.2. Antidiabetic Activity of *Polyscias fruticosa*

6.2.1. Type 2 Diabetes and the Need for New Therapies

Diabetes mellitus (DM) is a chronic, progressive metabolic disorder and one of the most urgent global health challenges of the 21st century. Data from the World Health Organization indicated a global prevalence of 2.8% in 2000, expected to reach 5.4% by 2025 [156]. More recent estimates suggest that by 2045, nearly 700 million individuals—approximately 10% of the global adult population—will be affected [157]. The burden is especially high in low- and middle-income countries, where urbanization, dietary changes, and limited healthcare access accelerate incidence.

Type 2 diabetes mellitus (T2DM), which represents over 90% of DM cases, is primarily characterized by insulin resistance and a relative deficiency in insulin secretion. Chronic hyperglycemia, the hallmark of T2DM, is a major driver of both microvascular complications (e.g., nephropathy, retinopathy, neuropathy) and macrovascular diseases (e.g., coronary artery disease, stroke, peripheral arterial disease) [158].

Pharmacological management of T2DM typically involves oral antihyperglycemic agents such as metformin, sulfonylureas, dipeptidyl peptidase-4 (DPP-4) inhibitors, sodium–glucose co-transporter 2 (SGLT2) inhibitors, glucagon-like peptide-1 (GLP-1) receptor agonists, and exogenous insulin therapy. Although effective for glycemic control, these drugs are associated with reduced long-term efficacy, adverse effects (e.g., hypoglycemia, gastrointestinal intolerance), and limited adherence [156,158]. In resource-limited settings, high cost and restricted access further hinder disease management [157].

These limitations have driven interest in plant-based therapies as adjuncts or alternatives. Numerous phytochemicals—including flavonoids, triterpenoids (notably oleanolic acid), saponins, phenolic acids, and coumarins—have been shown to exert antidiabetic effects through diverse mechanisms. These include insulin-mimetic activity, stimulation of pancreatic β-cell insulin secretion, inhibition of carbohydrate-digesting enzymes (e.g., α-glucosidase, α-amylase), enhancement of peripheral glucose uptake, and modulation of inflammation and oxidative stress [158].

Several species within the Araliaceae family, including *P. fruticosa*, have been traditionally used in the management of diabetes. These plants are rich in triterpenoid saponins, oleanolic acid derivatives, and a wide array of polyphenols, all of which have demonstrated antidiabetic properties in preclinical studies.

Thus, *P. fruticosa* is considered a promising candidate for developing affordable, multi-targeted phytotherapeutics to address the complex pathophysiology of T2DM.

6.2.2. Mechanisms of Action of Identified Compounds

Polyscias fruticosa, a medicinal plant widely utilized in traditional Southeast Asian practices, is a rich source of bioactive triterpenoid saponins primarily derived from oleanolic acid. Among these, the most extensively studied antidiabetic compound is 3-*O*-[β-D-glucopyranosyl-(1→4)-β-D-glucuronopyranosyl] oleanolic acid 28-*O*-β-D-glucopyranosyl ester, commonly referred to as PFS [57].

In vitro enzymatic assays have demonstrated that PFS exhibits potent inhibitory activity against two key carbohydrate-hydrolyzing enzymes: α-amylase and α-glucosidase. Kinetic studies showed mixed noncompetitive inhibition of α-amylase and noncompetitive inhibition of α-glucosidase [57]. These dual inhibitory effects delay the enzymatic breakdown of dietary carbohydrates in the small intestine, thereby reducing glucose absorption and attenuating postprandial glycemic elevation.

The antidiabetic effect of PFS has also been confirmed in vivo. In a diet-induced hyperglycemic mouse model, oral administration of PFS at 100 mg·kg^{-1} significantly reduced blood glucose levels in a sucrose tolerance test, as evidenced by a lower area under the curve (AUC) [57].

Together, these findings support the multitargeted antidiabetic mechanism of PFS, combining inhibition of key digestive enzymes with effective reduction in glycemic response in vivo.

In our opinion, the complexity of T2DM pathophysiology justifies the exploration of multi-targeted phytotherapeutics, such as *P. fruticosa*. Its rich phytochemical profile warrants further investigation in translational and clinical contexts.

6.2.3. In Vivo Evidence of Antidiabetic Activity

In vivo studies have substantiated the hypoglycemic properties of PFS isolated from *P. fruticosa*. In BALB/c mice subjected to a high-sucrose diet, oral administration of PFS (100 mg·kg^{-1} body weight) significantly reduced postprandial blood glucose levels following a sucrose challenge. This effect was reflected by a significant reduction in the area under the glucose curve (AUC), consistent with delayed digestion and absorption of carbohydrates due to enzymatic inhibition [57].

Moreover, Tran et al. [14] reported that co-administration of low-dose PFS with acarbose enhanced the inhibition of α-amylase, producing a synergistic effect superior to either agent alone. This suggests a potential adjuvant role of PFS, enabling lower doses of conventional antidiabetic drugs and minimizing side effects.

In our opinion, the observed in vivo effects of PFS demonstrate promising hypoglycemic activity via enzymatic inhibition and synergism with standard drugs. However, further studies are needed to elucidate the bioavailability, pharmacokinetics, and long-term safety of PFS. In addition, the specific saponins responsible for this effect remain to be identified and characterized in detail. These insights would enhance the translational potential of *P. fruticosa*-based formulations in T2DM management.

6.2.4. Structure–Activity Relationship and Glycosidic Considerations

Structure–activity relationship (SAR) studies of oleanolic saponins have shown that the position and type of sugar substitution strongly influence antidiabetic activity. Guo et al. [159] demonstrated that 28-O-monoglycosides display higher α-glucosidase inhibition than 3-O-substituted analogs, which may be sterically hindered. Additionally, the presence of a terminal α-L-rhamnose enhances potency, likely via improved enzyme binding.

Substitution at C-28 favors interaction with hydrophobic pockets of digestive enzymes, whereas large glycosidic chains at C-3 can hinder access to catalytic sites. [159].

In our opinion, these SAR insights are particularly relevant to *P. fruticosa*, which contains oleanolic acid-type saponins with diverse sugar moieties. However, the glycosylation patterns of PFS remain incompletely characterized, and structure-guided isolation of specific glycosides may help identify the most potent antidiabetic constituents. Future SAR studies on purified saponins from *P. fruticosa* are warranted to optimize their therapeutic efficacy.

6.2.5. Molecular Mechanisms in Diabetes: Anti-Inflammatory and Antioxidant Pathways

Increasing in vitro and in vivo data support the multimodal effects of *P. fruticosa* extracts in T2DM (T2DM). Le et al. [160] reported that co-administration of *P. fruticosa* and *Morus alba* alleviated diabetic complications, including neuropathy and retinopathy, indicating synergistic metabolic and vascular protection.

Among identified compounds, PFS remains the lead candidate due to its enzymatic inhibition profile, favorable tolerability, and the potential to optimize glycosidic moieties for enhanced bioactivity.

Although glycosylation increases aqueous solubility, it may compromise absorption by lowering lipophilicity and membrane permeability. Therefore, rational modification of glycosidic residues is a promising strategy to fine-tune pharmacokinetic and pharmacodynamic profiles of oleanolic saponins in antidiabetic therapy. In our opinion, targeted structural modifications of glycosidic moieties—particularly at C-3 and C-28 positions—could significantly improve the therapeutic performance of *P. fruticosa* saponins. Future studies should explore structure–absorption relationships and evaluate bioavailability using advanced in vivo models.

6.2.6. Pharmacokinetics and Bioavailability of PFS

Chronic low-grade inflammation and oxidative stress are major drivers of insulin resistance and pancreatic β-cell dysfunction in T2DM. Pro-inflammatory cytokines such as TNF-α, IL-1β, and IL-6 impair insulin signaling via downregulation of IRS-1 and inhibition of the PI3K/AKT pathway [57].

PFS, the oleanolic-acid-based saponin from *P. fruticosa*, exhibits anti-inflammatory effects by suppressing the NF-κB pathway, leading to decreased transcription of TNF-α, IL-1β, and IL-6 [57]. Concurrently, PFS activates the Nrf2-ARE signaling cascade, promoting the expression of antioxidant enzymes such as HO-1, catalase, and superoxide dismutase (SOD), thereby enhancing cellular defense against oxidative stress.

Through simultaneous modulation of inflammatory and redox-sensitive pathways, PFS demonstrates pleiotropic antidiabetic action, supporting its potential as a disease-modifying phytochemical in the management of T2DM.

In our opinion, the ability of PFS to simultaneously attenuate inflammatory signaling and enhance antioxidant defenses provides a mechanistic rationale for its use as a multi-target antidiabetic agent. Further studies are needed to confirm these effects in vivo and to assess their impact on insulin sensitivity and β-cell function.

6.2.7. Safety and Toxicity of *Polyscias fruticosa* Preparations

Preclinical safety data indicate a favorable toxicological profile for *P. fruticosa* extracts. In vitro cytotoxicity assays using mammalian cell lines showed no cytotoxic effects of aqueous and ethanolic extracts from leaves or roots, even at high concentrations [158].

Likewise, oral administration of PFS up to 100 $mg \cdot kg^{-1}$ in murine models produced no signs of hepatotoxicity, nephrotoxicity, or histological damage to major organs. Behavioral and metabolic parameters remained stable, supporting the extract's safety under subacute exposure conditions [158].

Traditional uses of *P. fruticosa* as food and herbal medicine across Southeast Asia, e.g., in teas, soups, and salads, offers ethnobotanical evidence of its tolerability. Its dietary application, without documented adverse events, further reinforces its safety [158].

However, the amphiphilic structure of triterpenoid saponins such as PFS may interact with erythrocyte membranes, posing a theoretical risk of hemolysis at supraphysiological concentrations [57].

Although no hemolytic effects have been observed at therapeutic doses, further studies are warranted to evaluate chronic toxicity, reproductive safety, and genotoxicity.

For clinical application, standardized formulations of *P. fruticosa* are essential, including detailed profiling of active saponins to ensure consistency and regulatory compliance.

In our opinion, further toxicological evaluation—particularly on chronic exposure, reproductive safety, and genotoxicity—is crucial for clinical translation. Future studies should also address herb–drug interactions and human metabolism of key saponins.

6.2.8. Comparison with Other Antidiabetic Plants

Among medicinal plants investigated for their antidiabetic activity, *P. fruticosa* emerges as a particularly promising candidate due to its multifaceted pharmacological profile. Its principal bioactive constituent—PFS, chemically defined as 3-*O*-[β-D-glucopyranosyl-(1→4)-β-D-glucuronopyranosyl] oleanolic acid 28-*O*-β-D-glucopyranosyl ester—exhibits potent dual inhibition of both α-amylase and α-glucosidase, key enzymes involved in postprandial glucose regulation [57]. This enzymatic inhibition is further complemented by the extract's anti-inflammatory properties, mediated via suppression of the NF-κB signaling cascade, and its stimulation of the Nrf2-dependent antioxidant response pathway [160].

In comparison, *Morus alba* (white mulberry) exerts its hypoglycemic effect primarily through 1-deoxynojirimycin (DNJ), a selective α-glucosidase inhibitor with limited or no activity against α-amylase. As a result, its ability to attenuate postprandial hyperglycemia may be less pronounced than that of multitarget agents such as PFS [160]. Moreover, *M. alba* lacks strong evidence of anti-inflammatory or antioxidant effects, which limits its utility in addressing the complex pathophysiology of T2DM.

Momordica charantia (bitter melon) contains insulin-mimetic compounds that promote glucose uptake and enhance glycemic control; however, marked variability in phytochemical composition among cultivars and geographic origins has been shown to affect the reproducibility of its hypoglycemic effects [156]. Similarly, *Panax notoginseng* exerts antidiabetic effects mainly through ginsenosides that improve insulin sensitivity and β-cell function, yet the overall magnitude and consistency of these effects remain variable, and the cost and standardization of ginsenoside-rich extracts present additional challenges [161].

A noteworthy comparison can be drawn with *Aralia elata*, a close relative of *P. fruticosa* within the Araliaceae family. This species contains oleanolic acid and triterpenoid saponins such as araloside A, which have demonstrated inhibition of aldose reductase, a key enzyme involved in diabetic complications, and enhancement of glucose homeostasis [157]. This suggests a conserved triterpenoid-based antidiabetic mechanism within the Araliaceae family.

The multitarget pharmacodynamic profile of *P. fruticose*—encompassing digestive enzyme inhibition, modulation of inflammatory signaling, and activation of redox-regulatory pathways—distinguishes it from other botanicals with more limited mechanisms of action. In addition to its low toxicity and traditional dietary use in Southeast Asia, these properties support its potential as a safe, culturally accepted, and biologically effective phytotherapeutic agent.

Unlike single-mechanism herbs such as *M. alba*, *P. fruticosa* may yield additive or synergistic effects when co-administered with conventional antidiabetic agents. For instance, co-administration with acarbose has demonstrated additive inhibitory effects on carbohydrate-digesting enzymes, supporting its role in combinatorial phytotherapy [14].

Further comparative studies in diabetic animal models and human trials are warranted to confirm the clinical relevance and superiority of *P. fruticosa* in managing type 2 diabetes mellitus.

In our opinion, the unique multitarget action of *P. fruticosa* positions it as a more comprehensive phytotherapeutic candidate compared to single-mechanism botanicals. Its synergy with standard drugs further increases its translational relevance in modern diabetes management.

6.3. Potential of Polyscias fruticosa in Neurodegenerative Diseases

Neurodegenerative diseases such as Parkinson's disease (PD) and Alzheimer's disease (AD) are characterized by progressive neuronal loss and currently lack effective disease-modifying therapies. Although pharmacological treatments such as levodopa and dopamine agonists offer symptomatic relief, their prolonged use is associated with significant side effects, including neurotoxicity, motor fluctuations, and dyskinesias [4,20,21,162]. These limitations have stimulated growing interest in medicinal plants such as *P. fruticosa* as potential alternative or adjunct therapies.

Multiple studies have shown that phytochemicals—particularly polyphenols, flavonoids, alkaloids, and saponins—can modulate oxidative stress, mitochondrial dysfunction, and neuroinflammation, which are central mechanisms underlying neurodegeneration [21,162]. *P. fruticosa*, a rich source of these bioactive compounds, has demonstrated antioxidant, anti-inflammatory, and neurotrophic properties relevant to neurodegenerative pathologies [20,21].

6.3.1. Molecular Mechanisms and Comparative Neuroprotective Potential of *Polyscias fruticosa*

The neuroprotective activity of *P. fruticosa* has been demonstrated in both in vivo and in vitro models. In a murine model of Parkinson's disease induced by MPTP, Ly et al. [20] reported that oral administration of ethanolic leaf extract significantly restored dopaminergic neuronal density in the substantia nigra and increased striatal dopamine levels. These effects were associated with activation of the AKT/CREB/BDNF signaling cascade, which supports neuronal survival and synaptic plasticity. Concurrently, the extract suppressed NF-κB activation and reduced the expression of pro-inflammatory cytokines, including IL-1β, IL-6, and TNF-α, as shown by Western blot and immunohistochemical analyses [20,163].

Supporting in vitro evidence was provided by Selvaraj et al. [21], who treated murine HT22 hippocampal neurons with a 75% ethanol extract of *P. fruticosa* roots (EEPF). At 50 $\mu g \cdot mL^{-1}$, EEPF markedly reduced glutamate-induced oxidative stress (assessed by DCF-DA fluorescence) and intracellular Ca^{2+} influx (measured with Fluo-3-AM). The extract also inhibited apoptosis by preventing AIF nuclear translocation and restored AKT and CREB phosphorylation and BDNF expression. Western blot analysis revealed modulation of MAPK phosphorylation and normalization of the Bax/Bcl-2 ratio, indicating mitochondrial pathway engagement.

Taken together, available evidence suggests that the neuroprotective effects of *P. fruticosa* are mediated by suppression of pro-inflammatory cytokines, ROS neutralization, mitochondrial stabilization, and activation of neurotrophic signaling pathways [8]. These multimodal mechanisms are relevant to the pathogenesis of disorders such as Parkinson's and Alzheimer's disease [20,21]. A meaningful comparison can be made with *Panax ginseng*, whose neuroprotective effects are mainly linked to ginsenosides like Rg3 acting via the PI3K/AKT pathway [20,164]. In contrast, *P. fruticosa* contains phenolic acids with potent antioxidant capacity (e.g., dehydroferulic acid, protocatechuic acid) and uniquely protects against glutamate excitotoxicity [21].

In our view, the broader mechanism of action of *P. fruticosa*, combining anti-inflammatory, antioxidant, and mitochondrial-stabilizing effects, may confer advantages over classical neuroprotective plants. Its distinct phytochemical profile supports further investigation as an alternative or complementary agent in neurodegenerative disease therapy.

6.3.2. Safety and Therapeutic Relevance

Toxicological assessments confirm the favorable safety profile of *P. fruticosa* extracts in preclinical models. Ly et al. [20] showed that repeated oral administration of ethanolic leaf extract at 100 $mg \cdot kg^{-1}$ for 14 days in MPTP-treated mice did not induce histopathological alterations in major organs. Hematological and biochemical parameters remained within normal ranges, suggesting systemic tolerability. This contrasts with synthetic dopaminergic agents that often induce hepatotoxicity and behavioral abnormalities upon chronic administration [20].

Selvaraj et al. [21] further demonstrated that co-treatment of HT22 neurons with *P. fruticosa* extract (50 $\mu g \cdot mL^{-1}$) and subtoxic doses of glutamate significantly enhanced cell viability compared to monotherapies, indicating potential synergism and a dose-sparing effect.

The multitarget pharmacological profile of *P. fruticosa*—encompassing antioxidant, anti-inflammatory, mitochondrial protective, and neurotrophic mechanisms—together with its low toxicity, supports its potential use as an adjunct neuroprotective agent. Further studies in translational animal models and clinical settings are warranted to validate its therapeutic utility in neurodegenerative disorders.

6.4. *Antibacterial Properties of Polyscias fruticosa*

The rapid emergence of antibiotic-resistant bacterial strains poses a serious threat to global health. The World Health Organization has identified antimicrobial resistance as one of the major public health challenges of the 21st century, with projections estimating up to 10 million annual deaths attributable to drug-resistant infections by 2050 [163]. The stagnation in the development of new antibiotics has intensified interest in alternative antimicrobial strategies, particularly those based on medicinal plants [165]. Medicinal plant-derived phytochemicals exhibit multitarget antibacterial activity and are increasingly explored as complementary agents against resistant pathogens. Plant-derived extracts constitute a rich reservoir of bioactive compounds capable of exerting broad-spectrum antibacterial effects through multiple mechanisms, such as membrane disruption, inhibition of macromolecular synthesis, and suppression of biofilm formation [166].

Within this context, *P. fruticosa*, a member of the Araliaceae family, has attracted interest due to its diverse phytochemical composition and experimentally validated antibacterial potential [16,17,94].

6.4.1. Phytochemical Composition and Antibacterial Potential

Polyscias fruticosa is known to contain a broad array of bioactive metabolites, including triterpenoid saponins (e.g., ladyginoside A, chikusetsusaponin IVa, polysciosides A–K), flavonoids (e.g., quercetin), phenolic acids (e.g., gallic acid), alkaloids, tannins, and polyacetylenes such as falcarinol and heptadeca-1,8(E)-diene-4,6-diyne-3,10-diol [10,94]. Among these, polyacetylenes have demonstrated particularly strong antibacterial activity, frequently surpassing that of saponin-rich fractions [10]. Comparative phytochemical analysis showed that ether-soluble fractions enriched in polyacetylenes (EPA) exhibited greater antibacterial potency than n-butanol fractions (NBHS) containing primarily triterpenoid saponins [10].

These findings suggest that polyacetylenes are likely the primary contributors to the antibacterial effects of *P. fruticosa*.

6.4.2. Comparative Antibacterial Efficacy

The antibacterial activity of *P. fruticosa* compares favorably with that of other medicinal plants. In the study by Titova et al. [17], extracts derived from *P. fruticosa* suspension cultures grown in bubble-type bioreactors exhibited minimum inhibitory concentration (MIC) values ranging from 250 to 2000 $\mu g \cdot mL^{-1}$, markedly lower than the MICs of 4000 $\mu g \cdot mL^{-1}$ reported for greenhouse-derived leaf extracts. These values also outperform those of *Thymus vulgaris* and *Syzygium aromaticum*, which exhibited MICs of approximately 3150 $\mu g \cdot mL^{-1}$ against *Bacillus cereus*, and *Rosmarinus officinalis*, which required >1000 $\mu g \cdot mL^{-1}$ to inhibit *E. coli* and *Staphylococcus aureus* [166].

In contrast, *Panax notoginseng*, a related Araliaceae species, displayed more limited antibacterial activity, primarily targeting *Streptococcus pyogenes*, with diminished efficacy against Gram-negative bacteria [167,168].

These comparisons underscore the broad-spectrum potential of *P. fruticosa*, particularly due to its polyacetylene-rich composition and favorable safety profile.

6.4.3. Evidence of Antibacterial Activity

Several studies have confirmed the antibacterial efficacy of *P. fruticosa* against clinically relevant pathogens, including *Staphylococcus aureus* (including methicillin-resistant *S. aureus*, MRSA), *E. coli*, *Pseudomonas aeruginosa*, and *Salmonella typhi* [16,17,94]. In particular, Titova et al. [17] reported superior activity of extracts obtained from in vitro suspension cultures, which produced significantly lower MICs than those derived from field-grown material.

Polyacetylene-rich fractions were consistently more effective than triterpenoid saponin fractions [10], suggesting that lipophilic compounds may better penetrate bacterial membranes or disrupt vital functions. Importantly, these extracts demonstrated no acute toxicity in murine models [10], supporting their potential safety as natural antimicrobial agents.

6.4.4. Mechanisms of Antibacterial Action

The antibacterial effects of *P. fruticosa* are believed to result from multiple synergistic mechanisms:

- Disruption of bacterial membrane integrity—both saponins and polyacetylenes can increase membrane permeability, leading to osmotic imbalance and cell lysis [165–168].
- Inhibition of protein and peptidoglycan biosynthesis—certain constituents may bind to ribosomal subunits or enzymes that are critical for bacterial cell wall synthesis, disrupting growth and replication [17].
- Alteration of membrane potential and intracellular pH—some extracts interfere with bacterial membrane electrochemical gradients, leading to acidification and metabolic dysfunction [165].
- Inhibition of biofilm formation—compounds such as falcarinol and flavonoids impair bacterial adhesion and prevent the establishment of protective biofilm matrices [17,94].

These multitarget mechanisms may enhance effectiveness against antibiotic-resistant strains and reduce the likelihood of resistance development. Further mechanistic studies using molecular and omics approaches are warranted to fully elucidate the antimicrobial pathways involved.

6.5. *Phytochemical Significance of Polyscias fruticosa in Green Synthesis of Anticancer Nanoparticles*

The use of plant-derived bioactive compounds in nanomedicine is gaining traction as a strategy to enhance the efficacy, selectivity, and safety of anticancer agents. *Polyscias fruticosa*, traditionally recognized for its anti-inflammatory and immunomodulatory properties, has recently gained attention as a valuable resource for the green synthesis of metal-based nanoparticles due to its content of triterpenoid saponins, polyphenols, and flavonoids [3,4,8,10,11,13].

These phytoconstituents play a dual role: (i) acting as natural reducing agents facilitating the conversion of metal ions into nanoparticles, and (ii) stabilizing the resulting nanostructures by improving colloidal stability and bioavailability [169,170].

Such dual functionality supports its use in environmentally sustainable nanotechnological approaches, particularly in biomedical applications such as cancer therapy.

6.5.1. Biosynthesis and Cytotoxicity of Nanoparticles

Recent studies have confirmed the feasibility of green synthesis of silver (AgNPs) and copper (CuNPs) nanoparticles using aqueous or ethanolic extracts from *P. fruticosa* leaves and roots [169,170]. These biosynthesized nanoparticles exhibit spherical morphology (50–120 nm), characteristic UV-Vis plasmon resonance peaks, and negative zeta potentials (−25 to −30 mV), indicating stability and uniformity.

Cytotoxicity assays demonstrated that Pfr-AgNPs reduced the viability of A549 human lung carcinoma cells by 47.3% at 100 $\mu g \cdot mL^{-1}$, while Pfr-CuNPs inhibited neuroblastoma cell proliferation by 55.5% at 125 $\mu g \cdot mL^{-1}$ [169,170]. Mechanistically, cytotoxic effects are associated with ROS generation, mitochondrial dysfunction, membrane depolarization, and caspase-mediated apoptosis.

Notably, brine shrimp lethality assays confirmed the low toxicity of the crude extract (LC_{50} > 1000 $\mu g \cdot mL^{-1}$), whereas the nanoparticles exhibited moderate toxicity (LC_{50} = 524 $\mu g \cdot mL^{-1}$), suggesting selective cytotoxicity toward cancer cells.

6.5.2. Mechanistic Insights and Therapeutic Prospects

Current evidence indicates that the cytotoxic effects of *P. fruticosa*-derived nanoparticles are mainly due to the release of Ag^+ or Cu^+ ions, which induce intracellular oxidative stress, apoptosis pathways, and inhibition of cellular proliferation [171]. Additionally, phytochemical surface coatings composed of saponins and flavonoids may facilitate cellular uptake and improve intracellular delivery.

Triterpenoid saponins present in the extract are hypothesized to influence multiple molecular targets, including MAPK signaling, topoisomerase inhibition, and regulation of cell cycle genes and metastasis-related pathways, offering a multimodal anticancer mechanism.

However, further studies are required to evaluate the in vivo efficacy, biodistribution, and long-term safety of these nanoparticles, as the current evidence is limited to in vitro models.

6.6. *Reproductive Effects of Polyscias fruticosa*

Medicinal plants have played a foundational role in the management of reproductive disorders within various traditional medical systems. Their phytochemical complexity, including phytoestrogens, alkaloids, flavonoids, and saponins, enables modulation of endocrine pathways and offers potential therapeutic alternatives to conventional hormone-based interventions [172]. Botanical species such as *Trifolium pratense* (red clover), *Withania somnifera* (ashwagandha), and *Panax ginseng* have demonstrated efficacy in regulating folliculogenesis, improving hormonal balance, and enhancing fertility parameters in both females and males [172].

In this context, *P. fruticosa*, widely recognized for its adaptogenic, anti-inflammatory, and immunomodulatory properties, has recently attracted attention for its potential reproductive effects. Emerging preclinical data suggest that its extracts modulate both ovarian and testicular function through phytohormonal and antioxidant pathways.

6.6.1. Female Reproductive Effects

Boye et al. [173] investigated the influence of *P. fruticosa* leaf extract (PFE) on ovarian function and implantation parameters in non-pregnant female rats. Oral administration of PFE at doses of 100 and 200 $mg \cdot kg^{-1}$ body weight significantly enhanced follicular development, as evidenced by increased counts of primordial and primary follicles. These outcomes mirrored the stimulatory effects of clomiphene citrate, a standard ovulation-inducing agent.

Corresponding increases in uterine weight and epithelial proliferation were also observed, suggesting estrogen receptor-mediated modulation of uterine tissue.

Hormonal assays revealed a decrease in serum follicle-stimulating hormone (FSH) levels and concomitant elevations in luteinizing hormone (LH) and estradiol, indicating potential activation of the hypothalamic–pituitary–gonadal (HPG) axis. However, administration of the highest tested dose (500 mg$\cdot$kg^{-1}) led to a significant increase in post-implantation loss, implying potential embryotoxic effects at elevated concentrations [173].

These findings emphasize the importance of identifying an optimal therapeutic window, as excessive stimulation may disrupt implantation and embryonic viability.

6.6.2. Male Reproductive Effects

A subsequent study by the same group [155] explored the effects of PFE on male reproductive parameters over a 21-day period. Rats treated with 100, 250, or 500 mg$\cdot$kg^{-1} of the extract demonstrated notable improvements in sperm count, motility, and morphological integrity. Histological examination of testicular tissues revealed well-preserved seminiferous tubule architecture at all doses, although mild vacuolization was detected at the highest dose.

Endocrinological analysis showed a dose-dependent decrease in serum testosterone levels, accompanied by elevated LH concentrations. This paradoxical profile may indicate disruption of Leydig cell steroidogenesis or compensatory upregulation of gonadotropin secretion due to altered negative feedback.

Despite this testosterone suppression, the improvements in spermatogenic indices indicate a favorable effect on spermatogenesis and sperm functionality [155].

6.6.3. Phytoestrogenic Mechanisms and Broader Context

The reproductive effects of *P. fruticosa* are likely mediated in part by its phytoestrogenic constituents, including flavonoids and triterpenoid saponins, which may bind to estrogen receptors and modulate gene expression along the HPG axis. Similar estrogenic mechanisms have been implicated in other phytoestrogen-rich botanicals used for treating menstrual irregularities, polycystic ovary syndrome (PCOS), and premature ovarian failure [172].

Furthermore, the adaptogenic and antioxidant properties of *P. fruticosa* may contribute to improved reproductive outcomes under stress conditions, oxidative load, or environmental insults. Its saponin profile shares pharmacodynamic similarities with ginsenosides from *Panax ginseng*, which are known to promote male sexual performance and regulate female endocrine homeostasis [172,174].

Of note, comparative analyses of triterpenoid structures support the hypothesis of shared receptor targets across Araliaceae-derived adaptogens.

Taken together, these findings position *P. fruticosa* as a promising multifunctional agent for reproductive health. Nonetheless, further investigations—including long-term toxicity, fertility, and teratogenicity studies—are essential to validate its safety and effectiveness in clinical use. The standardization of extract composition and dose–response characterization remain critical future directions.

6.7. Anti-Osteoclastogenic Potential of Polyscias fruticosa in Bone Health

The maintenance of skeletal homeostasis relies on a delicate balance between bone-forming osteoblasts and bone-resorbing osteoclasts. Disruption of this balance in favor of osteoclastic bone resorption underlies the pathogenesis of several skeletal disorders, including osteoporosis, rheumatoid arthritis, and Paget's disease [175].

Osteoclasts originate from monocyte/macrophage precursors and undergo differentiation in response to key cytokines—macrophage colony-stimulating factor (M-CSF) and receptor activator of nuclear factor kappa-B ligand (RANKL). Engagement of RANKL with its receptor RANK activates intracellular cascades, such as the mitogen-activated protein kinase (MAPK) pathways and nuclear factor kappa-light-chain-enhancer of activated B cells (NF-κB), which in turn upregulate essential transcription factors, including c-Fos and NFATc1, driving osteoclastogenesis [176].

Tran et al. [19] investigated the anti-osteoclastogenic effects of ethanol extract from *P. fruticosa* leaves (EEPL) in both bone marrow-derived macrophages (BMMs) and RAW264.7 murine macrophage cells. Treatment with EEPL at concentrations ranging from 12.5 to 100 $\mu g \cdot mL^{-1}$ markedly inhibited RANKL-induced osteoclast differentiation in a dose-dependent manner. At the highest tested concentration (100 $\mu g \cdot mL^{-1}$), the extract suppressed the formation of tartrate-resistant acid phosphatase-positive ($TRAP^{+}$) multinucleated cells by more than 85% relative to the RANKL-only control ($p < 0.001$).

EEPL also disrupted actin ring formation and significantly reduced the resorption pit area, indicative of impaired osteoclast function ($p < 0.01$ and $p < 0.001$ for higher doses).

This suppression of both osteoclastogenesis and resorptive capacity indicates functional inhibition beyond mere cytotoxicity.

These functional outcomes were accompanied by decreased mRNA and protein expression of osteoclast-associated markers, including TRAP, matrix metallopeptidase-9 (MMP-9), cathepsin K (CtsK), c-Fos, and NFATc1. Mechanistically, EEPL selectively inhibited the phosphorylation of p38 and JNK MAPKs while leaving ERK1/2 signaling unaffected, suggesting targeted interference with RANKL-mediated downstream signaling events [19,176].

The antiresorptive activity of *P. fruticosa* is comparable to that of other phytotherapeutics with known bone-protective properties. For example, ethanol extracts of *Osmanthus fragrans* have been shown to inhibit osteoclastogenesis by reducing intracellular reactive oxygen species and attenuating both NF-κB and MAPK signaling pathways [176].

Likewise, *Perilla frutescens* hexane leaf extract inhibited osteoclast differentiation through suppression of MMP-9 expression and RANKL pathway modulation in both cellular and animal models [177].

Such comparisons underscore the growing relevance of botanicals in bone health management, particularly those modulating osteoimmune crosstalk.

Given the adverse effects associated with conventional antiresorptive agents such as bisphosphonates, including osteonecrosis of the jaw and atypical femoral fractures, plant-based therapeutics like EEPL offer an attractive, multitarget alternative with a favorable safety profile.

Notably, *P. fruticosa* exhibits a broad pharmacological spectrum encompassing anti-inflammatory, antioxidant, neuroprotective, antidiabetic, and osteoprotective activities. The multitarget profile of *P. fruticosa* suggests potential benefits in complex pathologies such as postmenopausal osteoporosis, where inflammation, oxidative stress, and hormonal dysregulation coexist.

Its principal active compounds, triterpenoid saponins (e.g., PFS), flavonoids, and polyacetylenes, are implicated in these diverse biological effects.

In particular, saponins may modulate RANKL-induced transcription, while polyacetylenes could contribute to anti-inflammatory signaling inhibition.

However, challenges remain, particularly concerning the limited oral bioavailability of saponins and the potential for endocrine modulation at high doses. Further research, including in vivo validation in osteoporotic models, pharmacokinetic and toxicological profiling, and the development of targeted delivery systems such as nanocarriers, is necessary to fully elucidate and harness the anti-osteoclastogenic potential of *P. fruticosa* in clinical bone health management.

Moreover, standardization of extract composition and identification of active constituents are critical steps toward therapeutic development.

6.8. Author's Perspective on the Pharmacological Potential of *Polyscias fruticosa*

Polyscias fruticosa emerges as a pharmacologically versatile medicinal plant whose broad spectrum of biological activities—ranging from antidiabetic and anti-inflammatory to neuroprotective, antimicrobial, and osteoprotective—has been increasingly substantiated by preclinical evidence [10,11,13,15,17–21]. Unlike many botanical agents that exert isolated effects, *P. fruticosa* demonstrates a multitarget pharmacodynamic profile, largely attributed to its diverse phytochemical composition, including triterpenoid saponins, polyacetylenes, flavonoids, phenolic acids, and sterols [3,4,6,10,11,16].

A critical comparative analysis with related medicinal plants—such as *Panax ginseng*, *Morus alba*, and *Momordica charantia*—highlights *P. fruticosa*'s unique advantages, including dual enzyme inhibition in diabetes management, mitochondrial stabilization in neurodegeneration, and superior antibacterial activity due to polyacetylene-rich fractions [10,11]. Furthermore, its adaptogenic and immunomodulatory properties provide a theoretical basis for its use in hormone-sensitive conditions, such as reproductive disorders and postmenopausal osteoporosis.

However, despite these promising findings, significant knowledge gaps remain. First, many pharmacological studies rely on ethanolic or crude extracts without standardization, making reproducibility and dose extrapolation challenging. Second, the *oral bioavailability and pharmacokinetics* of key compounds, particularly saponins, remain poorly defined. Third, safety data from long-term and reproductive toxicity studies are scarce—particularly in relation to embryotoxicity observed at high doses in female rats [173].

Importantly, the recent application of *P. fruticosa*-derived phytochemicals in green synthesis of metal-based nanoparticles opens new avenues for targeted anticancer therapy [169,170]. Nevertheless, this nanomedical potential demands further optimization of formulation strategies, cytotoxicity profiling in non-cancerous cells, and in vivo validation.

To advance *P. fruticosa* toward evidence-based clinical application, the following priorities are recommended:

- Standardization and quantification of active fractions;
- Comparative efficacy studies in validated animal models;
- Mechanistic investigations using omics platforms;
- Toxicological profiling under chronic and reproductive exposure;
- Development of delivery systems to overcome bioavailability limitations.

In summary, *P. fruticosa* represents a phytotherapeutic candidate with strong applicative potential. Its complex pharmacological potential aligns with the multifactorial nature of chronic diseases, but systematic research efforts—both mechanistic and clinical—are required to unlock its full therapeutic promise.

7. Conclusions and Future Perspectives

Polyscias fruticosa emerges as a promising, yet underutilized, medicinal plant situated at the intersection of plant biotechnology, phytochemistry, and pharmacology. Its demonstrated amenability to in vitro propagation, structurally diverse array of secondary metabolites, and broad spectrum of pharmacological activities underscore its value as a candidate for phytotherapeutic and nutraceutical development.

In plant biotechnology, robust micropropagation protocols employing apical meristem cultures and somatic embryogenesis have been successfully established. Suspension cultures derived from callus tissues have demonstrated biosynthetic competence for various classes of secondary metabolites, including triterpenoid saponins and phenolic compounds. However, current investigations remain limited to the laboratory scale. Future efforts should prioritize the upscaling of biomass and metabolite production using semi-technical or industrial bioreactor systems. Optimization of culture media, the application of elicitors, control of physicochemical parameters, and the implementation of AI-assisted modeling of growth and metabolite dynamics represent key directions for future research. Notably, the absence of studies on genetically transformed root cultures in *P. fruticosa* presents an opportunity for the development of alternative, non-transgenic production platforms aligned with sustainable biotechnological standards.

Phytochemically, *P. fruticosa* exhibits a complex profile comprising triterpenoid saponins, flavonoids, phenolic acids, sterols, polyacetylenes, and fatty acid derivatives. Many of these compounds share structural similarities with ginsenosides and other metabolites characteristic of the Araliaceae family. However, further elucidation of stereochemical configurations and biosynthetic pathways remains a critical gap. Integrative metabolomic approaches combining UPLC-QTOF-MS/MS, GC×GC-MS, and NMR spectroscopy with transcriptomic profiling are essential to deepen our understanding of its metabolic landscape. In particular, the identification and functional characterization of key biosynthetic enzymes—such as cytochrome P450s, glycosyltransferases, and methyltransferases—would facilitate targeted metabolic engineering for enhanced compound production.

From a pharmacological standpoint, *P. fruticosa* has demonstrated anti-inflammatory, antidiabetic, antiasthmatic, neuroprotective, and antiresorptive activities in preclinical models. Nonetheless, most studies remain exploratory and lack comprehensive mechanistic and translational validation. Future research should incorporate systems pharmacology approaches, including molecular docking, multi-omics target validation, and disease-specific in vivo models. The pharmacodynamic interplay between compound classes, such as saponin–flavonoid synergy, should be investigated to uncover pleiotropic effects on interconnected signaling networks. Standardized extracts and purified fractions must be subjected to rigorous pharmacokinetic and toxicological assessments, followed by well-designed clinical trials, particularly in chronic metabolic and neuroinflammatory disorders.

In conclusion, *P. fruticosa* exemplifies a next-generation medicinal plant with strong translational potential. Its advancement demands a multidisciplinary framework integrating innovative plant tissue culture technologies, state-of-the-art analytical chemistry, and mechanistically driven pharmacological research. As an alternative source of Araliaceae-type saponins, *P. fruticosa* holds particular promise as a sustainable, bioactive reservoir for future phytopharmaceutical applications.

Author Contributions: Conceptualization, original draft preparation, reviewing, editing, and visualization: A.A.Ś.; literature assistance and manuscript support: K.T. All authors have read and agreed to the published version of the manuscript.

Funding: This research received no external funding.

Institutional Review Board Statement: Not applicable.

Informed Consent Statement: Not applicable.

Data Availability Statement: Data are contained within the article.

Acknowledgments: The authors gratefully acknowledge Maciej Obrębski for granting the license to use the graphical abstract Created with (Academic (Student Plan) version) BioRender.com. Obrębski, M. (2025). Available online: https://BioRender.com/r2qnh1h (accessed on 18 August 2025) [178] in this manuscript (agreement number: AF285G0WEJK). The authors also thank Rafał Kiełkiewicz for his assistance in preparing the graphical abstract.

Conflicts of Interest: The authors declare no conflicts of interest.

References

1. Lowry, P.P., II; Plunkett, G.M. Recircumscription of *Polyscias* (Araliaceae) to include six related genera, with a new infrageneric classification and a synopsis of species. *Plant Divers. Evol.* **2010**, *128*, 55–84. [CrossRef]

2. Hernández Peña, A.M.; Hernández Pérez, L.A. *Polyscias fruticosa* L. en Cuba. Valores de uso. *Agrisost* **2020**, *26*, 1–7.
3. Vo, D.H.; Yamamura, S.; Ohtani, K.; Kasai, R.; Yamasaki, K.; Chau, N.T.N.; Minh, H.M. Saponins from *Polyscias fruticosa*. *Phytochemistry* **1998**, *47*, 451–457. [CrossRef] [PubMed]
4. Ashmawy, N.S.; Gad, H.A.; Ashour, M.L.; El-Ahmady, S.H.; Singab, A.N.B. The genus *Polyscias* (Araliaceae): A phytochemical and biological review. *J. Herb. Med.* **2020**, *23*, 100377. [CrossRef]
5. Proliac, A.; Chaboud, A.; Rougny, A.; Gopalsamy, N.; Raynaud, J.; Cabalion, P. A oleanolic saponin from *Polyscias fruticosa* Harms var. yellow leaves. *Pharmazie* **1996**, *51*, 611–612.
6. Divakar, M.; Pillai, N.R.; Rao, S.B. Triterpene Saponins from *Polyscias fruticosa* Leaves and Roots. *Indian J. Nat. Prod.* **2005**, *21*, 7–13.
7. Do, V.M.; Tran, C.L.; Nguyen, T.P. Polysciosides J and K, two new oleanane-type triterpenoid saponins from the leaves of *Polyscias fruticosa* (L.) Harms. cultivating in An Giang Province, Viet Nam. *Nat. Prod. Res.* **2020**, *34*, 1250–1255. [CrossRef]
8. Do, V.M.; Tran, C.L.; Duong, T.H.; Phan, H.V.T.; Nguyen, H.H.; Nguyen, T.P.; Sichaem, J. Chemical Constituents of the Leaves of *Polyscias fruticosa*. *Chem. Nat. Compd.* **2021**, *57*, 1125–1127. [CrossRef]
9. Brophy, J.J.; Lassakt, E.V.; Suksamrarn, A. Constituents of the Volatile Leaf Oils of *Polyscias fruticosa* (L.) Harms. *Flavour Fragr. J.* **1990**, *5*, 179–182. [CrossRef]
10. Rarison, R.H.G.; Truong, V.L.; Yoon, B.H.; Park, J.W.; Jeong, W.S. Antioxidant and Anti-Inflammatory Mechanisms of Lipophilic Fractions from *Polyscias fruticosa* Leaves Based on Network Pharmacology, In Silico, and In Vitro Approaches. *Foods* **2023**, *12*, 3643. [CrossRef]
11. Lutomski, J.; Luan, T.C.; Hoa, T.T. Polyacetylenes in the Araliaceae Family. Part IV. *Herba Pol.* **1992**, *3*, 137–140.
12. Le, T.V.A.; Tran, N.T.A.; Duong, P.A.; Ha, T.B.C.; Dinh, T.H.D.; Mai, T.P.N. Influence of the elicitors on the accumulation of secondary metabolites and antioxidant activities in the *Polyscias fruticosa* (L.) Harms in vitro roots. *Acad. J. Biol.* **2024**, *46*, 91–102. [CrossRef] [PubMed]
13. Nguyen, M.P. Impact of Roasting to Total Phenolic, Flavonoid and Antioxidant Activities in Root, Bark and Leaf of *Polyscias fruticosa*. *J. Pharm. Res. Int.* **2020**, *32*, 13–17. [CrossRef]
14. Tran, T.H.H.; Nguyen, H.D.; Nguyen, T.D. α-Amylase and α-Glucosidase Inhibitory Saponins from *Polyscias fruticosa* Leaves. *J. Chem.* **2016**, *2016*, 2082946.
15. Asumeng Koffuor, G.; Boye, A.; Kyei, S.; Ofori-Amoah, J.; Akomanin Asiamah, E.; Barku, A.; Acheampong, J.; Amegashie, E.; Kumi Awuku, A. Anti-asthmatic property and possible mode of activity of an ethanol leaf extract of *Polyscias fruticosa*. *Pharm. Biol.* **2016**, *54*, 1354–1363. [CrossRef]
16. Bensita, M.B.; Nilani, P.; Sandhya, S.M. Studies on the adaptogenic and antibacterial properties of *Polyscias fructicosa* (L.) Harms. *Anc. Sci. Life* **1999**, *18*, 231–246.
17. Titova, M.V.; Kochkin, D.V.; Sukhanova, E.S.; Gorshkova, E.N.; Tyurina, T.M.; Ivanov, I.M.; Lunkova, M.K.; Tsvetkova, E.V.; Orlova, A.; Popova, E.V.; et al. Suspension Cell Culture of *Polyscias fruticosa* (L.) Harms in Bubble-Type Bioreactors—Growth Characteristics, Triterpene Glycosides Accumulation and Biological Activity. *Plants* **2023**, *12*, 3641. [CrossRef]
18. Asumeng Koffuor, G.; Boye, A.; Ofori-Amoah, J.; Kyei, S.; Nouoma, C.; Debrah, A. Evaluating Muco-suppressant, Anti-tussive and Safety Profile of *Polyscias fruticosa* (L.) Harms (Araliaceae) in Asthma Management. *Br. J. Med. Med. Res.* **2015**, *10*, 1–11. [CrossRef]
19. Tran, P.T.; Dang, N.H.; Kim, O.; Van Cuong, P.; Dat, N.T.; Hwangbo, C.; Van Minh, C.; Lee, J.H. Ethanol extract of *Polyscias fruticosa* leaves suppresses RANKL-mediated osteoclastogenesis in vitro and LPS-Induced Bone Loss in Vivo. *Phytomedicine* **2019**, *59*, 152908. [CrossRef]
20. Ly, H.T.; Nguyen, T.T.H.; Le, V.M.; Lam, B.T.; Mai, T.T.T.; Dang, T.P.T. Therapeutic Potential of *Polyscias fruticosa* (L.) Harms Leaf Extract for Parkinson's Disease Treatment by *Drosophila Melanogaster* Model. *Oxid. Med. Cell. Longev.* **2022**, *2022*, 5262677. [CrossRef]
21. Selvaraj, B.; Le, T.T.; Kim, D.W.; Jung, B.H.; Yoo, K.Y.; Ahn, H.R.; Thuong, P.T.; Tran, T.T.T.; Pae, A.N.; Jung, S.H.; et al. Neuroprotective Effects of Ethanol Extract of *Polyscias fruticosa* (EEPF) against Glutamate-Mediated Neuronal Toxicity in HT22 Cells. *Int. J. Mol. Sci.* **2023**, *24*, 3969. [CrossRef]
22. Pandya, D.; Mankad, A.; Pandya, H. Cost effective micropropagation of *Polyscias fruticosa* (L.) Harm. *Int. Assoc. Biol. Comput. Dig.* **2022**, *1*, 58–62.
23. Sakr, S.S.; Melad, S.S.; El-Shamy, M.A.; Elhafez, A.E.A. In vitro Propagation of *Polyscias fruticosa* Plant. *Int. J. Plant Soil Sci.* **2014**, *3*, 1254–1265. [CrossRef]
24. Phuong, T.T.B.; Trung, V.P.; An, N.H.; Tuan, N.D.; Nguyen, P.T.T. The Effects of 2,4-Dichlorophenoxyacetic Acid and α-Naphthaleneacetic Acid on Biomass Increment, Rhizogenesis and Somatic Embryogenesis of Suspension-cultured Dinh Lang Cells [*Polyscias fruticosa* (L.) Harms]. *Indian J. Agric. Res.* **2022**, *56*, 70–75. [CrossRef]
25. Kim, P.T.A.; An, L.T.B.; Chung, N.T.; Truong, N.T.; Thu, L.T.A.; Huan, L.V.T.; Loc, N.H. Growth and Oleanolic Acid Accumulation of *Polyscias fruticosa* Cell Suspension Cultures. *Curr. Pharm. Biotechnol.* **2020**, *22*, 1266–1272. [CrossRef]

26. Kim, P.T.Á.; Ngân, N.T.H.; Thư, L.T.A.; Huân, L.V.T. Effects of Carbon Sources and Elicitors on Growth of *Polyscias fruticosa* (L.) Harms Suspension Cells. *Hue Univ. J. Sci. Nat. Sci.* **2018**, *127*, 85–94.
27. Lyu, S.; Nosov, A.M.; Eugene, R.; Andrey, A.G.; Ling, Y. Effects of malonyl-ginsenosides on cell growth and saponin accumulation of *Polyscias fruticosa* and *Polyscias filicifolia*. *Chin. Tradit. Herb. Drugs* **2024**, *55*, 8171–8184.
28. Andrews, H.C. *The Botanist's Repository for New and Rare Plants*; Public Domain Illustration Contributed by Missouri Botanical Garden; Biodiversity Heritage Library: Chicago, IL, USA, 1809; Plate 595; Volume 9, ISBN 2013206534.
29. Rumphius, G.E. *Herbarium Amboinense*; Public Domain Illustration Contributed by Missouri Botanical Garden, St. Louis, USA; Biodiversity Heritage Library: Chicago, IL, USA, 1743; Plate XXXIII; Volume 4, p. 78. ISBN 2013206534.
30. Vu, T.H.; Tran, Q.L.; Nguyen, H.V.; Tran, V.O.; Pham, Y.A.; Tran, D.K. Analyses of Genetic Diversity and Relationships of Some *Polyscias* Samples Collected in Vietnam Using Morphological and Molecular Markers. *African J. Biol. Sci.* **2024**, *6*, 1965–1980.
31. Plants of the World Online. Facilitated by the Royal Botanic Gardens, Kew. Available online: https://powo.science.kew.org/taxon/urn:lsid:ipni.org:names:847351-1 (accessed on 27 April 2025).
32. Popova, E.V.; Nosov, A.V.; Titova, M.V.; Kochkin, D.V.; Fomenkov, A.A.; Kulichenko, I.E.; Nosov, A.M. Advanced Biotechnologies: Collections of Plant Cell Cultures as a Basis for Development and Production of Medicinal Preparations. *Russ. J. Plant Physiol.* **2021**, *68*, 385–400. [CrossRef]
33. Yuorieva, N.; Sinetova, M.; Messineva, E.; Kulichenko, I.; Fomenkov, A.; Vysotskaya, O.; Osipova, E.; Baikalova, A.; Prudnikova, O.; Titova, M.; et al. Plants, Cells, Algae, and Cyanobacteria In Vitro and Cryobank Collections at the Institute of Plant Physiology, Russian Academy of Sciences—A Platform for Research and Production Center. *Biology* **2023**, *12*, 838. [CrossRef]
34. Hasnain, A.; Naqvi, S.A.H.; Ayesha, S.I.; Khalid, F.; Ellahi, M.; Iqbal, S.; Hassan, M.Z.; Abbas, A.; Adamski, R.; Markowska, D.; et al. Plants in vitro propagation with its applications in food, pharmaceuticals and cosmetic industries; current scenario and future approaches. *Front. Plant Sci.* **2022**, *13*, 1009395. [CrossRef]
35. Ozyigit, I.I.; Dogan, I.; Hocaoglu-Ozyigit, A.; Yalcin, B.; Erdogan, A.; Yalcin, I.E.; Cabi, E.; Kaya, Y. Production of secondary metabolites using tissue culture-based biotechnological applications. *Front Plant Sci.* **2023**, *14*, 1132555. [CrossRef]
36. Amit; Rajkumar; Singh, N. In Vitro Propagation of an Economically Important Medicinal Plant *Lawsonia inermis* L. through Nodal Segments. *J. Appl. Nat. Sci.* **2021**, *13*, 897–906. [CrossRef]
37. Tomiczak, K.; Mikuła, A.; Niedziela, A.; Wójcik-Lewandowska, A.; Domżalska, L.; Rybczyński, J.J. Somatic Embryogenesis in the Family Gentianaceae and Its Biotechnological Application. *Front. Plant Sci.* **2019**, *10*, 762. [CrossRef] [PubMed]
38. Mihai, R.A.; Melo Heras, E.J.; Pinto Valdiviezo, E.A.; Espinoza Caiza, I.A.; Cubi Insuaste, N.S.; Mejía, J.P.; Catana, R.D.; Moldoveanu, M.M.; Florescu, L.I. Somatic Embryogenesis of Representative Medicinal Trees in South America-Current Status. *Forests* **2023**, *14*, 2066. [CrossRef]
39. Lee, J.W.; Kwon, N.; Kim, J.U.; Bang, K.H.; Jung, S.M.; Lee, S.W.; Kim, D.H.; Kim, Y.C.; Jo, I.H.; Park, Y.D. In Vitro Micropropagation of Commercial Ginseng Cultivars (*Panax ginseng* Meyer) via Somatic Embryogenesis Compared to Traditional Seed Production. *Horticulturae* **2023**, *9*, 435. [CrossRef]
40. Cheng, Y.; Liu, H.; Tong, X.; Liu, Z.; Zhang, X.; Jiang, X.; Yu, X. Somatic embryogenesis and triterpenoid saponin production in *Aralia elata* (Miq.) Seem. *Sci. Hortic.* **2021**, *285*, 110162. [CrossRef]
41. Yang, G.; Huang, L.J.; Jiang, D.; Huang, J.; Cui, C.; Li, N. Development of indirect somatic embryogenesis and plant regeneration system with immature embryos of the cultivated traditional Chinese medicinal herb *Polygonatum cyrtonema*. *Ind. Crops Prod.* **2024**, *214*, 118557. [CrossRef]
42. Duta-Cornescu, G.; Constantin, N.; Pojoga, D.-M.; Nicuta, D.; Simon-Gruita, A. Somaclonal Variation—Advantage or Disadvantage in Micropropagation of the Medicinal Plants. *Int. J. Mol. Sci.* **2023**, *24*, 838. [CrossRef]
43. Tram, T.T.N.; Yen, T.P.; Anh, T.T.; Tung, H.T.; Ngan, H.T.M.; Nhut, D.T.; Nong, S. Somatic Embryogenesis of *Polyscias fruticosa* L. Harms via Culturing Ex Vitro Leaf Explant. *Vietnam. J. Biotechnol.* **2020**, *18*, 497–506. [CrossRef]
44. Murashige, T.; Skoog, F.A. Revised Medium for Rapid Growth and Bio Assays with Tobacco Tissue Cultures. *Physiol. Plant.* **1962**, *15*, 474–497. [CrossRef]
45. Gamborg, O.L.; Miller, R.A.; Ojima, K. Nutrient Requirements of Suspension Cultures of Soybean Root Cells. *Exp. Cell Res.* **1968**, *50*, 151–158. [CrossRef]
46. Jiang, X.L.; Piao, X.C.; Gao, R.; Jin, M.Y.; Jiang, J.; Jin, X.H.; Lian, M.L. Improvement of bioactive compound accumulation in adventitious root cultures of an endangered plant species, *Oplopanax elatus*. *Acta Physiol. Plant.* **2017**, *39*, 226. [CrossRef]
47. Linh, N.T.N.; Cuong, L.K.; Tam, H.T.; Tung, H.T.; Luan, V.Q.; Hien, V.T.; Loc, N.H.; Nhut, D.T. Improvement of bioactive saponin accumulation in adventitious root cultures of *Panax vietnamensis* via culture periods and elicitation. *Plant Cell Tissue Organ Cult.* **2019**, *137*, 101–113. [CrossRef]
48. Gao, X.; Zhu, C.; Jia, W.; Gao, W.; Qiu, M.; Zhang, Y.; Xiao, P. Induction and characterization of adventitious roots directly from the explants of *Panax notoginseng*. *Biotechnol. Lett.* **2005**, *27*, 1771–1775. [CrossRef] [PubMed]

49. Lee, E.J.; Park, S.Y.; Paek, K.Y. Enhancement strategies of bioactive compound production in adventitious root cultures of *Eleutherococcus koreanum* Nakai subjected to methyl jasmonate and salicylic acid elicitation through airlift bioreactors. *Plant Cell Tissue Organ Cult.* **2015**, *120*, 1–10. [CrossRef]
50. Rout, G.R. Effect of Auxins on Adventitious Root Development from Single Node Cuttings of *Camellia sinensis* (L.) Kuntze and Associated Biochemical Changes. *Plant Growth Regul.* **2006**, *48*, 111–117. [CrossRef]
51. Zhao, Y.; Guo, W.H.; Sun, X.Y.; Li, K.H.; Liu, K.J.; Wang, J.; Wang, Y.; Tan, X.; You, X.L. A Culture system for the stable and high-efficiency proliferation of adventitious roots of *Panax notoginseng* and ginsenoside accumulation. *Ind. Crops Prod.* **2020**, *157*, 112882. [CrossRef]
52. Ling, A.P.K.; Chin, M.F.; Hussein, S. Adventitious Root Production of *Centella asiatica* in Response to Plant Growth Regulators and Sucrose Concentrations. *Med. Aromat. Plant Sci. Biotechnol.* **2009**, *3*, 36–41.
53. Sarropoulou, V.; Sarrou, E.; Angeli, A.; Martens, S.; Maloupa, E.; Grigoriadou, K. Developing an in vitro elicitation strategy for specialized secondary metabolites production in adventitious root cultures of *Primula veris* subsp. veris. *Ind. Crops Prod.* **2023**, *197*, 116618. [CrossRef]
54. Marsik, P.; Langhansova, L.; Dvorakova, M.; Cigler, P.; Hruby, M.; Vanek, T. Increased Ginsenosides Production by Elicitation of In Vitro Cultivated *Panax Ginseng* Adventitious Roots. *Med. Aromat. Plants* **2014**, *3*, 147.
55. Adil, M.; Younas, Z.; Ahmad, I.; Al Rohily, K.M.; Mashwani, Z.-u.-R. Elicitation of *Withania somnifera* adventitious roots: In-vitro cultures for enhanced secondary metabolites synthesis. *Hortic. Environ. Biotechnol.* **2025**, *66*, 587–597. [CrossRef]
56. Koffuor, G.A.; Boye, A.; Ofori-Amoah, J.; Kyei, S.; Abokyi, S.; Nyarko, R.A.; Bangfu, R.N. Anti-inflammatory and safety assessment of *Polyscias fruticosa* (L.) Harms (Araliaceae) leaf extract in ovalbumin-induced asthma. *J. Phytopharmacol.* **2014**, *3*, 337–342. [CrossRef]
57. Luyen, N.T.; Dang, N.H.; Binh, P.T.X.; Hai, N.T.; Dat, N.T. Hypoglycemic property of triterpenoid saponin PFS isolated from *Polyscias fruticosa* leaves. *An. Acad. Bras. Cienc.* **2018**, *90*, 2881–2886. [CrossRef] [PubMed]
58. Khoang, L.T.; Huyen, H.T.T.; Chung, H.V.; Duy, L.X.; Toan, T.Q.; Bich, H.T.; Minh, P.T.H.; Pham, D.T.N.; Hien, T.T. Optimization of Total Saponin Extraction from *Polyscias fruticosa* Roots Using the Ultrasonic-Assisted Method and Response Surface Methodology. *Processes* **2022**, *10*, 2034. [CrossRef]
59. Quoc, L.P.T.; Anh, H.N.Q. Ultrasound-Assisted Extraction of Phenolic Compounds from *Polyscias fruticosa* (L.) Harms Root. *Sci. Notes Kazan Univ. Ser. Nat. Sci.* **2023**, *165*, 58–67. [CrossRef]
60. Lộc, P.V.; Luân, N.T.; Ngân, L.T.; An, V.T.X. A Study on Adventitious Root Formation of Ming Aralia (*Polyscias Fruticosa* L. Harms) by in Vitro Culture. *Univ. Danang-J. Sci. Technol.* **2014**, *3*, 106–108.
61. Khalafalla, M.M. Plant Cell Suspension Culture for Plant Secondary Metabolite Production: Current Status, Constraints, and Future Solutions. *Pol. J. Environ. Stud.* **2025**, *XX*, 1–14. [CrossRef]
62. Yue, W.; Ming, Q.L.; Lin, B.; Rahman, K.; Zheng, C.J.; Han, T.; Qin, L.P. Medicinal plant cell suspension cultures: Pharmaceutical applications and high-yielding strategies for the desired secondary metabolites. *Crit. Rev. Biotechnol.* **2016**, *36*, 215–232. [CrossRef]
63. Ochoa-Villarreal, M.; Howat, S.; Hong, S.M.; Jang, M.O.; Jin, Y.W.; Lee, E.K.; Loake, G.J. Plant cell culture strategies for the production of natural products. *BMB Rep.* **2016**, *49*, 149–158. [CrossRef]
64. Pandya, D.; Mankad, A.; Pandya, H. Comparative Phytoremediation Capacity of In-vivo and In-vitro Produced Plants of *Polyscias fruticosa* (L.) Harm. *Res. J. Agric. Sci.* **2020**, *11*, 1420–1422.
65. Bildziukevich, U.; Wimmerová, M.; Wimmer, Z. Saponins of Selected Triterpenoids as Potential Therapeutic Agents: A Review. *Pharmaceuticals* **2023**, *16*, 386. [CrossRef]
66. Parveen, A.; Farooq, M.A.; Kyunn, W.W. A New Oleanane Type Saponin from the Aerial Parts of *Nigella sativa* with Anti-Oxidant and Anti-Diabetic Potential. *Molecules* **2020**, *25*, 2171. [CrossRef] [PubMed]
67. Liu, L.; Li, H.; Hu, K.; Xu, Q.; Wen, X.; Cheng, K.; Chen, C.; Yuan, H.; Dai, L.; Sun, H. Synthesis and anti-inflammatory activity of saponin derivatives of δ-oleanolic acid. *Eur. J. Med. Chem.* **2021**, *209*, 112932. [CrossRef]
68. Adekunle, Y.A.; Samuel, B.B.; Nahar, L.; Fatokun, A.A.; Sarker, S.D. Cytotoxic triterpenoid saponins from the root of *Olax subscorpioidea* Oliv. (Olacaceae). *Phytochemistry* **2023**, *215*, 113853. [CrossRef]
69. Chaboud, A.; Rougny, A.; Proliac, A.; Raynaud, J.; Cabalion, P. A new triterpenoid saponin from *Polyscias fruticosa*. *Pharmazie* **1995**, *50*, 371.
70. Patkhullaeva, M.; Mzhel'skaya, L.G.; Abubakirov, N.K. Triterpene glycosides of *Ladyginia bucharica* V. The structure of ladyginoside E. *Chem Nat Compd.* **1973**, *9*, 771–772. [CrossRef]
71. Borel, C.; Gupta, M.P.; Hostettmann, K. Molluscicidal saponins from *Swartzia simplex*. *Phytochemistry* **1987**, *26*, 2685–2689. [CrossRef]
72. Chuyen, H.V. Extraction of saponins, total soluble solids and antioxidant activity from *Polyscias fruticosa* roots. *Food Res.* **2023**, *7*, 42–47. [CrossRef]
73. Wang, H.; Qi, J.; Li, L.; Wu, T.; Wang, Y.; Wang, X.; Ning, Q. Inhibitory effects of Chikusetsusaponin IVa on lipopolysaccharide-induced proinflammatory responses in THP-1 Cells. *Int. J. Immunopathol. Pharmacol.* **2015**, *28*, 308–317. [CrossRef]

74. Liu, Q.; Ma, Y.; Fan, H.; Li, J.; Tang, J.; Wang, T.; Fan, Y.; Su, J.; Lei, H. Protective Effect of Chikusetsu Saponin IVa on Hydrogen Peroxide Induced Injury of IPEC-J2 Cells. *Nat. Prod. Commun.* **2024**, *19*, 1–11.
75. Wang, X.J.; Xie, Q.; Liu, Y.; Jiang, S.; Li, W.; Li, B.; Wang, W.; Liu, C.X. *Panax japonicus* and chikusetsusaponins: A review of diverse biological activities and pharmacology mechanism. *Chin. Herb. Med.* **2021**, *13*, 64–77. [CrossRef]
76. Li, Y.; Zhang, T.; Cui, J.; Jia, N.; Wu, Y.; Xi, M.; Wen, A. Chikusetsu saponin IVa regulates glucose uptake and fatty acid oxidation: Implications in antihyperglycemic and hypolipidemic effects. *J. Pharm. Pharmacol.* **2015**, *67*, 997–1007. [CrossRef]
77. Sayed, S.M.A.; Alseekh, S.; Siems, K.; Fernie, A.R.; Luyten, W.; Schmitz-Linneweber, C.; Saul, N. Identification of a Hydroxygallic Acid Derivative, Zingibroside R1 and a Sterol Lipid as Potential Active Ingredients of *Cuscuta chinensis* Extract That Has Neuroprotective and Antioxidant Effects in Aged *Caenorhabditis elegans*. *Nutrients* **2022**, *14*, 4199. [CrossRef]
78. Hasegawa, H.; Matsumiya, S.; Uchiyama, M.; Kurokawa, T.; Inouye, Y.; Kasai, R.; Ishibashi, S.; Yamasaki, K. Inhibitory effect of some triterpenoid saponins on glucose transport in tumor cells and its application to in vitro cytotoxic and antiviral activities. *Planta Med.* **1994**, *60*, 240–243. [CrossRef]
79. Lagunin, A.; Povydysh, M.; Ivkin, D.; Luzhanin, V.; Krasnova, M.; Okovityi, S.; Nosov, A.; Titova, M.; Tomilova, S.; Filimonov, D.; et al. Antihypoxic Action of *Panax japonicus, Tribulus terrestris* and *Dioscorea deltoidea* Cell Cultures: In Silico and Animal Studies. *Mol. Inform.* **2020**, *39*, e2000093. [CrossRef]
80. Le, T.H.; Tran, H.C.; Nguyen, H.A.; Nguyen, T.N.T.; Nga, H.T.T. Effects of storage conditions on polyphenol and triterpenoid saponin content and the antioxidant capacity of ethanolic extract from leaves of *Polyscias fruticosa* (L.) Harms. *J. Sci. Technol. Food* **2020**, *3*, 47–53.
81. Wang, Y.; Zhang, H.; Ri, H.C.; An, Z.; Wang, X.; Zhou, J.N.; Zheng, D.; Wu, H.; Wang, P.; Yang, J.; et al. Deletion and tandem duplications of biosynthetic genes drive the diversity of triterpenoids in *Aralia elata*. *Nat. Commun.* **2022**, *13*, 2224. [CrossRef] [PubMed]
82. Kiełkiewicz, R.M.; Obrębski, M.; Śliwińska, A.A.; Równicki, M.; Kawka, M.; Sykłowska-Baranek, K.; Granica, S. Detailed qualitative and quantitative UHPLC-DAD-ESI-MS^3 analysis of *Aralia spinosa* L. (Araliaceae) phytochemical profile to evaluate its potential as novel plant material for bioactive compounds acquisition using *in vitro* culture. *Ind. Crops Prod.* **2024**, *219*, 119123. [CrossRef]
83. Yao, L.; Lu, J.; Wang, J.; Gao, W.Y. Advances in biosynthesis of triterpenoid saponins in medicinalplants. *Chin. J. Nat. Med.* **2020**, *18*, 417–424. [PubMed]
84. Moses, T.; Papadopoulou, K.K.; Osbourn, A. Metabolic and functional diversity of saponins, biosynthetic intermediates and semi-synthetic derivatives. *Crit. Rev. Biochem. Mol. Biol.* **2014**, *49*, 439–462. [CrossRef]
85. Biswas, T.; Dwivedi, U.N. Plant triterpenoid saponins: Biosynthesis, in vitro production, and pharmacological relevance. *Protoplasma* **2019**, *256*, 1463–1486. [CrossRef]
86. Kakkar, S.; Bais, S. A Review on Protocatechuic Acid and Its Pharmacological Potential. *ISRN Pharmacol.* **2014**, *2014*, 952943. [CrossRef] [PubMed]
87. Adefegha, S.A.; Oboh, G.; Ejakpovi, I.I.; Oyeleye, S.I. Antioxidant and antidiabetic effects of gallic and protocatechuic acids: A structure–function perspective. *Comp. Clin. Path.* **2015**, *24*, 1579–1585. [CrossRef]
88. Cadena-Iñiguez, J.; Santiago-Osorio, E.; Sánchez-Flores, N.; Salazar-Aguilar, S.; Soto-Hernández, R.M.; Riviello-Flores, M.d.l.L.; Macías-Zaragoza, V.M.; Aguiñiga-Sánchez, I. The Cancer-Protective Potential of Protocatechuic Acid: A Narrative Review. *Molecules* **2024**, *29*, 1439. [CrossRef]
89. Nguyen, N.Q.; Nguyen, M.T.; Nguyen, V.T.; Le, V.M.; Trieu, L.H.; Le, X.T.; Khang, T.V.; Giang, N.T.L.; Thach, N.Q.; Hung, T.T. The effects of different extraction conditions on the polyphenol, flavonoids components and antioxidant activity of *Polyscias fruticosa* roots. *IOP Conf. Ser. Mater. Sci. Eng.* **2020**, *736*, 02206799. [CrossRef]
90. Rahman, M.; Rahaman, S.; Islam, R.; Rahman, F.; Mithi, F.M.; Alqahtani, T.; Almikhlafi, M.A.; Alghamdi, S.Q.; Alruwaili, A.S.; Hossain, S.; et al. Role of Phenolic Compounds in Human Disease : Current Knowledge and Future Prospects. *Molecules* **2022**, *27*, 233. [CrossRef]
91. Le Roy, J.; Huss, B.; Creach, A.; Hawkins, S.; Neutelings, G. Glycosylation Is a Major Regulator of Phenylpropanoid Availability and Biological Activity in Plants. *Front. Plant Sci.* **2016**, *7*, 735. [CrossRef]
92. Choi, J.; Shin, K.M.; Park, H.J.; Jung, H.J.; Kim, H.J.; Lee, Y.S.; Rew, J.H.; Lee, K.T. Anti-inflammatory and antinociceptive effects of sinapyl alcohol and Its glucoside syringin. *Planta Med.* **2004**, *70*, 1027–1032. [CrossRef] [PubMed]
93. Wei, X.; Cui, S.; Xie, Y. Synthesis and Antibacterial Properties of Oligomeric Dehydrogenation Polymer from Lignin Precursors. *Molecules* **2022**, *27*, 1466. [CrossRef] [PubMed]
94. Mawea, F.; Indrayati, A.; Rahmawati, I. Review: Antibacterial Activity of *Polyscias fruticosa* and Molecular Mechanism of Active Compounds. *Int. J. Health Med. Curr. Res.* **2021**, *6*, 2062–2087.
95. Kim, M.; Shin, S.; Ryu, D.; Cho, E.; Yoo, J.; Park, D.; Jung, E. Evaluating the Sun Protection Factor of Cosmetic Formulations Containing Afzelin. *Chem. Pharm. Bull.* **2021**, *69*, 1039–1044. [CrossRef] [PubMed]

96. Xia, L.; Xu, X.; Li, M.; Zhang, X.; Cao, F. Afzelin induces immunogenic cell death against lung cancer by targeting NQO2. *BMC Complement. Med. Ther.* **2023**, *23*, 381. [CrossRef]
97. Akter, M.; Parvin, M.S.; Hasan, M.M.; Rahman, M.A.A.; Islam, M.E. Anti-tumor and antioxidant activity of kaempferol-3-O-alpha-L-rhamnoside (Afzelin) isolated from *Pithecellobium dulce* leaves. *BMC Complement. Med. Ther.* **2022**, *22*, 169. [CrossRef]
98. Wang, C.; Liu, B.; Dan, W.; Wei, Y.; Li, M.; Guo, C.; Zhang, Y.; Xie, H. Liquiritigenin inhibits the migration, invasion, and EMT of prostate cancer through activating ER Stress. *Arch. Biochem. Biophys.* **2024**, *761*, 110184. [CrossRef]
99. Lee, D.; Kim, J.Y.; Qi, Y.; Park, S.; Lee, H.L.; Yamabe, N.; Kim, H.; Jang, D.S.; Kang, K.S. Phytochemicals from the flowers of *Prunus persica* (L.) Batsch: Anti-adipogenic effect of mandelamide on 3T3-L1 preadipocytes. *Bioorganic Med. Chem. Lett.* **2021**, *49*, 128326. [CrossRef] [PubMed]
100. Qiao, S.; Zhao, R.; He, S.; Fu, X.; An, J.; Xia, T. Quercitrin attenuates the progression of osteoarthritis via inhibiting NF-κB signaling pathways and enhancing glucose transport capacity. *Exp. Cell Res.* **2023**, *433*, 113854. [CrossRef]
101. Liu, Y.; Wang, Y.; Yang, Y.; Quan, Y.; Guo, M. Liquiritigenin Induces Cell Cycle Arrest and Apoptosis in Lung Squamous Cell Carcinoma. *Cell Biochem. Biophys.* **2024**, *82*, 1397–1407. [CrossRef]
102. Meng, X.; Xia, C.; Wu, H.; Gu, Q.; Li, P. Metabolism of quercitrin in the colon and its beneficial regulatory effects on gut microbiota. *J. Sci. Food Agric.* **2024**, *104*, 9255–9264. [CrossRef]
103. Xie, J.; Chen, X.; Tan, Y.; Li, W.; Yin, C.; Zhong, T.; Su, D.; Sun, J.; Tian, H.; Huang, W. Anti-Hyperlipidemic Components of the Leaves of *Synsepalum dulcificum* (Miracle Fruit). *Plant Foods Hum. Nutr.* **2024**, *79*, 451–459. [CrossRef]
104. Hong, Z.; Wang, J.; Hu, B.; Tu, X.; Yang, J.; Sun, W.; Duan, X. Esculetin inhibits liver cancer by targeting glucose-6-phosphate isomerase mediated glycolysis. *Biomed. Pharmacother.* **2025**, *188*, 118118. [CrossRef]
105. Wang, G.; Li, Z.; Ni, W.; Ye, H.; Liu, Y.; Chen, L.; Wang, L.; Liu, C.; Chen, J.; Wang, X.; et al. A small molecule esculetin accelerates postprandial lipid clearance involving activation of C/EBPβ and CD36-mediated phagocytosis by adipose tissue macrophages. *Theranostics* **2025**, *15*, 5910–5930. [CrossRef]
106. Kim, A.T.; Park, Y. Esculetin Inhibits Fat Accumulation Through Insulin/Insulin-like Growth Factor- and AMP-Activated Protein Kinase-Dependent Pathways in *Caenorhabditis elegans*. *Nutrients* **2025**, *17*, 1565. [CrossRef] [PubMed]
107. Qu, Z.; Zeng, J.; Zeng, L.; Li, X.; Zhang, F. Esculetin triggers ferroptosis via inhibition of the Nrf2-XCT/GPx4 axis in hepatocellular carcinoma. *Chin. J. Nat. Med.* **2025**, *23*, 443–456. [CrossRef]
108. Espíndola, K.M.M.; Ferreira, R.G.; Narvaez, L.E.M.; Silva Rosario, R.A.C.; Da Silva, M.A.H.; Silva, B.A.G.; Oliveira Vieira, A.P.; Chagas Monteiro, M. Chemical and Pharmacological Aspects of Caffeic Acid and Its Activity in Hepatocarcinoma. *Front. Oncol.* **2019**, *9*, 3–5. [CrossRef] [PubMed]
109. Gonçalves, A.C.; Falcão, A.; Alves, G.; Silva, L.R.; Flores-Félix, J.D. Antioxidant activity of the main phenolics found in red fruits: An in vitro and in silico study. *Food Chem.* **2024**, *452*, 139459. [CrossRef]
110. Wu, T.Y.; Chen, C.C.; Lin, J.Y. Anti-inflammatory in vitro activities of eleven selected caffeic acid derivatives based on a combination of pro-/anti-inflammatory cytokine secretions and principal component analysis—A comprehensive evaluation. *Food Chem.* **2024**, *458*, 140201. [CrossRef] [PubMed]
111. Lee, M.A.; Park, H.J.; Chung, H.J.; Kim, W.K.; Lee, S.K. Antitumor Activity of 2-Hydroxycinnamaldehyde for Human Colon Cancer Cells through Suppression of Β-Catenin Signaling. *J. Nat. Prod.* **2013**, *76*, 1278–1284. [CrossRef]
112. Nguyen, H.A.; Kim, S.A. 2′-Hydroxycinnamaldehyde induces apoptosis through HSF1-mediated BAG3 expression. *Int. J. Oncol.* **2017**, *50*, 283–289. [CrossRef]
113. Lee, S.H.; Lee, C.W.; Lee, J.W.; Choi, M.S.; Son, D.J.; Chung, Y.B.; Lee, C.K.; Oh, K.W.; Moon, D.C.; Kwon, B.M.; et al. Induction of apoptotic cell death by 2′-hydroxycinnamaldehyde is involved with ERK-dependent inactivation of NF-kappaB in TNF-alpha-treated SW620 colon cancer cells. *Biochem. Pharmacol.* **2005**, *70*, 1147–1157. [CrossRef]
114. Yang, X.W.; Li, Y.L.; Li, S.M.; Shen, Y.H.; Tian, J.M.; Zhu, Z.J.; Feng, L.; Wu, L.; Lin, S.; Wang, N.; et al. Mono- and sesquiterpenoids, flavonoids, lignans, and other miscellaneous compounds of *Abies georgei*. *Planta Med.* **2011**, *77*, 742–748. [CrossRef]
115. Yao, L.; Han, C.; Chen, G.; Song, X.; Chang, Y.; Zang, W. A new asymmetric diamide from the seed cake of *Jatropha curcas* L. *Fitoterapia* **2012**, *83*, 1318–1321. [CrossRef]
116. Rogowska, A.; Szakiel, A. The Role of Sterols in Plant Response to Abiotic Stress. *Phytochem. Rev.* **2020**, *19*, 1525–1538. [CrossRef]
117. Morgan, L.V.; Petry, F.; Scatolin, M.; de Oliveira, P.V.; Alves, B.O.; Zilli, G.A.L.; Volfe, C.R.B.; Oltramari, A.R.; de Oliveira, D.; Scapinello, J.; et al. Investigation of the anti-inflammatory effects of stigmasterol in mice: Insight into its mechanism of action. *Behav. Pharmacol.* **2021**, *32*, 640–651. [CrossRef] [PubMed]
118. Nguyen, T.T.T.; Huynh, D.T.; Quach, N.M. One Unsual Sterol From *Polyscias fruticosa* (L.) Harms (Araliaceace). *J. Innov. Sustain. Dev.* **2017**, *07*, 33–36.
119. Bakrim, S.; Benkhaira, N.; Bourais, I.; Benali, T.; Lee, L.H.; El Omari, N.; Sheikh, R.A.; Goh, K.W.; Ming, L.C.; Bouyahya, A. Health Benefits and Pharmacological Properties of Stigmasterol. *Antioxidants* **2022**, *11*, 1912. [CrossRef]
120. Li, J.; Zheng, X.; Qi, J. Research Progress on the Therapeutic Mechanisms of Stigmasterol for Multiple Diseases. *Molecules* **2025**, *30*, 1874. [CrossRef] [PubMed]

121. Percot, A.; Yalcin, A.; Aysel, V.; Erduğan, H.; Dural, B.; Güven, K.C. Loliolide in marine algae. *Nat. Prod. Res.* **2009**, *23*, 460–465. [CrossRef] [PubMed]
122. Ge, L.; Dai, C.L.; Ma, S.Y.; Liang, G.X.; Yang, K.D. Chemical Constituents from the Leaves of *Camellia ptilosperma* and Their Cytotoxicity. *Chem. Nat. Compd.* **2024**, *60*, 639–643. [CrossRef]
123. Kim, H.S.; Wang, L.; Fernando, I.P.S.; Kim, M.; Jeon, Y.J.; Ahn, G. Antioxidant Efficacy of (−)-loliolide isolated from *Sargassum horneri* against AAPH-induced oxidative damage in Vero cells and zebrafish models in vivo. *J. Appl. Phycol.* **2020**, *32*, 3341–3348. [CrossRef]
124. Murata, M.; Nakai, Y.; Kawazu, K.; Ishizaka, M.; Kajiwara, H.; Abe, H.; Takeuchi, K.; Ichinose, Y.; Mitsuhara, I.; Mochizuki, A.; et al. Loliolide, a Carotenoid Metabolite, Is a Potential Endogenous Inducer of Herbivore Resistance. *Plant Physiol.* **2019**, *179*, 1822–1833. [CrossRef] [PubMed]
125. Lee, Y.R.; Bae, S.; Kim, J.Y.; Lee, J.; Cho, D.H.; Kim, H.S.; An, I.S.; An, S. Monoterpenoid Loliolide Regulates Hair Follicle Inductivity of Human Dermal Papilla Cells by Activating the Akt/β-Catenin Signaling Pathway. *J. Microbiol. Biotechnol.* **2019**, *29*, 1830–1840. [CrossRef] [PubMed]
126. Kim, H.S.; Cheon, J.; Kirindage, K.G.I.S.; Jayasinghe, A.M.K.; Han, E.J.; Park, S.M.; Ahn, G.; Cha, S.H. Loliolide combats glutamate-induced neurotoxicity by oxidative stress through MAPK/Nrf2 pathway in hippocampal neuronal cells. *Algal Res.* **2025**, *85*, 103866. [CrossRef]
127. Shi, D.; Song, X.; Guo, Y.; Xu, J.; Liu, Y.; Zhang, J.; Cui, C.A.; Jin, D.Q. Alismol, a Sesquiterpenoid Isolated from Vladimiria souliei, Suppresses Proinflammatory Mediators in Lipopolysaccharide-Stimulated Microglia. *J. Mol. Neurosci.* **2017**, *62*, 106–113. [CrossRef]
128. Feng, L.; Liu, T.T.; Huo, X.K.; Tian, X.G.; Wang, C.; Lv, X.; Ning, J.; Zhao, W.Y.; Zhang, B.J.; Sun, C.P.; et al. *Alisma* genus: Phytochemical constituents, biosynthesis, and biological activities. *Phytother. Res.* **2021**, *35*, 1872–1886. [CrossRef]
129. Kim, K.H.; Kim, S.; Kwun, M.J.; Lee, J.Y.; Oh, S.R.; Choi, J.Y.; Joo, M. Alismol Purified from the Tuber of *Alisma orientale* Relieves Acute Lung Injury in Mice via Nrf2 Activation. *Int. J. Mol. Sci.* **2023**, *24*, 15573. [CrossRef]
130. Kouame, C.; Ouattara, Z.A.; Kambire, D.A.; Monteil, M.; Mamyrbekova, J.A.; Bighelli, A.; Tomi, F.; Lecouvey, M.; Bekro, Y.A. Chemical Composition and Biological Activity of *Guarea cedrata* (A. Chev.) Pellegr. Leaf and Root Bark Essential Oil. *Int. J. Biochem. Res. Rev.* **2022**, *31*, 27–35. [CrossRef]
131. Thinh, B.B.; Thanh, V.Q.; Hanh, D.H.; Thin, D.B.; Doudkin, R.V. Chemical Composition and Antioxidant Activity of Essential Oil from Fruit of *Schisandra perulata*. *Chem. Nat. Compd.* **2022**, *58*, 763–765. [CrossRef]
132. Li, Y.; Tan, W.L.; Guo, K.; Gao, X.W.; Wei, J.; Yi, D.; Zhang, C.; Wang, Q. Synthesis and Biological Evaluation of Falcarinol-Type Analogues as Potential Calcium Channel Blockers. *J. Nat. Prod.* **2021**, *84*, 2138–2148. [CrossRef]
133. Kim, T.W.; Ko, S.G. A Novel PPARγ Modulator Falcarindiol Mediates ER Stress-Mediated Apoptosis by Regulating NOX4 and Overcomes Radioresistance in Breast Cancer. *Antioxidants* **2024**, *13*, 1533. [CrossRef]
134. Patial, P.K.; Cannoo, D.S. Evaluation of volatile compounds, phenolic acids, antioxidant potential and DFT study of essential oils from different parts of *Araucaria columnaris* (G. Forst.) Hook. from India. *Food Chem. Toxicol.* **2020**, *141*, 111376. [CrossRef]
135. Doungchawee, J.; Kulsing, C.; Suekaew, N.; Na Pombejra, S.; Chavasiri, W.; Plabutong, N.; Thammahong, A.; Khotavivattana, T. Volatile Chemical Composition, Antibacterial and Antifungal Activities of Extracts from Different Parts of *Globba schomburgkii* Hook.F. *Chem. Biodivers.* **2019**, *16*, e1900057. [CrossRef] [PubMed]
136. Rontani, J.F.; Bonin, P.C.; Volkman, J.K. Biodegradation of free phytol by bacterial communities Isolated from marine sediments under aerobic and denitrifying conditions. *Appl. Environ. Microbiol.* **1999**, *65*, 5484–5492. [CrossRef] [PubMed]
137. Osman, W.; Shantier, S.; Mohamed, M. Evaluation of Anti-Inflammatory Activity and Identification of a Monoterpenoidhydroxylactone (-)-loliolide from *Tribulus terrestris* L.: In vivo and In silico Approaches. *Hacettepe Univ. J. Fac. Pharm.* **2024**, *44*, 131–142.
138. Chen, M.; Ghelfi, M.; Poon, J.F.; Jeon, N.; Boccalon, N.; Rubsamen, M.; Valentino, S.; Mehta, V.; Stamper, M.; Tariq, H.; et al. Antioxidant-independent activities of alpha-tocopherol. *J. Biol. Chem.* **2025**, *301*, 108327. [CrossRef]
139. Jiang, Q. Metabolism of natural forms of vitamin E and biological actions of vitamin E metabolites. *Free Radic. Biol. Med.* **2022**, *179*, 375–387. [CrossRef]
140. Alfurayhi, R.; Huang, L.; Brandt, K. Pathways Affected by Falcarinol-Type Polyacetylenes and Implications for Their Anti-Inflammatory Function and Potential in Cancer Chemoprevention. *Foods* **2023**, *12*, 1192. [CrossRef] [PubMed]
141. Gurkok, G.; Altanlar, N.; Suzen, S. Investigation of antimicrobial activities of indole-3-aldehyde hydrazide/hydrazone derivatives. *Chemotherapy* **2009**, *55*, 15–19. [CrossRef]
142. Marques, T.M.; Wall, R.; O'Sullivan, O.; Fitzgerald, G.F.; Cotter, P.D.; O'Toole, P.W.; Ross, R.P.; Stanton, C. Dietary *trans*-10, *cis*-12-conjugated linoleic acid alters fatty acid metabolism and microbiota composition in mice. *Br. J. Nutr.* **2015**, *113*, 728–738. [CrossRef]
143. Murphy, E.F.; Hooiveld, G.J.; Müller, M.; Calogero, R.A.; Cashman, K.D. The Effect of trans-10, cis-12 conjugated linoleic acid on gene expression profiles related to lipid metabolism in human intestinal-like Caco-2 cells. *Genes Nutr.* **2009**, *4*, 103–112. [CrossRef]

144. Herrera-Valencia, V.A.; Us-Vázquez, R.A.; Larqué-Saavedra, F.A.; Cárdenas-Chávez, D.L.; Montalvo-Rodríguez, R. Naturally occurring fatty acid methyl esters and ethyl esters in the green microalga *Chlamydomonas reinhardtii*. *Ann. Microbiol.* **2012**, *62*, 865–870. [CrossRef]
145. Jaudszus, A.; Foerster, M.; Kroegel, C.; Wolf, I.; Jahreis, G. Cis-9,trans-11-CLA exerts anti-inflammatory effects in human bronchial epithelial cells and eosinophils: Comparison to trans-10,cis-12-CLA and to linoleic acid. *Biochim. Biophys. Acta* **2005**, *1737*, 111–118. [CrossRef]
146. Ko, Y.; Choi, H.S.; Kim, S.; Yun, B.; Lee, D. Anti-Inflammatory Effects of (9Z,11E)-13-Oxooctadeca-9,11-dienoic Acid (13-KODE) Derived from *Salicornia herbacea* L. on Lipopolysaccharide-Stimulated Murine Macrophage via NF-KB and MAPK Inhibition and Nrf2/HO-1 Signaling Activation. *Antioxidants* **2022**, *11*, 180. [CrossRef]
147. Pehlić, M.; Dumančić, S.; Radan, M.; Galić, J.; Gruica, B.; Marijan, S.; Vulić, M. Untargeted Urinary Volatilomics Reveals Hexadecanal as a Potential Biomarker for Preeclampsia. *Int. J. Mol. Sci.* **2024**, *25*, 12371. [CrossRef]
148. Liu, K.; Chen, Q.; Liu, Y.; Zhou, X.; Wang, X. Isolation and Biological Activities of Decanal, Linalool, Valencene, and Octanal from Sweet Orange Oil. *J. Food Sci.* **2012**, *77*, C1156–C1161. [CrossRef]
149. Shaikh, H.Y.; Niazi, S.K.; Bepari, A.; Cordero, M.A.W.; Sheereen, S.; Hussain, S.A.; Rudrappa, M.; Nagaraja, S.K.; Agadi, S.N. Biological Characterization of *Cleome felina* L.f. Extracts for Phytochemical, Antimicrobial, and Hepatoprotective Activities in Wister Albino Rats. *Antibiotics* **2023**, *12*, 1506. [CrossRef]
150. Zelante, T.; Iannitti, R.G.; Fallarino, F.; Gargaro, M.; De Luca, A.; Moretti, S.; Bartoli, A.; Romani, L. Tryptophan Feeding of the IDO1-AhR Axis in Host-Microbial Symbiosis. *Front. Immunol.* **2014**, *5*, 640. [CrossRef] [PubMed]
151. Puccetti, M.; Pariano, M.; Borghi, M.; Barola, C.; Moretti, S.; Galarini, R.; Mosci, P.; Ricci, M.; Costantini, C.; Giovagnoli, S. Enteric formulated indole-3-carboxaldehyde targets the aryl hydrocarbon receptor for protection in a murine model of metabolic syndrome. *Int. J. Pharm.* **2021**, *602*, 120610. [CrossRef] [PubMed]
152. Nasrollahi, S.; Ghoreishi, S.M.; Ebrahimabadi, A.H.; Khoobi, A. Gas chromatography-mass spectrometry analysis and antimicrobial, antioxidant and anti-cancer activities of essential oils and extracts of Stachys schtschegleevii plant as biological macromolecules. *Int. J. Biol. Macromol.* **2019**, *128*, 718–723. [CrossRef]
153. Rajizadeh, M.A.; Najafipour, H.; Bejeshk, M.A. An Updated Comprehensive Review of Plants and Herbal Compounds with Antiasthmatic Effect. *Evid.-Based Complement. Altern. Med.* **2024**, *2024*, 5373117. [CrossRef] [PubMed]
154. Taur, D.J.; Patil, R.Y. Some medicinal plants with antiasthmatic potential: A current status. *Asian Pac. J. Trop. Biomed.* **2011**, *1*, 413–418. [CrossRef] [PubMed]
155. Boye, A.; Osei-Owusu, A.K.; Koffuor, G.A.; Barku, V.Y.A.; Asiamah, E.A.; Asante, E. Assessment of *Polyscias fruticosa* (L.) Harm (Araliaceae) leaf extract on male fertility in rats. *J. Intercult. Ethnopharmacol.* **2018**, *7*, 45–56. [CrossRef]
156. Singh, V.K.; Sahu, M.K. Antidiabetic Medicinal Plants Having Insulin Mimetic Property: A Review. *Kenkyu J. Pharm. Pract. Health Care* **2018**, *60*, 56–60.
157. Ardalani, H.; Hejazi Amiri, F.; Hadipanah, A.; Kongstad, K.T. Potential antidiabetic phytochemicals in plant roots: A review of in vivo studies. *J. Diabetes Metab. Disord.* **2021**, *20*, 1837–1854. [CrossRef]
158. Verma, N.; Raghuvanshi, D.S.; Singh, R.V. Recent advances in the chemistry and biology of oleanolic acid and its derivatives. *Eur. J. Med. Chem.* **2024**, *276*, 116619. [CrossRef]
159. Guo, T.; Wu, S.; Guo, S.; Bai, L.; Liu, Q.; Bai, N. Synthesis and Evaluation of a Series of Oleanolic Acid Saponins as α-Glucosidase and α-Amylase Inhibitors. *Arch. Pharm.* **2015**, *348*, 615–628. [CrossRef] [PubMed]
160. Le, Q.U.; Lay, H.L.; Le, T.T. A Science Opinion on *Polyscias fruticosa* And *Morus alba* L. Combination: Better Anti-Diabetic and Late Complication Inhibitory Properties? *Curr. Res. Diabetes Obes. J.* **2019**, *10*, 555798. [CrossRef]
161. Zhang, X.; Shi, C.; Wang, Z.; Dai, J.; Guan, C.; Sheng, J.; Tao, L.; Tian, Y. Separation, Purification, Structural Characterization, and In Vitro Hypoglycemic Activity of Polysaccharides from *Panax notoginseng* Leaves. *Molecules* **2025**, *30*, 830. [CrossRef] [PubMed]
162. Nguyen, N.T.A.; Selvaraj, B.; Vu, H.T.; Nguyen, Q.N.S.; Oanh, L.H.; Lee, H.; Tran, Q.L.; Oanh, V.T.; Jung, S.H.; Thuong, P.T.; et al. The Ethanol Extract of *Polyscias scutellaria* (EEPS) Shows Anti-Inflammatory Signaling Pathway Against LPS-Induced Inflammation in RAW 264.7 Macrophages. *Nat. Prod. Commun.* **2025**, *20*, 1–15. [CrossRef]
163. Zouine, N.; El Ghachtouli, N.; El Abed, S.; Ibnsouda Koraichi, S. A comprehensive review on medicinal plant extracts as antibacterial agents: Factors, mechanism insights and future prospects. *Sci. Afr.* **2024**, *26*, e02395. [CrossRef]
164. Moura, M.V.N.; Mesquita da Conceição Bahia, G.; Gonçalves Correa, M.; Araujo Sarges, M.A.; Lobão, T.A.; Sanches, E.M.; Oliveira, K.R.H.M.; Herculano, A.M.; Bahia, C.P. Neuroprotective effects of crude extracts, compounds, and isolated molecules obtained from plants in the central nervous system injuries: A systematic review. *Front. Neurosci.* **2023**, *17*, 1249685. [CrossRef]
165. Gonelimali, F.D.; Lin, J.; Miao, W.; Xuan, J.; Charles, F.; Chen, M.; Hatab, S.R. Antimicrobial Properties and Mechanism of Action of Some Plant Extracts Against Food Pathogens and Spoilage Microorganisms. *Front. Microbiol.* **2018**, *9*, 1639. [CrossRef] [PubMed]
166. Zhang, L.; Piao, H.; Zang, H. A Comprehensive Review of Traditional Medicinal Uses, Geographical Distribution, Botanical Characterization, Phytochemistry, and Pharmacology of *Aralia continentalis* Kitag. *Molecules* **2024**, *29*, 3529. [CrossRef]

167. Wajima, T.; Kinugawa, R.; Yamada, T.; Ikoshi, H.; Noguchi, N. *Panax Notoginseng* Extract Possesses Significant Antibacterial Activity Against Pathogenic Streptococci. *Pharmacology* **2019**, *103*, 221–227. [CrossRef]
168. Wang, L.; Huang, Y.; Yin, G.; Wang, J.; Wang, P.; Chen, Z.Y.; Wang, T.; Ren, G. Antimicrobial activities of Asian ginseng, American ginseng, and notoginseng. *Phytother. Res.* **2020**, *34*, 1226–1236. [CrossRef]
169. Divakar, M.C.; Nikethen, G.S.; Yuvaraj, S.; Sumitha, E. Investigations on the Anti-Neoplastic Ability of *Polyscias fruticosa* (L) Harms Root CuNPs on Neuroblastoma Cell Lines. *NVEO* **2021**, *8*, 13697–13702.
170. Divakar, M.C.; Nikethen, G.S. Screening of the Anti-Proliferative Activity of *Polyscias fruticosa* (L) Harms Leaf AgNPs on Lung Cancer Cell Line. *J. Popul. Ther. Clin. Pharmacol.* **2024**, *29*, 304–310.
171. Divakar, M.C.; Nikethen, G.S.; Jeffrin, J.; Kaviarasan, R.; Dino, K.A.; Vishwapal, S.S.; Nivedha, K.; Ravindran, S.; Minu, G. Evaluation of the Cytotoxic and Anti-Cancer Activities of *Polyscias fruticosa* (L) Harms Root Phytosome on Neuroblastoma Cell Line. *J. Popul. Ther. Clin.* **2024**, *31*, 22–29.
172. Akbaribazm, M.; Goodarzi, N.; Rahimi, M. Female infertility and herbal medicine: An overview of the new findings. *Food Sci. Nutr.* **2021**, *9*, 5869–5882. [CrossRef] [PubMed]
173. Boye, A.; Mensah, L.; Barku, V.; Acheampong, D.; Asiamah, E. Maternal toxicity and post-implantation assessments in rats gestationally exposed to *Polyscias fruticosa* leaf extract. *J. Complement. Med. Res.* **2018**, *7*, 178–189. [CrossRef]
174. Swathi Krishna, S.; Kuriakose, B.B.; Lakshmi, P.K. Effects of phytoestrogens on reproductive organ health. *Arch. Pharm. Res.* **2022**, *45*, 849–864. [CrossRef] [PubMed]
175. Erkhembaatar, M.; Choi, E.J.; Lee, H.Y.; Lee, C.H.; Lee, Y.R.; Kim, M.S. Attenuated RANKL-induced cytotoxicity by *Portulaca oleracea* ethanol extract enhances RANKL-mediated osteoclastogenesis. *BMC Complement. Altern. Med.* **2015**, *15*, 226. [CrossRef]
176. Seo, Y.S.; Lim, H.I.; Seo, J.Y.; Kang, K.R.; Kim, D.K.; Lee, H.H.; Oh, D.S.; Kim, J.S. The Ethanol Extracts of *Osmanthus fragrans* Leaves Ameliorate the Bone Loss via the Inhibition of Osteoclastogenesis in Osteoporosis. *Plants* **2023**, *12*, 253. [CrossRef] [PubMed]
177. Phromnoi, K.; Yodkeeree, S.; Pintha, K.; Mapoung, S.; Suttajit, M.; Saenjum, C.; Dejkriengkraikul, P. Anti-Osteoporosis Effect of *Perilla frutescens* Leaf Hexane Fraction through Regulating Osteoclast and Osteoblast Differentiation. *Molecules* **2022**, *27*, 824. [CrossRef] [PubMed]
178. Obrębski, M. Created with BioRender.com. 2025. Available online: https://BioRender.com/r2qnh1h (accessed on 18 August 2025).

molecules

MDPI

Article

Anticancer Effects of Withanolides: In Silico Prediction of Pharmacological Properties

Gustavo Werneck de Souza e Silva [1], André Mesquita Marques [2] and André Luiz Franco Sampaio [1,*]

1 Laboratório de Farmacologia Molecular, Farmanguinhos, Fundação Oswaldo Cruz (FIOCRUZ), Rua Sizenando Nabuco 100, Manguinhos, Rio de Janeiro 21041-250, Brazil; gustavo.werneck@fiocruz.br

2 Laboratório de Tecnologia Para Biodiversidade em Saúde/TecBio, Farmanguinhos, Fundação Oswaldo Cruz (FIOCRUZ), Rua Sizenando Nabuco 100, Manguinhos, Rio de Janeiro 21041-250, Brazil; andre.marques@fiocruz.br

* Correspondence: andre.sampaio@fiocruz.br; Tel.: +55-21-39772443

Abstract: Withanolides are a class of naturally occurring C-28 ergostane steroidal lactones with an abundance of biological activities, and their members are promising candidates for antineoplastic drug development. The ADMET properties of withanolides are still largely unknown, and in silico predictions can play a crucial role highlighting these characteristics for drug development, shortening time and resources spent on the development of a drug lead. In this work, ADMET properties of promising antitumoral withanolides were assessed. Each chemical structure was submitted to the prediction tools: SwissADME, pkCSM–pharmacokinetics, admetSAR v2.0, and Molinspiration Cheminformatics. The results indicate a good gastrointestinal absorption rate, inability to cross the blood–brain barrier, CYP3A4 metabolization, without inhibition of other P450 cytochromes, high interaction with nuclear receptors, and a low toxicity. It was also predicted for the inhibition of pharmacokinetics transporters and some ecotoxicity. This demonstrates a viability for oral drug development, with low probabilities of side effects.

Keywords: withanolides; ADMET; withaferin; drug development; cancer; natural products

1. Introduction

Cancer is a worldwide health challenge that affects millions of patients every year. Environmental and genetic factors both increase the risk of developing cancer, compromising life expectancy and the patients' quality of life [1]. The adverse effects of anticancer drugs can be a major factor of the impairment of the patients' quality of life, where some of these effects can be irreversible [2]. The complexity and heterogeneity of cancer demand innovative and multifaceted approaches to combat its relentless progression [3]. Thus, in the last decades, despite the availability of several approved anticancer drugs, the ongoing research and development of new antitumoral agents is always a constant need as a foremost public health demand [4].

Naturally occurring plant secondary metabolites have been successfully used as natural-based templates by offering some structural advantages, in comparison with conventional synthetic molecules as drug leads. Regarding medicinal plants, their use in traditional medicine may provide some insights regarding efficacy and safety [5]. The interest in natural products as potential sources for drug discovery lies not only in their proven track record as therapeutics, but in their inherent chemical diversity. The metabolites complex scaffold structures and possible multiple chiral centers were fine-tuned over millions of years of evolution, that challenge traditional drug design paradigms and are the result of an interplay between living organisms and their environments [6]. These natural compounds have demonstrated a valuable ability to interact with a wide range of biological pathways involved in human health and disease, often acting by multiple modes of action and an inherent ability to engage multiple cellular targets simultaneously. This capacity makes them valuable assets in combating drug-resistant diseases with complex etiologies, including those involved in cancer initiation, cell proliferation, angiogenesis, and metastasis [7].

Historically, natural products were a major contributor to the development of new drugs, with more than 50% of anticancer drugs relating to this source [8]. The evolution of cancer drug discovery has witnessed phases of intense focus on synthetic compounds, which have temporarily overshadowed the exploration of natural products. However, in the wake of persistent challenges posed by drug resistance, systemic toxicity, and limited efficacy of conventional therapies, the scientific community has rediscovered the value of nature's pharmacopeia [9]. The potential for natural products to modulate key signaling cascades and interact with specific molecular targets has been validated in preclinical studies, paving the way for several promising candidates to enter clinical trials [10].

Withanolides are a class of naturally occurring C-28 ergostane steroidal lactones with more than 600 compounds isolated and characterized from various plant species, particularly from the Solanaceae family [11]. Primary pharmacological studies involving the withanolide class have shown a plethora of biological activities, including in vitro antineoplastic effects [12–14].

Recent investigations into the molecular mechanisms underlying withanolide-mediated anticancer effects have unveiled their ability to interfere with various signaling pathways crucial for cancer cell survival, proliferation, and metastasis [15,16]. The inhibition of key inflammatory signaling pathways, such as NF-κB, JAK/STAT, AP-1, PPARγ, Hsp90 Nrf2, and HIF-1, highlights their potential to attenuate inflammation-mediated chronic diseases, including cancer-promoting cascades, while inducing tumor cell apoptosis and cell cycle arrest [17,18]. Additionally, withanolides also have been shown to sensitize cancer cells to conventional chemotherapy and radiotherapy, potentially overcoming drug resistance and enhancing treatment outcomes [19].

In preclinical studies, withanolides have exhibited promising efficacy against a broad spectrum of cancers, including breast, prostate, lung, colon, pancreatic, and ovarian cancers, among others [20]. Their ability to selectively target cancer cells while sparing normal cells holds great promise in minimizing the adverse effects associated with conventional therapies. Moreover, their anti-metastatic properties and potential to inhibit angiogenesis may underpin their effects on cancer progression [21]. However, despite several pharmacological activities already reported, the ADMET properties of many withanolides are largely unknown. In this work, we have selected withanolides with antitumoral in vitro effects to predict in silico their toxicological effects, their safety for biological systems, their interactions with important proteins that affect drug pharmacokinetic, their metabolism, and whether or not they may grant tumor resistance to chemotherapy.

Pharmacological studies with withanolides have demonstrated anticancer properties on human cancer cells in vitro, as well as in vivo, inhibiting tumor growth and inducing metastasis suppression [22–24]. Recently, pharmacological investigations have suggested withanolides' possible mechanisms of action, including production of ROS, cell cycle disturbance, and cytoskeleton alterations [25,26]. However, the precise molecular mechanism and receptor(s) involved in withanolides' actions on cancer cells is still largely unknown.

In this context, in silico predictions may play a crucial role in streamlining the drug discovery process. In silico virtual screening techniques can efficiently assess the interactions between natural metabolites and target proteins, helping prioritize the most promising candidates for further experimental validation [27]. This approach significantly reduces the number of compounds that need to be synthesized, and tested in vitro or in vivo, prevents the duplication of efforts and enables researchers to focus on compounds with higher probabilities of activity on specific diseases. In silico studies also contribute for structure optimization for activity, selectivity, and improvement of pharmacological properties, reducing the time and resources spent on less promising leads [28].

The application of in silico predictions has become an important component of pharmaceutical research and development that can shorten and cheapen the process by using previous data of known molecules, and comparing them to new structures [29,30]. The use of computer modeling, to predict the absorption, distribution, metabolism, and excretion (ADME), to predict and understand structure–properties relationships of the pharmacokinetics and drug metabolism properties for novel compounds, is widely used in the development of new drug candidates [31]. A variety of computational techniques make it possible to predict the toxicity (T) of a given chemical compound and is one of the alternatives to animal testing, being widely used in design and drug discovery and development [32].

Despite the relevance of in silico predictions and their role in drug discovery and medicinal chemistry, it is important to note some limitations to the accuracy of prediction tools. Substances have a variety of characteristics that can interfere with pharmacological properties and biological responses depending on the organ, tissue, or cell type. Each predictive tool has its own database and training method (built based on experimental data), and the size and the quality of the data used for training can alter the results from its usage. Thus, it is important to use more than one prediction tool to evaluate ADMET characteristics for accurate prediction. The integration of in silico predictions and their confirmation with an experimental approach, can accelerate the identification of lead compounds and increase the efficiency of discovering novel drugs from natural sources [33].

2. Results

2.1. *Withanolides Structures and ADMET Studies*

Withanolides are steroidal molecules with 28 carbons, with a wide range of biological activities. These compounds are predominantly found in species of the Solanaceae family, their first member was isolated from *Withania somnifera* (Withaferin A) and are scarcely found in plants of other families.

The selected withanolides (Figures 1–3) are intended to represent a plethora of subtypes, to better understand the ADMET properties among the different structures. In the past years, in silico predictions, coupled with computational approaches, have played an important role in advancing the study of withanolides and their potential applications in drug discovery and development. Here, we present some key aspects of selected antitumoral withanolides for in silico ADMET predictions.

To better visualize the in silico ADMET predictions, data were expressed as a probability and organized in a heatmap (Figure 4) and tables for binary and other predictions. Data for each withanolide are available in the supplementary materials (Tables S3–S6).

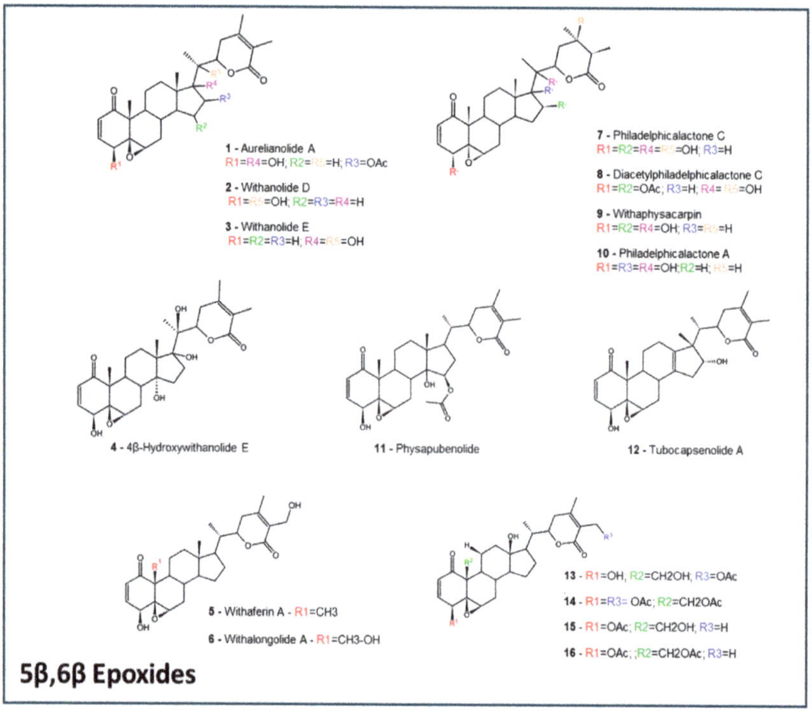

Figure 1. The 5β,6β epoxides withanolides. The structures were designed using the software ACD/ChemSketch 2020.2.0 (ACD/Labs).

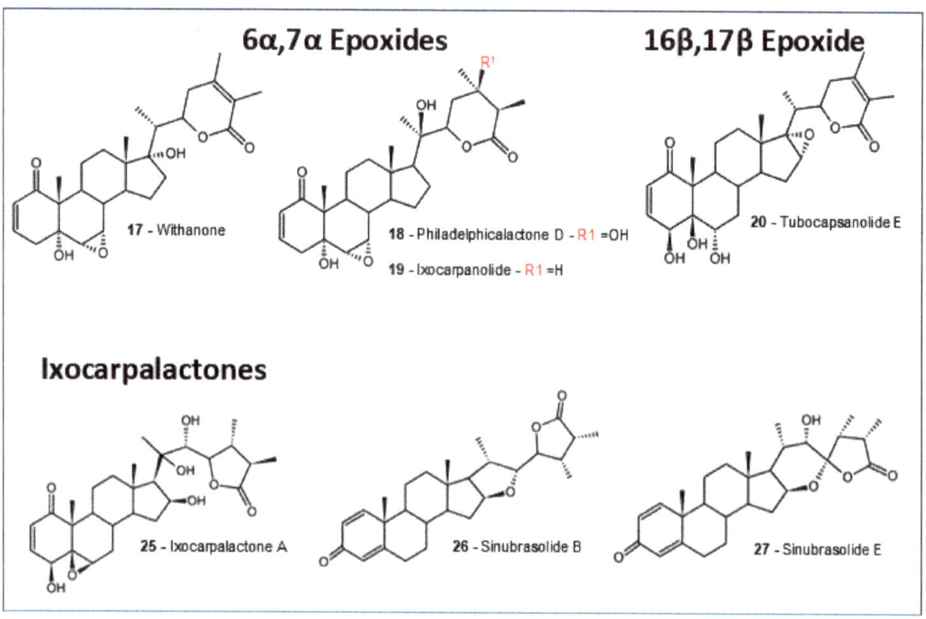

Figure 2. The 6α,7α epoxides, 16β,17β epoxides, and ixocarpalactones withanolides. The structures were designed using the software ACD/ChemSketch 2020.2.0 (ACD/Labs).

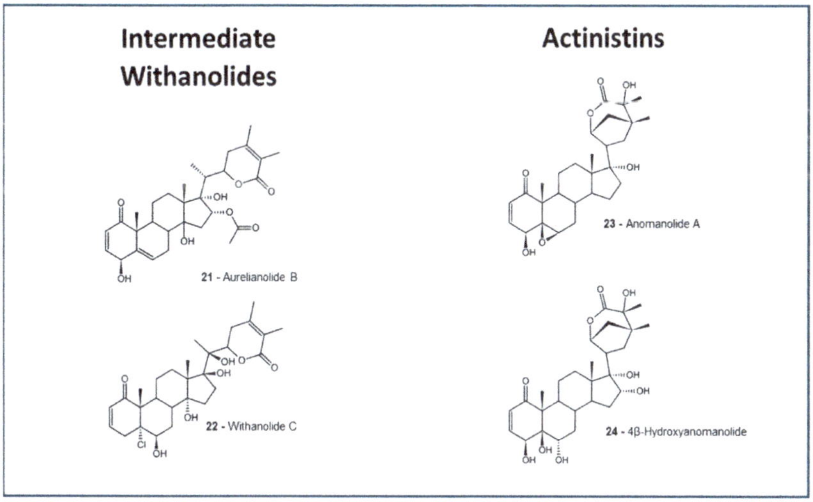

Figure 3. Actinistins and intermediate withanolides. The structures were designed using the software ACD/ChemSketch 2020.2.0 (ACD/Labs).

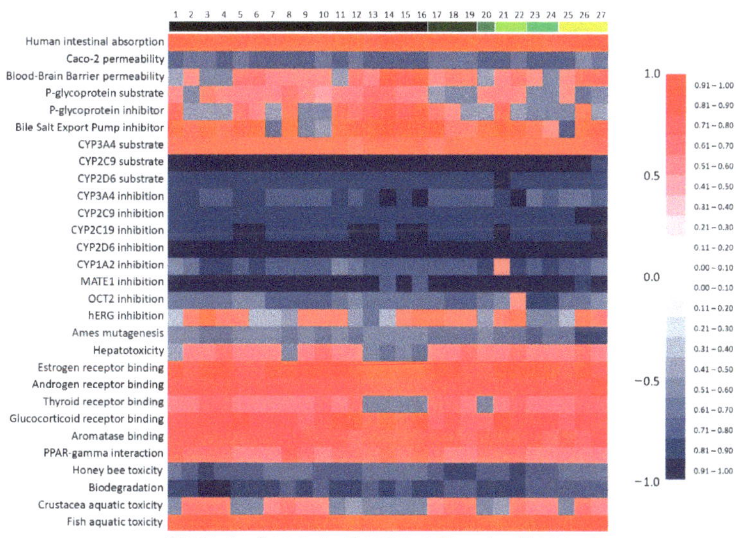

Figure 4. Heatmap constructed from admetSAR predictions. A total of 27 withanolides were assessed for their ADMET properties. Results range from 1.0 (+) to 1.0 (−), and were plotted following a color intensity scheme.

2.2. Oral Absorption

2.2.1. Lipinski's Rule of Five

Lipinski's rule of five is a set of guidelines used in medicinal chemistry and drug discovery to assess the likelihood of a compound's oral bioavailability and permeability. In his work [34], Lipinski has categorized some desired drug properties as good absorption and permeation through the gastrointestinal tract. These properties, known as "Lipinski's rule of 5" were described based on the characteristics of drugs in clinical use with the following criteria: molecular weight (MW) $\leq$ 500 Daltons; octanol–water partition coefficient

(LogP) ≤ 5; hydrogen bond donors (HBD) ≤ 5; and hydrogen bond acceptors (HBA) ≤ 10. As shown in Table 1, of the 27 withanolides analyzed, 26 fit the rule of five, and could be predicted with good oral absorption and permeation. Among them, 13 withanolides violated no rule, and 13 withanolides violated one rule, and only 4β-Hydroxyanomanolide violated two rules.

Table 1. Absorption related properties of withanolides. The parameters were assessed in four prediction tools and compiled in a table. TPSA was calculated using Molinspiration Cheminformatics. SwissADME provided Lipinki's rule violation and pkCSM predicted the withanolides as yes or no for P-gp substrate. For the admetSAR prediction tool, a probability was obtained, and 0.5 was the threshold between positives and negatives. Values in parenthesis mean the number of withanolides with that characteristic/total number of withanolides. Results are expressed as a mean ± SEM.

	Molinspiration		SwissADME	pkCSM	admetSAR			
Compound Group	TPSA	% Absorption [a]	Lipinski's Rule of Five (Violations)	P-gp Substrate	Human Intestinal Absorption	Caco-2 Permeability	Blood–Brain Barrier Permeability	P-gp Substrate
5β,6β epoxides	118.2 ± 3.96	68.23 ± 1.37	0 (7/16); 1 (9/16)	Yes (13/16); No (3/16)	0.9062 ± 0.0115	0.2785 ± 0.0127	0.6125 ± 0.0306	0.5832 ± 0.0108
6α,7α epoxides	103.1 ± 8.74	73.47 ± 2.33	0 (3/3)	Yes (3/3)	0.9391 ± 0.0093	0.3424 ± 0.0128	0.6333 ± 0.0167	0.4871 ± 0.0029
16β,17β epoxide	116.59	68.8	0	Yes	0.8657	0.265	0.5000	0.5123
Intermediate Withanolides	117.2 ± 7.08	68.55 ± 2.45	1 (2/2)	Yes (2/2)	0.9489 ± 0.0204	0.2888 ± 0.0243	0.6250 ± 0.0500	0.5536 ± 0.0098
Actinistins	140.7 ± 24.08	60.50	0 (1/2); 2(1/2)	Yes (2/2)	0.8943 ± 0.0528	0.2268 ± 0.0333	0.5125 ± 0.0876	0.4371 ± 0.0218
Ixocarpalactones	87.42 ± 25.38	78.83 ± 8.75	0 (1/3); 1 (2/3)	Yes (2/3); No (1/3)	0.9471 ± 0.0423	0.3182 ± 0.0602	0.6833 ± 0.0417	0.4561 ± 0.0683

[a] 109-[0.345xTPSA].

Furthermore, the topological polar surface area (TPSA) obtained in Molinspiration can be used to predict the percentage of absorption, using the equation 109-[0,345xTPSA] [35]. The results, as shown in Table 1, indicate that the ixocarpanolides have the highest percentage of absorption, as both sinubrasolides assessed showed high individual values, with 90.8% and 83.9%, for Sinubrasolide B and Sinubrasolide E, respectively. The majority of withanolides are predominantly around 70% of absorption, whereas two withanolides showed a lower absorption of less than 60% (Diacetylphiladelphicalactone C and 4β-Hydroxyanomanolide).

2.2.2. BOILED-Egg Prediction

The BOILED-Egg system is a graphic plot (Figure 5), that can predict and show in a visual way, the capability of molecules to surpass both the gastrointestinal barrier and the blood–brain barrier [36]. This model consists of plotting two properties: the Wildman and Crippen LogP (WLogP) and the Topological Polar Surface Area (TPSA) of the chemical structure of the molecules. In a generated image, we can define two zones, one that predicts a good gastrointestinal barrier permeation, and an inside zone that predicts a good blood–brain barrier permeation. These two zones form a shape similar to a boiled egg, therefore its model name.

We have observed, using the BOILED-Egg prediction system, that 25 withanolides would be unable to cross the BBB. However, the two sinubrasolides were plotted inside the BBB permeability area. This suggests an ability for these two ixocarpalactones to cross the BBB, making them potentially harmful for the central nervous system. This fact can be correlated with the higher hydrophobic character of those compounds in comparison to the other withanolides. The Sinubrasolide E structure has only one hydroxyl group, while in Sinubrasolide B, the OH is absent, which limits the hydrogen bond interactions and ionization of the molecule, thus favoring the passage through the BBB.

Also, three of the withanolides would not have good gastrointestinal permeability, whilst the majority would.

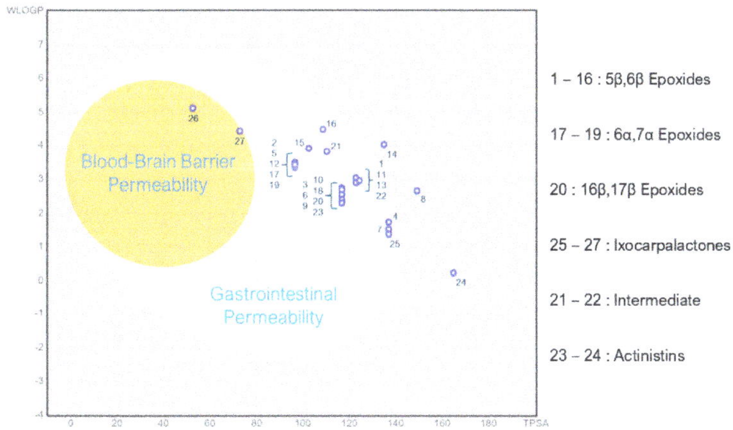

Figure 5. The BOILED-Egg scheme adapted from SwissADME. This plot of TPSA and WLOGP represents two major areas, whereas the withanolides are predicted to cross the gastrointestinal barrier (larger area), the blood–brain (smaller area), or none (outside both areas). Numbers correspond to the chemical structures shown in Figures 1–3.

2.2.3. AdmetSAR Barrier Predictions

The software admetSAR was able to predict the intestinal barrier and the BBB permeability of withanolides (Table 1; Figure 4). The predicted human intestinal absorption was highly positive for all withanolides, corroborating with the BOILED-Egg and Lipinski's rule predictions that withanolides could have good intestinal absorption and permeability.

Caco-2 is a cell line, derived from a colorectal adenocarcinoma, commonly utilized as an in vitro model of a human intestinal epithelial barrier for human intestinal absorption studies [37]. The predictions did not show that withanolides could traverse the Caco-2 cells, being strangely opposite to the fact that all predictions for oral permeability and intestinal absorption were positive.

In opposition to the BOILED-Egg, admetSAR predicted that withanolides, in general, have a high chance of surpassing the blood brain barrier, with only six withanolides being predicted as unable to surpass this barrier: Aurelianolide A, Withanolide E, 4β-Hydroxywithanolide E, Physapubenolide, Ixocarpanolide, and 4β-Hydroxyanomanolide. All groups have shown at least 50% probability for accessing the central nervous system (Table 1). This opposite result shows that the different methods of prediction can vary the results, and the real properties should be further investigated using biological systems.

2.3. Toxicity Predictions

2.3.1. Hepatotoxicity

Among withanolides analyzed by the admetSAR software, five displayed a probability above the 0.6 tier for hepatotoxicity, being one ixocarpalactone (Sinubrasinolide B), one intermediate withanolide (Withanolide C), the 6a, 7a epoxide Ixocarpanolide, and the 5β,6β epoxides Philadelphicalactone A and 4β-Hydroxyanomanolide. On the other hand, two withanolides were predicted with probability higher than 0.61 to be non-hepatotoxics (Withanolides 14 and 16). The other withanolides displayed probabilities between the 0.51–0.6 tiers (Figure 4), both positively and negatively, with lower variation (Table 2). Chemotherapeutic drugs had a higher score for hepatotoxicity, which agrees with real data for most of these molecules.

Table 2. Toxicity related predictions for withanolides. Cardiotoxicity is represented in the hERG channel inhibition potential and genotoxicity in the Ames mutagenicity test, while hepatotoxicity is represented in a general manner. The pkCSM predicted the withanolides toxicity as yes or no. For the admetSAR prediction tool, a probability was obtained, and 0.5 was the threshold between positives and negatives. Values in parenthesis mean the number of withanolides with that characteristic/total number of withanolides. Results are expressed as a mean ± SEM.

	PREDICTION TOOL					
	pkCSM			admetSAR		
Compound Group	**Hepatotoxicity**	**hERG Inhibitor**	**Ames Mutagenicity**	**Hepatotoxicity**	**hERG Inhibition**	**Ames Mutagenicity**
5β,6β epoxides	Yes (1/16); No (15/16)	No (16/16)	Yes (1/16); No (15/16)	0.5295 ± 0.0244	0.6403 ± 0.0250	0.4177 ± 0.0118
6α,7α epoxides	No (3/3)	No (3/3)	No (3/3)	0.5884 ± 0.0252	0.6921 ± 0.0183	0.3131 ± 0.0060
16β,17β epoxide	No	No	No	0.5717	0.5774	0.4100
Intermediate Withanolides	No (2/2)	No (2/2)	No (2/2)	0.6163 ± 0.0661	0.7452 ± 0.0801	0.3447 ± 0.0283
Actinistins	No (2/2)	No (2/2)	No (2/2)	0.5929 ± 0.0021	0.4366 ± 0.0246	0.3089 ± 0.0589
Ixocarpalactones	No (3/3)	No (3/3)	No (3/3)	0.5844 ± 0.0290	0.6722 ± 0.0525	0.2387 ± 0.0759

The pkCSM prediction tool was used to predict the hepatotoxicity of withanolides. The results, which are shown only as positive or negative, consider the probability of the hepatotoxic effects of withanolides, increasing the robustness of the prediction. This software predicted that 26 of the withanolides are non-hepatotoxic, including those previously predicted as positive by admetSAR (Table 2).

Together, these data suggest that some of the withanolides may be considered safe for liver function, whilst further experimental data is necessary to confirm the possibility of liver tissue damage.

2.3.2. Cardiotoxicity

When analyzed for cardiotoxicity by pkCSM (via interaction with hERG potassium channels), chosen withanolides (Table 2) seem not to interfere in hERG channels, indicating that these molecules are safe for the cardiovascular system.

However, the admetSAR prediction showed a balanced probability between positives and negatives. Eleven withanolides were predicted as non-cardiotoxic, while sixteen were predicted as cardiotoxic. Even though most groups had at least a 0.60 probability to be cardiotoxic, most of the results were all on the borderline between positivity and negativity, thus not being able to define a major profile of cardiotoxicity for the antitumoral withanolides chosen (Table 2).

However, we can associate actinistins to a lower probability of hERG inhibition, with a 0.4366 probability, while intermediate withanolides had the higher probabilities, which could be associated with the absence of epoxide groups (Table 2).

2.3.3. Ames Mutagenesis

Withanolides were predicted to be unable to promote the mutagenicity observed at the Ames mutagenesis test by admetSAR (Table 2; Figure 4), while only one of them was predicted to be mutagenic by pkCSM (Table 2). From this data, we can infer that withanolides are predicted, in a general manner, to be unable to promote mutagenicity.

2.4. Metabolism and Excretion Predictions

2.4.1. Cytochrome Interactions

Data obtained using in silico predictions indicate that CYP3A4 is probably the main CYP responsible for withanolide metabolism. Predictions suggest that withanolides do not interact with CYP2D6, another cytochrome responsible for metabolizing xenobiotics. The software also predicted that the majority of withanolides could not inhibit the CYPs available for calculation: CYP3A4, CYP2D6, CYP2C9, CYP2C19, and CYP1A2 (Table 3).

Table 3. Withanolides interactions with cytochrome P450 interactions. Substrate and inhibition probabilities were assessed with the admetSAR prediction tool. Results are expressed as a mean ± SEM. A probability of 0.5 was the threshold between positives and negatives.

admetSAR CYP Predictions								
		Substrate				Inhibition		
Compound Group	**CYP3A4 Substrate**	**CYP2C9 Substrate**	**CYP2D6 Substrate**	**CYP3A4 Inhibition**	**CYP2C9 Inhibition**	**CYP2C19 Inhibition**	**CYP2D6 Inhibition**	**CYP1A2 Inhibition**
5β,6β epoxides	0.7375 ± 0.0038	0	0.1026 ± 0.0010	0.1766 ± 0.0173	0.1323 ± 0.0062	0.1032 ± 0.0067	0.0486 ± 0.0012	0.2498 ± 0.0186
6α,7α epoxides	0.7128 ± 0.0108	0	0.0921 ± 0.0005	0.2445 ± 0.0027	0.1190 ± 0.0112	0.1116 ± 0.0019	0.03907 ± 0.0025	0.2613 ± 0.0075
16β,17β epoxide	0.7111	0	0.1016	0.2184	0.1072	0.0935	0.0495	0.1412
Intermediate Withanolides	0.7362 ± 0.0076	0	0.0902 ± 0.0070	0.1314 ± 0.0534	0.1188 ± 0.0145	0.1085 ± 0.0248	0.0661 ± 0.0174	0.3473 ± 0.1894
Actinistins	0.7196 ± 0.0032	0	0.1018 ± 0.0051	0.2853 ± 0.0287	0.1048 ± 0.0129	0.1254 ± 0.0111	0.0372 ± 0.0009	0.1902 ± 0.0195
Ixocarpalactones	0.7485 ± 0.0108	0.0607 ± 0.0607	0.1034 ± 0.0057	0.3099 ± 0.0438	0.0863 ± 0.0304	0.0867 ± 0.0324	0.0456 ± 0.0031	0.2653 ± 0.0607

2.4.2. P-Glycoprotein Interaction

Except for four, the pkCSM prediction tool predicted withanolides as P-glycoprotein (P-gp) substrates (Table 1). The admetSAR predictions also corroborated with the positiveness of many compounds, excluding eight that were predicted as non-substrate: all the 6α,7α epoxides, the actinistins, the sinubrasolides, and a single 5β,6β epoxide. The different structures of these groups may deny the P-gp efflux effect.

2.4.3. OCT-2 and MATE-1 Inhibition

Withanolides have shown a homogenous prediction concerning the MATE-1 inhibition. All withanolides were predicted, with high probability, to be unable to inhibit the functioning of the MATE-1 protein. This finding is corroborated by the fact that our system has predicted Imatinib [38] to be a MATE-1 inhibitor (Figure 4). The OCT-2 inhibition was also predicted as negative for the vast majority of withanolides. Withanolide C was the only compound predicted to be an inhibitor of the OCT-2.

2.4.4. BSEP Inhibition

Data obtained from the predictions show a potential of BSEP inhibition by withanolides. A total of 23 of the 27 withanolides were predicted to be BSEP inhibitors; the exceptions were the 5β,6β epoxides Philadelphicalactone C, Withaphysacarpin, Philadelphicalactone A, and Ixocarpalactone A.

2.5. Nuclear Receptor Binding

In this work, we have predicted the binding of withanolides to some members of this superfamily: estrogen, androgen, thyroid, glucocorticoid, aromatase, and PPAR-gamma receptors. In a general manner, withanolides are predicted to interact with the NR, with higher frequency to estrogen, androgen, glucocorticoid, aromatase, and PPAR-gamma receptors (Figure 4).

The thyroid receptor binding followed a similar pattern, but with negative binding results for the 16β,17β epoxide Tubocapsanolide E, and the 5β,6β epoxides, compounds **13**, **14**, **15**, and **16**.

2.6. Ecotoxicity Predictions

Our findings using the admetSAR predictions (Table 4) showed that withanolides are harmless for honeybees, an important agent in ecological systems. However, all compounds are predicted to be dangerous to aquatic environments, with high fish toxicity and low biodegradability probabilities. Also, the majority of withanolides are predicted to be potentially harmful to Crustacea. The pkCSM tool predicted toxicity concentrations for minnows, which were high, reaching higher than 4 log mM (>10,000 mM). As we have selected potent withanolides, with IC_{50} lower than 10 μM, they can be, in their majority, considered not toxic for minnows. For *Tetrahymena pyriformis* toxicity, the predicted concentrations are also above the potential therapeutic concentrations for withanolides, characterizing them as potentially safe for water environments, according to the pkCSM data.

Table 4. Withanolides' ecotoxicity predictions by the pkCSM and admetSAR tools. Log of toxic concentrations for *Tetrahymena* and minnows are shown in the pkCSM tool. For admetSAR prediction tool, probabilities of toxic effects are evaluated, and 0.5 was the threshold between positives and negatives. Results are expressed as a mean ± SEM.

Prediction of Ecotoxicity						
	pkCSM		admetSAR			
Compound Group	*Tetrahymena pyriformis* Toxicity (log μg/L)	Minnow Toxicity (log mM)	Honey Bee Toxicity	Biodegradation	Crustacea Aquatic Toxicity	Fish Aquatic Toxicity
5β,6β epoxides	0.288 ± 0.002	2.350 ± 0.317	0.2830 ± 0.0150	0.1594 ± 0.0139	0.5281 ± 0.0195	0.9745 ± 0.0024
6α,7α epoxides	0.290 ± 0.004	1.664 ± 0.3495	0.1777 ± 0.0082	0.1917 ± 0.0221	0.5967 ± 0.0433	0.9722 ± 0.0029
16β,17β epoxide	0.285	1.663	0.2019	0.1000	0.4700	0.9730
Intermediate Withanolides	0.290 ± 0.004	1.956 ± 0.5645	0.2219 ± 0.0375	0.1500 ± 0.0250	0.5800 ± 0.0800	0.9906 ± 0.0013
Actinistins	0.285 ± 0.001	3.231 ± 0.3735	0.2507 ± 0.0328	0.2125 ± 0.0125	0.5900 ± 0.0100	0.9767 ± 0.0010
Ixocarpalactones	0.3193 ± 0.024	0.8740 ± 1.226	0.3357 ± 0.0204	0.2167 ± 0.0167	0.5800 ± 0.0577	0.9871 ± 0.0044

3. Discussion

3.1. Absorption and Distribution

Oral drug administration is the preferable non-invasive route for drug delivery to conscious and cooperating patients. However, there are molecules that do not possess physicochemical properties to ensure good bioavailability in the gastrointestinal tract [39].

If a given compound fills in the characteristics predicted in Lipinsky's rule of five, based in the chemical structure, that molecule may be developed as an oral drug. Every rule has exceptions, and it is no different for Lipinsky's rule of five. In a general manner, molecules can violate up to one parameter and still be able to have a good prediction. However, Lipinski et al. [34] described some drugs that violate the parameters of the "rule of 5", such as antibiotics, antifungals, vitamins, and cardiac glycosides, which have pharmaceutical formulations for oral administration, as their chemical structures allow them to act as substrates for natural transporters. In this study we have observed that predicted characteristics of antitumor withanolides fit Lipinsky's rule of five, suggesting that these molecules may be used as drug development candidates or lead molecules for further development using medicinal chemistry.

It is not uncommon for anticancer drugs to violate two or more of "Lipinski's rule of 5"; therefore, these drugs may be suitable for the development of intravenous medicines, such as Vincristine, Vinblastine, Doxorubicin, Daunorubicin, and Paclitaxel, among others.

Regarding withanolide compounds, it is observed that many have molecular weights greater than 500 Daltons, due to their complex structure and functional groups. This might make them larger and potentially less likely to meet the molecular weight criterion For example, Aurelianolide A and B, 4β-Hydroxywithanolide E, Physapubenolide, Withanolide C, and Philadelphicalactone C and D, as well as its diacetyl derivative have presented an MW > 500 Da. The n-octanol–water partition coefficient (Kow) is a partition coefficient for the two-phase system consisting of n-octanol and water. Kow serves as a measure of the relationship between lipophilicity and hydrophilicity of a compound. If the Kow value is greater than one, the substance is more soluble in fat-like solvents, such as n-octanol, and less than one if it is more soluble in water. Despite its steroidal scaffold, withanolides often have complex structures with multiple functional groups, including lactones, acetyls, conjugated ketones, hydroxyls, and glycosyls, which give the molecules a greater possibility for carrying out interactions via hydrogen bonds, and thus increasing their hydrophilic character. These features can lead to relatively low LogPow values, which favor some withanolides to meet these criteria. Among the chosen substances in this study, most withanolides presented more than two hydroxyl groups in the structure. The compound 4β-Hydroxyanomanolide is considered to be the most hydrophilic compound endowed by the six OH groups, while Sinubrasolide E and Sinubrasolide B were the most hydrophobic compounds with one and no hydroxyl group, respectively. It is known that the presence of oxygen covalently bonded to hydrogen in the hydroxyl groups (-OH) in the structure of withanolides can act as hydrogen bond donors. Usually, most of the chosen withanolide compounds have hydroxyl groups on C4, C5, C6, C14, C15, and C20. However, one withanolide exceeds the HBD limit of five, the 4β-Hydroxyanomanolide (6-OH groups). Withanolide metabolites are also commonly endowed by several strong electronegative atoms, such as oxygen, that contains a lone pair in functional groups, including hydroxyls, ketones, and esters, that can act as hydrogen bond acceptors. Despite the presence of several hydrogen bond acceptors in the selected compounds, it was not observed that any withanolides exceed the HBA limit of nine, respecting the ten HBA limit criterion.

Overall, due to their complex and often larger structures, many withanolides might not strictly adhere to "Lipinski's rule of 5". However, it is important to note that these rules are not absolute predictors of a compound's bioavailability of drug-likeness. There are many successful drugs that do not meet all these criteria, and exceptions can be made based on additional considerations, such as the specific therapeutic target and mechanism of action. Researchers and drug developers often use Lipinski's rule of five as a guideline rather than a strict rule, and they consider other factors when assessing the potential of a compound for drug development.

Chemotherapeutics are usually delivered via the parenteral route, with some exceptions, such as the imatinib mesylate, anastrozole, letrozole, and tamoxifen citrate, which were developed as oral drugs. Studies on the ability of withanolides to pass the gastrointestinal barrier may be useful for specific applications and pharmaceutical development. Among the tested withanolides in the BOILED-Egg prediction system, only 4β-Hydroxyanomanolide, Diacetylphiladelphicalactone C, and compound 14 would not be able to pass the gastrointestinal barrier (Figure 5), suggesting that most withanolides would be absorbed by the gastrointestinal system making them optimal candidates for oral administration to patients, an advantage that usually increases the adherence to the treatment.

A very important parameter that can be obtained from the BOILED-Egg plot is the capability of the molecules to surpass the blood–brain barrier and therefore reach the central nervous system. This information will help us to address the possible side effects of these molecules, and to suggest strategies for a better and more specific delivery system/route.

The blood–brain barrier (BBB) is a characteristic feature of the central nervous system blood vessels, that controls the permeability/flux of molecules between the blood and the central nervous system [40], protecting the brain against toxic substances [41]. Therefore, this barrier is extremely important to maintain the cell function and central nervous system homeostasis. Cancer chemotherapy is known to have several side effects, including the cognitive side effects caused by drugs that can cross the blood–brain barrier, affecting homeostasis and cell function, and compromising neuropsychological behavior [42].

Our conflicting findings show that the majority of withanolides are unable to cross the BBB by the BOILED-Egg method, while admetSAR predicted withanolides to be majorly positive. Looking closely at the prediction tools, we can deduct what to take from these results. The BOILED-Egg method shows a high cross-validated accuracy of 0.8775 [36]. While the admetSAR method presents a 0.85 accuracy, it has a 0.66 positive predictive value [43], meaning it has a higher number of false positives, which could be the case for our study, and may account for this discrepancy between models.

Based on the BOILED-Egg method (Figure 5), the majority of withanolides are probably safe for the central nervous system as they do not cross the BBB, reducing the adverse effects of chemotherapy when treating peripheral tumors, such as leukemias. Moreover, delivery strategies must be developed for the treatment of central nervous system tumors with these compounds. The results also suggest that sinubrasolides should be treated separately, as they can access the central nervous system. However, further experimental studies should be carried out to support this suggestion.

Some in silico observations were validated in an ex vivo permeability study [44] that was carried out to investigate the absorption pattern of some withanolides present in *W. somnifera*. A time-dependent absorption of withanolides was observed, including the major withanolides Withaferin A and Withanone, through the intestinal barrier, like BCS class I drugs with high solubility and permeability. In this study, Withanone was detected in plasma [44]. In another study on Withaferin A oral bioavailability in rats [45], it was demonstrated that Withaferin A oral bioavailability was 32.4 $\pm$ 4.8% based on intravenous (5 mg/kg) and oral (10 mg/kg) administrations in male rats. According to the authors, the in vitro results showed that Withaferin A could be easily transported across Caco-2 cells and, apparently, it is not a substrate for P-glycoprotein. It was reported that the first-pass metabolism of this withanolide might be the main barrier in achieving good oral bioavailability, since it rapidly decreased, and 27.1% remained within 1 h in a rat intestine–liver in situ perfusion system [45].

3.2. *Toxicity*

The liver is an organ involved in many metabolic pathways and xenobiotic transformations and elimination. However, hepatotoxicity is a common problem observed in antitumor drugs, with many examples of chemotherapics that cause hepatic tissue damage, such as the platinum-based chemical cisplatin, cyclophosphamide, mercaptopurine, and other commonly used drugs. The hepatic damage is often hard to detect and cure [46,47]. Therefore, it is important to find safer antitumoral molecules that cause no hepatic damage or malfunction, that will also be very useful to be introduced as chemotherapeutic agents for patients suffering from hepatic illness or conditions.

AdmetSAR predictions for hepatotoxicity have an accuracy of 0.833 and a sensibility of 0.943, meaning that it is a good tool to discover true hepatotoxic substances, but its low sensitivity of 0.255 can infer many false positives [48]. On the other hand, pkCSM has a low accuracy of 0.658 [49], indicating that the major non-hepatotoxic prediction need to be evaluated further.

The withanolide compounds are known to contain multiple electrophilic groups (two Michael acceptors and an epoxide) in their scaffold, which are associated with adverse drug reactions. The presence of conjugated ketone, lactone, and epoxide groups, generally termed as toxicophores or structural alerts, can often be correlated to some toxicity potential [50]. Found as main metabolites from the medicinal plant *Withania somnifera*, the withanolides, Withaferin A and Withanone, are considered to be the responsible agents for many known pharmacological properties of the Ashwagandha medicinal plant. The hepatoprotective potential has been investigated in animal models using the APAP-induced acute liver injury model. It was suggested that Withaferin A was able to attenuate APAP-induced hepatotoxicity accompanied by hepatic NRF2 activation. The hepatoprotective activity of a crude extract of *W. somnifera* was also found to significantly reduce several elevated hepatotoxicity biomarkers [51]. However, despite the suggested medicinal benefits of *W. somnifera*, recently, several cases of liver toxicity have been reported after the use of commercially available Ashwagandha products. It is suggested that the use of a higher concentrated extract could increase the risk of liver toxicity when compared to the traditional use of Ashwagandha, such as in a tonic, for example. The investigation of the withanolide, Withanone, suggested some toxicophores or structural alerts that are commonly associated with adverse drug reactions. The authors suggested that Withanone can form non-labile adducts with the nucleosides dG, dA, and dC. The Withanone effect can be detoxified by GSH in limited amounts; however, when the GSH system is overwhelmed, severe liver injury occurs, and it can cause DNA damage [52].

Cardiotoxicity is a major issue during preclinical and clinical drug development, a friction factor that leads to failure of lead molecules and projects. An assessment of cardiotoxicity in the early stages of drug development is particularly relevant for drugs that would be used continuously or for an extended period of time in the treatment of chronic diseases or cancer [53]. Cardiotoxicity evaluation and prediction rely on the ionic potassium channels, known as hERG, that are crucial to cardiac function. Molecules that inhibit hERG function can cause severe arrhythmias and sudden death [54]. Doxorubicin and Daunorubicin are representative of the anthracyclines that are known to cause irreversible cardiotoxicity [55], but do not block the hERG channels [56]. Imatinib is a cardiotoxic drug [57], and an hERG inhibitor [58]. In our findings, Imatinib was predicted to inhibit the hERG channels only by admetSAR, while Doxorubicin was not, corroborating to the accuracy of the test.

Withania somnifera extracts, which contains Withaferin A, were evaluated in vivo for its cardiotoxic potential. A study has demonstrated that a prior treatment with an extract containing 1.5% of withanolides can attenuate the cardiotoxic effects of Doxorubicin [59]. In another study, extracts could promote cardiotoxicity in neonatal cardiomyocytes, while adult cardiomyocytes remained unharmed by the extracts, providing a cardiotonic effect [60].

The Ames mutagenesis test is a bacterial method, which can be utilized as a preclinical method to assess both the mutagenicity and carcinogenicity of compounds [61]. Mutagenesis is an issue that can cause cell damage and possibly evolve into a tumor or fetus malformation. Therefore, many regulatory agencies require data for the mutagenicity and carcinogenicity of drug candidates to proceed in the drug development process [62]. Being developed as a cancer treatment, which is an extended treatment, this data can be utilized in a beneficial way to support safety of withanolide usage.

Concerning the potential of antitumor withanolides for drug development, our findings related to the toxicology of withanolides predict that they are overall relatively safe for major biological systems, including the liver and cardiac function. As a long term antitumoral drug candidate, it also shows low mutagenicity probability. Therefore, withanolides can be promising substances to be included in cancer drug development programs for their safety alongside their good absorption.

3.3. Metabolism and Excretion

Withanolides are often metabolized in the liver through enzymatic processes. The liver contains various enzymes, including cytochrome P450 (CYP) enzymes, which play a crucial role in breaking down foreign substances, including drugs and natural compounds. These enzymes help convert withanolides into metabolites that are more water-soluble and can be easily eliminated from the body.

Derived from the phytosterol pathway, withanolides are generally highly oxidized metabolites derived via cycloartenol, which undergo various biochemical transformations, such as hydroxylation, dealkylation, epoxidations, and glycosylation, and are postulated to be catalyzed by cytochrome P450 enzymes (CYP450) [63]. The cytochrome P450 family (CYP) are responsible for the metabolization of approximately 70% of clinical use drugs. CYP3A4 is the main enzyme that accounts for the metabolism of xenobiotics, and is expressed in almost all liver tissue [64]. Because of this role, CYP interaction is one of the mechanisms that undergo drug–drug interactions [65]. Utilizing in silico predictions, we were able to identify possible interactions with CYPs (Table 3).

Recently, a study about the CYP mediated herb–drug interactions of the Ashwagandha medicinal plant, along with case examples of remdesivir, showed that the aqueous extract of Ashwagandha did not show any inhibitory activity towards CYP3A4, CYP2C8, and CYP2D6, and therefore seems to be safe to co-administer with respective substrates [66].

The P-glycoprotein (P-gp) is a transmembrane protein of the ABC (ATP-binding cassette) transporter superfamily. It is decoded by the MDR1 gene and promotes the extrusion of drugs and xenobiotics from cells, granting them resistance to some therapies [67]. We have predicted the susceptibility of withanolides to the effect of these transporters, to see how they would fare in a situation of a multidrug resistant tumor super expressing the MDR1 gene. We used Imatinib and Ibrutinib as positive control drugs, that are known to be P-gp substrates, with a decrease of effectiveness against MDR1 positive tumors [68,69]. The lower effectiveness observed in multidrug resistant tumors can be extrapolated to a withanolide resistance, based on the predictions of P-gp interactions. Supporting this evidence, we have recently demonstrated [18] a higher cytotoxic IC_{50} for Aurelianolide A and B on K562 Lucena-1 leukemia cells that are MDR phenotype due to P-gp increased activity [70]. However, there is in vitro evidence where Withanolide D did not inhibit P-gp activity. Moreover, by blocking the efflux, the cytotoxicity in myeloma cells remained the same [71].

The organic cation transporter 2 (OCT-2) and the multidrug and toxin extrusion protein 1 (MATE-1) are transporters from the ATP-binding cassette (ABC) superfamily. They are abundant in the kidney, controlling the efflux and influx of many molecules, varying from endogenous organic molecules to exogenous drugs and xenobiotics [72]. The interaction with these transporters plays an important role in drug toxicity, drug–drug interactions, and pharmacokinetics [73]. These findings show that withanolides possibly do not interact with the OCT-2 and MATE-1, decreasing the possibility of drug interactions via these kidney transporters.

The bile salt export pump (BSEP) is an ABC transporter localized in the membrane of hepatocytes, transporting bile acids from these cells to the bile. The inhibition of BSEP can lead to a toxic increase of intracellular bile acids, leading to severe liver injury [74]. Albeit the hepatotoxicity data for these findings suggest a possibility of hepatotoxicity from the inhibition of bile acid transporters, and therefore this toxicity should be assessed in future in vitro and in vivo studies.

The nuclear receptor (NR) superfamily are transcription factors that play an important role in biological homeostasis, such as metabolism, reproduction, and inflammation [75]. As a drug candidate, the possible capability of withanolides to bind with nuclear receptors can be a two-edged sword, as this binding can be deleterious by disbalancing homeostasis, causing serious toxic effects. On the other hand, hormone blocking therapies are very valuable to treat hormone responsive tumors, such as prostate and breast cancers, suggesting that withanolides that block hormone receptors may be a very useful tool for the treatment of hormone-sensitive tumors [76,77].

Regarding the in vitro data, there is a study which associates the effects of Withanolide A with glucocorticoid receptors, which are a part of the nuclear receptor superfamily [78]. Alongside our findings, this can indicate the interaction of withanolides with nuclear receptors.

3.4. Ecotoxicity

Ecotoxicity refers to the potential harmful effects that chemicals or substances can have on ecosystems and/or the organisms within them. There has been a growing concern for the anthropogenic impacts on the environment, with a rising concern on the impact of drugs and drug wastes in household and industry effluents [79,80]. Therefore, the ecotoxicology of drug candidates can be evaluated to reduce the environmental effects of potentially harmful compounds [81]. Natural bioactive compounds produced by plants or microorganisms can be just as toxic as any anthropogenically-produced chemicals. However, unlike the industrially produced chemicals, such as pesticides, food chemicals, and pharmaceutical chemicals, they are rarely regulated or have their environmental toxicity predicted using QSAR models [82]. The effects of isolated compounds on nature can range from acute toxicity, where high concentrations of a substance lead to immediate harm or death of organisms, to chronic toxicity, where lower concentrations of a substance over a longer period can cause sublethal effects, disrupt reproductive capabilities, and have long-term impacts on the ecosystem's health. Thus, ecotoxicity studies are conducted to assess the potential risks that substances pose to the environment. The studies involve exposing various organisms, such as aquatic species, plants, and microorganisms, to different concentrations of the substance in question. In this context, a toxicity assessment through computational methods provides knowledge of the chemicals lacking experimental data, and may guide early screening studies for development of safer drugs, and may also serve as an alternative to toxicity studies on animal models [83].

In the current study, all compounds are predicted to have some degree of toxicity in aquatic environments, with high fish toxicity and low biodegradability probabilities. These findings altogether raise an alert and suggest studies on the best production practices and correct waste disposal for withanolides, enlightening scientists and regulators to understand the potential impact of these substances on the environment, guiding decisions on their use and regulation.

4. Materials and Methods

4.1. Databases

To select and search for the structures and characteristics of withanolides and antineoplastic drugs, we have used databases from the National Institutes of Health (NIH), such as PubMed®, the U.S. National Institutes of Health, and PubChem (National Library of Medicine, National Center of Biotechnology Information). To find further information about clinical usage of antineoplastic chemotherapics compounds, searches on DrugBank Online were performed.

4.2. Withanolides Selection Criteria

For this work, we have selected 27 withanolides with reported in vitro antitumoral activity with IC_{50} lower than 10 μM [71,84–92]. See Supplementary Material Table S1. A plethora of withanolides that represented some of the known types were selected, and allocated by their groups: 5β,6β epoxides (Figure 1), 6α,7α epoxides, 16β,17β epoxides, ixocarpalactones (Figure 2), intermediate withanolides, and actinistins (Figure 3). All withanolides selected were analyzed for in silico predictions in all platforms previously described.

4.3. Antineoplastic Drugs

To compare selected antitumoral withanolides to already described molecules and clinical use drugs, we selected 17 widely used antitumor drugs. The selection tried to be representative of drugs with different molecular targets used in clinics for several tumor types; see Supplementary Material Table S2.

4.4. ADMET: Physicochemical Descriptors

The structures were designed using the software ACD/ChemSketch 2020.2.0 (ACD/Labs), and the SMILES notations were generated for use in studies; see Supplementary Material Table S1. Each chemical structure from the SMILES notation was submitted for predicting physicochemical and pharmacokinetic properties and toxicity properties using the websites SwissADME (Swiss Institute of Bioinformatics) [93], pkCSM–pharmacokinetics [49], admetSAR v2 [48], and Molinspiration Cheminformatics. All the platforms are free access.

5. Conclusions

Withanolides are molecules with good antitumoral potential, being studied as drug candidates worldwide. Considering some limitations, the in silico predictions demonstrated good oral absorption, possibly a low toxicity, a common CYP3A4 metabolization, low inhibition of pharmacokinetics transporters, high probability of nuclear receptor interactions, and a high alert for aquatic environments ecotoxicity.

In summary, the predictions evaluated some positive characteristics that need to be further investigated and confirmed using in vitro and in vivo assays during the drug development process. Our predictions can guide and stimulate the research process for the pharmacological characteristics of withanolides.

Supplementary Materials: The following supporting information can be downloaded at: https://www.mdpi.com/article/10.3390/molecules30112457/s1, Table S1: Compound names, Smiles notations used for predictions and references for antitumoral activity; Table S2: Antineoplastic drugs used as standard compounds in predictions and their clinical indication. Table S3: Absorption related properties of withanolides. The parameters were assessed in four prediction tools and compiled in a table. TPSA was calculated using Molinspiration Cheminformatics. SwissADME provided Lipinki's rule violation and pkCSM predicted the withanolides as yes or no for P-gp substrate. For admetSAR prediction tool, (+) = positive probability, (-) = negative probability. Table S4: Toxicity related predictions for the withanolides. Cardiotoxicity is represented in the hERG channel inhibition potential and genotoxicity in the Ames mutagenicity test, while hepatotoxicity is represented in a general manner. pkCSM predicted the withanolides toxicity as yes or no. For admetSAR prediction tool, (+) = positive probability, (-) = negative probability. Table S5: Withanolides interactions with cytocrome P450 interactions. Subtrate and inhibition probabilities were assessed with the admetSAR prediction tool. (+) = positive probability, (-) = negative probability. Table S6: Withanolides ecotoxicity predictions by the pkCSM and admetSAR tools. Log of toxic concentrations for *Tetrahymena* and minnow are shown in the pkCSM tool. For admetSAR prediction tool, probabilities of toxic effects are evaluated. (+) = positive probability, (-) = negative probability.

Author Contributions: Conceptualization, G.W.d.S.e.S., A.M.M. and A.L.F.S.; methodology, G.W.d.S.e.S.; validation, A.M.M. and A.L.F.S.; formal analysis, G.W.d.S.e.S., A.M.M. and A.L.F.S.; investigation, G.W.d.S.e.S. and A.M.M.; resources, A.L.F.S.; data curation, G.W.d.S.e.S. and A.L.F.S.; writing—original draft preparation, G.W.d.S.e.S.; writing—review and editing, G.W.d.S.e.S., A.M.M. and A.L.F.S.; visualization, G.W.d.S.e.S. and A.M.M.; supervision, A.L.F.S.; project administration, A.L.F.S.; funding acquisition, A.L.F.S. All authors have read and agreed to the published version of the manuscript.

Funding: This work was supported by the CNPq PROEPFAR under Grant 440018/2022-6 and Grant 447630/2024-5.

Institutional Review Board Statement: Not applicable.

Informed Consent Statement: Not applicable.

Data Availability Statement: The original contributions presented in this study are included in the article/Supplementary Material. Further inquiries can be directed to the corresponding author(s).

Acknowledgments: We would like to express our gratitude to Magdalena Nascimento Rennó for its contribution to the guidance on the use of prediction tools and data analysis.

Conflicts of Interest: The authors declare no conflicts of interest.

Abbreviations

The following abbreviations are used in this manuscript:

ABC	ATP-binding cassette
ADMET	Absorption, Distribution, Metabolism, Excretion and Toxicity
BBB	Blood–Brain Barrier
BSEP	Bile Salt Export Pump
MATE-1	Multidrug and Toxin Extrusion protein 1
NR	Nuclear Receptors
OCT-2	Organic Cation Transporter 2
P-gp	P-glycoprotein
TPSA	Topological Polar Surface Area

References

1. Sung, H.; Ferlay, J.; Siegel, R.L.; Laversanne, M.; Soerjomataram, I.; Jemal, A.; Bray, F. Global Cancer Statistics 2020: GLOBOCAN Estimates of Incidence and Mortality Worldwide for 36 Cancers in 185 Countries. *CA Cancer J Clin* **2021**, *71*, 209–249. [CrossRef] [PubMed]
2. Qi, L.; Luo, Q.; Zhang, Y.; Jia, F.; Zhao, Y.; Wang, F. Advances in Toxicological Research of the Anticancer Drug Cisplatin. *Chem Res. Toxicol.* **2019**, *32*, 1469–1486. [CrossRef] [PubMed]
3. Dong, B.; Miao, J.; Wang, Y.; Luo, W.; Ji, Z.; Lai, H.; Zhang, M.; Cheng, X.; Wang, J.; Fang, Y.; et al. Single-Cell Analysis Supports a Luminal-Neuroendocrine Transdifferentiation in Human Prostate Cancer. *Commun. Biol.* **2020**, *3*, 778. [CrossRef]
4. Magalhães, H.; Fontes-Sousa, M.; Machado, M. Immunotherapy in Advanced Gastric Cancer: An Overview of the Emerging Strategies. *Can. J. Gastroenterol. Hepatol.* **2018**, *2018*, 2732408. [CrossRef]
5. Dzobo, K. The Role of Natural Products as Sources of Therapeutic Agents for Innovative Drug Discovery. In *Comprehensive Pharmacology*; Elsevier: Amsterdam, The Netherlands, 2022; pp. 408–422.
6. Atanasov, A.G.; Zotchev, S.B.; Dirsch, V.M.; International Natural Product Sciences Taskforce; Supuran, C.T. Natural Products in Drug Discovery: Advances and Opportunities. *Nat. Rev. Drug Discov.* **2021**, *20*, 200–216. [CrossRef]
7. Thomford, N.E.; Senthebane, D.A.; Rowe, A.; Munro, D.; Seele, P.; Maroyi, A.; Dzobo, K. Natural Products for Drug Discovery in the 21st Century: Innovations for Novel Drug Discovery. *Int. J. Mol. Sci.* **2018**, *19*, 1578. [CrossRef]
8. Newman, D.J.; Cragg, G.M. Natural Products as Sources of New Drugs over the Nearly Four Decades from 01/1981 to 09/2019. *J. Nat. Prod.* **2020**, *83*, 770–803. [CrossRef]

9. Huang, M.; Lu, J.-J.; Ding, J. Natural Products in Cancer Therapy: Past, Present and Future. *Nat. Prod. Bioprospect.* **2021**, *11*, 5–13. [CrossRef]
10. Gielecińska, A.; Kciuk, M.; Mujwar, S.; Celik, I.; Kołat, D.; Kałuzińska-Kołat, Ż.; Kontek, R. Substances of Natural Origin in Medicine: Plants vs. Cancer. *Cells* **2023**, *12*, 986. [CrossRef]
11. Hussain, H.; Csuk, R.; Green, I.R.; Ur Rehman, N.; Abbas, G.; Hussain, W. Journey Describing the Cytotoxic Potential of Withanolides: A Patent Review. *Recent. Pat. Anticancer Drug Discov.* **2018**, *13*, 411–421. [CrossRef]
12. Chen, L.-X.; Xia, G.-Y.; He, H.; Huang, J.; Qiu, F.; Zi, X.-L. New Withanolides with TRAIL-Sensitizing Effect from *Physalis pubescens* L. *RSC Adv.* **2016**, *6*, 52925–52936. [CrossRef]
13. Huang, M.; He, J.-X.; Hu, H.-X.; Zhang, K.; Wang, X.-N.; Zhao, B.-B.; Lou, H.-X.; Ren, D.-M.; Shen, T. Withanolides from the Genus Physalis: A Review on Their Phytochemical and Pharmacological Aspects. *J. Pharm. Pharmacol.* **2020**, *72*, 649–669. [CrossRef] [PubMed]
14. Samadi, A.K. Potential Anticancer Properties and Mechanisms of Action of Withanolides. *Enzymes* **2015**, *37*, 73–94. [CrossRef]
15. Chirumamilla, C.S.; Pérez-Novo, C.; Van Ostade, X.; Vanden Berghe, W. Molecular Insights into Cancer Therapeutic Effects of the Dietary Medicinal Phytochemical Withaferin A. *Proc. Nutr. Soc.* **2017**, *76*, 96–105. [CrossRef] [PubMed]
16. Atteeq, M. Evaluating Anticancer Properties of Withaferin A-a Potent Phytochemical. *Front. Pharmacol.* **2022**, *13*, 975320. [CrossRef]
17. White, P.T.; Subramanian, C.; Motiwala, H.F.; Cohen, M.S. Natural Withanolides in the Treatment of Chronic Diseases. *Adv. Exp. Med. Biol.* **2016**, *928*, 329–373. [CrossRef] [PubMed]
18. De Souza E Silva, G.W.; Marques, A.M.; Fontão, A.P.G.A.; DE Moura Lima, S.C.; Kaplan, M.A.C.; Figueiredo, M.R.; Sampaio, A.L.F. Aurelianolides from Aureliana Fasciculata Var. Fasciculata Trigger Apoptosis With Caspase Activation in Human Leukemia Cells. *Anticancer Res.* **2023**, *43*, 1245–1253. [CrossRef]
19. Lem, F.F.; Yong, Y.S.; Goh, S.; Chin, S.N.; Chee, F.T. Withanolides, the Hidden Gem in Physalis Minima: A Mini Review on Their Anti-Inflammatory, Anti-Neuroinflammatory and Anti-Cancer Effects. *Food Chem.* **2022**, *377*, 132002. [CrossRef]
20. Singh, A.; Raza, A.; Amin, S.; Damodaran, C.; Sharma, A.K. Recent Advances in the Chemistry and Therapeutic Evaluation of Naturally Occurring and Synthetic Withanolides. *Molecules* **2022**, *27*, 886. [CrossRef]
21. Kashyap, V.K.; Peasah-Darkwah, G.; Dhasmana, A.; Jaggi, M.; Yallapu, M.M.; Chauhan, S.C. Withania Somnifera: Progress towards a Pharmaceutical Agent for Immunomodulation and Cancer Therapeutics. *Pharmaceutics* **2022**, *14*, 611. [CrossRef]
22. Paul, S.; Chakraborty, S.; Anand, U.; Dey, S.; Nandy, S.; Ghorai, M.; Saha, S.C.; Patil, M.T.; Kandimalla, R.; Proćków, J.; et al. *Withania somnifera* (L.) Dunal (Ashwagandha): A Comprehensive Review on Ethnopharmacology, Pharmacotherapeutics, Biomedicinal and Toxicological Aspects. *Biomed. Pharmacother.* **2021**, *143*, 112175. [CrossRef]
23. Chen, Y.-M.; Xu, W.; Liu, Y.; Zhang, J.-H.; Yang, Y.-Y.; Wang, Z.-W.; Sun, D.-J.; Li, H.; Liu, B.; Chen, L.-X. Anomanolide C Suppresses Tumor Progression and Metastasis by Ubiquitinating GPX4-Driven Autophagy-Dependent Ferroptosis in Triple Negative Breast Cancer. *Int. J. Biol. Sci.* **2023**, *19*, 2531–2550. [CrossRef] [PubMed]
24. Hahm, E.-R.; Kim, S.-H.; Singh, S.V. Withaferin A Inhibits Breast Cancer-Induced Osteoclast Differentiation. *Mol. Carcinog.* **2023**, *62*, 1051–1061. [CrossRef]
25. Almeida, A.A.; Lima, G.D.A.; Eiterer, M.; Rodrigues, L.A.; do Vale, J.A.A.; Zanatta, A.C.; Bressan, G.C.; de Oliveira, L.L.; Leite, J.P.V. A Withanolide-Rich Fraction of Athenaea Velutina Induces Apoptosis and Cell Cycle Arrest in Melanoma B16F10 Cells. *Planta Med.* **2022**, *88*, 429–439. [CrossRef] [PubMed]
26. Nishikawa, Y.; Okuzaki, D.; Fukushima, K.; Mukai, S.; Ohno, S.; Ozaki, Y.; Yabuta, N.; Nojima, H. Withaferin A Induces Cell Death Selectively in Androgen-Independent Prostate Cancer Cells but Not in Normal Fibroblast Cells. *PLoS ONE* **2015**, *10*, e0134137. [CrossRef]
27. Agamah, F.E.; Mazandu, G.K.; Hassan, R.; Bope, C.D.; Thomford, N.E.; Ghansah, A.; Chimusa, E.R. Computational/in Silico Methods in Drug Target and Lead Prediction. *Brief. Bioinform.* **2020**, *21*, 1663–1675. [CrossRef]
28. Sadybekov, A.V.; Katritch, V. Computational Approaches Streamlining Drug Discovery. *Nature* **2023**, *616*, 673–685. [CrossRef]
29. Rayan, A.; Raiyn, J.; Falah, M. Nature Is the Best Source of Anticancer Drugs: Indexing Natural Products for Their Anticancer Bioactivity. *PLoS ONE* **2017**, *12*, e0187925. [CrossRef]
30. Ferreira, L.L.G.; Andricopulo, A.D. ADMET Modeling Approaches in Drug Discovery. *Drug Discov. Today* **2019**, *24*, 1157–1165. [CrossRef]
31. Lombardo, F.; Desai, P.V.; Arimoto, R.; Desino, K.E.; Fischer, H.; Keefer, C.E.; Petersson, C.; Winiwarter, S.; Broccatelli, F. In Silico Absorption, Distribution, Metabolism, Excretion, and Pharmacokinetics (ADME-PK): Utility and Best Practices. An Industry Perspective from the International Consortium for Innovation through Quality in Pharmaceutical Development. *J. Med. Chem.* **2017**, *60*, 9097–9113. [CrossRef]
32. Alqahtani, S. In Silico ADME-Tox Modeling: Progress and Prospects. *Expert. Opin. Drug Metab. Toxicol.* **2017**, *13*, 1147–1158. [CrossRef] [PubMed]

33. Shaker, B.; Ahmad, S.; Lee, J.; Jung, C.; Na, D. In Silico Methods and Tools for Drug Discovery. *Comput. Biol. Med.* **2021**, *137*, 104851. [CrossRef] [PubMed]
34. Lipinski, C.A.; Lombardo, F.; Dominy, B.W.; Feeney, P.J. Experimental and Computational Approaches to Estimate Solubility and Permeability in Drug Discovery and Development Settings. *Adv. Drug Deliv. Rev.* **2001**, *46*, 3–26. [CrossRef]
35. Zhao, Y.H.; Abraham, M.H.; Le, J.; Hersey, A.; Luscombe, C.N.; Beck, G.; Sherborne, B.; Cooper, I. Rate-Limited Steps of Human Oral Absorption and QSAR Studies. *Pharm. Res.* **2002**, *19*, 1446–1457. [CrossRef]
36. Daina, A.; Zoete, V. A BOILED-Egg To Predict Gastrointestinal Absorption and Brain Penetration of Small Molecules. *ChemMedChem* **2016**, *11*, 1117–1121. [CrossRef]
37. Lea, T. Caco-2 Cell Line. In *The Impact of Food Bioactives on Health: In Vitro and Ex Vivo Models*; Verhoeckx, K., Cotter, P., López-Expósito, I., Kleiveland, C., Lea, T., Mackie, A., Requena, T., Swiatecka, D., Wichers, H., Eds.; Springer: Cham, Switzerland, 2015; ISBN 978-3-319-15791-7.
38. Kajiwara, M.; Ban, T.; Matsubara, K.; Nakanishi, Y.; Masuda, S. Urinary Dopamine as a Potential Index of the Transport Activity of Multidrug and Toxin Extrusion in the Kidney. *Int. J. Mol. Sci.* **2016**, *17*, 1228. [CrossRef] [PubMed]
39. Fasinu, P.; Pillay, V.; Ndesendo, V.M.K.; du Toit, L.C.; Choonara, Y.E. Diverse Approaches for the Enhancement of Oral Drug Bioavailability. *Biopharm. Drug Dispos.* **2011**, *32*, 185–209. [CrossRef]
40. Daneman, R.; Prat, A. The Blood-Brain Barrier. *Cold Spring Harb. Perspect. Biol.* **2015**, *7*, a020412. [CrossRef]
41. Emmerová, R.; Engelová, J.; Vinakurau, S.; Ondrová, B. CNS Tumors—Clinical and Radiological Aspects. *Cesk Patol.* **2022**, *58*, 150–160.
42. Cascella, M.; Di Napoli, R.; Carbone, D.; Cuomo, G.F.; Bimonte, S.; Muzio, M.R. Chemotherapy-Related Cognitive Impairment: Mechanisms, Clinical Features and Research Perspectives. *Recenti Prog. Med.* **2018**, *109*, 523–530. [CrossRef]
43. Shaker, B.; Lee, J.; Lee, Y.; Yu, M.-S.; Lee, H.-M.; Lee, E.; Kang, H.-C.; Oh, K.-S.; Kim, H.W.; Na, D. A machine learning-based quantitative model (LogBB_Pred) to predict the blood-brain barrier permeability (logBB value) of drug compounds. *Bioinformatics* **2023**, *39*, btad577. [CrossRef]
44. Modi, S.J.; Tiwari, A.; Ghule, C.; Pawar, S.; Saste, G.; Jagtap, S.; Singh, R.; Deshmukh, A.; Girme, A.; Hingorani, L. Pharmacokinetic Study of Withanosides and Withanolides from Withania Somnifera Using Ultra-High Performance Liquid Chromatography-Tandem Mass Spectrometry (UHPLC-MS/MS). *Molecules* **2022**, *27*, 1476. [CrossRef] [PubMed]
45. Dai, T.; Jiang, W.; Guo, Z.; Wang, Z.; Huang, M.; Zhong, G.; Liang, C.; Pei, X.; Dai, R. Studies on Oral Bioavailability and First-Pass Metabolism of Withaferin A in Rats Using LC-MS/MS and Q-TRAP. *Biomed. Chromatogr.* **2019**, *33*, e4573. [CrossRef]
46. Floyd, J.; Mirza, I.; Sachs, B.; Perry, M.C. Hepatotoxicity of Chemotherapy. *Semin. Oncol.* **2006**, *33*, 50–67. [CrossRef]
47. Oun, R.; Moussa, Y.E.; Wheate, N.J. The Side Effects of Platinum-Based Chemotherapy Drugs: A Review for Chemists. *Dalton Trans.* **2018**, *47*, 6645–6653. [CrossRef]
48. Yang, H.; Lou, C.; Sun, L.; Li, J.; Cai, Y.; Wang, Z.; Li, W.; Liu, G.; Tang, Y. admetSAR 2.0: Web-Service for Prediction and Optimization of Chemical ADMET Properties. *Bioinformatics* **2019**, *35*, 1067–1069. [CrossRef]
49. Pires, D.E.V.; Blundell, T.L.; Ascher, D.B. pkCSM: Predicting Small-Molecule Pharmacokinetic and Toxicity Properties Using Graph-Based Signatures. *J. Med. Chem.* **2015**, *58*, 4066–4072. [CrossRef]
50. Dar, N.J.; Hamid, A.; Ahmad, M. Pharmacologic Overview of Withania Somnifera, the Indian Ginseng. *Cell Mol. Life Sci.* **2015**, *72*, 4445–4460. [CrossRef]
51. Xia, Y.; Yan, M.; Wang, P.; Hamada, K.; Yan, N.; Hao, H.; Gonzalez, F.J.; Yan, T. Withaferin A in the Treatment of Liver Diseases: Progress and Pharmacokinetic Insights. *Drug Metab. Dispos.* **2022**, *50*, 685–693. [CrossRef]
52. Siddiqui, S.; Ahmed, N.; Goswami, M.; Chakrabarty, A.; Chowdhury, G. DNA Damage by Withanone as a Potential Cause of Liver Toxicity Observed for Herbal Products of Withania Somnifera (Ashwagandha). *Curr. Res. Toxicol.* **2021**, *2*, 72–81. [CrossRef]
53. Ferri, N.; Siegl, P.; Corsini, A.; Herrmann, J.; Lerman, A.; Benghozi, R. Drug Attrition during Pre-Clinical and Clinical Development: Understanding and Managing Drug-Induced Cardiotoxicity. *Pharmacol. Ther.* **2013**, *138*, 470–484. [CrossRef] [PubMed]
54. Vandenberg, J.I.; Perry, M.D.; Perrin, M.J.; Mann, S.A.; Ke, Y.; Hill, A.P. hERG K(+) Channels: Structure, Function, and Clinical Significance. *Physiol. Rev.* **2012**, *92*, 1393–1478. [CrossRef] [PubMed]
55. Dong, J.; Chen, H. Cardiotoxicity of Anticancer Therapeutics. *Front. Cardiovasc. Med.* **2018**, *5*, 9. [CrossRef]
56. Ducroq, J.; Moha ou Maati, H.; Guilbot, S.; Dilly, S.; Laemmel, E.; Pons-Himbert, C.; Faivre, J.F.; Bois, P.; Stücker, O.; Le Grand, M. Dexrazoxane Protects the Heart from Acute Doxorubicin-Induced QT Prolongation: A Key Role for I(Ks). *Br. J. Pharmacol.* **2010**, *159*, 93–101. [CrossRef]
57. Tiribelli, M.; Medeot, M. Cardiotoxicity of Imatinib: At the Heart of the Problem. *Leuk. Res.* **2011**, *35*, 36–37. [CrossRef]
58. Dong, Q.; Fu, X.-X.; Du, L.-L.; Zhao, N.; Xia, C.-K.; Yu, K.-W.; Cheng, L.-X.; Du, Y.-M. Blocking of the Human Ether-à-Go-Go-Related Gene Channel by Imatinib Mesylate. *Biol. Pharm. Bull.* **2013**, *36*, 268–275. [CrossRef]
59. Hamza, A.; Amin, A.; Daoud, S. The Protective Effect of a Purified Extract of Withania Somnifera against Doxorubicin-Induced Cardiac Toxicity in Rats. *Cell Biol. Toxicol.* **2008**, *24*, 63–73. [CrossRef]

60. Poindexter, B.J.; Allison, A.W.; Bick, R.J.; Dasgupta, A. Ginseng: Cardiotonic in Adult Rat Cardiomyocytes, Cardiotoxic in Neonatal Rat Cardiomyocytes. *Life Sci.* **2006**, *79*, 2337–2344. [CrossRef]
61. Zeiger, E. The Test That Changed the World: The Ames Test and the Regulation of Chemicals. *Mutat. Res. Genet. Toxicol. Environ. Mutagen.* **2019**, *841*, 43–48. [CrossRef]
62. Mortelmans, K.; Zeiger, E. The Ames Salmonella/Microsome Mutagenicity Assay. *Mutat. Res.* **2000**, *455*, 29–60. [CrossRef]
63. Dhar, N.; Razdan, S.; Rana, S.; Bhat, W.W.; Vishwakarma, R.; Lattoo, S.K. A Decade of Molecular Understanding of Withanolide Biosynthesis and In Vitro Studies in Withania Somnifera (L.) Dunal: Prospects and Perspectives for Pathway Engineering. *Front. Plant Sci.* **2015**, *6*, 1031. [CrossRef] [PubMed]
64. Werk, A.N.; Cascorbi, I. Functional Gene Variants of CYP3A4. *Clin. Pharmacol. Ther.* **2014**, *96*, 340–348. [CrossRef]
65. Zhang, Z.-Y.; Wong, Y.N. Enzyme Kinetics for Clinically Relevant CYP Inhibition. *Curr. Drug Metab.* **2005**, *6*, 241–257. [CrossRef]
66. Shilpashree, H.B.; Sudharshan, S.J.; Shasany, A.K.; Nagegowda, D.A. Molecular Characterization of Three CYP450 Genes Reveals Their Role in Withanolides Formation and Defense in Withania Somnifera, the Indian Ginseng. *Sci. Rep.* **2022**, *12*, 1602. [CrossRef] [PubMed]
67. Mollazadeh, S.; Sahebkar, A.; Hadizadeh, F.; Behravan, J.; Arabzadeh, S. Structural and Functional Aspects of P-Glycoprotein and Its Inhibitors. *Life Sci.* **2018**, *214*, 118–123. [CrossRef]
68. Czyzewski, K.; Styczynski, J. Imatinib Is a Substrate for Various Multidrug Resistance Proteins. *Neoplasma* **2009**, *56*, 202–207. [CrossRef] [PubMed]
69. van Hoppe, S.; Rood, J.J.M.; Buil, L.; Wagenaar, E.; Sparidans, R.W.; Beijnen, J.H.; Schinkel, A.H. P-Glycoprotein (MDR1/ABCB1) Restricts Brain Penetration of the Bruton's Tyrosine Kinase Inhibitor Ibrutinib, While Cytochrome P450-3A (CYP3A) Limits Its Oral Bioavailability. *Mol. Pharm.* **2018**, *15*, 5124–5134. [CrossRef]
70. Maia, R.C.; Silva, E.A.; Harab, R.C.; Lucena, M.; Pires, V.; Rumjanek, V.M. Sensitivity of Vincristine-Sensitive K562 and Vincristine-Resistant K562-Lucena 1 Cells to Anthracyclines and Reversal of Multidrug Resistance. *Braz. J. Med. Biol. Res.* **1996**, *29*, 467–472.
71. Issa, M.E.; Wijeratne, E.M.K.; Gunatilaka, A.a.L.; Cuendet, M. Withanolide D Exhibits Similar Cytostatic Effect in Drug-Resistant and Drug-Sensitive Multiple Myeloma Cells. *Front. Pharmacol.* **2017**, *8*, 610. [CrossRef]
72. Arruda, A.C.; Perilhão, M.S.; Santos, W.A.; Gregnani, M.F.; Budu, A.; Neto, J.C.R.; Estrela, G.R.; Araujo, R.C. PPARα-Dependent Modulation by Metformin of the Expression of OCT-2 and MATE-1 in the Kidney of Mice. *Molecules* **2020**, *25*, 392. [CrossRef]
73. Koepsell, H. Organic Cation Transporters in Health and Disease. *Pharmacol. Rev.* **2020**, *72*, 253–319. [CrossRef]
74. Kis, E.; Ioja, E.; Rajnai, Z.; Jani, M.; Méhn, D.; Herédi-Szabó, K.; Krajcsi, P. BSEP Inhibition: In Vitro Screens to Assess Cholestatic Potential of Drugs. *Toxicol. In Vitro* **2012**, *26*, 1294–1299. [CrossRef] [PubMed]
75. Weikum, E.R.; Liu, X.; Ortlund, E.A. The Nuclear Receptor Superfamily: A Structural Perspective. *Protein Sci.* **2018**, *27*, 1876–1892. [CrossRef] [PubMed]
76. Tan, M.H.E.; Li, J.; Xu, H.E.; Melcher, K.; Yong, E. Androgen Receptor: Structure, Role in Prostate Cancer and Drug Discovery. *Acta Pharmacol. Sin.* **2015**, *36*, 3–23. [CrossRef]
77. Saatci, O.; Huynh-Dam, K.-T.; Sahin, O. Endocrine Resistance in Breast Cancer: From Molecular Mechanisms to Therapeutic Strategies. *J. Mol. Med.* **2021**, *99*, 1691–1710. [CrossRef] [PubMed]
78. Soh, S.; Ong, W.-Y. Effect of Withanolide A on 7-Ketocholesterol Induced Cytotoxicity in hCMEC/D3 Brain Endothelial Cells. *Cells* **2022**, *11*, 457. [CrossRef]
79. Duan, W.; Meng, F.; Cui, H.; Lin, Y.; Wang, G.; Wu, J. Ecotoxicity of Phenol and Cresols to Aquatic Organisms: A Review. *Ecotoxicol. Environ. Saf.* **2018**, *157*, 441–456. [CrossRef]
80. Duan, W.; Cui, H.; Jia, X.; Huang, X. Occurrence and Ecotoxicity of Sulfonamides in the Aquatic Environment: A Review. *Sci. Total Environ.* **2022**, *820*, 153178. [CrossRef]
81. Barrick, A.; Châtel, A.; Bruneau, M.; Mouneyrac, C. The Role of High-Throughput Screening in Ecotoxicology and Engineered Nanomaterials. *Environ. Toxicol. Chem.* **2017**, *36*, 1704–1714. [CrossRef]
82. Sripriya, J.; Dash, A. Analytical Study of Kharif Food Grain Production in Odisha. *Int. J. Plant Soil Sci.* **2021**, *33*, 78–85. [CrossRef]
83. Rim, K.-T. In Silico Prediction of Toxicity and Its Applications for Chemicals at Work. *Toxicol. Environ. Health Sci.* **2020**, *12*, 191–202. [CrossRef] [PubMed]
84. Wang, H.-C.; Tsai, Y.-L.; Wu, Y.-C.; Chang, F.-R.; Liu, M.-H.; Chen, W.-Y.; Wu, C.-C. Withanolides-Induced Breast Cancer Cell Death Is Correlated with Their Ability to Inhibit Heat Protein 90. *PLoS ONE* **2012**, *7*, e37764. [CrossRef]
85. Hassannia, B.; Logie, E.; Vandenabeele, P.; Vanden Berghe, T.; Vanden Berghe, W. Withaferin A: From Ayurvedic Folk Medicine to Preclinical Anti-Cancer Drug. *Biochem. Pharmacol.* **2020**, *173*, 113602. [CrossRef]
86. Wang, T.; Subramanian, C.; Yu, M.; White, P.T.; Kuai, R.; Sanchez, J.; Moon, J.J.; Timmermann, B.N.; Schwendeman, A.; Cohen, M.S. Mimetic sHDL Nanoparticles: A Novel Drug-Delivery Strategy to Target Triple-Negative Breast Cancer. *Surgery* **2019**, *166*, 1168–1175. [CrossRef]

87. Maldonado, E.; Pérez-Castorena, A.L.; Garcés, C.; Martínez, M. Philadelphicalactones C and D and Other Cytotoxic Compounds from Physalis Philadelphica. *Steroids* **2011**, *76*, 724–728. [CrossRef]
88. Ma, T.; Fan, B.-Y.; Zhang, C.; Zhao, H.-J.; Han, C.; Gao, C.-Y.; Luo, J.-G.; Kong, L.-Y. Metabonomics Applied in Exploring the Antitumour Mechanism of Physapubenolide on Hepatocellular Carcinoma Cells by Targeting Glycolysis through the Akt-P53 Pathway. *Sci. Rep.* **2016**, *6*, 29926. [CrossRef]
89. Wadegaonkar, V.P.; Wadegaonkar, P.A. Withanone as an Inhibitor of Survivin: A Potential Drug Candidate for Cancer Therapy. *J. Biotechnol.* **2013**, *168*, 229–233. [CrossRef] [PubMed]
90. Yu, T.-J.; Tang, J.-Y.; Lin, L.-C.; Lien, W.-J.; Cheng, Y.-B.; Chang, F.-R.; Ou-Yang, F.; Chang, H.-W. Withanolide C Inhibits Proliferation of Breast Cancer Cells via Oxidative Stress-Mediated Apoptosis and DNA Damage. *Antioxidants* **2020**, *9*, 873. [CrossRef]
91. Wang, S.-B.; Zhu, D.-R.; Nie, B.; Li, J.; Zhang, Y.-J.; Kong, L.-Y.; Luo, J.-G. Cytotoxic withanolides from the aerial parts of Tubocapsicum anomalum. *Bioorg. Chem.* **2018**, *81*, 396–404. [CrossRef]
92. Huang, C.-Y.; Liaw, C.-C.; Chen, B.-W.; Chen, P.-C.; Su, J.-H.; Sung, P.-J.; Dai, C.-F.; Chiang, M.Y.; Sheu, J.-H. Withanolide-Based Steroids from the Cultured Soft Coral Sinularia Brassica. *J. Nat. Prod.* **2013**, *76*, 1902–1908. [CrossRef]
93. Daina, A.; Michielin, O.; Zoete, V. SwissADME: A Free Web Tool to Evaluate Pharmacokinetics, Drug-Likeness and Medicinal Chemistry Friendliness of Small Molecules. *Sci. Rep.* **2017**, *7*, 42717. [CrossRef] [PubMed]

molecules

MDPI

Article

Characteristics, Antioxidant Activity Stability, and Anti-Fatigue Activity of Hydrolysates from *Cucumaria frondosa* Tentacles

Mingbo Li [1,†], Juan Chen [2,†], Qiuting Wang [1], Chuyi Liu [3,4], Wenkui Song [5] and Leilei Sun [1,*]

1 Yantai Key Laboratory of Characteristic Agricultural Bioresource Conservation & Germplasm Innovative Utilization, School of Life Sciences, Yantai University, Yantai 264005, China; limingbo1711@163.com (M.L.); wqt1981979471@163.com (Q.W.)
2 College of Health, Yantai Nanshan University, Yantai 265713, China; chenjuan8796@126.com
3 Marine Biomedical Research Institute of Qingdao, Qingdao 266073, China; liucy@ouc.edu.cn
4 College of Food Science and Engineering, Ocean University of China, Qingdao 266003, China
5 Guangdong Provincial Key Laboratory of Aquatic Products Processing and Safety, National Research and Development Branch Center for Shellfish Processing (Zhanjiang), Guangdong Provincial Engineering Technology Research Center of Seafood, Guangdong Province Engineering Laboratory for Marine Biological Products, College of Food Science and Technology, Guangdong Ocean University, Zhanjiang 524088, China; songwk@gdou.edu.cn
* Correspondence: leilei.198966@163.com; Tel.: +86-0535-6902638
† These authors contributed equally to this work.

Abstract: This study aimed to assess the impact of alcalase, trypsin, flavourzyme, and neutrase on the characteristics, antioxidant activity stability, and anti-fatigue activity of hydrolysates derived from *Cucumaria frondosa* tentacles (CFTHs). The results demonstrate that favourzyme hydrolysates exhibited the highest degree of hydrolysis (DH). Zeta potential and particle size measurements indicated that hydrolyzed peptides treated with favourzyme appeared aggregated and exhibited larger particle sizes. The antioxidant properties of CFTHs demonstrated good thermal stability, pH stability, and enhanced simulated gastrointestinal digestive stability. The anti-fatigue activity of CFTHs was examined using an acute exercise fatigue model. The results indicate that CFTHs extended the exhaustive swimming time of mice to 17.81 min. Additionally, CFTHs significantly elevated ($p < 0.01$) blood glucose (Glu) and liver glycogen (LG) levels, while also decreasing ($p < 0.05$) the concentrations of metabolites such as lactic acid (LA), urea nitrogen (BUN), creatine kinase (CK), lactate dehydrogenase (LDH), and ammonia (NH3). This reduction contributed to the alleviation of fatigue in the body. Furthermore, the levels of superoxide dismutase (SOD) and glutathione peroxidase (GSH-Px) were significantly increased ($p < 0.05$), which aided in mitigating oxidative damage induced by strenuous exercise. These findings strongly support the potential utilization of CFTHs in food products as natural antioxidant and anti-fatigue alternatives.

Keywords: *Cucumaria frondosa* tentacle; hydrolysate; characteristic; antioxidant activity; anti-fatigue activity

1. Introduction

Currently, humanity is confronting the challenges posed by COVID-19 [1], while the fast-paced lifestyle has led to various health issues, including fatigue, low immunity, anxiety, insomnia, and various chronic diseases such as hypertension, diabetes, obesity, and even cancer. As a result, there is an increasing emphasis on enhancing and maintaining good health. Fatigue, which can escalate to exhaustion, is typically triggered by a significant decrease in energy during physical exertion [2]. High-intensity and excessive exercise generally result in the production and accumulation of substantial amounts of free radicals, which are closely associated with oxidative damage and fatigue [3]. The antioxidant activities of peptides have been extensively investigated, with numerous studies emphasizing the potential for generating antioxidant peptides through the in vitro enzymatic digestion of marine protein resources. Liu et al. [1] confirmed that abalone visceral peptides exhibited significant in vitro antioxidant activity and cytoprotective effects against oxidative damage. Research has demonstrated that food-derived bioactive peptides can also exert their anti-fatigue effects by increasing glycogen reserves, enhancing the activity of antioxidant enzymes, reducing the accumulation of metabolites, and protecting tissue cells. Ye et al. [4] prepared peptides from the sea cucumber (*Stichopus japonicus*) and suggested that these peptides exhibited anti-fatigue activity in an endurance swimming rat model. They proposed that the anti-fatigue effects may be attributed to the normalization of energy metabolism, as well as the alleviation of oxidative damage and inflammatory responses.

Cucumaria frondosa, commonly referred to as the orange-footed sea cucumber, is the most abundant and widely distributed species in the cold waters of the North Atlantic Ocean, and is classified within the Cucurbitaceae family. *Cucumaria frondosa* is of commercial significance in eastern Canada [5]. It can grow to a maximum length of 40 to 50 cm, a width of 10 to 15 cm, and a weight ranging from 100 to 500 g. This species is a suspension feeder that employs its tentacles to capture phytoplankton, zooplankton, and organic materials. Certain enterprises market the dehydrated tentacles, referred to as "flower" [5]. *Cucumaria frondosa* thrives in a distinct growth environment and possesses a prolonged growth cycle, resulting in minimal pollutant accumulation and a rich nutrient profile [6]. Consequently, its quality is superior to that of other sea cucumber varieties. Following capture, *Cucumaria frondosa* is typically processed into various forms, including ready-to-eat sea cucumbers, dried sea cucumbers, and salted sea cucumbers. The primary product obtained from sea cucumbers is the body wall. This processing generates substantial by-products such as tentacles, intestines, and ovum, constituting approximately 50% of the sea cucumber's total weight. Currently, the by-products of *Cucumaria frondosa* are entirely discarded, leading to environmental pollution and a waste of resources [7]. Hossain et al. [8] conducted a study on the free, esterified, and insoluble-bound phenolics found in the tentacles of *Cucumaria frondosa* and their antioxidant activity. However, there is a paucity of research regarding the structure and biological activity of its protein hydrolysates. Consequently, future research should focus on the utilization of *Cucumaria frondosa* by-products for the extraction of value-added products and their potential applications as nutraceuticals and functional food ingredients.

The physicochemical properties and biological activity of hydrolysates are predominantly influenced by the specific proteases employed and the method of hydrolysis applied [9,10]. Nevertheless, there is limited research on the effects of various proteases on the physicochemical and biological activities of hydrolysates derived from *Cucumaria frondose* tentacles. Therefore, this research aimed to explore the influences of different proteases on the physicochemical properties and antioxidant characteristics of hydrolysates derived from *Cucumaria frondose* tentacles (CFTHs), as well as their stability in antioxidant activity. Additionally, the research assessed the anti-fatigue effects of CFTHs by investigating their impact on biochemical indicators, including exhaustive swimming time, energy reserves, related metabolite accumulation, and oxidative stress in mice. The findings offer theoretical support for the utilization of by-products derived from *Cucumaria frondose*.

2. Results and Discussion

2.1. Degree of Hydrolysis of Hydrolysates Derived from Cucumaria frondosa Tentacles

The hydrolysis of CFTHs was investigated using various proteases, and the degree of hydrolysis (DH) of CFTHs is illustrated in Figure 1a. The type of protease employed exhibited a significant impact on the DH of the product ($p < 0.05$) [11]. As shown in

Figure 1a, the DH achieved with flavourzyme was significantly higher compared to the other three proteases. The results indicate that, with the exception of flavourzyme, the DH attained by the other proteases was below 30%. The difference arises from the fact that flavourzyme functions as both exopeptidases and endopeptidases, specifically as a cysteine protease with leucine aminopeptidase activity [12].

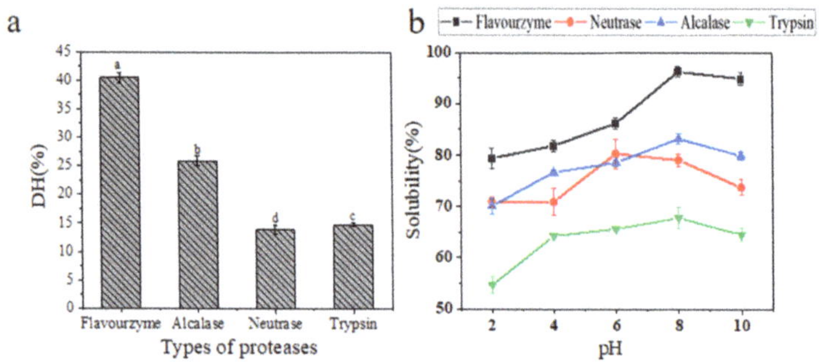

Figure 1. (**a**) DH of the CFTHs obtained by different proteases; (**b**) solubility of the CFTHs obtained by different proteases (n = 5). Different letters indicate significant differences ($p < 0.05$).

2.2. Solubility of Hydrolysates Derived from *Cucumaria frondosa* Tentacles

The solubility of protein hydrolysates is a critical factor that significantly influences their physicochemical and functional characteristics [13]. As illustrated in Figure 1b, among all the samples, the flavourzyme hydrolysate exhibited the highest solubility, while the solubility of the other three protease hydrolysates also surpassed 50%. The lower solubility observed in the trypsin hydrolysate may be attributed to its lower DH. This finding aligns with those of the study reported by Hau et al. [14], which suggested that a higher DH corresponded to smaller hydrolysate sizes. Smaller peptide molecules tend to form stronger hydrogen bonds with water compared to intact proteins, resulting in the increased solubility of CFTHs. Interestingly, Senadheera et al. [15] indicated that protein hydrolysates derived from different parts of the North Atlantic sea cucumber exhibited similar solubility characteristics. Notably, solubility improves with a shift towards more basic pH conditions.

2.3. Particle Size, Polydispersity Index, and Zeta Potential

The particle size, polydispersity index (PDI), and zeta potential of each hydrolysate are exhibited in Figure 2. Among the proteases examined, flavourzyme exhibited the largest particle size, whereas neutrase demonstrated the smallest. Contrary to expectations that the hydrolysate from flavourzyme would yield a smaller particle size compared to the other proteases, Figure 2 indicated that it was actually the largest. This phenomenon may be attributed to the aggregation of peptides and amino acids into larger fragments or particles due to the formation of chemical bonds [16].

The PDI serves as a crucial metric for assessing the dispersion properties of macromolecular polymers. A lower PDI value indicates improved dispersion in water [17]. Various protease treatments resulted in distinct dispersion characteristics among the hydrolysates, with flavourzyme demonstrating the most effective dispersion.

Furthermore, a higher absolute value of zeta potential diminishes the flocculation and aggregation caused by attractive forces, thereby enhancing the stability of the solution [18]. The hydrolysates derived from alcalase exhibited significantly greater absolute zeta potentials compared to the other treatments ($p < 0.05$). An elevated zeta potential promotes electrostatic repulsion between molecules and facilitates the diffusion of the hydrolysate, ultimately leading to improved dispersion [19].

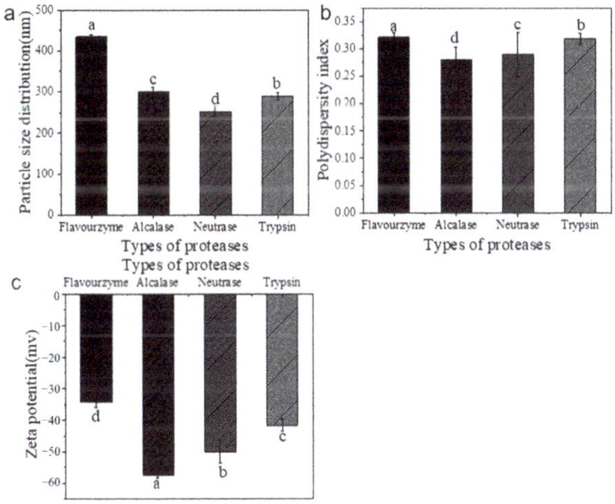

Figure 2. (**a**) The particle sizes of CFTHs obtained by different proteases; (**b**) the PDI of CFTHs obtained by different proteases; (**c**) the zeta potential of CFTHs obtained by different proteases (n = 5). Different letters indicate significant differences ($p < 0.05$).

2.4. *Effects of Protease on Antioxidant Activity of Hydrolysates Derived from Cucumaria frondosa Tentacles*

2.4.1. DPPH Radical Scavenging Capacity

DPPH is widely utilized to assess the antioxidant activity and capability of bioactive substances due to its stability as a free radical [20]. As illustrated in Figure 3a, the scavenging capacity of CFTHs on the DPPH radical exhibited a significant ($p < 0.05$) dose-dependent effect. Among the hydrolysates generated by the four proteases, the hydrolysate derived from flavourzyme demonstrated a significantly higher ($p < 0.05$) DPPH free radical scavenging capacity compared to the other three proteases. This finding suggests that flavorzyme was particularly effective in generating peptides with potent capabilities to scavenge DPPH free radicals, exhibiting an IC_{50} of 5.34 mg/mL, which is consistent with that in the study by Yu et al. [21].

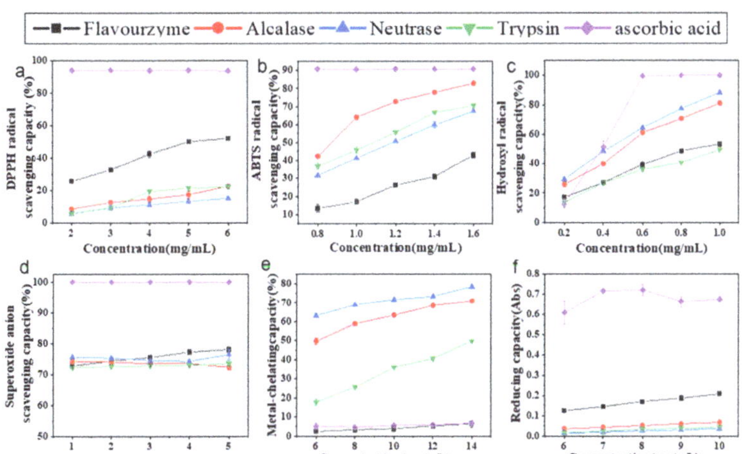

Figure 3. (**a**) DPPH radical scavenging capacity of CFTHs; (**b**) ABTS radical scavenging capacity of CFTHs; (**c**) hydroxyl radical scavenging capacity; (**d**) superoxide anion scavenging capacity of CFTHs; (**e**) metal-chelating capacity of CFTHs; (**f**) reducing capacity of CFTHs (n = 5).

2.4.2. ABTS Radical Scavenging Capacity

The ABTS method is a highly sensitive technique employed to confirm the free radical activity of samples [22]. Consistent with the findings of Hernández-Ruiz et al. [20], the scavenging capacity of CFTHs increased with concentration (Figure 3b). In comparison, the scavenging capacity of alcalase hydrolysate was significantly stronger than that of the other three proteases, with an IC_{50} of 0.82 mg/mL, which aligned with that in the study conducted by Karami et al. [9]. Additionally, the alcalase hydrolysate exhibited a higher content of aromatic amino acids, which can convert free radicals into stable molecules by acting as electron donors. This mechanism enhances the ABTS radical scavenging capacity [23].

2.4.3. Hydroxyl Radical Scavenging Capacity

The hydroxyl radical, known for its high reactivity with biological tissue proteins, can induce cellular damage and contribute to various physiological disorders when it interacts with endogenous biomolecules such as proteins [24]. This study demonstrated that the hydroxyl radical scavenging capacity of CFTHs increased with concentration, ranging from 0.2 to 1.0 mg/mL (Figure 3c). Notably, at lower concentrations, CFTHs exhibited higher scavenging activity compared to ascorbic acid, with the hydrolysate from neutrase displaying the strongest scavenging capacity, characterized by an IC_{50} of 0.44 mg/mL. Furthermore, CFTHs demonstrated a greater hydroxyl radical scavenging capacity than both mung bean protein hydrolysate [23] and hydrolysates of milk protein concentrate [24]. Therefore, CFTHs show promise as a potent scavenger in the food industry.

2.4.4. Superoxide Anion Scavenging Capacity

The superoxide anion scavenging capacity of CFTHs was significantly lower ($p < 0.05$) compared to that of ascorbic acid. Additionally, no significant differences ($p > 0.05$) were observed in the scavenging activity among the four proteases (Figure 3d). The presence of inactive polypeptides in CFTHs may contribute to the reduced clearance activity [25].

2.4.5. Metal-Chelating Capacity

Metal ions play a significant role in promoting lipid peroxidation. Therefore, the removal of these ions from food systems can effectively mitigate oxidation reactions [26]. Hydrolysates produced by alcalase, neutrase, and trypsin exhibited higher chelating activity compared to ascorbic acid, whereas flavourzyme demonstrated a chelating activity comparable to that of ascorbic acid. Alcalase, an endopeptidase with broad specificity, efficiently cleaves polypeptide bonds, thereby increasing the abundance of acidic and basic amino acids, especially phenylalanine (Phe), tyrosine (Tyr), and lysine (Lys). This enhancement in negative charge density accounts for the enhanced chelation activity of polypeptides following enzymatic hydrolysis [27].

2.4.6. Reducing Capacity

The reducing capacity of protein hydrolysates is commonly utilized as an indicator of their potential antioxidant and electron-donating abilities [28]. A higher absorbance at 700 nm indicates a stronger reducing capacity. In comparison to ascorbic acid (Figure 3f), CFTHs exhibited a higher reducing capacity, although it was lower than that of yellowfin tuna skin (*Thunnus albacares*) hydrolysate [29]. The pronounced reducing capacity of flavourzyme may be attributed to the release and exposure of amino acids such as Phe, tryptophan (Try), aspartic acid (Asp), and glutamic acid (Glu). The exposure of these amino acid side chain groups during hydrolysis can provide an additional supply of electrons and protons, thereby maintaining the reducing capacity [30].

2.5. Antioxidant Activity Stability of Hydrolysates Derived from Cucumaria frondosa Tentacles

Considering the potential use of CFTHs as a functional food ingredient, it is crucial to account for appropriate food processing and storage conditions when incorporating them into functional foods. This study examined the antioxidant activity of CFTHs during in vitro simulated digestion. As depicted in Figure 4, the DPPH radical scavenging capacity, ABTS radical scavenging capacity, and reducing capacity of CFTHs decreased following in vitro simulated gastrointestinal digestion. These results align with the findings derived by Lee et al. [31]. However, the hydroxyl radical scavenging capacity and metal-chelating capacity of CFTHs significantly increased, while the superoxide anion scavenging capacity remained unchanged, after in vitro simulated gastrointestinal digestion. This phenomenon can be attributed to the breakdown of larger proteins into hydrolysates, which may result in a persistence of, reduction in or enhancement of antioxidant properties due to the production of smaller peptides and the release of free amino acids [32]. The enhanced antioxidant properties observed after gastrointestinal digestion can be ascribed to the release of peptides and amino acids through the action of pepsin and pancreatic enzymes. A study conducted by Morais et al. [33] reported that small peptides exhibited resistance to hydrolysis by digestive enzymes, and were readily absorbed in the gut. This finding may elucidate why flavourzyme hydrolysates demonstrate greater resistance to gastrointestinal digestion compared to the other three proteases.

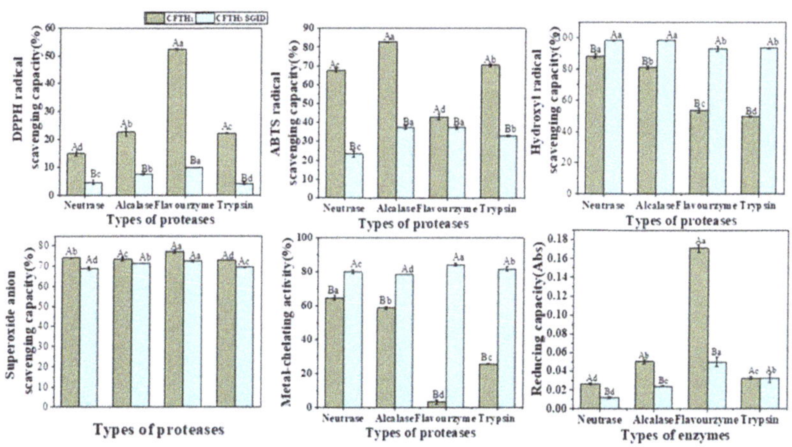

Figure 4. Antioxidant activity stability of CFTHs after in vitro simulated gastrointestinal digestion (n = 5). The uppercase letters indicate significant differences in the activity of CFTHs obtained by the same protease hydrolysis before and after in vitro simulated gastrointestinal digestion, and the lowercase letters indicate significant differences in the activity of CFTHs obtained by different protease hydrolysis.

The effect of pH on the antioxidant activity of CFTHs is illustrated in Figure 5. pH is a crucial factor influencing the stability of active peptides. Generally, the DPPH radical scavenging capacity, superoxide anion scavenging capacity, metal-chelating capacity, and reducing capacity were optimal in a neutral environment, which is consistent with the findings of Sheng et al. [34]. In contrast, the ABTS radical scavenging capacity and hydroxyl radical scavenging capacity were not significantly affected by variations in pH. Nevertheless, changes in pH can influence the biological activity of the hydrolysate, potentially related to the presence of specific amino acids. For instance, acidic conditions may lead to the degradation of glutamine and asparagine residues, while alkaline conditions can result in the degradation of threonine, serine, and cysteine residues, thereby altering their biological activity [35].

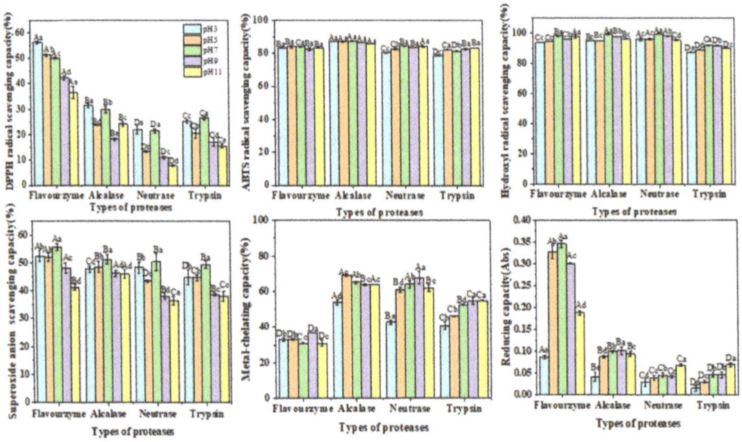

Figure 5. Effects of varying pH levels on the antioxidant activity of CFTHs (n = 5). The uppercase letters indicate significant differences in the antioxidant activity of CFTHs at the same pH level, and the lowercase letters indicate significant differences in the antioxidant activity of CFTHs at different pH levels.

As illustrated in Figure 6, the antioxidant activity of CFTHs displayed slight fluctuations across varying temperatures but remained relatively stable, indicating good thermal stability. These findings are consistent with those reported by Zhang et al. [12]. It is plausible that the low molecular mass of the samples utilized in this experiment contributes to their reduced sensitivity to temperature, resulting in the minimal structural denaturation of the peptides when exposed to temperatures below a certain threshold. Consequently, the observed changes in activity were less pronounced [36].

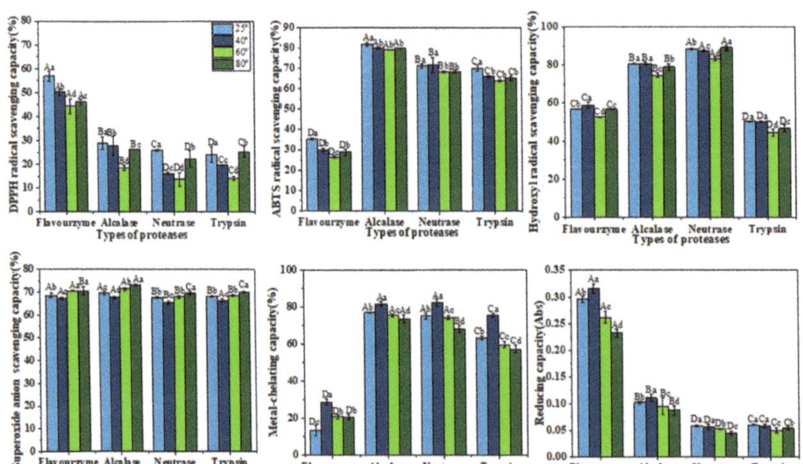

Figure 6. Effects of different temperatures on the antioxidant activity of CFTHs (n = 5). The uppercase letters indicate significant differences in antioxidant activity of CFTHs at the same temperature, and the lowercase letters indicate significant differences in antioxidant activity of CFTHs at different temperatures.

2.6. Effects of Hydrolysates Derived from Cucumaria frondosa Tentacles on Body Weight and Visceral Index in Mice

Changes in the body weight of mice during gavage can reflect the effects of CFTHs on appetite and overall health status [37]. The body weights of mice after 30 days of continuous gavage are presented in Figure 7. As the duration of intragastric administration increased, the body weight of the mice gradually increased. However, there was no significant difference in the growth rate of body weight among the various groups of mice during the administration period, indicating that CFTHs did not have a notable effect on appetite or health status. Furthermore, there were no significant differences in the coefficients of the liver, kidney, spleen, and thymus between the experimental group and the blank control group ($p > 0.05$). This suggests that the administration of CFTHs at different doses did not impact the visceral index of the mice.

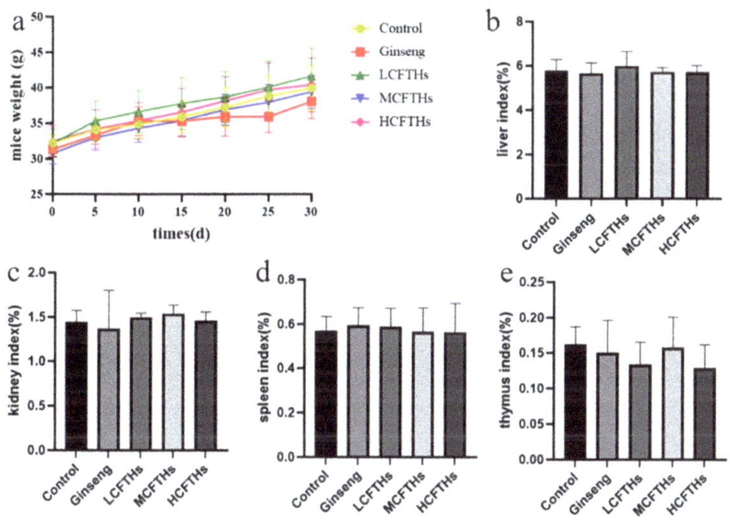

Figure 7. Effects of CFTHs on body weight and visceral index in mice (n = 9). (**a**) Changes in body weight of mice; (**b**) liver index; (**c**) kidney index; (**d**) spleen index; (**e**) thymus index.

2.7. Effects of Hydrolysates Derived from Cucumaria frondosa Tentacles on Mice Liver Tissue Morphology

Following exhaustive swimming, the liver tissue structure of the mice exhibited varying degrees of damage. In the control group, cell boundaries were indistinct, the cytoplasm appeared fused and swollen, and the nuclei exhibited signs of shrinkage (Figure 8). In contrast, supplementation with CFTHs demonstrated a protective effect on the livers of mice subjected to exhaustive swimming.

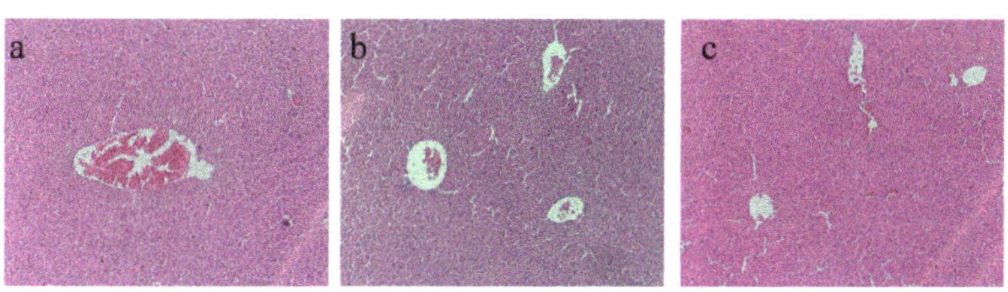

Figure 8. Liver histomorphology of mice. (**a**) Control group; (**b**) positive control group; (**c**) CFTHs group.

2.8. Effects of Hydrolysates Derived from Cucumaria frondosa Tentacles on Weight-Loaded Swimming Capacity

The forced swimming test is a widely utilized method for assessing the anti-fatigue effects of biologically active substances. Systemic changes induced by exercise-related fatigue can be observed in mice, including immune deficiencies and metabolic disorders. This study employed an exercise swimming test to evaluate the physical fatigue experienced by mice and to assess the anti-fatigue effects of CFTHs. Our results indicate that MCFTHs significantly prolonged the forced swimming time ($p < 0.05$) compared to the control group, with a mean duration of 17.81 min (Figure 9). These findings demonstrate that the MCFTHs-treated groups exhibited enhanced swimming endurance.

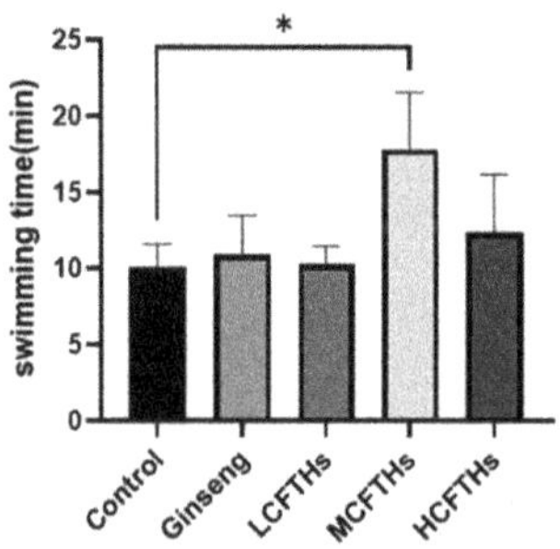

Figure 9. Swimming time of mice (n = 9). * $p < 0.05$.

2.9. Effects of Hydrolysates Derived from Cucumaria frondosa Tentacles on Liver Glycogen and Blood Glucose in Mice

Glycogen content serves as a crucial indicator of physical fatigue. As illustrated in Figure 10a, the serum liver glycogen (LG) content in mice was measured, revealing that CFTHs elevated LG levels in a dose-dependent manner compared to the control group, with HCFTHs demonstrating the most pronounced effect, increasing LG by 83.49%. These results indicate that CFTHs could enhance LG reserves, thereby providing energy for the body, alleviating physical fatigue, improving exercise endurance, and exhibiting significant anti-fatigue properties. Glucose serves as the primary energy-supplying substance in the human body, and maintaining stable blood glucose levels is essential for normal physiological functioning and resistance to fatigue. As depicted in Figure 10b, CFTHs significantly increased blood glucose (Glu) levels ($p < 0.05$) compared to the blank control group, with LCFTHs, MCFTHs, and HCFTHs showing increases of 31.82%, 80.52%, and 85.92%, respectively. This indicates that CFTHs could provide glucose to the body, thereby contributing to the alleviation of fatigue.

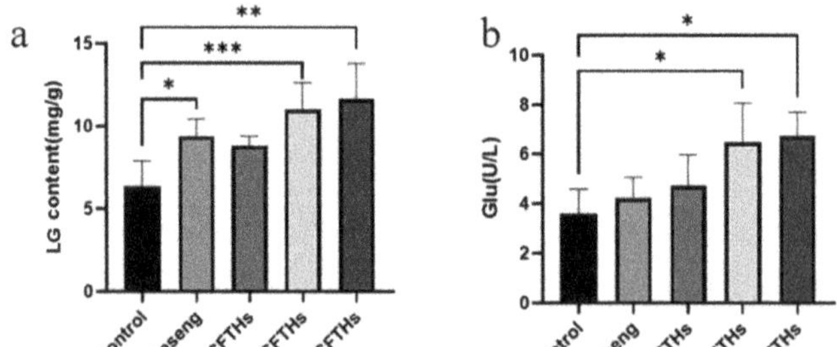

Figure 10. Effects of CFTHs on LG and Glu in mice (n = 9). (**a**) LG content; (**b**) Glu content. * $p < 0.05$, ** $p < 0.01$, *** $p < 0.001$.

2.10. *Effects of Hydrolysates Derived from Cucumaria frondosa Tentacles on Metabolite Accumulation*

The metabolite accumulation theory posits that, as athletes consume greater amounts of energy substrates, the production of metabolites increases, particularly during high-intensity exercise compared to rest. These metabolites accumulate in the blood and skeletal muscle, disrupting the dynamic balance of the internal environment, which subsequently leads to a decline in muscle tissue motor function and results in exercise-induced fatigue [38]. During strenuous exercise, the body experiences the significant depletion of adenosine triphosphate (ATP), accompanied by elevated levels of ammonia (NH_3) in skeletal muscle. This condition promotes glycolytic reactions, resulting in increased concentrations of lactic acid (LA) and urea nitrogen (BUN). Such disruptions to normal dynamic homeostasis contribute to fatigue. To assess the effects of CFTHs on metabolite accumulation, we measured serum levels of LA, BUN, and NH_3 in mice. As illustrated in Figure 11, compared to the blank control group, the administration of CFTHs resulted in significant decreases in LA, BUN, and NH_3 levels, effectively reversing the accumulation of these metabolites. Among the sample groups, the HCFTHs group exhibited the lowest levels of BUN and NH_3, while the MCFTHs group showed the lowest levels of LA.

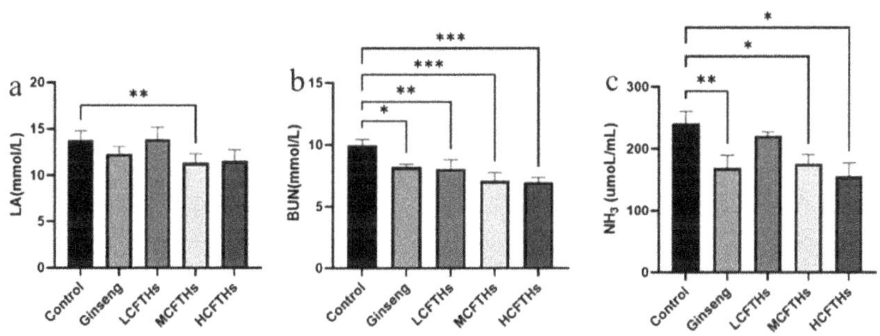

Figure 11. Effects of CFTHs on metabolite accumulation (n = 9). (**a**) LA content; (**b**) BUN content; (**c**) NH_3 content. * $p < 0.05$, ** $p < 0.01$, *** $p < 0.001$.

2.11. *Protective Effects of Hydrolysates Derived from Cucumaria frondosa Tentacles on Muscle*

Creatine kinase (CK) activity is a crucial marker of exercise-induced muscle damage, as CK is prevalent in various muscle cells types, including skeletal, smooth, and cardiac muscles. An increase in CK activity in the bloodstream typically indicates damage to muscle cells, resulting in the release of CK into the circulation [39]. Additionally, lactate dehydrogenase (LDH) serves as an indicator of muscle fiber damage and is primarily located in muscle tissue. Elevated LDH levels often occur following prolonged exercise, leading to its leakage into the bloodstream [40]. As illustrated in Figure 12, CK activity was reduced in the CFTHs group compared to the control group. Furthermore, CFTHs markedly ($p < 0.01$) inhibited the increase in blood LDH concentration induced by forced swimming, suggesting that CFTHs effectively mitigate muscle fiber rupture. These findings suggest that CFTHs can substantially lower CK and LDH levels in the blood, thereby aiding recovery from physical fatigue and providing muscle protection.

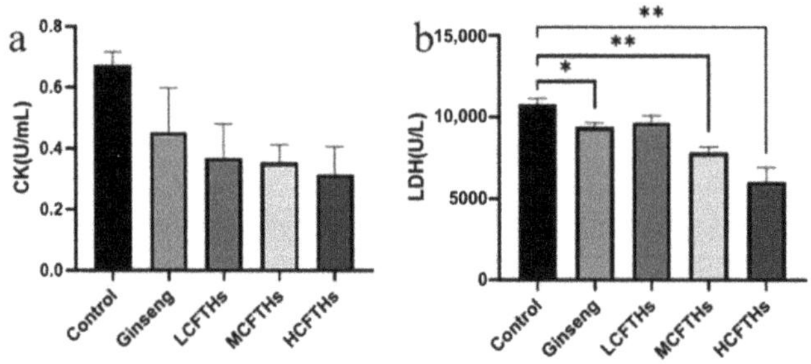

Figure 12. Protective effects of CFTHs on muscle (n = 9). (**a**) CK activity; (**b**) LDH activity. * $p < 0.05$, ** $p < 0.01$.

2.12. *Effects of Hydrolysates Derived from Cucumaria frondosa Tentacles on Antioxidant Levels in Mice Liver*

Oxidative stress induced by strenuous exercise may contribute to exercise-related fatigue [41]. Superoxide dismutase (SOD) plays a critical role among antioxidant enzymes in combating oxidative stress. Glutathione peroxidase (GSH-Px) catalyzes the formation of glutathione, which is the primary non-protein thiol in organisms, and is essential for enhancing antioxidant defenses and reacting with ROS to mitigate oxidative damage and lipid peroxidation. Additionally, GSH-Px facilitates the decomposition of hydrogen peroxide into water and oxygen, thereby preventing the deleterious effects of excess hydrogen peroxide on tissues and organs [42]. As illustrated in Figure 13, CFTHs significantly increased the activities of SOD and GSH-Px in mice. Compared to the control group, HCFTHs enhanced the activities of SOD and GSH-Px by 16.91% and 18.29%, respectively. These findings suggest that CFTHs could elevate antioxidant enzyme activities, thereby protecting the body from oxidative damage associated with strenuous exercise.

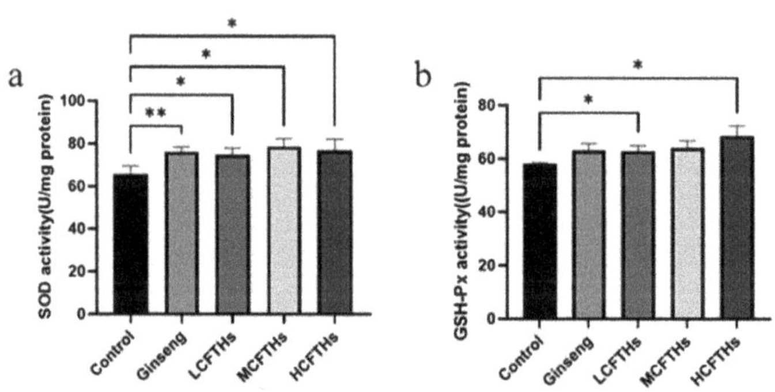

Figure 13. Effects of CFTHs on antioxidant levels in mice liver (n = 9). (**a**) SOD activity; (**b**) GSH-Px activity. * $p < 0.05$, ** $p < 0.01$.

3. Materials and Methods

3.1. *Materials and Reagents*

Recently harvested *Cucumaria frondosa* tentacles were acquired from the Haizhongbao seafood market in Yantai, China. Food-grade neutrase (5.0×10^4 U/g), alcalase (2.0×10^5 U/g), flavourzyme (1.5×10^4 U/g), and trypsin (2.5×10^5 U/g) were sourced from Solarbio biotechnology Co. Ltd. in Beijing, China. All other reagents used in this study were of analytical grade.

3.2. Preparation of Hydrolysates Derived from Cucumaria frondosa Tentacles

As shown in Table 1, the tentacles of *Cucumaria frondosa* were subjected to hydrolysis through the addition of proteases to the prepared CFTHs. This hydrolysis process was conducted in a water bath shaker set to a speed of 100 rpm. Following the incubation period, the mixture was heated in a water bath at a temperature of 90 ± 2 °C for 15 min to terminate the hydrolysis process. The resulting CFTHs were then rapidly chilled in ice water and subsequently centrifuged at 10,000 rpm for 15 min at a temperature of 4 °C. The supernatant obtained from centrifugation was freeze-dried to yield the CFTHs.

Table 1. Optimal enzymatic hydrolysis conditions of different proteases.

Proteases	Temperature (°C)	pH	Solid–Liquid Ratio (*w*/*v*)	Proteases Addition (U/g Protein)	Time (h)
Flavourzyme	40	5.8	1:6	10,000	7
Alcalase	55	9.5	1:8	8500	7
Trypsin	55	8	1:4	9500	4
Neutrase	45	7.2	1:10	7500	5

3.3. Determination of the Degree of Hydrolysis

The DH value of CFTHs was determined using a slightly modified ninhydrin colorimetric method [43]. In this procedure, 2 mL of the sample was mixed with 1 mL of the ninhydrin solution in a test tube. The tubes were subsequently heated in a boiling water bath for 15 min. Following rapid cooling in cold water, 5 mL of a 40% ethanol solution was added to the tube. The solution was then vigorously shaken until the brownish-red color faded, after which it was allowed to stand at room temperature for 10 min. The absorbance of the solution was measured at 570 nm, with the baseline established using distilled water. The DH was calculated using the following equation:

$$\mathrm{DH}(\%) = \frac{h}{h_{\mathrm{tot}}} \times 100 \tag{1}$$

where h represents the millimoles of peptide bonds cleaved per gram of sample (mmol) and h_{tot} represents the millimoles of peptide bonds present per gram of sample (mmol). The h_{tot} value used in this experiment was 8.56 mmol/g, determined based on the amino acid composition of *Cucumaria frondose* tentacles.

3.4. Determination of the Solubility

The solubility of CFTHs was determined using the refined method described by Vásquez et al. [44]. Solutions of CFTHs (20 mL at a concentration of 1%, *w*/*v*) were prepared, and their pH values were adjusted to 2.0, 4.0, 6.0, 8.0, and 10.0 using 1 mol/L NaOH or 1 mol/L HCl. Following incubation, the hydrolysate solution was centrifuged at 4000 rpm for 15 min, and the resulting supernatant was collected. The protein content of the supernatant was assessed using the method established by Lowry et al. [45], and the solubility of the samples was calculated as a percentage according to the following equation:

$$\text{Solubility (\%)} = (\text{Protein content of the supernatant})/(\text{Protein content of the sample}) \times 100 \tag{2}$$

3.5. Determination of the Particle Size, Polydispersity Index, and Zeta Potential

The particle size, PDI, and zeta potential of CFTHs were determined using a modified version of the method described by Wang et al. [17]. Prior to measurement, each sample was dispersed in 0.01 M sodium dihydrogen phosphate buffer (pH 7.0) at a concentration of

0.3 mg/mL. The dispersion was subsequently analyzed using a laser particle size analyzer (Malvern Mastersizer, Malvern Instruments, Malvern, UK).

3.6. Antioxidant Activity

3.6.1. DPPH Radical Scavenging Capacity

The DPPH radical scavenging capacity of CFTHs was measured following the method outlined by Du et al. [46]. Various concentrations of samples (2.0, 3.0, 4.0, 5.0, and 6.0 mg/mL) were combined with DPPH (0.2 mM) in equal proportions and incubated at 25 °C for 30 min in the dark. Following the incubation period, the absorbance was measured at 517 nm, with vitamin C (VC) serving as a positive control. Anhydrous ethanol of the same volume was utilized as a blank control. The DPPH radical scavenging capacity was calculated using the following formula

$$\text{DPPH radical scavenging capacity (\%)} = [1 - (A_1 - A_2)/A_0] \times 100 \quad (3)$$

where A_0 represents the absorbance values of anhydrous ethanol and DPPH, A_1 represents the absorbance values of the sample and DPPH, and A_2 represents the absorbance values of anhydrous ethanol and the sample.

3.6.2. Hydroxyl Radical Scavenging Capacity

The hydroxyl radical scavenging capacity was assessed using the method described by Zhou et al. [47], with minor modifications. Samples at concentrations of 0.2, 0.4, 0.6, 0.8, and 1.0 mg/mL were mixed with $FeSO_4$ (2 mM) and a salicylic acid–ethanol solution (6 mM) in a 1:1:1 ratio. Subsequently, 1.0 mL of H_2O_2 (6 mM) was added to the mixture, which was then incubated in a water bath at 37 °C for 30 min. The absorbance of the mixture was measured immediately at 510 nm using a microplate reader, with VC serving as a positive control. The hydroxyl radical scavenging activity was calculated using the following equation:

$$\text{Hydroxyl radical scavenging capacity (\%)} = [1 - (A_2 - A_1)/A_0)] \times 100 \quad (4)$$

where A_0 represents the absorbance value of the blank group, A_1 represents the absorbance value of the sample after replacing H_2O_2 with water, and A_2 represents the absorbance value of the sample group.

3.6.3. Superoxide Anion Scavenging Capacity

The scavenging capacity of the superoxide anion was evaluated using a modified version of the method described by Xie et al. [48]. CFTHs were prepared in solutions with concentrations of 1.0, 2.0, 3.0, 4.0, and 5.0 mg/mL. A volume of 0.5 mL from each concentration of the samples was transferred into a test tube, followed by the addition of 5 mL of Tris-HCl buffer (50 mM, pH 8.2). The mixture was incubated at 25 °C for 20 min. For the blank group, an equivalent volume of distilled water was added. In the determination tube, the VC standard was substituted with the sample solution. Subsequently, 0.3 mL of a 10 mM pyrogallol solution was introduced. After a reaction period of 3 min, the absorbance was measured at 325 nm. The scavenging capacity of the superoxide anion (O^{2-}) was calculated using the following formula:

$$\text{Superoxide anion radical scavenging capacity (\%)} = (1 - A_1/A_0) \times 100 \quad (5)$$

where A_1 represents the absorbance value of the sample group and A_0 represents the absorbance value of the blank group.

3.6.4. Reducing Capacity

The reducing capacity was determined according to the method described by Liu et al. [49], with several modifications. Samples of varying concentrations (1.0 mL, 6.0–10.0 mg/mL) were incubated with 1.0 mL of 1% $K_3Fe(CN)_6$ and 1.0 mL of 0.2 M PBS buffer (pH 6.8). Following a reaction at 50 °C for 20 min, 1.0 mL of 10% TCA solution was added to the mixture. The resulting solution was then centrifuged at 5000 rpm for 10 min, and 2.5 mL of the supernatant was extracted. Following this, 2.5 mL of deionized water and 1.2 mL of 0.1% $FeCl_3$ solution were added sequentially. The absorbance of the resulting complex was measured at 700 nm, with higher absorbance values indicating a stronger reducing capacity.

3.6.5. Metal-Chelating Capacity

The metal-chelating capacity was evaluated using the method outlined by Gao et al. [50], with some modifications. A 0.50 mL sample of CFTHs, with concentrations ranging from 6.0 to 14.0 mg/mL, was mixed with 2 mL of water, 5 μL of $FeCl_2$ (2 mM), and 100 μL of ferrozine (5 mM). The mixture was shaken and allowed to stand at 25 °C for 10 min. Subsequently, the absorbance was measured at 562 nm. The absorbance of the blank was determined using the same procedure, substituting distilled water for the sample. The metal-chelating ability was calculated as follows:

$$\text{Metal-chelating capacity (\%)} = [1 - A_1/A_0] \times 100 \quad (6)$$

where A_1 represents the absorbance value of the sample group, and A_0 represents the absorbance value of the blank group.

3.6.6. ABTS Radical Scavenging Capacity

According to Liu et al. [49], CFTHs at various concentrations (0.2, 0.4, 0.6, 0.8, and 1 mg/mL) were mixed with the ABTS diluent in a ratio of 1:8 and incubated at 37 °C for 10 min. The absorbance was measured at 734 nm using a microplate reader (Thermo Scientific, Waltham, MA, USA). The ABTS radical scavenging capacity was calculated using the following formula:

$$\text{ABTS radical scavenging capacity (\%)} = (1 - A_1/A_0) \times 100 \quad (7)$$

where A_0 represents the absorbance value of the blank group, and A_1 represents the absorbance value after the addition of the sample.

3.7. Determination of Antioxidant Activity Stability

3.7.1. Simulated Digestion In Vitro

According to Minekus et al. [51], the method of in vitro simulated digestion of hydrolysates was employed. All hydrolysate solutions were maintained at an equivalent protein concentration.

Gastric digestion stage: The sample was dissolved in water (520 mg/5 mL) and combined with 7.5 mL of simulated gastric juice, 1.6 mL of pepsin (resulting in a final enzyme concentration of 2000 U/mL, as configured by the simulated gastric juice), 5 μL of 0.3 M $CaCl_2$, and 695 μL of water. The pH of the mixture was adjusted to 3.0 ± 0.1 using 1 M HCl. The beaker was then placed on a magnetic stirrer at 37 °C and 200 rpm for 2 h. Upon completion of the simulated digestion, the pH was adjusted to 7 to terminate the action of the protease.

Simulated intestinal digestion stage: A 20 mL aliquot of the gastric phase digestion mixture was combined with 11 mL of simulated intestinal fluid, 5 mL of trypsin (resulting in a final enzyme concentration of 100 U/mL, as configured by the simulated intestinal fluid), 2.5 mL of bile salt (10 mM), 40 μL of 0.3 M $CaCl_2$, and 1.31 mL of water. The pH of this mixture was adjusted to 7.0 ± 0.1 using either 1 M NaOH or 1 M HCl. The beaker was again placed on a magnetic stirrer at 37 °C and 200 rpm for 2 h. Following the reaction, the mixture was precooled in ice water for 10 min and subsequently frozen at −40 °C for an additional 10 min to halt the trypsin reaction.

3.7.2. Temperature and pH Stability Test

The stability of the antioxidant activity of the hydrolysates was evaluated using a modified method based on the work of Xiang et al. [52]. The hydrolysate solutions, maintained at an equivalent protein concentration, were incubated at temperatures of 25, 40, 60, and 80 °C for a duration of 2 h. Following incubation, the samples were cooled to room temperature, and their antioxidant activity was evaluated. To investigate the impact of pH on the stability of antioxidant activity, the pH of the hydrolysate was initially adjusted to a range of 3.0 to 11.0 and allowed to incubate at room temperature for 2 h. Following this incubation period, the pH was readjusted to 7.0, and the antioxidant activity was subsequently assessed.

3.8. Animal Experiments

Ninety male ICR mice, each weighing 26 ± 2 g, were purchased from Jinan Pengyue experimental animal breeding Co., Ltd. (Jinan, China). The environmental conditions were maintained at a room temperature of 25 ± 2 °C, with a relative humidity of 50 ± 5%, and a 12 h light/12 h dark cycle. The mice were routinely fed a standard diet and had free access to food and water. During the week of adaptive feeding, the mice underwent training sessions twice to acclimatize them to swimming for 5 min each on days 2 and 5, respectively. Following a one-week adaptation period, all mice successfully learned to swim and were then randomly divided into five groups, with 18 mice in each group, distributed across four or five cages. The five experimental groups included a blank control group (receiving distilled water of the same volume), a positive control group (receiving ginseng at a dosage of 0.5 mg/g body weight/day), a low-dose CFTHs group (LCFTHs, 0.25 mg/g body weight/day), a medium-dose CFTHs group (MCFTHs, 0.5 mg/g body weight/day), and a high-dose CFTHs group (HCFTHs, 1 mg/g body weight/day). Each mouse was administered the corresponding dose of the test substance daily, based on its body weight, using a gavage volume of 0.01 mL/g. This was conducted once a day for 30 consecutive days with the aid of oral gavage needles. The body weight of the mice was measured daily throughout the trial. At the conclusion of the study, cervical dislocation was performed for euthanasia following blood collection from all mice. Additionally, the weights of the liver, kidney, spleen, and thymus were recorded, and the visceral index was calculated by dividing the visceral weight (in grams) by the body weight of each mouse (in grams).

3.9. The Exhaustive Swimming Experiment

Thirty minutes after the last administration, nine mice were randomly selected from each group, and their body surface grease was removed using soapy water. A 5% body weight lead weight was affixed to the base of each mouse's tail, after which the mice were placed in a constant temperature water bath. The swimming test was conducted in a bathtub maintained at 25 °C with a length of 100 cm, 75 cm in width, and filled with water to a depth of 60 cm. Timing commenced as the mice began to swim and concluded when a mouse exhibited exhaustion, defined as a noticeable loss of coordinated movements and an inability to return to the water surface within at least 10 s. At this point, timing was stopped to record the exhaustive swimming time. During the swimming period, if any mouse ceased or suspended its movement, a glass rod was employed to stir the surrounding water to encourage continuous movement. At the conclusion of the study, cervical dislocation was performed for euthanasia.

3.10. Hematoxylin–Eosin Staining

The liver sample from the mouse was excised and immediately placed in 4% formalin for 24 h. Following fixation, the sample underwent dehydration through a series of gradient ethanol solutions, ranging from 70% to 100%. It was then embedded in paraffin using a tissue embedding technique. Subsequently, the tissue was sectioned into 4 μm slices using a microtome and stained with hematoxylin and eosin. Photographs were captured using an optical microscope equipped with a camera (Nikon Eclipse CI, Tokyo, Japan).

3.11. Determination of Serum and Liver Biochemical Parameters

Thirty minutes after the final administration, the mice were placed in a swimming box with a water temperature maintained at 25 ± 1 °C and a minimum water depth of 30 cm. Following 30 min of swimming, blood samples were collected and centrifuged to obtain serum, which was subsequently analyzed for Glu content, LDH, CK, LA, BUN, and NH_3.

Following serum collection, the mice were immediately sacrificed. A suitable amount of mouse liver was combined with an appropriate volume of normal saline to prepare a 10% liver tissue homogenate. This homogenate was ground and then centrifuged at 4000 rpm for 20 min to obtain the supernatant. A kit was utilized to assess the levels of LG in the mouse liver, as well as the activities of SOD and GSH-Px in the liver tissue.

3.12. Statistical Analysis

All experimental data are presented as mean ± standard deviation. One-way ANOVA, followed by Tukey's test (for equal variances) or Dunnett's T3 test (for different variances), was employed when the samples were normally distributed. In contrast, the Kruskal–Wallis test was utilized for samples that were not normally distributed. Statistical analyses were conducted using GraphPad Prism 9.0, and a p-value of less than 0.05 was deemed statistically significant. Graphs were generated using Origin 2018 (Origin Lab Corporation, Northampton, MA, USA).

4. Conclusions

This study investigated the characteristics, antioxidant activity stability, and anti-fatigue effects of hydrolysates derived from the tentacles of *Cucumaria frondosa* using four different proteases—flavourzyme, alcalase, neutrase, and trypsin. The results indicate that the hydrolysates produced by flavourzyme exhibited a higher DH compared to those generated by the other proteases. Additionally, the alcalase hydrolysate displayed decreased dispersibility in aqueous solution. The hydrolysates obtained through protease hydrolysis demonstrated significant antioxidant capacity, with flavourzyme hydrolysates showing enhanced stability during gastrointestinal digestion. Furthermore, the CFTHs exhibited no toxic effects on mice, with a consistent increase in body weight observed during intragastric administration. The anti-fatigue effect of the CFTHs was significant, as evidenced by an extension in the exhaustive swimming time of the mice. The CFTHs also enhanced the levels of LG and Glu. Moreover, the CFTHs provided a protective effect on muscle tissue and reduced the accumulation of metabolites such as LA, BUN, NH_3, CK, and LDH. The levels of SOD and GSH-Px in the CFTHs groups were elevated, indicating that the CFTHs inhibited exercise-induced fatigue. These findings offer substantial reference value for the development of CFTHs as functional foods with significant anti-fatigue properties. Additionally, they present potential opportunities for the high-value utilization of *Cucumaria frondosa* tentacles, which could yield considerable ecological and economic benefits.

Author Contributions: Conceptualization, M.L. and J.C.; methodology, L.S. and J.C.; software, M.L.; formal analysis, M.L., J.C. and Q.W.; investigation, C.L. and W.S.; data curation, M.L., Q.W. and C.L.; writing—original draft preparation, M.L., J.C. and Q.W.; writing—review and editing, L.S.; funding acquisition, L.S. and W.S. All authors have read and agreed to the published version of the manuscript.

Funding: This research was funded by the Natural Science Foundation of Shandong Province, No. ZR2021QD030, National Natural Science Foundation of China, No. 42106111 and the Doctoral Startup Project of Guangdong Ocean University funded by W.S, No. R20076.

Institutional Review Board Statement: The animal study protocol was approved by the Ethical Committee of Yantai University (protocol code 20230615s149, approved on 15 June 2023).

Informed Consent Statement: Not applicable.

Data Availability Statement: The datasets generated and analyzed during the current study are available from the corresponding authors upon reasonable request.

Conflicts of Interest: The authors declare no conflicts of interest.

References

1. Liu, J.; Wu, G.; Yang, J.; He, C.; Xiong, H.; Ma, Y. Abalone visceral peptides containing Cys and Tyr exhibit strong in vitro antioxidant activity and cytoprotective effects against oxidative damage. *Food Chem. X* **2023**, *17*, 100582. [CrossRef] [PubMed]
2. Berger, A.M.; Mitchell, S.A.; Jacobsen, P.B.; Pirl, W.F. Screening, evaluation, and management of cancer-related fatigue: Ready for implementation to practice? *CA Cancer J. Clin.* **2015**, *65*, 190–211. [CrossRef] [PubMed]
3. Jiang, P.; Ji, X.; Xia, J.; Xu, M.R.; Hao, F.; Tong, H.B.; Jiao, L.L. Structure and potential anti-fatigue mechanism of polysaccharides from *Bupleurum chinense* DC. *Carbohydr. Polym.* **2023**, *306*, 120608. [CrossRef]
4. Ye, J.; Shen, C.H.; Huang, Y.Y.; Zhang, X.Q.; Xiao, M.T. Anti-fatigue activity of sea cucumber peptides prepared from *Stichopus japonicus* in an endurance swimming rat model. *J. Sci. Food Agric.* **2017**, *97*, 4548–4556. [CrossRef]
5. Hossain, A.; Dave, D.; Shahidi, F. Northern Sea Cucumber (*Cucumaria frondosa*): A Potential Candidate for Functional Food, Nutraceutical, and Pharmaceutical Sector. *Mar. Drugs* **2020**, *18*, 274. [CrossRef]
6. Bordbar, S.; Anwar, F.; Saari, N. High-value components and bioactives from sea cucumbers for functional food—A review. *Mar. Drugs* **2011**, *9*, 1761–1805. [CrossRef]
7. Mamelona, J.; Saint-Louis, R.; Pelletier, E. Proximate composition and nutritional profile of by-products from green urchin and Atlantic sea cucumber processing plants. *Int. J. Food Sci. Technol.* **2010**, *45*, 2119–2126. [CrossRef]
8. Hossain, A.; Senadheera, T.R.L.; Dave, D.; Shahidi, F. Phenolic profiles of Atlantic sea cucumber (*Cucumaria frondosa*) tentacles and their biological properties. *Food Res. Int.* **2023**, *163*, 112262. [CrossRef]
9. Karami, Z.; Butkinaree, C.; Yingchutrakul, Y.; Simanon, N.; Duangmal, K. Comparative study on structural, biological and functional activities of hydrolysates from Adzuki bean (*Vigna angularis*) and mung bean (*Vigna radiata*) protein concentrates using Alcalase and Flavourzyme. *Food Res. Int.* **2022**, *161*, 111797. [CrossRef]
10. Zheng, Z.; Li, J.; Li, J.; Sun, H.; Liu, Y. Physicochemical and antioxidative characteristics of black bean protein hydrolysates obtained from different enzymes. *Food Hydrocoll.* **2019**, *97*, 105222. [CrossRef]
11. Fathollahy, I.; Farmani, J.; Kasaai, M.R.; Hamishehkar, H. Characteristics and functional properties of Persian lime (*Citrus latifolia*) seed protein isolate and enzymatic hydrolysates. *LWT-Food Sci. Technol.* **2021**, *140*, 110765. [CrossRef]
12. Zhang, X.D.; Dai, Z.Y.; Zhang, Y.Q.; Dong, Y.; Hu, X.J. Structural characteristics and stability of salmon skin protein hydrolysates obtained with different proteases. *LWT-Food Sci. Technol.* **2022**, *153*, 112460. [CrossRef]
13. Sharma, S.; Pradhan, R.; Manickavasagan, A.; Tsopmo, A.; Thimmanagari, M.; Dutta, A. Corn distillers solubles by two-step proteolytic hydrolysis as a new source of plant-based protein hydrolysates with ACE and DPP4 inhibition activities. *Food Chem.* **2023**, *401*, 134120. [CrossRef] [PubMed]
14. Hau, E.H.; Teh, S.S.; Yeo, S.K.; Mah, S.H. Physicochemical and functional properties of Alcalase-extracted protein hydrolysate from oil palm leaves. *J. Sci. Food Agric.* **2022**, *102*, 233–240. [CrossRef] [PubMed]
15. Senadheera, T.R.L.; Dave, D.; Shahidi, F. Antioxidant potential and physicochemical properties of protein hydrolysates from body parts of North Atlantic sea cucumber (*Cucumaria frondosa*). *Food Prod. Process. Nutr.* **2021**, *3*, 3. [CrossRef]
16. Ai, M.; Tang, T.; Zhou, L.; Ling, Z.; Guo, S.; Jiang, A. Effects of different proteases on the emulsifying capacity, rheological and structure characteristics of preserved egg white hydrolysates. *Food Hydrocoll.* **2019**, *87*, 933–942. [CrossRef]
17. Wang, Y.Y.; Wang, C.Y.; Wang, S.T.; Li, Y.Q.; Mo, H.Z.; He, J.X. Physicochemical properties and antioxidant activities of tree peony (*Paeonia suffruticosa Andr.*) seed protein hydrolysates obtained with different proteases. *Food Chem.* **2021**, *345*, 128765. [CrossRef]

18. Tong, X.; Cao, J.; Sun, M.; Liao, P.; Dai, S.; Cui, W.; Wang, H. Physical and oxidative stability of oil-in-water (O/W) emulsions in the presence of protein (peptide): Characteristics analysis and bioinformatics prediction. *LWT-Food Sci. Technol.* **2021**, *149*, 111782. [CrossRef]
19. Du, X.; Jing, H.; Wang, L.; Huang, X.; Wang, X.; Wang, H. Characterization of structure, physicochemical properties, and hypoglycemic activity of goat milk whey protein hydrolysate processed with different proteases. *LWT-Food Sci. Technol.* **2022**, *159*, 113257. [CrossRef]
20. Hernández-Ruiz, K.L.; López-Cervantes, J.; Sánchez-Machado, D.I.; Campas-Baypoli, O.N.; Quintero-Guerrero, A.A.; de Lourdes Grijalva-Delgado, M.; Chávez-Almanza, A.F. Collagen peptide fractions from tilapia (*Oreochromis aureus Steindachner*, 1864) scales: Chemical characterization and biological activity. *Food Biosci.* **2023**, *53*, 102658. [CrossRef]
21. Yu, X.; Chen, Y.; Qi, Z.; Chen, Q.; Cao, Y.; Kong, Q. Preparation and identification of a novel peptide with high antioxidant activity from corn gluten meal. *Food Chem.* **2023**, *424*, 136389. [CrossRef] [PubMed]
22. Ahmed, S.A.; Taie, H.A.A.; Abdel Wahab, W.A. Antioxidant capacity and antitumor activity of the bioactive protein prepared from orange peel residues as a by-product using fungal protease. *Int. J. Biol. Macromol.* **2023**, *234*, 123578. [CrossRef]
23. Liu, F.F.; Li, Y.Q.; Wang, C.Y.; Liang, Y.; Zhao, X.Z.; He, J.X.; Mo, H.Z. Physicochemical, functional and antioxidant properties of mung bean protein enzymatic hydrolysates. *Food Chem.* **2022**, *393*, 133397. [CrossRef]
24. Cui, Q.; Duan, Y.; Zhang, M.; Liang, S.; Sun, Y.; Cheng, J.; Guo, M. Peptide profiles and antioxidant capacity of extensive hydrolysates of milk protein concentrate. *J. Dairy Sci.* **2022**, *105*, 7972–7985. [CrossRef]
25. Xie, J.; Du, M.; Shen, M.; Wu, T.; Lin, L. Physico-chemical properties, antioxidant activities and angiotensin-I converting enzyme inhibitory of protein hydrolysates from Mung bean (*Vigna radiate*). *Food Chem.* **2019**, *270*, 243–250. [CrossRef]
26. Sarabandi, K.; Jafari, S.M. Improving the antioxidant stability of flaxseed peptide fractions during spray drying encapsulation by surfactants: Physicochemical and morphological features. *J. Food Eng.* **2020**, *286*, 110131. [CrossRef]
27. Cian, R.E.; Martínez-Augustin, O.; Drago, S.R. Bioactive properties of peptides obtained by enzymatic hydrolysis from protein byproducts of Porphyra columbina. *Food Res. Int.* **2012**, *49*, 364–372. [CrossRef]
28. Mongkonkamthorn, N.; Malila, Y.; Yarnpakdee, S.; Makkhun, S.; Regenstein, J.M.; Wangtueai, S. Production of protein hydrolysate containing antioxidant and angiotensin -i-converting enzyme (ACE) inhibitory activities from Tuna (*Katsuwonus pelamis*) blood. *Processes* **2020**, *8*, 1518. [CrossRef]
29. Wardani, D.W.; Ningrum, A.; Manikharda; Vanidia, N.; Munawaroh, H.S.H.; Susanto, E.; Show, P.L. In silico and in vitro assessment of yellowfin tuna skin (*Thunnus albacares*) hydrolysate antioxidation effect. *Food Hydrocoll. Health* **2023**, *3*, 100126. [CrossRef]
30. Chin, Y.L.; Chai, K.F.; Chen, W.N. Upcycling of brewers' spent grains via solid-state fermentation for the production of protein hydrolysates with antioxidant and techno-functional properties. *Food Chem. X* **2022**, *13*, 100184. [CrossRef]
31. Lee, S.Y.; Lee, D.Y.; Hur, S.J. Changes in the stability and antioxidant activities of different molecular weight bioactive peptide extracts obtained from beef during in vitro human digestion by gut microbiota. *Food Res. Int.* **2021**, *141*, 110116. [CrossRef] [PubMed]
32. Bustamante, S.Z.; González, J.G.; Sforza, S.; Tedeschi, T. Bioactivity and peptide profile of whey protein hydrolysates obtained from Colombian double-cream cheese production and their products after gastrointestinal digestion. *LWT-Food Sci. Technol.* **2021**, *145*, 111334. [CrossRef]
33. Morais, H.A.; Silve, M.P.C.; Silva, V.D.M.; Silva, M.R.; Silveir, J.N. Correlation between the degree of hydrolysis and the peptide profile of whey protein concentrate hydrolysates: Effect of the Enzyme Type and Reaction Time. *Am. J. Food Tech.* **2013**, *8*, 1–16. [CrossRef]
34. Sheng, Y.; Wang, W.Y.; Wu, M.F.; Wang, Y.M.; Zhu, W.Y.; Chi, C.F.; Wang, B. Eighteen novel bioactive peptides from Monkfish (*Lophius litulon*) swim bladders: Production, identification, antioxidant activity, and stability. *Mar. Drugs* **2023**, *21*, 169. [CrossRef]
35. Kristinsson, H.G.; Hultin, H.O. Effect of low and high pH treatment on the functional properties of cod muscle proteins. *J. Arg. Food Chem.* **2003**, *51*, 5103. [CrossRef]
36. Arcan, I.; Yemenicioglu, A. Antioxidant activity of protein extracts from heat-treated or thermally processed chickpeas and white beans. *Food Chem.* **2007**, *103*, 301–312. [CrossRef]
37. Chen, J.; Lu, X.; Chen, P.; Shen, Y.; Zheng, B.; Guo, Z. Anti-fatigue effect of glycoprotein from hairtail (*Trichiurus lepturus*) by-products in a behavioral mouse model. *Food Chem. X* **2023**, *18*, 100645. [CrossRef]
38. Ament, W.; Verkerke, G.J. Exercise and Fatigue. *Sports Med.* **2009**, *39*, 389–422. [CrossRef]
39. Li, Z.L.; Zhu, H.K.; Hua, H.Y.; Liu, C.; Cheng, Y.L.; Guo, Y.H.; Du, P.; Qian, H. Anti-fatigue activity of Brassica rapa L. extract and correlation among biochemical changes in forced swimming mice. *Food Bio* **2022**, *47*, 101633. [CrossRef]
40. Zhang, D.; Xiong, J.; Zhao, X.; Gan, Y. Anti-fatigue activities of γ-aminobutyric acid-enriched soymilk in an acute exercise-treated mouse model via regulating AMPK/PGC-1α pathway. *Food Bio* **2023**, *55*, 103060. [CrossRef]
41. Lu, Z.; Sun, N.; Dong, L.; Gao, Y.; Lin, S. Production of Bioactive Peptides from Sea Cucumber and Its Potential Health Benefits: A Comprehensive Review. *J. Agric. Food Chem.* **2022**, *70*, 7607–7625. [CrossRef] [PubMed]

42. He, J.R.; Zhu, J.J.; Yin, S.W.; Yang, X.Q. Bioaccessibility and Intracellular Antioxidant Activity of Phloretin Embodied by Gliadin/Sodium Carboxymethyl Cellulose Nanoparticles. *Food Hydrocoll.* **2021**, *4*, 107076. [CrossRef]
43. Wu, W.F.; Li, B.F.; Hou, H.; Zhang, H.W.; Zhao, X. Identification of iron-chelating peptides from Pacific cod skin gelatin and the possible binding mode. *J. Funct. Foods* **2017**, *35*, 418–427. [CrossRef]
44. Vásquez, P.; Sepúlveda, C.T.; Zapata, J.E. Functional properties of rainbow trout (*Oncorhynchus mykiss*) viscera protein hydrolysates. *Biocatal. Agric. Biotechnol.* **2022**, *39*, 102268. [CrossRef]
45. Lowry, O.; Rosebrough, N.; Farr, A.L.; Randall, R. Protein Measurement with the Folin Phenol Reagent. *J. Biol. Chem.* **1951**, *193*, 265–275. [CrossRef]
46. Du, M.X.; Xie, J.H.; Gong, B.; Xu, X.; Tang, W.; Li, X.; Xie, M.Y. Extraction, physicochemical characteristics and functional properties of Mung bean protein. *Food Hydrocoll.* **2018**, *76*, 131–140. [CrossRef]
47. Zhou, C.; Mi, S.; Li, J.; Gao, J.; Wang, X.H.; Sang, Y.X. Purification, characterisation and antioxidant activities of chondroitin sulphate extracted from Raja porosa cartilage. *Carbohydr. Polym.* **2020**, *241*, 116306. [CrossRef]
48. Xie, J.H.; Wang, Z.J.; Shen, M.Y.; Nie, S.P.; Gong, B.; Li, H.S.; Xie, M.Y. Sulfated modification, characterization and antioxidant activities of polysaccharide from Cyclocarya paliurus. *Food Hydrocoll.* **2016**, *53*, 7–15. [CrossRef]
49. Liu, J.B.; Jin, Y.; Lin, S.Y.; Jones, G.S.; Chen, F. Purification and identification of novel antioxidant peptides from egg white protein and their antioxidant activities. *Food Chem.* **2015**, *175*, 258–266. [CrossRef]
50. Gao, J.; Li, T.; Chen, D.; Gu, H.; Mao, X. Identification and molecular docking of antioxidant peptides from hemp seed protein hydrolysates. *LWT-Food Sci. Technol.* **2021**, *147*, 111453. [CrossRef]
51. Minekus, M.; Alminger, M.; Alvito, P.; Ballance, S.; Bohn, T.; Bourlieu, C.; Brodkorb, A. A standardised static in vitro digestion method suitable for food—An international consensus. *Food Funct.* **2014**, *5*, 1113–1124. [CrossRef] [PubMed]
52. Xiang, H.; Waterhouse, D.S.; Liu, P.; Waterhouse, G.I.N.; Li, J.; Cui, C. Pancreatic lipase-inhibiting protein hydrolysate and peptides from seabuckthorn seed meal: Preparation optimization and inhibitory mechanism. *LWT-Food Sci. Technol.* **2020**, *134*, 109870. [CrossRef]

molecules

MDPI

Review

Mechanism of Action and Therapeutic Potential of Xanthohumol in Prevention of Selected Neurodegenerative Diseases

Anna Długosz [1,*], Błażej Błaszak [1,*], Damian Czarnecki [2] and Joanna Szulc [1]

1 Faculty of Chemical Technology and Engineering, Department of Food Industry Technology and Engineering, Bydgoszcz University of Science and Technology, 85-326 Bydgoszcz, Poland; joanna.szulc@pbs.edu.pl

2 Faculty of Health Sciences, Department of Preventive Nursing, Collegium Medicum in Bydgoszcz, Nicolaus Copernicus University in Torun, 85-821 Bydgoszcz, Poland; czarneckidamian@cm.umk.pl

* Correspondence: anna.dlugosz@pbs.edu.pl (A.D.); blazej.blaszak@pbs.edu.pl (B.B.)

Abstract: Xanthohumol (XN), a bioactive plant flavonoid, is an antioxidant, and as such, it exhibits numerous beneficial properties, including anti-inflammatory, antimicrobial, and antioxidative effects. The main dietary source of XN is beer, where it is introduced through hops. Although the concentration of XN in beer is low, the large quantities of hop-related post-production waste present an opportunity to extract XN residues for technological or pharmaceutical purposes. The presented study focuses on the role of XN in the prevention of neurodegenerative diseases, analyzing its effect at a molecular level and including its signal transduction and metabolism. The paper brings up XN's mechanism of action, potential effects, and experimental and clinical studies on Alzheimer's disease (AD), Parkinson's disease (PD), and amyotrophic lateral sclerosis (ALS). Additionally, challenges and future research directions on XN, including its bioavailability, safety, and tolerance, have been discussed.

Keywords: Alzheimer's disease; amyotrophic lateral sclerosis; anti-inflammatory; antioxidant; neurodegenerative diseases; Parkinson's disease; xanthohumol

1. Introduction

In recent years, neurodegenerative diseases have emerged as one of the most frequently discussed and analyzed health challenges. This increased attention is largely due to the aging global population and the corresponding rise in the prevalence of these conditions. It is estimated that 1% of individuals aged 60 years have Alzheimer's disease (AD), with the prevalence rising to as high as 50% among those aged 90 years and older. For Parkinson's disease (PD), approximately 0.15% of the general population is affected, while the prevalence increases to 1.5–2% among individuals aged over 70 years [1].

Neurodegenerative diseases are commonly classified based on their pathophysiological characteristics. They include conditions that impair cognitive functions and memory, as well as those that affect movement, communication, and respiratory abilities. Examples of neurodegenerative diseases include AD, PD, Huntington's disease, amyotrophic lateral sclerosis (ALS), frontotemporal dementia, and spinocerebellar ataxias [2]. The progression of these diseases is influenced by various factors, including specific protein accumulations, anatomical vulnerabilities, and fundamental neuronal processes such as progressive neuronal dysfunction and death, oxidative stress, programmed cell death, neuroinflammation, proteotoxic stress, and abnormalities in the ubiquitin–proteasome and autophagosomal/lysosomal systems [3].

 https://doi.org/10.3390/molecules30030694

Oxidative stress is a common factor contributing to the progression of neurodegenerative diseases. This is attributable to the brain's high oxygen consumption coupled with its relatively low antioxidant levels, making it particularly susceptible to oxidative damage. Oxidative stress occurs when the balance between pro-oxidants and antioxidants shifts in favor of pro-oxidants. Under normal physiological conditions, reactive oxygen species (ROS) (including O_2, •OH, H_2O_2, and O_2^{-}•) play essential roles in cellular signaling pathways and transcription activation. However, when their levels exceed the cell's antioxidant capacity, ROS can damage biological macromolecules, disrupt cellular functions, stimulate the production of pro-apoptotic proteins, and ultimately induce neuronal apoptosis [4,5].

Plants are a rich source of compounds that serve both nutritional purposes and act as specific plant responses to adverse environmental conditions or threats from pathogens (secondary metabolites). In medicine, plant secondary metabolites have found widespread applications due to their health-promoting properties, including anti-inflammatory, antimicrobial, antiaging, antioxidant, and anticancer activities [6]. Owing to the wide range of compounds and their impact on human health, both natural compounds and their chemically synthesized analogs are currently being investigated for their potential in preventing and treating various diseases, including neurodegenerative disorders. Confirmed activity in this regard has been demonstrated by isocumarins, which are derivatives of the widely distributed plant compound coumarin. These compounds, among other mechanisms, may positively influence the inhibition of disease progression by stimulating specific receptors [7,8]. Another compound with similar properties is xanthohumol (XN). XN (3′-[3,3-dimethylallyl]-2′,4′,4-trihydroxy-6′-methoxychalcone) is a natural chalcone belonging to the prenylflavonoid group, primarily found in the β-hard resin of female hop cones. In these cones, XN accounts for 0.1–1.0% of the dry mass [9,10]. Numerous derivatives of XN have been identified, with the basic compound structure and isoxanthohumol being the most well-known representatives (Figure 1).

The main dietary source of XN is beer, where it is introduced through hops. However, steps such as filtration, fermentation, and thermal treatment—during which isomerization of XN to isoxanthohumol occurs—result in a low final concentration of XN in beer. It is estimated that beer contains up to 0.69 mg/L of XN and as much as 3.44 mg/L of isoxanthohumol [9,11]. Despite this low concentration, the significant global production of beer and the large quantities of hop-related post-production waste present an opportunity to extract XN residues. This extraction could support the production of dietary supplements based on hop extracts. Consequently, research into XN has increasingly focused on methods for its efficient extraction [11].

Numerous scientific studies, conducted both in vitro and in animal models, have attributed various health-promoting properties to XN (Figure 2). These include its positive effects on metabolic processes (e.g., in the context of overweight/obesity and glucose metabolism), anticancer properties through inhibition of procarcinogens, angiogenesis, and cancer cell growth—and even induction of apoptosis in cancer cells. Additionally, XN demonstrates antiatherosclerotic and neuroprotective effects [9,11–13]. Due to its beneficial health effects and the fact that it is easily available from plants and food industry byproducts, XN has the potential to be used in medicine, especially in neurodegenerative disease prevention. Thus, the therapeutic potential of XN requires a summary providing an insight into the research conducted to date, especially into its impact on biochemical mechanisms and expression of enzymes and proteins, which is the main objective of this paper.

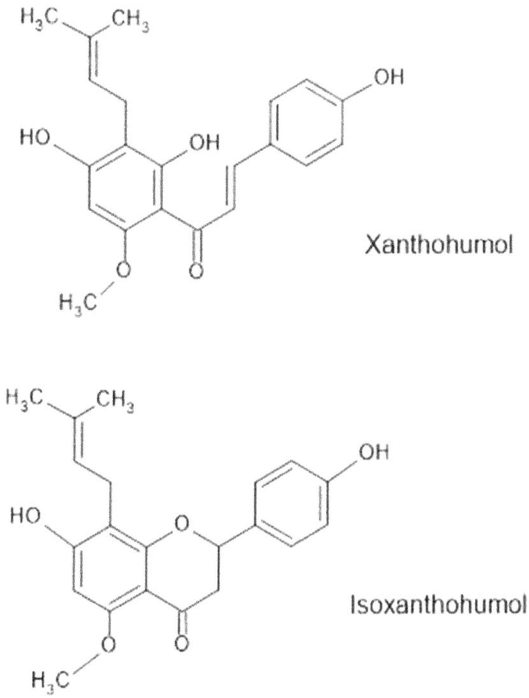

Figure 1. Structure of xanthohumol and isoxanthohumol [9].

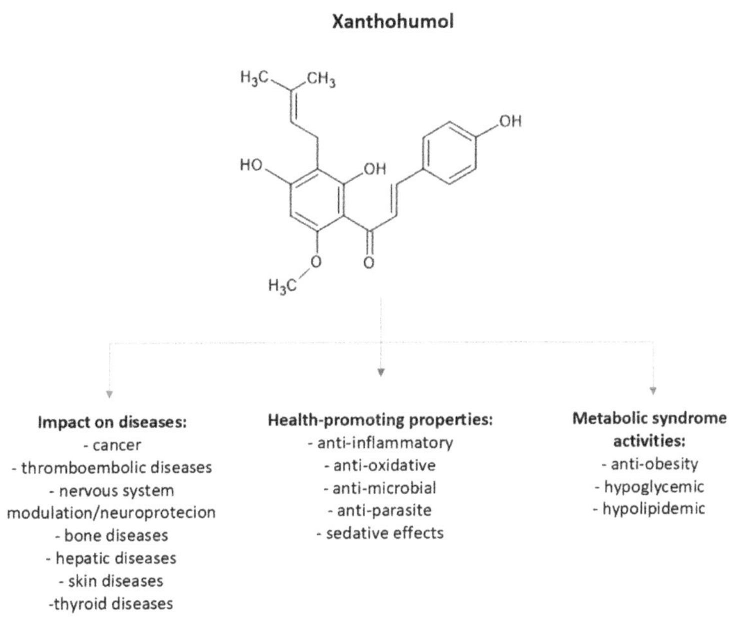

Figure 2. Pro-health properties of XN [9].

2. Methods

We conducted an extensive literature search using the ISI Web of Science, Pub-Med, ScienceDirect, and Google Scholar databases to gather information on the mechanism of action and therapeutic potential of XN in the prevention of neurodegenerative diseases, including AD, PD, and ALS. The following keywords were used in the data search: ("xanthohumol" and "neurodegenerative diseases"); ("xanthohumol" and "antioxidant"); ("xanthohumol" and "anti-inflammatory"); ("xanthohumol" and "Parkinson's disease"); ("xanthohumol" and "Alzheimer's disease"); ("xanthohumol" and "amyotrophic lateral sclerosis"); ("neuroprotection" and "xanthohumol"); ("oxi-dative stress" and "neurodegenerative diseases"); ("neurodegenerative diseases" and "xanthohumol" and "oxidative stress"); ("inflammation" and "xanthohumol" and "neurodegenerative diseases"). There were no restrictions on data collection, and no language restrictions were applied during the search. We focused primarily on articles published in the last 15 years. After performing the initial search, we further examined the full text of identified studies to assess their eligibility for inclusion in this review. Editorials, conference abstracts, and studies with incomplete or unavailable data were excluded. Additionally, priority was given to studies that investigated the biochemical pathways involved in XN's neuroprotective effects, specifically its antioxidant, anti-inflammatory, and anti-apoptotic properties. We included studies that provided evidence from both in vitro and in vivo experiments, as well as those exploring the efficacy of XN in preclinical models of PD, AD, and ALS. Meta-analyses, when available, were also considered to provide a quantitative overview of the available data.

3. Mechanism of Action of Xanthohumol

Xanthohumol has garnered significant attention in research due to its potent antioxidant properties. XN exhibits antioxidative effects primarily through its ability to scavenge ROS and RNS, thereby mitigating oxidative stress [14,15]. This free radical scavenging ability is largely attributed to the presence of hydroxyl groups in its structure [16], which can donate electrons to neutralize free radicals, thus preventing cellular damage. Additionally, XN influences intracellular signaling pathways, such as the Nrf2 pathway, which upregulates the expression of endogenous antioxidant enzymes like SOD, catalase, and glutathione peroxidase. Beyond direct radical scavenging, XN also modulates the redox state by chelating transition metals, thereby inhibiting metal-catalyzed oxidative reactions. These multifaceted mechanisms contribute to its protective role against oxidative damage, underpinning its potential therapeutic applications in managing diseases linked to oxidative stress, such as cancer, neurodegeneration, and cardiovascular disorders [14,17].

Chemical compounds with free radical scavenging activity typically neutralize reactive free radicals through several reaction mechanisms [18,19]. The primary mechanisms include HAT, which is characterized by a single-step process where the antioxidant, XN, donates a hydrogen atom to the free radical, neutralizing it. This results in the formation of a relatively stable antioxidant radical due to the delocalization of the unpaired electron [20]. Another mechanism is SET, where XN transfers a single electron to the free radical, neutralizing its unpaired electron and converting it into a more stable species. Additionally, a two-step mechanism called SPLET can occur, where the antioxidant first loses a proton, forming an anion, which then donates an electron to the free radical [20–22]. Tošovič et al. [23] investigated the antioxidative properties of XN, observing its behavior with selected free radicals and evaluating the effectiveness of various neutralizing mechanisms, including HAT, SET, and SPLET. Their study found that the HAT mechanism was most favorable for neutralizing $CH_3O\bullet$ and $HOO\bullet$ radicals.

Different antioxidant mechanisms through which XN can react lead to varying activity and antioxidant power when laboratory methods are applied. These methods assess a substance's ability to scavenge free radicals or inhibit oxidative processes [24]. Common assays include the DPPH assay, which measures the ability of antioxidants to donate electrons and reduce the DPPH radical to a colorless form [25]. The ABTS assay is another widely used method that detects the ability of antioxidants to scavenge the ABTS radical cation, resulting in a color change [26]. The FRAP assay, which evaluates the reduction of ferric ions (Fe^{3+}) to ferrous ions (Fe^{2+}), is also commonly used to assess antioxidant activity [27]. Additionally, the ORAC assay is a fluorescence-based method that measures the ability of a substance to quench free radicals in a controlled environment [28]. These laboratory methods, along with others such as the total phenolic content assay, help evaluate and compare the antioxidant efficacy of various substances, providing insight into their potential for preventing oxidative stress-related diseases.

The results obtained from antioxidant assays, such as DPPH, ABTS, FRAP, and ORAC, can be influenced by several factors that should be carefully controlled. Variability in results between different methods is affected by various conditions, including reaction time, pH, temperature, solvent type, matrix interference, XN extraction procedures, and the properties of the raw material (e.g., variety, cultivation location). Kontek et al. [29] pointed out that simple antiradical methods with artificial stable radicals, such as DPPH and ABST, have limitations when assessing the antioxidant potential of plant extracts or compounds, and it is not recommended to compare results evaluated with these tests to other antioxidant activity assays. Table 1 presents the antiradical activity of XN and hops-derived extracts using different antioxidant activity assays.

Table 1. Antiradical activity of xanthohumol, hops-derived extracts, and selected compounds using a variety of antioxidant activity assays.

Sample	Type of Antiradical Activity Assay	Antioxidant Activity	Antioxidant Activity Compared to Ascorbic Acid (IC_{50}sample/IC_{50}AA)	References
Hops-derived hexane extract	ABTS	IC_{50} = 0.499 mg/mL	nd.	[29]
Hops-derived hexane extract	DPPH	IC_{50} = 0.294 mg/mL	91.9	[29]
Xanthohumol (reagent ≥ 99%)	ABTS	IC_{50} = 0.660 mg/mL	nd.	[29]
Xanthohumol (reagent ≥ 99%)	DPPH	IC_{50} > 1.2 mg/mL	>375	[29]
Hops-derived methanolic extract	ABTS	IC_{50} = 0.535 mg/mL	nd.	[29]
Hops-derived methanolic extract	DPPH	IC_{50} = 0.484 mg/mL	151	[29]
Xantohumol (reagent > 98%)	ORAC	23.447 mM TE/g	nd.	[30]
Xantohumol (reagent > 98%)	HORAC	72.245 mM TE/g	nd.	[30]
Xanthohumol-rich extract (Xantho-Flav, 90% XN)	ORAC	22.107 mM TE/g	nd.	[30]
Xanthohumol-rich extract (Xantho-Flav, 90% XN)	HORAC	55.662 mM TE/g	nd.	[30]
Hops-derived acetone extract	ABTS	0.31 mM TE/L	nd.	[31]
Hops-derived acetone extract	FRAP	0.27 mM TE/L	nd.	[31]
Hop leaves-derived methanolic extract (98% *v*/*v*, extraction time 60 min)	DPPH	3.72 mg TE/g	nd.	[32]
Hop leaves-derived methanolic extract (98% *v*/*v*, extraction time 60 min)	FRAP	8.55 mg TE/g	nd.	[32]
Hop leaves-derived ethanolic extract (70% *v*/*v*, extraction time 60 min)	DPPH	3.61 mg TE/g	nd.	[32]
Hop leaves-derived ethanolic extract (70% *v*/*v*, extraction time 60 min)	FRAP	6.18 mg TE/g	nd.	[32]

Table 1. *Cont.*

Sample	Type of Antiradical Activity Assay	Antioxidant Activity	Antioxidant Activity Compared to Ascorbic Acid (IC_{50}sample/IC_{50}AA)	References
Hops-derived acetone extracts (90% *v*/*v*)	FRAP	63.5 ÷ 101.6 μM TE/g DW	nd.	[33]
Hops-derived acetone extracts (90% *v*/*v*)	ORAC	1069 to 1910 μM TE/g DW	nd.	[33]
Xanthohumol (reagent > 96%)	ORAC	24,745.1 μM TE/g DW	nd.	[23]
Xanthohumol (reagent > 96%)	FRAP	12,689.1 μM TE/g DW	nd.	[23]
Hops-derived extracts (different varieties)	DPPH	33.6 ÷ 77.7%	nd.	[34]
Xanthohumol	ORAC	4.2 TE	nd.	[35]
Xanthohumol	SOAC (vitamin E equivalent)	14.1	nd.	[35]
Quercetin	DPPH	IC_{50} = 0.0085 mg/mL	2.7	[35]
Resveratrol	DPPH	IC_{50} = 0.013 mg/mL	4.1	[36]
Butylated hydroxytoluene (BHT)	DPPH	IC_{50} = 0.0083 mg/mL	2.6	[37]
Isoxanthohumol	DPPH	IC_{50} = 2.971 mg/mL	928	[38]
Naringenin	DPPH	IC_{50} = 6.234 mg/mL	1948	[38]
Ascorbic acid	DPPH	IC_{50} = 0.0032 mg/mL	1.0	[38]

Abbreviations: 2,2′-azinobis(3-ethylbenzothiazoline-6-sulfonic acid) (ABTS); 2,2-diphenyl-1-picrylhydrazyl (DPPH); oxygen radical absorbance capacity (ORAC); hydroxyl radical antioxidant capacity (HORAC); ferric reducing antioxidant power (FRAP); singlet oxygen absorbance capacity (SOAC); half-maximal inhibitory concentration (IC_{50}); Trolox equivalent antioxidant capacity (TE); dry weight (DW); half-maximal inhibitory concentration of Ascorbic Acid (IC_{50}AA); no data (nd.).

Antioxidant activity is commonly expressed in several units depending on the assay method used. The most frequently used units are TEAC, typically given in micromoles of Trolox equivalent per gram (μmol TE/g) or per milliliter (μmol TE/mL) of the sample. Another unit to describe antioxidant activity in Percent Inhibition or Percent Scavenging (%), which is a common unit used, is assays with DPPH or ABST as a free radical. FRAP is typically expressed in micromoles of Fe^{2+} per gram (μmol Fe^{2+}/g) or per milliliter (μmol Fe^{2+}/mL), but it can also be referred to as the Trolox equivalent. Similar to TEAC, ORAC values are often expressed in micromoles of Trolox equivalent per gram (μmol TE/g) or per milliliter (μmol TE/mL) of the sample. ORAC measures the ability of an antioxidant to quench peroxyl radicals in a controlled system. Antioxidant activity can also be presented as IC_{50}. IC_{50} refers to the concentration of the antioxidant required to scavenge 50% of the radicals or inhibit 50% of a specific oxidative process [19–22]. Such a multitude of methods and ways of expressing antioxidant activity makes quantitative comparison of this property difficult. Nevertheless, the results presented in Table 1 indicate that both pure XN (reagent), XN extracted from hops, and hops-derived extracts obtained by various methods have high antioxidant potential. Depending on the solvent used for extraction, hop extracts rich in XN were characterized by different antioxidant activity and evaluated using the same method [32]. The same situation is observed in the case of XN. It is worth mentioning that the XN SOAC value was about 14 times higher than that of vitamin E, recognized as one of the strongest antioxidants [35]. When compared to other water-soluble antioxidants, XN has a lower antioxidant capacity. For example, quercetin is characterized by an IC_{50} value that is 35 times lower than that of XN, at 0.0085 mg/mL and 0.294 mg/mL, respectively [29,39]. Similar findings can be observed in the case of ascorbic acid, a powerful antioxidant. XN and hops extracts exhibit antioxidant activity that is 91 to 375 times lower than that of ascorbic acid (Table 1). However, XN is a stronger antioxidant than isoxanthohumol or naringenin and is still considered a bioactive compound with significant potential in diseases triggered by oxidative stress.

The above-mentioned studies and their results demonstrate the antioxidative potential of XN and extracts rich in this compound. This creates many possibilities for application, especially in preventing oxidative stress-related diseases.

The molecular mechanism of action of XN includes very complex pathways (Figure 3). XN reduces oxidative stress and regulates the activity of antioxidant enzymes [14,17,20]. XN is also a factor that impacts the cell cycle, e.g., inhibiting cell proliferation (particularly controlling cell cycle transcription during G1 and S phases in cancer cells) and inducing apoptosis (promoting cancerous cell death). XN is known for the inhibition of pro-inflammatory pathways. Blocking these pathways reduces the production of pro-inflammatory cytokines such as TNF-α and IL-6 [40] due to evidence that neurodegenerative diseases are related to the occurrence of oxidative stress, resulting in free radicals presence. More detailed mechanisms related to this group of diseases, especially AD, are presented in the following paragraphs.

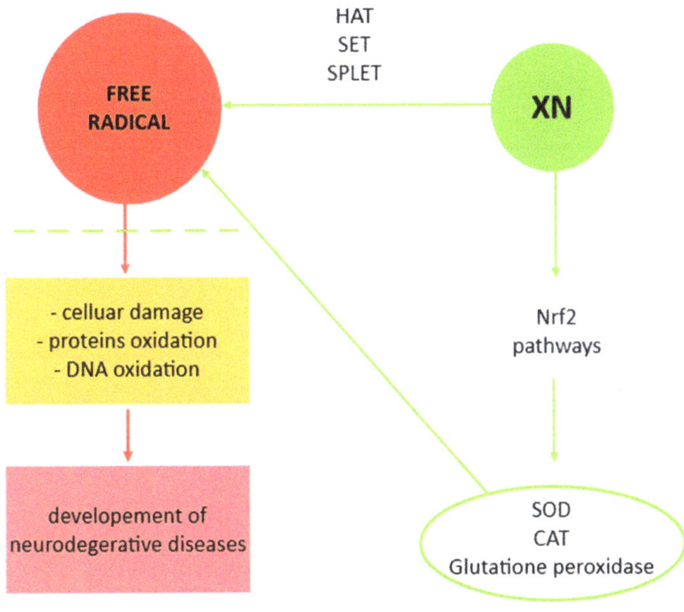

Figure 3. Mechanism of action of XN. Abbreviations: catalase (CAT); hydrogen atom transfer (HAT); nuclear respiratory factor 2 (Nrf2); sequential proton loss electron transfer (SPLET); single electron transfer (SET); superoxide dismutase (SOD).

4. Therapeutic Potential of Xanthohumol in Selected Neurodegenerative Diseases

4.1. Alzheimer's Disease

Alzheimer's disease is one of the most widespread neurodegenerative diseases, characterized by the accumulation of Aβ plaques and hyperphosphorylated tau protein in the brain, leading to the loss of cognitive functions. In recent years, research on XN has suggested that this natural flavonoid may possess neuroprotective properties that could counteract the pathological mechanisms of AD [41,42]. The hypothesis of mitochondrial cascade posits that damaged mitochondria increase the production of Aβ as a toxic oxidative stressor [43]. The free radicals damage DNA. Free radicals occur in histone-free mitochondrial DNA. There is a significant increase in double-strand breaks in the brain of people with AD, and dysfunctional DNA repair contributes to the progression [43].

In vitro studies have shown that XN exhibits strong antioxidant and anti-inflammatory properties. In cellular models, XN has been found to protect neuronal cells from oxidative stress, which is a key factor in the pathogenesis of AD [13,44,45]. One study conducted on human neuronal cells demonstrated that XN reduces the production of ROS, leading to decreased lipid peroxidation and cellular damage induced by Aβ [46–48]. Additionally, research has shown that XN inhibits the activity of the enzyme AChE, which may enhance cholinergic transmission, crucial for learning and memory processes [46,49].

In vivo studies on animal models, such as transgenic mice overexpressing amyloid, have also provided evidence of the therapeutic potential of XN. In one such study, long-term administration of XN to mice resulted in a significant reduction of Aβ deposits in the brain, which was correlated with improved performance in behavioral tests assessing cognitive functions, such as the Morris water maze test [42,50]. XN not only reduced Aβ accumulation but also lowered levels of inflammatory markers in the brain, such as IL-6 and TNF-α, suggesting its anti-inflammatory effects [51,52].

Additionally, XN is able to initiate the process of improving cognitive impairment by removing the inhibition of miRNA as miR-532-3p on Mpped1 in the mouse hippocampus [53]. However, it is miR-532-5p that has the most significant correlation with AD [54].

The molecular mechanisms by which XN may exert its protective effects in AD are diverse and complex [55–57]. One of the primary mechanisms is the modulation of oxidative stress, which plays a crucial role in the pathogenesis of AD. XN acts as a potent antioxidant, neutralizing ROS and reducing oxidative damage to DNA, proteins, and lipids. Additionally, XN may influence signaling pathways related to cellular stress responses, such as the Nrf2/ARE pathway (the nuclear factor E2-related factor 2—Nrf2; Nrf2-ARE pathway is an intrinsic mechanism of defense against oxidative stress), which regulates the expression of antioxidant and detoxifying enzymes. Activation of this pathway by XN can lead to enhanced protection of neurons against oxidative stress [58–60].

Another important mechanism is XN's ability to inhibit neuroinflammation. Brain inflammation, triggered by the activation of microglia and astrocytes in response to Aβ accumulation, is one of the key processes contributing to the progression of AD. XN reduces the production of pro-inflammatory cytokines such as TNF-α, IL-1β, and IL-6 by inhibiting the activation of the NF-κB pathway, which is a major regulator of the inflammatory response [61].

Additionally, XN exhibits the ability to directly inhibit beta-amyloid aggregation. Studies suggest that XN may bind to Aβ monomers, stabilizing them and preventing their aggregation into neurotoxic oligomers and fibrils. This property could be particularly relevant in the context of AD prevention, where inhibiting the early stages of Aβ aggregation may slow the progression of the disease [41,62].

XN has yet to be extensively explored in the preclinical phases [63].

All these mechanisms suggest that XN may act in multiple ways, inhibiting key pathogenetic processes in AD, making it a promising candidate for further research on its potential use as a therapeutic agent in AD.

4.2. Parkinson's Disease

Parkinson's disease is a progressive neurodegenerative disorder primarily characterized by the loss of dopaminergic neurons in the substantia nigra, a critical area of the brain involved in motor control. This neurodegeneration leads to a decrease in dopamine levels, resulting in the hallmark motor symptoms of PD: tremors, bradykinesia (slowness of movement), rigidity, and postural instability [64]. The pathophysiology of PD also involves the formation of Lewy bodies, which are intracellular aggregates primarily composed of alpha-synuclein protein. The accumulation of these Lewy bodies is associated with further neuronal damage and contributes to the progression of the disease [65,66].

Accumulating evidence implicates oxidative stress as a key driver of the complex degenerating cascade underlying dopaminergic neurodegeneration in all forms of PD [67].

Additionally, inflammation is a factor contributing to the progressive neurodegenerative mechanism observed in PD [68].

In the context of PD, XN has been explored for its potential neuroprotective properties through a variety of experimental studies, including both cellular models and animal models. Cellular studies have demonstrated that XN exhibits potent antioxidant properties, which are crucial in countering oxidative stress associated with PD. For example, XN has been shown to mitigate the effects of oxidative stress in dopaminergic cell lines exposed to neurotoxins such as 6-OHDA and MPP+. These studies reveal that XN can reduce the production of ROS and protect against cellular damage induced by these toxins [69]. Studies using rodent models of Parkinson's disease, such as those induced by 6-OHDA or MPTP, have shown that XN administration can significantly improve motor function and reduce neurodegeneration in the substantia nigra, a key area affected in PD. These findings suggest that XN exerts protective effects on dopaminergic neurons and mitigates the loss of dopaminergic terminals [70,71].

XN's neuroprotective mechanisms in PD involve several key processes.

XN's strong antioxidant properties are critical in neutralizing ROS and protecting dopaminergic neurons from oxidative damage. By scavenging free radicals and reducing oxidative stress, XN helps to preserve neuronal integrity and function [47,72].

XN has been shown to inhibit apoptotic pathways in dopaminergic neurons, reducing cell death that is commonly observed in PD. It achieves this by modulating key apoptotic signaling proteins, such as caspases, and by enhancing the expression of anti-apoptotic factors [55].

By reducing oxidative stress, XN helps to prevent damage to neuronal cells and tissues, contributing to overall neuroprotection. It modulates several oxidative stress-related pathways, including the Nrf2/ARE pathway, which enhances cellular defenses against oxidative damage [55].

XN's anti-inflammatory effects are mediated through the inhibition of pro-inflammatory cytokines and the reduction of neuroinflammation. It influences the expression and activity of inflammatory mediators, such as TNF-α and IL-1β, thereby reducing neuroinflammatory responses in PD [73].

Preliminary clinical research into XN's effects on PD is limited but promising. Recent studies are beginning to explore the potential therapeutic benefits of XN in human patients. Early-phase clinical trials are evaluating the safety and efficacy of XN in patients with Parkinson's disease. These studies are focused on assessing XN's ability to improve motor symptoms and quality of life in PD patients. Initial results indicate that XN is well-tolerated and may offer potential benefits in reducing disease severity and improving motor function [55,63,73]. These studies and findings collectively suggest that XN holds promise as a neuroprotective agent in PD through multiple mechanisms, including its antioxidant, antiapoptotic, and anti-inflammatory properties. Further research, especially larger clinical trials, will be essential to fully understand its therapeutic potential and efficacy in humans.

4.3. Amyotrophic Lateral Sclerosis

Amyotrophic lateral sclerosis is a progressive neurodegenerative disorder that primarily affects motor neurons, leading to muscle weakness, paralysis, and eventually respiratory failure. Current research into potential treatments for ALS has increasingly focused on natural compounds with neuroprotective properties, including XN [74–76].

Recent studies have explored the role of XN in treating ALS, particularly through preclinical research using animal models. These studies aim to understand how XN can influence the progression of ALS by protecting motor neurons from degeneration. In rodent models of ALS, such as those involving mutations in the SOD1 gene (a common genetic cause of ALS), XN has shown promise in enhancing motor neuron survival and delaying disease progression [55,77]. The SOD1 gene provides instructions for making an enzyme called superoxide dismutase, which is abundant in cells throughout the body. This enzyme attaches to molecules of zinc and copper to break down toxic, charged oxygen molecules called superoxide radicals. The molecules are byproducts of natural cell processes, and they should be broken down to avoid damaging cells [78]. For example, a study conducted on SOD1-G93A transgenic mice (a well-established ALS model) demonstrated that XN administration led to a significant increase in motor neuron survival and improved motor function. The study highlighted the compound's ability to reduce oxidative stress markers and attenuate neuroinflammatory responses, which are critical factors in ALS pathology [79].

Additionally, emerging evidence from in vitro studies using motor neuron cell lines suggests that XN can modulate cellular stress responses, such as ER stress, and prevent apoptosis in motor neurons, further supporting its potential as a therapeutic agent in ALS [80].

Using XN as an Nrf2 modulator may have significant clinical potential in ALS therapy. The study suggests that natural polyphenols (e.g., XN) protect cortical cells against corticosterone-induced cytotoxicity and enhance cell survival via modulation of the Nrf2 pathway [81–83].

4.4. Potential Therapeutic Benefits in Selected Neurodegenerative Diseases

Oxidative stress plays a central role in ALS pathogenesis, contributing to the degeneration of motor neurons. XN's potent antioxidant properties have been shown to neutralize ROS and reduce oxidative damage in neuronal cells. This reduction in oxidative stress helps to preserve motor neuron function and delay the onset of symptoms in ALS models [84,85].

Inflammation is another critical factor in ALS, with activated microglia and astrocytes releasing pro-inflammatory cytokines that exacerbate motor neuron damage. XN has demonstrated anti-inflammatory effects by downregulating the production of cytokines such as TNF-α and IL-1β, thereby mitigating the inflammatory responses in the CNS. This modulation of the immune response could slow the progression of ALS and improve patient outcomes [86,87].

XN's neuroprotective effects extend to enhancing the survival and function of motor neurons. In experimental models, XN has been shown to protect against glutamate-induced excitotoxicity, a major driver of motor neuron death in ALS. By stabilizing cellular homeostasis and preventing excessive calcium influx, XN helps maintain motor neuron integrity and supports neuromuscular function [88,89]. XN is emerging as a promising candidate for ALS treatment due to its multifaceted neuroprotective properties. While current research is primarily preclinical, the findings provide a strong rationale for further investigation, including clinical trials to evaluate XN's therapeutic potential in ALS patients. Future studies should focus on optimizing dosage and delivery methods and understanding the long-term effects of XN treatment in ALS.

Preclinical results indicate the high efficacy of XN in reducing neuronal damage and delaying the progression of neurodegenerative diseases in animals. For instance, a study conducted on a rat model of AD demonstrated that XN significantly improved cognitive function, as assessed by the Morris water maze test, which is commonly used to evaluate spatial learning and memory in animals. This study also reported a marked reduction in Aβ plaque accumulation, a hallmark of AD pathology [90]. Another example comes from research on PD, where XN administration in a mouse model led to a decrease in oxidative stress, as evidenced by lower levels of MDA and increased activity of antioxidant enzymes such as SOD and CAT [91,92]. These findings highlight the potential of XN in mitigating the oxidative damage associated with neurodegeneration.

Moreover, studies have shown that XN can modulate neuroinflammation, which plays a crucial role in the progression of neurodegenerative diseases. In a recent experiment involving a model of multiple sclerosis (EAE), XN treatment resulted in reduced expression of pro-inflammatory cytokines like TNF-α, IL-6, and IL-1β in brain tissue, alongside improvements in motor function [93,94]. This anti-inflammatory action underscores its potential as a therapeutic agent in diseases characterized by chronic inflammation. One study suggested that XN has the potential to develop into a therapeutic agent for improving glutamate-related nervous system diseases. This is important because toxicity induced by excessive glutamate has been implicated in many brain disorders [95].

XN exhibits neuroprotective properties and supports neuroregeneration, making it a promising compound for neurological health applications [96–98]. This process is important in the induction of neuronal differentiation for regenerative medical approaches based on multipotent NSCs. These cells are present in the adult human brain throughout life [99,100] and are capable of self-renewal and differentiation into cell types of the brain. Neural stem cells respond to external stimuli such as the learning process [100,101], physical activity [100,102], and molecules like XN [103]. XN, as a small molecule, may have the potential to induce the body's own regenerative mechanisms and support healing after ischemic insults and other neurotoxic events [100].

The study suggests that oral ingestion of low doses of XN can be sufficient to alter lipoteichoic acid-dependent immune responses of monocytes in the peripheral blood of healthy humans. This outcome further showed that the beneficial effects of XN are related to a suppression of the CD14-/TLR2-dependent activation of cells [104].

The findings from these preclinical studies suggest that XN may play a key role in preventing neurodegenerative processes, particularly by reducing oxidative damage, inhibiting Aβ accumulation, and decreasing neuroinflammation. However, further research, including well-designed clinical trials, is necessary to confirm these effects in humans and determine the appropriate therapeutic dosing. Despite the promising animal data, human studies are still limited, and the pharmacokinetics of XN in the human brain remain to be fully elucidated.

5. Challenges and Future Research Directions on Xanthohumol

5.1. Issues Related to Bioavailability

One of the key challenges in harnessing the full therapeutic potential of XN is its limited bioavailability. Despite promising preclinical results demonstrating its wide range of biological activities—such as antioxidant, anti-inflammatory, anticancer, and antimicrobial properties—the translation of these findings into effective clinical applications is hindered by several pharmacokinetic limitations. Understanding and addressing these challenges is crucial for advancing XN-based therapies [46,105].

XN, like many hydrophobic polyphenols, exhibits poor water solubility, which significantly impairs its absorption in the gastrointestinal tract. This low solubility restricts the dissolution of the compound in the aqueous environment of the digestive system, leading to suboptimal absorption through passive diffusion. According to recent studies, enhancing the solubility of XN is a critical area for future research. Approaches such as the use of cyclodextrin complexes, micellar formulations, or nano-encapsulation have shown promise in improving the solubility and overall bioavailability of XN in experimental models [46,106,107].

Following ingestion, XN undergoes extensive biotransformation in the liver and intestines, which limits its presence in the bloodstream. Phase I and Phase II metabolic processes, including oxidation, reduction, and conjugation reactions (such as glucuronidation and sulfation), lead to the formation of various metabolites, including isoxanthohumol and 8-prenylnaringenin. These metabolites, while bioactive in some cases, may have different pharmacokinetic profiles and may not fully retain the biological potency of the parent compound. A study by Legette et al. [108] highlights that XN is rapidly converted to isoxanthohumol upon ingestion, which poses a challenge for achieving therapeutic concentrations of the parent compound in the systemic circulation. Future research should focus on strategies to modulate the metabolic pathways of XN to preserve its bioactivity. This could involve the development of prodrugs, enzyme inhibitors, or metabolic pathway modulation to reduce the rate of biotransformation [109–111].

In addition to rapid metabolism, XN has a relatively short half-life, which further reduces its therapeutic efficacy. Studies have indicated that the plasma half-life of XN is limited to a few hours post-ingestion, necessitating frequent dosing to maintain therapeutic levels in the body. However, such frequent dosing may not be feasible or desirable, particularly in chronic treatment settings. To address this issue, future research should investigate delivery systems that provide controlled or sustained release of XN, ensuring more stable plasma concentrations over an extended period. Nanotechnology-based delivery platforms, such as liposomes and polymeric nanoparticles, hold the potential for improving the pharmacokinetics of XN, enhancing both its bioavailability and half-life [112,113]. However, attempts are being made to develop formulas to increase the bioavailability of XN [114].

Nanoparticles, liposomes, and nanoemulsions have been explored as carriers to improve the absorption, stability, and distribution of XN. These systems can protect the compound from degradation in the digestive tract, facilitate its absorption, and extend its circulation time in the body [115–117]. Co-administration with absorption enhancers, such as piperine or other bioactive compounds, has been shown to improve the intestinal absorption of poorly soluble compounds like XN. This strategy could be investigated further to determine its applicability in enhancing XN bioavailability [118,119]. Cyclodextrin complexes have been reported to improve the solubility and stability of hydrophobic compounds. Cyclodextrin-based inclusion complexes with XN may improve its aqueous solubility, thus enhancing gastrointestinal absorption and systemic bioavailability [46,120]. Designing prodrugs that undergo enzymatic or chemical conversion to XN in the body can provide a controlled release mechanism that improves the compound's stability and reduces its rapid metabolism [121].

5.2. *Safety and Tolerance of Xanthohumol*

Preclinical and clinical research indicates that XN, a prenylated flavonoid derived from hops, is generally well tolerated at moderate doses. In vitro and in vivo studies have not reported significant toxic effects at doses commonly tested for therapeutic purposes.

For instance, rodent studies demonstrated safety at doses up to 1000 mg/kg, while human clinical trials observed no serious adverse events at doses between 12 mg and 24 mg daily [122]. To facilitate understanding, Figures 4 and 5 illustrate the relationship between XN concentrations and observed effects, highlighting safe dosage ranges for both preclinical and clinical studies. The graphs delineate effective therapeutic doses (e.g., neuro-protection, metabolic benefits) and identify areas where safety data remain insufficient, such as chronic high-dose exposures.

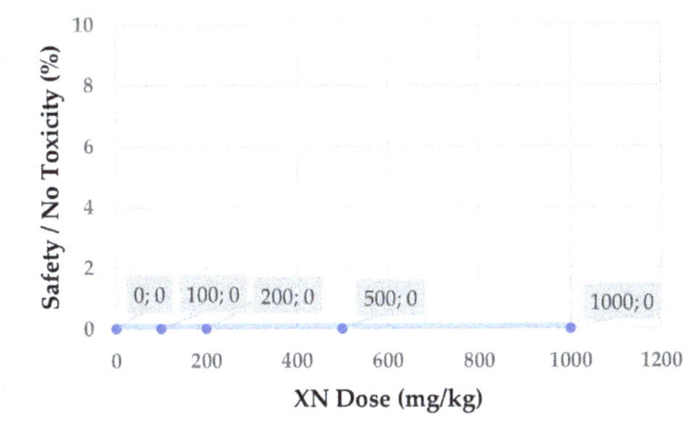

Figure 4. XN dose and safety/no toxicity in preclinical studies.

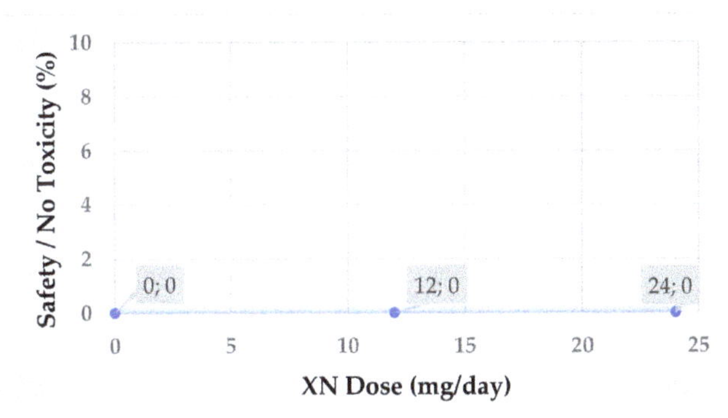

Figure 5. XN dose and safety/no toxicity in clinical studies.

However, while these findings are promising, the long-term safety of XN has not been thoroughly investigated. Most clinical trials have been limited to short durations, and the effects of chronic exposure remain uncertain. The potential for cumulative effects, particularly on liver and kidney function, as well as on metabolic pathways, warrants further investigation in both preclinical and clinical settings [108].

Although XN exhibits low toxicity at moderate doses, higher concentrations could potentially pose risks, as suggested by its structural similarity to other flavonoids, which can influence estrogenic and anti-estrogenic activity in some tissues [122]. Prolonged high-dose exposure might also interact with cytochrome P450 enzymes, affecting drug metabolism pathways and leading to potential drug interactions. This calls for further studies to determine the safety threshold and to explore any long-term metabolic or hormonal effects of XN supplementation.

Individuals with pre-existing liver conditions or those on medications metabolized by the liver should exercise caution with XN supplementation. Additionally, patients undergoing treatment for hormone-related cancers should consult a healthcare provider before using XN due to its potential to modulate estrogen pathways.

In conclusion, while current evidence supports the general safety of XN in moderate doses, long-term, and higher-dose studies are necessary to fully understand its safety profile and potential interactions, particularly for individuals using concurrent medications.

Authors of a study in mice models referred to equivalent doses in humans, stating that applications of XN can be expected to be safe in humans [123]. Human studies have confirmed the safety of XN. After standardizing an extract of spent hops to these marker compounds, an escalating dose study was carried out in menopausal women to evaluate safety and pharmacokinetics. There was no effect on selected hormones and blood clotting. The maximum serum concentrations of the prenylated phenols (including XN) reached 2 to 7 h, indicating slow absorption. Slow absorption and enterohepatic recirculation contributed to half-lives exceeding 20 h. The authors' study confirms that short-term consumption of a standardized preparation of spent hops (containing, among others, XN) is safe for patients (women) and that once daily dosing might be appropriate [124].

Studies in the different areas of medicine (therapy for patients in intensive care), where XN was administered enterally three times a day every 8 h at a dose of 1.5 mg/kg body weight (4.5 mg/kg body weight/day) for 7 days [125], showed that treatment with XN improved the clinical course and lower the severity of the inflammatory response and mortality rate [126].

5.3. Future Research Directions

Despite the promising therapeutic potential of XN, significant gaps remain in the understanding of its pharmacokinetics, long-term safety, and clinical efficacy, particularly in treating complex diseases. Future research should prioritize improving XN's bioavailability, exploring its potential in neurodegenerative diseases, and conducting more extensive long-term safety studies [122]. Only through these efforts can XN transition from promising preclinical findings to effective clinical therapies.

Recent research [127] in humans shows that 24 mg daily XN taken over an eight-week period was safe and well-tolerated by healthy adults and did not find abnormal values in clinical biomarkers, including those of renal and hepatic function, electrolytes, fasting glucose, and blood counts. It suggests safety and a lack of harm to major organs of the body. There were no severe or Food and Drug Administration-defined serious adverse events, but non-serious adverse events were documented in both the placebo and XN groups. Findings related to tolerability suggested that XN did not negatively influence quality of life.

XN continues to garner interest for its broad-spectrum biological activities, extending beyond its well-documented antioxidant and anti-inflammatory properties. Emerging research highlights its potential in the treatment of various diseases, including cancer, cardiovascular disorders, diabetes, and metabolic syndromes, as well as its neuroprotective effects.

XN's potential as an anticancer agent has been extensively studied. Its chemopreventive effects are linked to its ability to induce apoptosis, inhibit cancer cell proliferation, and interfere with angiogenesis. XN has been shown to suppress the growth of various cancer cell lines, including breast, colon, prostate, and liver cancers, by modulating key signaling pathways such as NF-κB and PI3K/Akt/mTOR [122]. XN can interfere with the initiation, promotion, and progression phase of carcinogenesis by a variety of inhibitory mechanisms [128]. Furthermore, its ability to enhance the effectiveness of conventional chemotherapeutics and mitigate drug resistance positions XN as a promising adjunct in cancer treatment.

XN demonstrates cardioprotective effects, largely attributed to its antioxidant activity and ability to reduce inflammation. It has been shown to improve endothelial function, reduce oxidative stress, and inhibit the oxidation of LDL, a key factor in atherosclerosis development. Studies also suggest that XN can modulate lipid metabolism, reduce cholesterol levels, and improve overall cardiovascular risk profiles, making it a candidate for treating cardiovascular diseases [122].

In preclinical models, XN has exhibited the ability to improve insulin sensitivity, regulate blood glucose levels, and ameliorate lipid profiles, positioning it as a potential therapeutic for type 2 diabetes and metabolic syndrome. It influences several key metabolic pathways, including AMPK activation and PPARγ modulation, which are crucial for regulating glucose homeostasis and lipid metabolism. These findings suggest that XN may help prevent complications associated with diabetes, such as cardiovascular disease and liver dysfunction [129].

The neuroprotective properties of XN stem from its potent antioxidant, anti-inflammatory, and antiapoptotic effects. XN's neuroprotective properties are driven by its antioxidant, anti-inflammatory, and antiapoptotic effects. It has demonstrated potential in protecting against neurodegenerative diseases such as AD and PD by reducing oxidative damage, inhibiting neuroinflammation, and preventing neuronal death. This makes XN a candidate for future therapies aimed at slowing the progression of these debilitating disorders, although more clinical research is required to confirm these effects in humans [41,130]. The neuroprotective effects of XN showed that XN is a promising supplement for ischemic stroke protection. The experimental studies showed that XN could revive neuronal apoptosis induced by oxygen–glucose deprivation by preventing oxidative stress injury (effects of the inhibition of phosphorylation of p38-MAPK and the mediation of nuclear Nrf2 activation) [47].

Due to its robust anti-inflammatory and antioxidant capabilities, XN may also have therapeutic applications in the treatment of metabolic and autoimmune diseases. Its ability to modulate immune responses, coupled with its effect on lipid metabolism, positions it as a potential candidate for managing conditions like rheumatoid arthritis and lupus. Research into its role in regulating immune cell activity, particularly in reducing pro-inflammatory cytokines, suggests that it could be a novel therapeutic approach for chronic inflammatory diseases [131,132].

Great hopes are placed on the lack of negative impact of XN on the microbiome and mental health [127].

The wide-ranging biological activities of XN make it a promising candidate for various therapeutic applications, from cancer and cardiovascular disease to diabetes and neurodegeneration. However, further clinical research is essential to fully validate its efficacy and safety in humans, as well as to optimize its bioavailability for therapeutic use.

6. Conclusions

Xanthohumol (XN), a bioactive flavonoid found in hops, has emerged as a promising candidate for the prevention and treatment of neurodegenerative diseases, thanks to its diverse mechanisms of action. The experimental evidence highlights XN's potent antioxidant capabilities, which play a crucial role in mitigating oxidative stress—a key factor in the pathogenesis of conditions such as Alzheimer's, Parkinson's, and Huntington's diseases. By scavenging free radicals and upregulating the body's endogenous antioxidant defenses, XN protects neurons from oxidative damage. Notably, in amyotrophic lateral sclerosis (ALS), preclinical studies suggest that XN can help preserve motor neurons, even in the presence of SOD1 gene mutations.

Moreover, XN exhibits significant anti-inflammatory properties, which are particularly important given the central role of neuroinflammation in many neurodegenerative disorders. By inhibiting pro-inflammatory mediators such as NF-κB, TNF-α, and IL-1β, XN effectively reduces the chronic activation of microglia and astrocytes, thereby preventing further neuronal damage. This multifaceted anti-inflammatory action aligns with current trends emphasizing the importance of controlling inflammation to maintain neuronal health.

In addition, XN influences key neuroprotective pathways, notably the Nrf2/ARE pathway. Activation of Nrf2 leads to the expression of antioxidant and cytoprotective genes, enhancing neuronal resilience to various stressors. This is particularly relevant in Alzheimer's disease, where the accumulation of amyloid-beta (Aβ) and hyperphosphorylated tau proteins contributes to cognitive decline. Experimental results indicate that XN reduces Aβ production and aggregation and inhibits tau hyperphosphorylation, thus potentially slowing the progression of the disease.

Another critical aspect of XN's action is its role in supporting mitochondrial function, a vital factor in neurodegenerative diseases. By maintaining ATP production, reducing mitochondrial oxidative damage, and promoting mitochondrial biogenesis, XN helps sustain neuronal energy metabolism, which is crucial for cognitive function and overall brain health. This aligns with the current scientific focus on preserving mitochondrial health as a strategy to combat neurodegenerative disorders.

Finally, studies have demonstrated that XN positively impacts synaptic plasticity, enhances memory, and prevents cognitive impairment, which underscores its potential as a therapeutic agent. However, despite these promising findings, the bioavailability of XN in humans remains a challenge. Early clinical trials, such as those conducted in 2021, suggest that XN supplementation is safe and beneficial for gut microbiota and overall quality of life. Future research should aim to optimize delivery methods and dosages to fully realize XN's therapeutic potential.

Author Contributions: Conceptualization, A.D. and D.C.; writing—original draft preparation, A.D., D.C., B.B. and J.S.; writing—review and editing, B.B., J.S. and A.D., visualization, B.B. and J.S.; supervision, A.D. All authors have read and agreed to the published version of the manuscript.

Funding: This research received no external funding.

Institutional Review Board Statement: Not applicable.

Informed Consent Statement: Not applicable.

Data Availability Statement: No new data were created.

Conflicts of Interest: The authors declare no conflicts of interest.

Abbreviations

1-methyl-4-phenyl-1,2,3,6-tetrahydropyridine	MPTP
1-methyl-4-phenylpyridinium	MPP+
2,2′-azinobis(3-ethylbenzothiazoline-6-sulfonic acid)	ABTS
2,2-diphenyl-1-picrylhydrazyl	DPPH
5′AMP-activated protein kinase	AMPK
6-hydroxydopamine	6-OHDA
acetylcholinesterase	AChE
adenosine triphosphate	ATP

Alzheimer's disease	AD
amyotrophic lateral sclerosis	ALS
antioxidant response element	ARE
beta-amyloid	Aβ
catalase	CAT
central nervous system	CNS
cluster of differentiation 14	CD14
endoplasmic reticulum	ER
experimental autoimmune encephalomyelitis	EAE
ferric reducing antioxidant power	FRAP
half-maximal inhibitory concentration	IC_{50}
hydrogen atom transfer	HAT
hydrogen peroxide	H_2O_2
hydroperoxy radical	HOO•
hydroxyl radical	•OH
hydroxyl radical antioxidant capacity	HORAC
interleukin-1β	IL-1β
interleukin-6	IL-6
low-density lipoprotein	LDL
malondialdehyde	MDA
mammalian target of rapamycin	mTOR
metallophosphoesterase domain containing 1	Mpped1
methoxy radical	CH_3O•
neuronal stem cells	NSCs
nuclear factor-κB	NF-κB
nuclear respiratory factor 2	Nrf2
oxygen radical absorbance capacity	ORAC
p38 mitogen-activated protein kinases	p38-MAPK
Parkinson's disease	PD
peroxisome proliferator-activated receptor gamma	PPARγ
phosphoinositide 3-kinase	PI3K
protein kinase B	Akt
reactive nitrogen species	RNS
reactive oxygen species	ROS
sequential proton loss electron transfer	SPLET
single electron transfer	SET
singlet oxygen absorbance capacity	SOAC
superoxide anion	$O_2^{\bullet -}$
superoxide dismutase	SOD
superoxide dismutase 1	SOD1
toll-like receptor 2	TLR2
Trolox equivalent antioxidant capacity	TEAC or TE
tumor necrosis factor-alpha	TNF-α
xanthohumol	XN

References

1. Gaweł, M.; Potulska-Chromik, A. Neurodegenerative diseases: Alzheimer's and Parkinson's disease. *Postępy Nauk Med.* **2015**, *7*, 468–476.
2. Gitler, A.D.; Dhillon, P.; Shorter, J. Neurodegenerative Disease: Models, Mechanisms, and a New Hope. *Dis. Models Mech.* **2017**, *10*, 499–502. [CrossRef] [PubMed]
3. Dugger, B.N.; Dickson, D.W. Pathology of Neurodegenerative Diseases. *Cold Spring Harb. Perspect. Biol.* **2017**, *9*, a028035. [CrossRef] [PubMed]
4. Bai, R.; Guo, J.; Ye, X.-Y.; Xie, Y.; Xie, T. Oxidative Stress: The Core Pathogenesis and Mechanism of Alzheimer's Disease. *Ageing Res. Rev.* **2022**, *77*, 101619. [CrossRef]

5. Sies, H.; Berndt, C.; Jones, D.P. Oxidative Stress. *Annu. Rev. Biochem.* **2017**, *86*, 715–748. [CrossRef]
6. Szulc, J.; Czaczyk, K.; Dobrowolska, A.; Gozdecka, G.; Błaszak, B. Elicitation as a Process of Enhancing Bioactive Compounds Concentration in Sprouts. *Processes* **2024**, *12*, 174. [CrossRef]
7. Ramanan, M.; Sinha, S.; Sudarshan, K.; Aidhen, I.S.; Doble, M. Inhibition of the Enzymes in the Leukotriene and Prostaglandin Pathways in Inflammation by 3-Aryl Isocoumarins. *Eur. J. Med. Chem.* **2016**, *124*, 428–434. [CrossRef]
8. Sudarshan, K.; Boda, A.K.; Dogra, S.; Bose, I.; Yadav, P.N.; Aidhen, I.S. Discovery of an Isocoumarin Analogue That Modulates Neuronal Functions via Neurotrophin Receptor TrkB. *Bioorg. Med. Chem. Lett.* **2019**, *29*, 585–590. [CrossRef]
9. Neumann, H.F.; Frank, J.; Venturelli, S.; Egert, S. Bioavailability and Cardiometabolic Effects of Xanthohumol: Evidence from Animal and Human Studies. *Mol. Nutr. Food Res.* **2022**, *66*, 2100831. [CrossRef]
10. Stevens, J.F.; Page, J.E. Xanthohumol and Related Prenylflavonoids from Hops and Beer: To Your Good Health! *Phytochemistry* **2004**, *65*, 1317–1330. [CrossRef]
11. Silva, G.V.d.A.; Arend, G.D.; Zielinski, A.A.F.; Di Luccio, M.; Ambrosi, A. Xanthohumol Properties and Strategies for Extraction from Hops and Brewery Residues: A Review. *Food Chem.* **2023**, *404*, 134629. [CrossRef] [PubMed]
12. Aggarwal, D.; Upadhyay, S.K.; Singh, R.; Tuli, H.S. Recent Patents on Therapeutic Activities of Xanthohumol: A Prenylated Chalconoid from Hops (*Humulus lupulus* L.). *Pharm. Pat. Anal.* **2021**, *10*, 37–49. [CrossRef] [PubMed]
13. Liu, M.; Hansen, P.E.; Wang, G.; Qiu, L.; Dong, J.; Yin, H.; Qian, Z.; Yang, M.; Miao, J. Pharmacological Profile of Xanthohumol, a Prenylated Flavonoid from Hops (*Humulus lupulus*). *Molecules* **2015**, *20*, 754–779. [CrossRef] [PubMed]
14. Zugravu, C.-A.; Bohiltea, R.-E.; Salmen, T.; Pogurschi, E.; Otelea, M.R. Antioxidants in Hops: Bioavailability, Health Effects and Perspectives for New Products. *Antioxidants* **2022**, *11*, 241. [CrossRef]
15. Salehi, B.; Martorell, M.; Arbiser, J.L.; Sureda, A.; Martins, N.; Maurya, P.K.; Sharifi-Rad, M.; Kumar, P.; Sharifi-Rad, J. Antioxidants: Positive or Negative Actors? *Biomolecules* **2018**, *8*, 124. [CrossRef]
16. Verzele, M.; Stockx, J.; Fontijn, F.; Anteunis, M. Xanthohumol, a New Natural Chalkone. *Bull. Des. Sociétés Chim. Belg.* **1957**, *66*, 452–475. [CrossRef]
17. Jiang, C.-H.; Sun, T.-L.; Xiang, D.-X.; Wei, S.-S.; Li, W.-Q. Anticancer Activity and Mechanism of Xanthohumol: A Prenylated Flavonoid from Hops (*Humulus lupulus* L.). *Front. Pharmacol.* **2018**, *9*, 530. [CrossRef]
18. Lü, J.-M.; Lin, P.H.; Yao, Q.; Chen, C. Chemical and Molecular Mechanisms of Antioxidants: Experimental Approaches and Model Systems. *J. Cell. Mol. Med.* **2010**, *14*, 840–860. [CrossRef]
19. Munteanu, I.G.; Apetrei, C. Analytical Methods Used in Determining Antioxidant Activity: A Review. *Int. J. Mol. Sci.* **2021**, *22*, 3380. [CrossRef]
20. Apak, R.; Özyürek, M.; Güçlü, K.; Çapanoğlu, E. Antioxidant Activity/Capacity Measurement. 1. Classification, Physicochemical Principles, Mechanisms, and Electron Transfer (ET)-Based Assays. *J. Agric. Food Chem.* **2016**, *64*, 997–1027. [CrossRef]
21. Litwinienko, G.; Mulder, P. Comment on "Temperature and Solvent Effects on Radical Scavenging Ability of Phenols". *J. Phys. Chem. A* **2009**, *113*, 14014–14016. [CrossRef] [PubMed]
22. Shahidi, F.; Zhong, Y. Measurement of Antioxidant Activity. *J. Funct. Foods* **2015**, *18*, 757–781. [CrossRef]
23. Tošović, J.; Kolenc, Z.; Hostnik, G.; Bren, U. Exploring Antioxidative Properties of Xanthohumol and Isoxanthohumol: An Integrated Experimental and Computational Approach with Isoxanthohumol pKa Determination. *Food Chem.* **2025**, *463*, 141377. [CrossRef] [PubMed]
24. Antolovich, M.; Prenzler, P.D.; Patsalides, E.; McDonald, S.; Robards, K. Methods for Testing Antioxidant Activity. *Analyst* **2002**, *127*, 183–198. [CrossRef]
25. Brand-Williams, W.; Cuvelier, M.E.; Berset, C. Use of a Free Radical Method to Evaluate Antioxidant Activity. *LWT-Food Sci. Technol.* **1995**, *28*, 25–30. [CrossRef]
26. Malta, L.G.; Liu, R.H. Analyses of Total Phenolics, Total Flavonoids, and Total Antioxidant Activities in Foods and Dietary Supplements. In *Encyclopedia of Agriculture and Food Systems*; Van Alfen, N.K., Ed.; Academic Press: Oxford, UK, 2014; pp. 305–314, ISBN 978-0-08-093139-5.
27. Benzie, I.F.F.; Strain, J.J. The Ferric Reducing Ability of Plasma (FRAP) as a Measure of "Antioxidant Power": The FRAP Assay. *Anal. Biochem.* **1996**, *239*, 70–76. [CrossRef]
28. Nenadis, N.; Tsimidou, M.Z. Assessing the Activity of Natural Food Antioxidants. In *Oxidation in Foods and Beverages and Antioxidant Applications*; Decker, E.A., Ed.; Woodhead Publishing Series in Food Science, Technology and Nutrition; Woodhead Publishing: Cambridge, UK, 2010; pp. 332–367, ISBN 978-1-84569-648-1.
29. Kontek, B.; Jedrejek, D.; Oleszek, W.; Olas, B. Antiradical and Antioxidant Activity in vitro of Hops-Derived Extracts Rich in Bitter Acids and Xanthohumol. *Ind. Crops Prod.* **2021**, *161*, 113208. [CrossRef]
30. Van Hoyweghen, L.; Biendl, M.; Heyerick, A. Radical Scavenging Capacity of Hop-Derived Products. *Brew. Sci.* **2010**, *63*, 1–5.
31. Zhang, X.-L.; Zhang, Y.-D.; Wang, T.; Guo, H.-Y.; Liu, Q.-M.; Su, H.-X. Evaluation on Antioxidant Effect of Xanthohumol by Different Antioxidant Capacity Analytical Methods. *J. Chem.* **2014**, *2014*, 249485. [CrossRef]

32. Muzykiewicz, A.; Nowak, A.; Zielonka-Brzezicka, J.; Florkowska, K.; Duchnik, W.; Klimowicz, A. Comparison of Antioxidant Activity of Extracts of Hop Leaves Harvested in Different Years. *Herba Pol.* **2019**, *65*, 1–9. [CrossRef]
33. Kolenc, Z.; Hribernik, T.; Langerholc, T.; Pintarič, M.; Prevolnik Povše, M.; Bren, U. Antioxidant Activity of Different Hop (*Humulus lupulus* L.) Genotypes. *Plants* **2023**, *12*, 3436. [CrossRef] [PubMed]
34. Krofta, K.; Mikyška, A.; Hašková, D. Antioxidant Characteristics of Hops and Hop Products. *J. Inst. Brew.* **2008**, *114*, 160–166. [CrossRef]
35. Yamaguchi, N.; Satoh-Yamaguchi, K.; Ono, M. In Vitro Evaluation of Antibacterial, Anticollagenase, and Antioxidant Activities of Hop Components (*Humulus lupulus*) Addressing Acne Vulgaris. *Phytomedicine* **2009**, *16*, 369–376. [CrossRef] [PubMed]
36. Constantinescu, T.; Mihis, A.G. Resveratrol as a Privileged Molecule with Antioxidant Activity. *Food Chem. Adv.* **2023**, *3*, 100539. [CrossRef]
37. Jumina, J.; Siswanta, D.; Zulkarnain, A.K.; Triono, S.; Priatmoko, P.; Yuanita, E.; Fatmasari, N.; Nursalim, I. Development of C-Arylcalix[4]Resorcinarenes and C-Arylcalix[4]Pyrogallolarenes as Antioxidant and UV-B Protector. *Indones. J. Chem.* **2019**, *19*, 273–284. [CrossRef]
38. Potaniec, B.; Grabarczyk, M.; Stompor, M.; Szumny, A.; Zieliński, P.; Żołnierczyk, A.K.; Anioł, M. Antioxidant Activity and Spectroscopic Data of Isoxanthohomol Oxime and Related Compounds. *Spectrochim. Acta Part A Mol. Biomol. Spectrosc.* **2014**, *118*, 716–723. [CrossRef]
39. Majewska, M.; Skrzycki, M.; Podsiad, M.; Czeczot, H. Evaluation of Antioxidant Potential of Flavonoids: An in Vitro Study. *Acta Pol. Pharm.* **2011**, *68*, 611–615.
40. Piekara, J.; Piasecka-Kwiatkowska, D. Antioxidant Potential of Xanthohumol in Disease Prevention: Evidence from Human and Animal Studies. *Antioxidants* **2024**, *13*, 1559. [CrossRef]
41. Wang, X.; Ho, S.-L.; Poon, C.-Y.; Yan, T.; Li, H.-W.; Wong, M.S. Amyloid-β Aggregation Inhibitory and Neuroprotective Effects of Xanthohumol and Its Derivatives for Alzheimer's Diseases. *Curr. Alzheimer Res.* **2019**, *16*, 836–842. [CrossRef]
42. Liu, W.; Chen, X.; Zhao, J.; Yang, C.; Huang, G.; Zhang, Z.; Liu, J. Protective Signature of Xanthohumol on Cognitive Function of APP/PS1 Mice: A Urine Metabolomics Approach by Age. *Front. Pharmacol.* **2024**, *15*, 1423060. [CrossRef]
43. Ionescu-Tucker, A.; Cotman, C.W. Emerging Roles of Oxidative Stress in Brain Aging and Alzheimer's Disease. *Neurobiol. Aging* **2021**, *107*, 86–95. [CrossRef] [PubMed]
44. Bordoloi, S.; Pathak, K.; Devi, M.; Saikia, R.; Das, J.; Kashyap, V.H.; Das, D.; Ahmad, M.Z.; Abdel-Wahab, B.A. Some Promising Medicinal Plants Used in Alzheimer's Disease: An Ethnopharmacological Perspective. *Discov. Appl. Sci.* **2024**, *6*, 215. [CrossRef]
45. Huang, X.; Wang, J.; Chen, X.; Liu, P.; Wang, S.; Song, F.; Zhang, Z.; Zhu, F.; Huang, X.; Liu, J.; et al. The Prenylflavonoid Xanthohumol Reduces Alzheimer-Like Changes and Modulates Multiple Pathogenic Molecular Pathways in the Neuro2a/APPswe Cell Model of AD. *Front. Pharmacol.* **2018**, *9*, 199. [CrossRef] [PubMed]
46. Oledzka, E. Xanthohumol—A Miracle Molecule with Biological Activities: A Review of Biodegradable Polymeric Carriers and Naturally Derived Compounds for Its Delivery. *Int. J. Mol. Sci.* **2024**, *25*, 3398. [CrossRef]
47. Jiao, Y.; Cao, Y.; Lu, X.; Wang, J.; Saitgareeva, A.; Kong, X.; Song, C.; Li, J.; Tian, K.; Zhang, S.; et al. Xanthohumol Protects Neuron from Cerebral Ischemia Injury in Experimental Stroke. *Mol. Biol. Rep.* **2020**, *47*, 2417–2425. [CrossRef]
48. Lee, K.H.; Cha, M.; Lee, B.H. Neuroprotective Effect of Antioxidants in the Brain. *Int. J. Mol. Sci.* **2020**, *21*, 7152. [CrossRef]
49. Arya, A.; Chahal, R.; Rao, R.; Rahman, M.H.; Kaushik, D.; Akhtar, M.F.; Saleem, A.; Khalifa, S.M.A.; El-Seedi, H.R.; Kamel, M.; et al. Acetylcholinesterase Inhibitory Potential of Various Sesquiterpene Analogues for Alzheimer's Disease Therapy. *Biomolecules* **2021**, *11*, 350. [CrossRef]
50. Xia, T.; Zhang, J.; Guo, Y.; Jiang, Y.; Qiao, F.; Li, K.; Wang, N.; Han, T.; Xin, H. *Humulus lupulus* L. Extract Protects against Senior Osteoporosis through Inhibiting Amyloid β Deposition and Oxidative Stress in APP/PS1 Mutated Transgenic Mice and Osteoblasts. *Molecules* **2023**, *28*, 583. [CrossRef]
51. Jung, F.; Staltner, R.; Baumann, A.; Burger, K.; Halilbasic, E.; Hellerbrand, C.; Bergheim, I. A Xanthohumol-Rich Hop Extract Diminishes Endotoxin-Induced Activation of TLR4 Signaling in Human Peripheral Blood Mononuclear Cells: A Study in Healthy Women. *Int. J. Mol. Sci.* **2022**, *23*, 12702. [CrossRef]
52. Wang, W.; Zhang, J.; Liu, Z.; Zhu, Y.; Mei, L.; Tao, Y.; Jiang, L. Xanthotoxol from Saussurea Obvallata Attenuates LPS-Induced RAW 264.7 Cells Inflammatory Responses through NF-κB Pathway. *Russ. J. Bioorg Chem.* **2022**, *48*, 300–309. [CrossRef]
53. Liu, Y.; Shao, J.; Qiao, R.; Li, J.; Li, C.; Cao, W. Xanthohumol Improves Cognitive Impairment by Regulating miRNA-532-3p/Mpped1 in Ovariectomized Mice. *Psychopharmacology* **2023**, *240*, 1169–1178. [CrossRef] [PubMed]
54. Klyucherev, T.O.; Olszewski, P.; Shalimova, A.A.; Chubarev, V.N.; Tarasov, V.V.; Attwood, M.M.; Syvänen, S.; Schiöth, H.B. Advances in the Development of New Biomarkers for Alzheimer's Disease. *Transl. Neurodegener.* **2022**, *11*, 25. [CrossRef] [PubMed]
55. Awouafack, M.D.; Lee, Y.-E.; Morita, H. Xanthohumol: Recent Advances on Resources, Biosynthesis, Bioavailability and Pharmacology. In *Handbook of Dietary Flavonoids*; Xiao, J., Ed.; Springer International Publishing: Cham, Switzerland, 2023; pp. 1–23, ISBN 978-3-030-94753-8.

56. Hu, F.; Gao, Q.; Zheng, C.; Zhang, W.; Yang, Z.; Wang, S.; Zhang, Y.; Lu, T. Encapsulated Lactiplantibacillus Plantarum Improves Alzheimer's Symptoms in APP/PS1 Mice. *J. Nanobiotechnol.* **2024**, *22*, 582. [CrossRef] [PubMed]
57. Láng, L.; McArthur, S.; Lazar, A.S.; Pourtau, L.; Gaudout, D.; Pontifex, M.G.; Müller, M.; Vauzour, D. Dietary (Poly)Phenols and the Gut–Brain Axis in Ageing. *Nutrients* **2024**, *16*, 1500. [CrossRef]
58. Hammad, M.; Salma, R.; Balosso, J.; Rezvani, M.; Haghdoost, S. Role of Oxidative Stress Signaling, Nrf2, on Survival and Stemness of Human Adipose-Derived Stem Cells Exposed to X-Rays, Protons and Carbon Ions. *Antioxidants* **2024**, *13*, 1035. [CrossRef]
59. Thiruvengadam, M.; Venkidasamy, B.; Subramanian, U.; Samynathan, R.; Ali Shariati, M.; Rebezov, M.; Girish, S.; Thangavel, S.; Dhanapal, A.R.; Fedoseeva, N.; et al. Bioactive Compounds in Oxidative Stress-Mediated Diseases: Targeting the NRF2/ARE Signaling Pathway and Epigenetic Regulation. *Antioxidants* **2021**, *10*, 1859. [CrossRef]
60. Buendia, I.; Michalska, P.; Navarro, E.; Gameiro, I.; Egea, J.; León, R. Nrf2-ARE Pathway: An Emerging Target against Oxidative Stress and Neuroinflammation in Neurodegenerative Diseases. *Pharmacol. Ther.* **2016**, *157*, 84–104. [CrossRef]
61. Sun, E.; Motolani, A.; Campos, L.; Lu, T. The Pivotal Role of NF-kB in the Pathogenesis and Therapeutics of Alzheimer's Disease. *Int. J. Mol. Sci.* **2022**, *23*, 8972. [CrossRef]
62. Sharoar, M.G.; Thapa, A.; Shahnawaz, M.; Ramasamy, V.S.; Woo, E.-R.; Shin, S.Y.; Park, I.-S. Keampferol-3-O-Rhamnoside Abrogates Amyloid Beta Toxicity by Modulating Monomers and Remodeling Oligomers and Fibrils to Non-Toxic Aggregates. *J. Biomed. Sci.* **2012**, *19*, 104. [CrossRef]
63. Phukan, B.C.; Roy, R.; Gahatraj, I.; Bhattacharya, P.; Borah, A. Therapeutic Considerations of Bioactive Compounds in Alzheimer's Disease and Parkinson's Disease: Dissecting the Molecular Pathways. *Phytother. Res.* **2023**, *37*, 5657–5699. [CrossRef]
64. Wang, Y.; Cui, L.; Zhao, H.; He, H.; Chen, L.; Song, X.; Liu, D.; Qiu, J.; Sun, Y. Exploring the Connectivity of Neurodegenerative Diseases: Microglia as the Center. *J. Inflamm. Res.* **2023**, *16*, 6107–6121. [CrossRef] [PubMed]
65. Maiti, P.; Manna, J.; Dunbar, G.L. Current Understanding of the Molecular Mechanisms in Parkinson's Disease: Targets for Potential Treatments. *Transl. Neurodegener.* **2017**, *6*, 28. [CrossRef] [PubMed]
66. Zhou, Z.D.; Yi, L.X.; Wang, D.Q.; Lim, T.M.; Tan, E.K. Role of Dopamine in the Pathophysiology of Parkinson's Disease. *Transl. Neurodegener.* **2023**, *12*, 44. [CrossRef] [PubMed]
67. Trist, B.G.; Hare, D.J.; Double, K.L. Oxidative Stress in the Aging Substantia Nigra and the Etiology of Parkinson's Disease. *Aging Cell* **2019**, *18*, e13031. [CrossRef]
68. Lee, S.Y.H.; Yates, N.J.; Tye, S.J. Inflammatory Mechanisms in Parkinson's Disease: From Pathogenesis to Targeted Therapies. *Neuroscientist* **2022**, *28*, 485–506. [CrossRef]
69. Hor, S.L.; Teoh, S.L.; Lim, W.L. Plant Polyphenols as Neuroprotective Agents in Parkinson's Disease Targeting Oxidative Stress. *Curr. Drug Targets* **2020**, *21*, 458–476. [CrossRef]
70. Barata-Antunes, S.; Teixeira, F.G.; Mendes-Pinheiro, B.; Domingues, A.V.; Vilaça-Faria, H.; Marote, A.; Silva, D.; Sousa, R.A.; Salgado, A.J. Impact of Aging on the 6-OHDA-Induced Rat Model of Parkinson's Disease. *Int. J. Mol. Sci.* **2020**, *21*, 3459. [CrossRef]
71. Hernandez-Baltazar, D.; Nadella, R.; Rovirosa-Hernandez, M.D.J.; Zavala-Flores, L.M.; Jarquin, C.D.J.R. Animal Model of Parkinson Disease: Neuroinflammation and Apoptosis in the 6-Hydroxydopamine-Induced Model. In *Experimental Animal Models of Human Diseases: An Effective Therapeutic Strategy*; Bartholomew, I., Ed.; InTech: Rijeka, Croatia, 2018.
72. Huangfu, Y.; Yu, X.; Wan, C.; Zhu, Y.; Wei, Z.; Li, F.; Wang, Y.; Zhang, K.; Li, S.; Dong, Y.; et al. Xanthohumol Alleviates Oxidative Stress and Impaired Autophagy in Experimental Severe Acute Pancreatitis through Inhibition of AKT/mTOR. *Front. Pharmacol.* **2023**, *14*, 1105726. [CrossRef]
73. Bradley, R.; Langley, B.O.; Ryan, J.J.; Phipps, J.; Hanes, D.A.; Stack, E.; Jansson, J.K.; Metz, T.O.; Stevens, J.F. Xanthohumol Microbiome and Signature in Healthy Adults (the XMaS Trial): A Phase I Triple-Masked, Placebo-Controlled Clinical Trial. *Trials* **2020**, *21*, 835. [CrossRef]
74. Brown, R.H.; Al-Chalabi, A. Amyotrophic Lateral Sclerosis. *N. Engl. J. Med.* **2017**, *377*, 162–172. [CrossRef]
75. Nabavi, S.F.; Daglia, M.; D'Antona, G.; Sobarzo-Sánchez, E.; Talas, Z.S.; Nabavi, S.M. Natural Compounds Used as Therapies Targeting to Amyotrophic Lateral Sclerosis. *Curr. Pharm. Biotechnol.* **2015**, *16*, 211–218. [CrossRef] [PubMed]
76. Kiernan, M.C.; Vucic, S.; Cheah, B.C.; Turner, M.R.; Eisen, A.; Hardiman, O.; Burrell, J.R.; Zoing, M.C. Amyotrophic Lateral Sclerosis. *Lancet* **2011**, *377*, 942–955. [CrossRef] [PubMed]
77. Ortiz, D.A.; Peregrín, N.; Valencia, M.; Vinueza-Gavilanes, R.; Marín-Ordovas, E.; Ferrero, R.; Nicolás, M.J.; González-Aseguinolaza, G.; Arrasate, M.; Aragón, T. GCN2 Inhibition Reduces Mutant SOD1 Clustering and Toxicity and Delays Disease Progression in an Amyotrophic Lateral Sclerosis Mouse Model. *Transl. Neurodegener.* **2024**, *13*, 49. [CrossRef] [PubMed]
78. SOD1 Gene: MedlinePlus Genetics. Available online: https://medlineplus.gov/genetics/gene/sod1/ (accessed on 22 November 2024).
79. Mead, R.J.; Shan, N.; Reiser, H.J.; Marshall, F.; Shaw, P.J. Amyotrophic Lateral Sclerosis: A Neurodegenerative Disorder Poised for Successful Therapeutic Translation. *Nat. Rev. Drug Discov.* **2023**, *22*, 185–212. [CrossRef]

80. Shi, M.; Chai, Y.; Zhang, J.; Chen, X. Endoplasmic Reticulum Stress-Associated Neuronal Death and Innate Immune Response in Neurological Diseases. *Front. Immunol.* **2021**, *12*, 794580. [CrossRef]
81. Mancuso, R.; del Valle, J.; Modol, L.; Martinez, A.; Granado-Serrano, A.B.; Ramirez-Núñez, O.; Pallás, M.; Portero-Otin, M.; Osta, R.; Navarro, X. Resveratrol Improves Motoneuron Function and Extends Survival in SOD1(G93A) ALS Mice. *Neurotherapeutics* **2014**, *11*, 419–432. [CrossRef]
82. Donoso, F.; Ramírez, V.T.; Golubeva, A.V.; Moloney, G.M.; Stanton, C.; Dinan, T.G.; Cryan, J.F. Naturally Derived Polyphenols Protect Against Corticosterone-Induced Changes in Primary Cortical Neurons. *Int. J. Neuropsychopharmacol.* **2019**, *22*, 765–777. [CrossRef]
83. Donoso, F.; Ramírez, V.T.; Golubeva, A.V.; Moloney, G.; Stanton, C.; Dinan, T.G.; Cryan, J.F. Corrigendum to: Naturally Derived Polyphenols Protect Against Corticosterone-Induced Changes in Primary Cortical Neurons. *Int. J. Neuropsychopharmacol.* **2023**, *26*, 151–153. [CrossRef]
84. Barber, S.C.; Shaw, P.J. Oxidative Stress in ALS: Key Role in Motor Neuron Injury and Therapeutic Target. *Free Radic. Biol. Med.* **2010**, *48*, 629–641. [CrossRef]
85. Carrì, M.T.; D'Ambrosi, N.; Cozzolino, M. Pathways to Mitochondrial Dysfunction in ALS Pathogenesis. *Biochem. Biophys. Res. Commun.* **2017**, *483*, 1187–1193. [CrossRef]
86. Beers, D.R.; Appel, S.H. Immune Dysregulation in Amyotrophic Lateral Sclerosis: Mechanisms and Emerging Therapies. *Lancet Neurol.* **2019**, *18*, 211–220. [CrossRef] [PubMed]
87. Butovsky, O.; Weiner, H.L. Microglial Signatures and Their Role in Health and Disease. *Nat. Rev. Neurosci.* **2018**, *19*, 622–635. [CrossRef] [PubMed]
88. Arnold, F.J.; Putka, A.F.; Raychaudhuri, U.; Hsu, S.; Bedlack, R.S.; Bennett, C.L.; La Spada, A.R. Revisiting Glutamate Excitotoxicity in Amyotrophic Lateral Sclerosis and Age-Related Neurodegeneration. *Int. J. Mol. Sci.* **2024**, *25*, 5587. [CrossRef] [PubMed]
89. Verma, M.; Lizama, B.N.; Chu, C.T. Excitotoxicity, Calcium and Mitochondria: A Triad in Synaptic Neurodegeneration. *Transl. Neurodegener.* **2022**, *11*, 3. [CrossRef]
90. Zamzow, D.R.; Elias, V.; Legette, L.L.; Choi, J.; Stevens, J.F.; Magnusson, K.R. Xanthohumol Improved Cognitive Flexibility in Young Mice. *Behav. Brain Res.* **2014**, *275*, 1–10. [CrossRef]
91. Chen, M.; He, X.; Fan, Y.; Xia, L.; Dong, Z. Sofalcone Attenuates Neurodegeneration in MPTP-Induced Mouse Model of Parkinson's Disease by Inhibiting Oxidative Stress and Neuroinflammation. *Mol. Biol. Rep.* **2024**, *51*, 908. [CrossRef]
92. Wang, K.; Han, C.; Yang, J.; Xu, W.; Wang, L.; Li, H.; Wang, Y. Benfotiamine Protects MPTP-Induced Parkinson's Disease Mouse Model via Activating Nrf2 Signaling Pathway. *PLoS ONE* **2024**, *19*, e0307012. [CrossRef]
93. Nociti, V.; Romozzi, M. The Role of BDNF in Multiple Sclerosis Neuroinflammation. *Int. J. Mol. Sci.* **2023**, *24*, 8447. [CrossRef]
94. An, J.; Chen, B.; Kang, X.; Zhang, R.; Guo, Y.; Zhao, J.; Yang, H. Neuroprotective Effects of Natural Compounds on LPS-Induced Inflammatory Responses in Microglia. *Am. J. Transl. Res.* **2020**, *12*, 2353–2378.
95. Wang, C.C.; Ho, Y.H.; Hung, C.F.; Kuo, J.R.; Wang, S.J. Xanthohumol, an Active Constituent from Hope, Affords Protection against Kainic Acid-Induced Excitotoxicity in Rats. *Neurochem. Int.* **2020**, *133*, 104629. [CrossRef]
96. Urmann, C.; Bieler, L.; Priglinger, E.; Aigner, L.; Couillard-Despres, S.; Riepl, H.M. Neuroregenerative Potential of Prenyl- and Pyranochalcones: A Structure–Activity Study. *J. Nat. Prod.* **2021**, *84*, 2675–2682. [CrossRef] [PubMed]
97. Bieler, L.; Vogl, M.; Kirchinger, M.; Urmann, C.; Riepl, H.; Bandtlow, C.; Klimaschewski, L.; Aigner, L.; Couillard-Despres, S. The Prenylflavonoid ENDF1 Overrules Central Nervous System Growth Inhibitors and Facilitates Regeneration of DRG Neurons. *Front. Cell Neurosci.* **2019**, *13*, 332. [CrossRef] [PubMed]
98. Oberbauer, E.; Urmann, C.; Steffenhagen, C.; Bieler, L.; Brunner, D.; Furtner, T.; Humpel, C.; Bäumer, B.; Bandtlow, C.; Couillard-Despres, S.; et al. Chroman-like Cyclic Prenylflavonoids Promote Neuronal Differentiation and Neurite Outgrowth and Are Neuroprotective. *J. Nutr. Biochem.* **2013**, *24*, 1953–1962. [CrossRef] [PubMed]
99. Eriksson, P.S.; Perfilieva, E.; Björk-Eriksson, T.; Alborn, A.M.; Nordborg, C.; Peterson, D.A.; Gage, F.H. Neurogenesis in the Adult Human Hippocampus. *Nat. Med.* **1998**, *4*, 1313–1317. [CrossRef] [PubMed]
100. Urmann, C.; Bieler, L.; Hackl, M.; Chia-Leeson, O.; Couillard-Despres, S.; Riepl, H. Semi-Synthesis of Different Pyranoflavonoid Backbones and the Neurogenic Potential. *Molecules* **2023**, *28*, 4023. [CrossRef]
101. Gould, E.; Beylin, A.; Tanapat, P.; Reeves, A.; Shors, T.J. Learning Enhances Adult Neurogenesis in the Hippocampal Formation. *Nat. Neurosci.* **1999**, *2*, 260–265. [CrossRef]
102. van Praag, H.; Schinder, A.F.; Christie, B.R.; Toni, N.; Palmer, T.D.; Gage, F.H. Functional Neurogenesis in the Adult Hippocampus. *Nature* **2002**, *415*, 1030–1034. [CrossRef]
103. Urmann, C.; Riepl, H. Semi-Synthetic Approach Leading to 8-Prenylnaringenin and 6-Prenylnaringenin: Optimization of the Microwave-Assisted Demethylation of Xanthohumol Using Design of Experiments. *Molecules* **2020**, *25*, 4007. [CrossRef]
104. Jung, F.; Staltner, R.; Tahir, A.; Baumann, A.; Burger, K.; Halilbasic, E.; Hellerbrand, C.; Bergheim, I. Oral Intake of Xanthohumol Attenuates Lipoteichoic Acid-Induced Inflammatory Response in Human PBMCs. *Eur. J. Nutr.* **2022**, *61*, 4155–4166. [CrossRef]

105. Harish, V.; Haque, E.; Śmiech, M.; Taniguchi, H.; Jamieson, S.; Tewari, D.; Bishayee, A. Xanthohumol for Human Malignancies: Chemistry, Pharmacokinetics and Molecular Targets. *Int. J. Mol. Sci.* **2021**, *22*, 4478. [CrossRef]
106. Christaki, S.; Spanidi, E.; Panagiotidou, E.; Athanasopoulou, S.; Kyriakoudi, A.; Mourtzinos, I.; Gardikis, K. Cyclodextrins for the Delivery of Bioactive Compounds from Natural Sources: Medicinal, Food and Cosmetics Applications. *Pharmaceuticals* **2023**, *16*, 1274. [CrossRef] [PubMed]
107. Mahli, A.; Seitz, T.; Freese, K.; Frank, J.; Weiskirchen, R.; Abdel-Tawab, M.; Behnam, D.; Hellerbrand, C. Therapeutic Application of Micellar Solubilized Xanthohumol in a Western-Type Diet-Induced Mouse Model of Obesity, Diabetes and Non-Alcoholic Fatty Liver Disease. *Cells* **2019**, *8*, 359. [CrossRef] [PubMed]
108. Legette, L.; Ma, L.; Reed, R.L.; Miranda, C.L.; Christensen, J.M.; Rodriguez-Proteau, R.; Stevens, J.F. Pharmacokinetics of Xanthohumol and Metabolites in Rats after Oral and Intravenous Administration. *Mol. Nutr. Food Res.* **2012**, *56*, 466–474. [CrossRef] [PubMed]
109. Kores, K.; Kolenc, Z.; Furlan, V.; Bren, U. Inverse Molecular Docking Elucidating the Anticarcinogenic Potential of the Hop Natural Product Xanthohumol and Its Metabolites. *Foods* **2022**, *11*, 1253. [CrossRef]
110. Żołnierczyk, A.K.; Baczyńska, D.; Potaniec, B.; Kozłowska, J.; Grabarczyk, M.; Woźniak, E.; Anioł, M. Antiproliferative and Antioxidant Activity of Xanthohumol Acyl Derivatives. *Med. Chem. Res.* **2017**, *26*, 1764–1771. [CrossRef]
111. Moens, E.; Bolca, S.; Van de Wiele, T.; Van Landschoot, A.; Goeman, J.L.; Possemiers, S.; Verstraete, W. Exploration of Isoxanthohumol Bioconversion from Spent Hops into 8-Prenylnaringenin Using Resting Cells of Eubacterium Limosum. *AMB Express* **2020**, *10*, 79. [CrossRef]
112. Li, Q.; Li, X.; Zhao, C. Strategies to Obtain Encapsulation and Controlled Release of Small Hydrophilic Molecules. *Front. Bioeng. Biotechnol.* **2020**, *8*, 437. [CrossRef]
113. Peng, S.; Li, P. Applications of Nanomaterials and Nanotechnology in Biomedicine. In *Nanomaterials and Nanotechnology: Basic, Preparation and Applications*; Peng, S., Li, P., Eds.; Springer Nature: Singapore, 2024; pp. 411–451, ISBN 978-981-97-8433-2.
114. Kirchinger, M.; Bieler, L.; Tevini, J.; Vogl, M.; Haschke-Becher, E.; Felder, T.K.; Couillard-Després, S.; Riepl, H.; Urmann, C. Development and Characterization of the Neuroregenerative Xanthohumol C/Hydroxypropyl-β-Cyclodextrin Complex Suitable for Parenteral Administration. *Planta Med.* **2019**, *85*, 1233–1241. [CrossRef]
115. Dhiman, N.; Awasthi, R.; Sharma, B.; Kharkwal, H.; Kulkarni, G.T. Lipid Nanoparticles as Carriers for Bioactive Delivery. *Front. Chem.* **2021**, *9*, 580118. [CrossRef]
116. Ranjbar, S.; Emamjomeh, A.; Sharifi, F.; Zarepour, A.; Aghaabbasi, K.; Dehshahri, A.; Sepahvand, A.M.; Zarrabi, A.; Beyzaei, H.; Zahedi, M.M.; et al. Lipid-Based Delivery Systems for Flavonoids and Flavonolignans: Liposomes, Nanoemulsions, and Solid Lipid Nanoparticles. *Pharmaceutics* **2023**, *15*, 1944. [CrossRef]
117. Ashfaq, R.; Rasul, A.; Asghar, S.; Kovács, A.; Berkó, S.; Budai-Szűcs, M. Lipid Nanoparticles: An Effective Tool to Improve the Bioavailability of Nutraceuticals. *Int. J. Mol. Sci.* **2023**, *24*, 15764. [CrossRef] [PubMed]
118. Tripathi, A.K.; Ray, A.K.; Mishra, S.K. Molecular and Pharmacological Aspects of Piperine as a Potential Molecule for Disease Prevention and Management: Evidence from Clinical Trials. *Beni Suef Univ. J. Basic. Appl. Sci.* **2022**, *11*, 16. [CrossRef] [PubMed]
119. Sa, S.; Sa, C.; Sb, S.; Ra, D. Potential of Piperine as a Bioavailability Enhancer. *Int. J. Biol. Res.* **2019**, *4*, 3–6.
120. Dhiman, P.; Bhatia, M. Pharmaceutical Applications of Cyclodextrins and Their Derivatives. *J. Incl. Phenom. Macrocycl. Chem.* **2020**, *98*, 171–186. [CrossRef]
121. Łój, D.; Janeczko, T.; Bartmańska, A.; Huszcza, E.; Tronina, T. Biotransformation of Xanthohumol by Entomopathogenic Filamentous Fungi. *Int. J. Mol. Sci.* **2024**, *25*, 10433. [CrossRef]
122. Stevens, J.F. Xanthohumol and Structurally Related Prenylflavonoids for Cancer Chemoprevention and Control. In *Natural Products for Cancer Chemoprevention: Single Compounds and Combinations*; Pezzuto, J.M., Vang, O., Eds.; Springer International Publishing: Cham, Switzerland, 2020; pp. 319–350, ISBN 978-3-030-39855-2.
123. Vanhoecke, B.W.; Delporte, F.; Van Braeckel, E.; Heyerick, A.; Depypere, H.T.; Nuytinck, M.; De Keukeleire, D.; Bracke, M.E. A Safety Study of Oral Tangeretin and Xanthohumol Administration to Laboratory Mice. *In Vivo* **2005**, *19*, 103–107.
124. van Breemen, R.B.; Yuan, Y.; Banuvar, S.; Shulman, L.P.; Qiu, X.; Alvarenga, R.F.R.; Chen, S.-N.; Dietz, B.M.; Bolton, J.L.; Pauli, G.F.; et al. Pharmacokinetics of Prenylated Hop Phenols in Women Following Oral Administration of a Standardized Extract of Hops. *Mol. Nutr. Food Res.* **2014**, *58*, 1962–1969. [CrossRef]
125. Legette, L.; Karnpracha, C.; Reed, R.L.; Choi, J.; Bobe, G.; Christensen, J.M.; Rodriguez-Proteau, R.; Purnell, J.Q.; Stevens, J.F. Human Pharmacokinetics of Xanthohumol, an Antihyperglycemic Flavonoid from Hops. *Mol. Nutr. Food Res.* **2014**, *58*, 248–255. [CrossRef]
126. Dabrowski, W.; Gagos, M.; Siwicka-Gieroba, D.; Piechota, M.; Siwiec, J.; Bielacz, M.; Kotfis, K.; Stepulak, A.; Grzycka-Kowalczyk, L.; Jaroszynski, A.; et al. Humulus Lupus Extract Rich in Xanthohumol Improves the Clinical Course in Critically Ill COVID-19 Patients. *Biomed. Pharmacother.* **2023**, *158*, 114082. [CrossRef]

127. Langley, B.O.; Ryan, J.J.; Hanes, D.; Phipps, J.; Stack, E.; Metz, T.O.; Stevens, J.F.; Bradley, R. Xanthohumol Microbiome and Signature in Healthy Adults (the XMaS Trial): Safety and Tolerability Results of a Phase I Triple-Masked, Placebo-Controlled Clinical Trial. *Mol. Nutr. Food Res.* **2021**, *65*, e2001170. [CrossRef]
128. Grudzień, M.; Pawlak, A.; Tronina, T.; Kutkowska, J.; Kruszyńska, A.; Popłoński, J.; Huszcza, E.; Rapak, A. The Effect of Xanthohumol Derivatives on Apoptosis Induction in Canine Lymphoma and Leukemia Cell Lines. *Int. J. Mol. Sci.* **2023**, *24*, 11724. [CrossRef] [PubMed]
129. Choi, S.-S.; Kim, E.-S.; Jung, J.-E.; Marciano, D.P.; Jo, A.; Koo, J.Y.; Choi, S.Y.; Yang, Y.R.; Jang, H.-J.; Kim, E.-K.; et al. PPARγ Antagonist Gleevec Improves Insulin Sensitivity and Promotes the Browning of White Adipose Tissue. *Diabetes* **2016**, *65*, 829–839. [CrossRef] [PubMed]
130. Tavan, M.; Hanachi, P.; de la Luz Cádiz-Gurrea, M.; Segura Carretero, A.; Mirjalili, M.H. Natural Phenolic Compounds with Neuroprotective Effects. *Neurochem. Res.* **2024**, *49*, 306–326. [CrossRef] [PubMed]
131. Alunno, A.; Carubbi, F.; Giacomelli, R.; Gerli, R. Cytokines in the Pathogenesis of Rheumatoid Arthritis: New Players and Therapeutic Targets. *BMC Rheumatol.* **2017**, *1*, 3. [CrossRef]
132. Qiu, J.; Wu, B.; Goodman, S.B.; Berry, G.J.; Goronzy, J.J.; Weyand, C.M. Metabolic Control of Autoimmunity and Tissue Inflammation in Rheumatoid Arthritis. *Front. Immunol.* **2021**, *12*, 652771. [CrossRef]

molecules

MDPI

Review

Exploring the Therapeutic Value of Some Vegetative Parts of *Rubus* and *Prunus*: A Literature Review on Bioactive Profiles and Their Pharmaceutical and Cosmetic Interest

Andreea Georgiana Roșcan [1], Irina-Loredana Ifrim [2,*], Oana-Irina Patriciu [2] and Adriana-Luminița Fînaru [2,*]

1 Doctoral School in Environmental Engineering, "Vasile Alecsandri" University of Bacau, 157 Marasesti Str., 600115 Bacau, Romania; anroscan99@yahoo.ro

2 Department of Chemical and Food Engineering, "Vasile Alecsandri" University of Bacau, 157 Marasesti Str., 600115 Bacau, Romania; oana.patriciu@ub.ro

* Correspondence: irinaifrim@ub.ro (I.-L.I.); adrianaf@ub.ro (A.-L.F.)

Abstract

The resulting plant waste from *R. idaeus*, *P. serotina*, *P. avium*, and *P. cerasus* exhibits a complex chemical composition, depending on the variety from which it originates, with applications in multiple fields such as the food, pharmaceutical or dermato-cosmetic industry due to the presence of phytochemical compounds such as flavonoids, flavonols, tannins, cyanogenic glycosides, vitamins, aldehyde, and phenolic acids. The aim of this review was to summarize and analyze the most recent and significant data from literature on the importance of plant waste resulting from the pruning process of trees and shrubs, in the context of applying circular economy principles, with a focus on the pharmacological importance (antimicrobial, antioxidant, anti-inflammatory, anticoagulant, antiviral, and antitumoral) of some bioactive compounds identified in these species. Their applicability in various industries is closely linked to both the bioavailability of the final products and the study of their toxicity. The literature indicates that the isolation of these compounds can be carried out using conventional or modern methods, the last ones being favored due to the increased efficiency of the processes, as well as from the perspective of environmental protection. This review increases the attention and perspective of using plant waste as a linked source of pharmaceutical and dermato-cosmetic agents.

Keywords: plant waste; extraction; phytochemicals; biological activity; synergistic effect

1. Introduction

The concept of the circular economy can be effectively applied in the management of plant waste by valorizing by-products in alternative industrial processes [1]. Specialized literature highlights that the plant waste resulting from orchard maintenance work can be utilized by mulching the land, thus supporting the principle of the circular economy, and, in addition to the benefit of ecological fertilization, financial sustainability is also added [2]. Although current technologies for their valorization are promising, their large-scale applicability is still limited and requires further studies on the technical-economic viability of the methods [3].

Additionally, there are other methods for valorizing these wastes, but not all of them have a minimally invasive or even positive impact on the environment. For example, the use of woody biomass as an energy source has a negative ecological impact on the environment, highlighting the need to research more ecological and efficient alternatives for its valorization [4].

Gas emissions and fine particles resulting from combustion contribute to global warming, but human health is also impacted by air pollution [2,5]. A study from the USA highlighted that emissions from the bioenergy sector contribute a maximum of 17% to total emissions from all energy [6].

A viable method of valorization on cherry and sour cherry woody biomass resulting from orchard renewal is to use the wood to make barrels that are used in the food industry for aging distillates, wines, or vinegar [7]. In addition, in the food industry, the use of cherry wood for smoking cheeses, such as Cheddar, is notable [8], as well as in smoking pork preparations [9]. However, this preservation method can promote contamination of food with carcinogenic polycyclic aromatic hydrocarbons [10].

Recent studies suggest that plant waste can significantly contribute to the development of sustainable alternatives in various industries, even as a substitute for lignocellulos. For example, Öncül et al. demonstrated the viability of replacing filler materials with woody biomass of *P. avium* to obtain environmentally sustainable polymeric materials. The results showed that the biocomposite containing only 5% filler material exhibits optimal mechanical properties [11].

Cherry trees and raspberries, plants belonging to the *Rosaceae* family, have a distinct distribution: genus *Prunus* ssp. is found across all continents except Antarctica, and genus *Rubus* ssp. is mainly distributed throughout the temperate zone of the northern hemisphere. These species, easily adaptable to different environmental conditions (climate, soil, etc.), with a variable chemical composition depending on numerous factors such as cultivation techniques, region, ripening, harvesting, and storage, are well represented in the northeastern area of Romania [12].

Plant waste from species such as red raspberry (*Rubus idaeus*) and cherry trees (*Prunus avium*—sweet cherry, *Prunus serotina*—bitter black cherry, *Prunus cerasus*—sour cherry) exhibits significant pharmacological potential, representing a path for sustainable and ecological valorization. Red raspberry stems contain compounds with antioxidant, anti-inflammatory [13], and antitumoral [14] actions, making them attractive to the pharmaceutical industry. According to specialized literature, calcium and magnesium are the most representative minerals, in terms of quantity, found in red raspberry stems [15]. Additionally, the twigs of bitter black cherry and sweet cherry are rich in phytochemical compounds [16] with beneficial effects on health, including antioxidant and anti-inflammatory activities [17,18]. These plant wastes can be transformed into valuable ingredients in the pharmaceutical and cosmetic industries, having applicability in medical treatments as well as in the development of new products [19].

Up to now, all the results suggest that *Rubus* and *Prunus* wastes possess significant potential for further research to generate value-added products which can be applied in multiple industries, offering both economic and health benefits.

However, there is a need for more in-depth research to fully understand the potential of these resources and to optimize the extraction and utilization process of bioactive compounds.

This review summarizes the research progress related to the bioactive compound content of certain *Rubus* and *Prunus* species, their extraction and isolation, as well as information regarding their pharmacological applicability and limitations. Also, aspects presented in the specialized literature regarding the structure–activity relationship of bioactive compounds and the synergistic effect they can have are highlighted, which could open the way to new applications.

2. Research Methodology

The selection of specialized literature was carried out with particular care, applying clear criteria to guarantee both thematic relevance and the scientific quality of the sources used in the following databases: PubMed, Science Direct, and SpringerLink.

Only those studies that specifically explored the chemical composition, the possibilities of valorization, and the practical uses of plant waste from the four investigated species were included in the analysis, with a special emphasis on twigs and shoots—plant residues frequently resulting from maintenance or harvesting activities. In addition, priority was given to works that provided detailed characterizations of the plant material and/or proposed solutions applicable in various fields, such as the pharmaceutical, food, cosmetic, or agricultural industries.

The initial documentation generated a considerable volume of information, exceeding 50,000 scientific articles. A large part of this resulted from the combination of different search terms such as:

- the expression "*Rubus idaeus* + shoots + bioactive compounds" produced over 1570 relevant results;
- the search "*Prunus avium* + twigs + bioactive compounds" provided approximately 2400 studies;
- "*Prunus serotina* + twigs + bioactive compounds" led to the identification of 540 articles;
- and the formula "*Prunus cerasus* + twigs + bioactive compounds" returned more than 1000 works.

More general terms, such as plant waste, twigs, biomass, or extraction of phenolic compounds, generated a very large number of results (over 26,000 for prunus woody biomass and over 16,000 for *Rubus* woody biomass). However, only those sources that were directly related to the species analyzed were retained for evaluation.

The narrowing of the search period was determined by the relatively recent interest of researchers in the sustainable valorization of plant waste. Also, the desire to present the latest experimental observations regarding the extraction and isolation of bioactive compounds, which are also viable from an ecological point of view, was also the basis for limiting the search interval.

Considering the graph presented in Figure 1, there is an upward trend in recent years in the interest shown by specialists in the field for the four previously mentioned species.

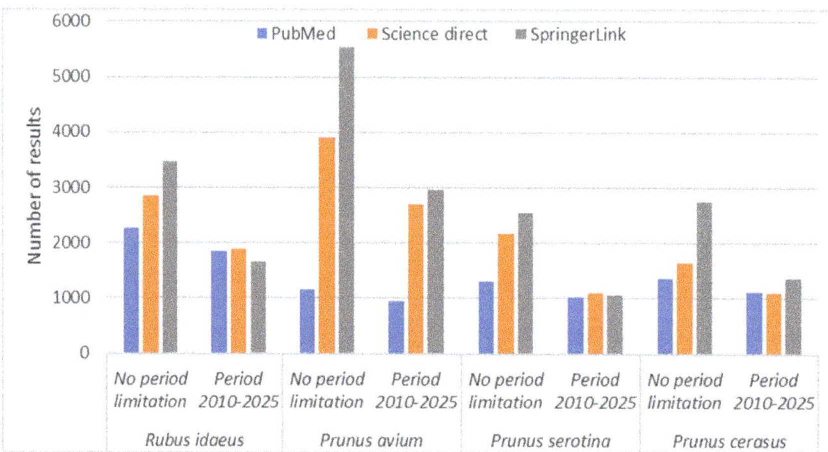

Figure 1. The distribution of articles by species published between 2010 and 2025.

After applying all the selection filters-which targeted the relevance of the subject, methodological clarity, applicative value, and the elimination of redundancies-over 300 scientific sources were finally retained, with less than 10% of these published before 2010. This rigorous approach was the basis for a well-founded synthesis, which highlights the real potential for valorization of twigs and shoots from the *R. idaeus*, *P. avium*, *P. serotina*, and *P. cerasus* species, contributing to the promotion of sustainable practices and the consolidation of the circular economy in the agricultural and industrial sectors.

3. Bioactive Compounds from Plant Waste of *Rubus idaeus*, *Prunus serotina*, *Prunus avium*, and *Prunus cerasus*

From both an ecological and economic perspective, plant waste, a diverse mixture of woody and vegetable by-products generated mainly through deforestation and landscape maintenance, orchards, etc., requires appropriate management to transform it into a valuable and sustainable resource.

It is worth noting that woody biomass, a heterogeneous material, which is mainly considered a source of three natural polymers (cellulose, hemicelluloses and lignin), also contains an extractable fraction, which, although minor (<9%), includes important classes of compounds with potential biological activity (terpenoids, phenolic compounds, tannins, glycosides, vitamins, fatty acids, minerals, etc.).

A recent study by Newman and Cragg [20] on the impact of natural substances on pharmaceutical products introduced on the market between 1981 and 2019 highlights that over 37% of the 1881 molecules marketed during this period are based on natural sources: 71 are strictly natural, 356 are derivatives of natural substances obtained by semi-synthesis, and 272 are obtained by organic synthesis, having a pharmacophore inspired by natural substances. These data confirm the importance of focusing on the efficient valorization of the vegetative parts of *Rubus* and *Prunus* as sources of bioactive compounds (Figure 2).

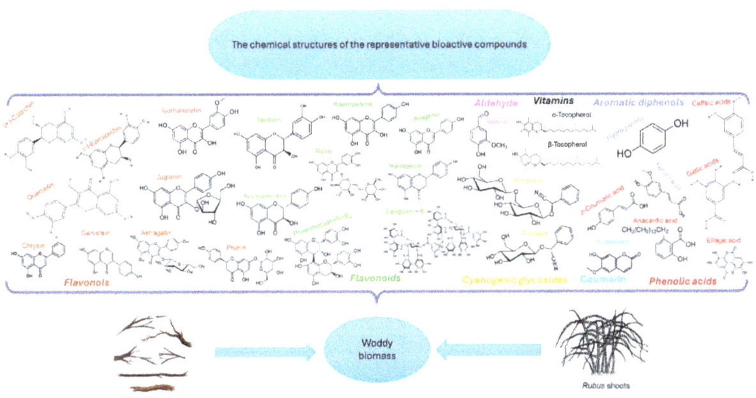

Figure 2. The chemical structures of the representative bioactive compounds from *Prunus* and *Rubus* woody biomass with health benefits.

The studied literature showed that there is a relative similarity in the chemical composition of the three *Prunus* species, but specific bioactive compounds have also been identified, such as juglanin [17] and prunasin [19] in *P. serotina*, taxifolin and vanillin [7] in *P. avium*, and phlorizin [21] and galangin [22] in *P. cerasus*. On the other hand, *R. idaeus* stands out due to its content of sanguiin H6 [23] and casuarinin [24]. Among the biologically active chemical compounds identified in all plant sources are caffeic acid and p-coumaric acid, among others [25–27].

In the following table, several bioactive compounds found in the four plant sources are presented, for which concentrations have also been identified in the specialized literature.

According to the data presented in Table 1, it is observed that *R. idaeus* exhibits a higher concentration of bioactive compounds common with *Prunus* species, but there are also exceptions, such as chlorogenic and *p*-coumaric acids, which are found in higher concentrations in *P. avium*, as well as ferulic acid, which has a higher concentration in *P. serotina*.

Table 1. Representative classes/bioactive compounds found in different plant parts of *R. idaeus*, *P. serotina*, *P. avium*, and *P. cerasus*.

Bioactive Compound	Source	Content	References
	Flavonols		
Catechin	*P. serotina* (dry leaves)	605–2342 mg/kg	[27]
	R. idaeus (Willlamette: non-lignified dry shoots)	129.3 mg/100 g	[23]
	P. avium (wood)	0.32–30.15 mg/g	[7]
	P. avium (dry leaves and branches)	6.879 mg/g and 0.42–3.74 mg/g	[28]
	P. cerasus (resin)	1.91 mg/L	[22]
	P. avium (resin)	0.33 mg/L	[22]
Epicatechin	*R. idaeus* (non-lignified dry shoots)	10.9–85.3 mg/100 g	[23]
	P. avium (wood)	0.36 mg/g	[7]
	P. avium (dry branches)	0.0873–0.1102 mg/g	[28]
Quercetin	*P. avium* (resin)	1.77 mg/L	[22]
	P. cerasus (resin)	0.63 mg/L	[22]
Quercetin derivates	*R. idaeus* (non-lignified dry shoots)	10.3–67.4 mg/100 g	[23]
Quercetin 3-*O*-rutinoside	*P. avium* (dry branches)	404.39–767 μg/g	[29]
Quercetin 3-*O*-hexosides	*P. avium* (dry branches)	665.76–1025.78 μg/g	[29]
Chrysin	*P. avium* (resin)	1.57 mg/L	[22]
	P. cerasus (resin)	0.16 mg/L	[22]
Genistein (genistein-7-*O*-glucoside)	*P. avium* (dry branches)	0.42–3.74 mg/g	[28]
	Flavonoids		
Kaempferol-3-*O*-rutinoside	*R. idaeus* (dry leaves)	37.92 mg/g	[24]
	P. avium (dry leaves and branches)	6.6 mg/g and 0.88 mg/g	[28]
Kaempeferol	*R. idaeus* (dry leaves)	1.88–82.28 g/100 g	[30]
	P. cerasus (resin)	1.04 mg/L	[22]
	P. avium (resin)	0.22 mg/L	[22]
Rutin	*P. cerasus* (resin)	0.22 mg/L	[22]
	P. avium (resin)	0.19 mg/L	[22]
Apigenin hidroxihexoside	*P. serotina* (dry leaves)	57.4–63.4 mg/kg	[27]
Apigenin	*P. avium* (dry branches)	0.033 mg/g	[28]
Aromadendrin	*P. avium* (wood)	0.08–4.54 g/kg	[7]
Aromadendrin-7-*O*-hexoside	*P. avium* (dry branches)	0.86–2.66 mg/g	[28]

Table 1. *Cont.*

Bioactive Compound	Source	Content	References
Naringenin	*P. avium* (resin) *P. cerasus* (resin) *P. avium* (dry leaves) *P. avium* (wood) *P. serotina* (lyophilized leaves)	5.01 mg/L 4.73 mg/L 0.74 mg/g 0.17–0.41 mg/g 0.13 mg/100 g	[22] [22] [28] [7] [16]
Naringenin-7-*O*-hexoside	*P. avium* (dry branches)	1482.67–1940.77 µg/g	[29]
Taxifolin	*P. avium* (wood) *P. avium* (dry branches)	0.09–8.46 mg/g 0.19–0.79 mg/g	[7] [28]
	Tannins		
Proanthocyanidin B_1	*R. idaeus* (Willlamette: non-lignified dry shoots) *P. avium* (wood)	229 mg/100 g 0.15 mg/g	[23] [7]
Proanthocyanidin B_2	*R. idaeus* (Willlamette: non-lignified dry shoots) *P. avium* (wood)	646 mg/100 g 0.72 mg/g	[23] [7]
Proanthocyanidin dimer B type 2	*P. avium* (dry branches)	7149.5–8810.67 µg/g	[29]
Proanthocyanidin dimer type B	*P. avium* (wood)	3.65 mg/g	[7]
Proanthocyanidin trimer type B	*P. avium* (wood)	1.25 mg/g	[7]
Sanguiin H-6	*R. idaeus* (non-lignified dry shoots)	139.2–633.1 mg/100 g	[23]
	Cyanogenic glycosides		
Prunasin	*P. serotina* (leaves)	59.49 mg/g	[16]
Amigdalin	*P. serotina* (leaves)	20.95 mg/g	[16]
	Vitamins		
α-Tocopherol	*P. avium* (lyophilized branches)	512.58 µg/100 g	[31]
β-Tocopherol	*P. avium* (lyophilized branches)	31.94 µg/100 g	[31]
γ-Tocopherol	*P. avium* (lyophilized branches)	23.58 µg/100 g	[31]
	Aldehyde		
Vanillin	*P. avium* (wood)	4.68 mg/g	[7]
	P. avium (dry branches)	0.079 mg/g	[28]
	Phenolic acids		
Ellagic acid	*R. idaeus* (non-lignified dry shoots) *P. avium* (wood)	26.1–106.8 mg/100 g 0.27 mg/g	[23] [7]
Chlorogenic acid	*R. idaeus* (Willlamette: non-lignified dry shoots) *P. serotina* (lyophilized leaves) *P. avium* (dry leaves) *P. avium* (resin) *P. cerasus* (resin)	177.4 mg/100 g 29.5 mg/100 g 17.06 mg/g 0.62 mg/L 0.27 mg/L	[23] [16] [28] [22] [22]

Table 1. *Cont.*

Bioactive Compound	Source	Content	References
Gallic acid	*R. idaeus* (Willlamette: non-lignified dry shoots)	72.2 mg/100 g	[23]
	P. serotina (lyophilized leaves)	19.56 mg/100 g	[16]
	P. avium (dry branches)	0.041–0.05 mg/g	[28]
Caffeic acid	*R. idaeus* (dry leaves)	0.64–7.21 mg/g	[32]
	P. serotina (dry leaves)	75–158.8 mg/kg	[27]
Ferulic acid	*P. serotina* (lyophilized leaves)	185.3 mg/100 g	[16]
	P. avium (dry branches)	0.22–0.23 mg/g	[28]
	R. idaeus (dry leaves)	0.1–0.49 mg/g	[32]
p-Coumaric acid	*P. serotina* (lyophilized leaves)	103.6 mg/100 g	[16]
	P. avium (wood)	26.3 mg/g	[7]
	R. idaeus (dry leaves)	0.07–0.95 mg/g	[32]
	P. avium (dry branches)	0.038–0.161 mg/g	[28]

The polyphenol concentration was investigated in 11 varieties of *R. idaeus;* the presence of pentoside quercetin was identified in a single variety, with a concentration of 23.9 g/100 g dry shoot sample, while the compound sanguiin was identified in 10 out of 11 varieties [23]. The rarity of quercetin pentoside may be justified by different climatic growing conditions or the earlier character of the variety. A specialized study aimed at identifying the impact of covering fruit trees with anti-hail netting on the phytochemical profile revealed that direct exposure to sunlight can lead to a lower content of quercetin pentoside compared to the content when the crop is covered [33]. The stems are notable for their content of chlorogenic acid and proanthocyanidin B1, but smaller amounts of catechin, salicylic acid, and astragalin are also present [15]. The dominant component in the leaf extract of *R. idaeus* is casuarinin, which constitutes 83% of all identified polyphenolic compounds in the extract [24]. Although the studies consulted did not explicitly highlight the presence of casuarinine in the extracts, it was noted that ellagitannins, a class to which casuarinine also belongs, are found in high concentrations in the leaf extract [34].

In contrast to *Rubus*, *Prunus* species show divergent trends in phenolic distribution. The total phenolic content, expressed in mg gallic acid/g dry sample, is significantly higher in *P. avium* branches (301.98) compared to leaves (100.71) or flowers (81.2). On the other hand, the flavonoid content is lower in branch samples, whether it is hydroethanolic extract or infusion [28].

Among the organic acids mentioned by various studies [31,35], the significant presence, both in fruits and in plant waste, of malic and quinic acids is noteworthy, while tartaric, citric, succinic, or oxalic acids showed a marginal content.

In a study that includes a comparative chemical analysis of the fruits and branches of *P. avium*, it was highlighted that the amount of oxalic acid in the branches is double that of the content in cherries, and the citric acid content is approximately 35 times higher in the branches. Significant differences were also identified in the tocopherol content, with γ-tocopherol being identified only in the branches [31].

Wojdyło et al. [35] demonstrated through the analysis of extracts obtained from fruits and leaves of *P. avium* and *P. cerasus* that there is a higher concentration of polyphenolic compounds in leaves compared to fruits, regardless of the analyzed variety. However, it is worth mentioning that anthocyanins were identified only in fruit extracts.

The polyphenolic compounds in the leaves were quite diverse; therefore, it can be considered that the leaves may represent an alternative, unconventional, and cheap source of antioxidants and preservatives, with various uses in the pharmaceutical, cosmetic, and food industries [35].

Overall, these results (Table 1) clearly indicate that the accumulation of bioactive compounds is closely dependent on the plant part analyzed.

Also, the differences between the results reported in various studies regarding the presence/absence of some compounds and their quantity could be explained by the stage of development of the analyzed parts, as well as by the different applied extraction/separation and identification methodologies.

4. Extraction and Isolation Methods

4.1. Extraction

The methods for extracting bioactive compounds from the woody biomass of various trees and shrubs are extremely diverse. The literature highlights that a number of solvents used for the extraction of compounds from different parts of berry plants are also effective for red raspberries: acidified ethanol–water extraction to obtain anthocyanidins, procyanidins, or caffeoylquinic acids [36]; methanolic extraction to obtain polyphenolic compounds and flavonoids; acetone–water mixture extraction to isolate tannins and methanol-hydrochloric acid solution for anthocyanins [37]. Considering that some extracts may have applicability in the food industry, the use of solvents such as methanol is not safe; therefore, the adoption of green technologies, such as subcritical water extraction, is necessary [38].

Regarding the extraction of bioactive compounds from cherry branches, a study comparing conventional extraction with ethanol (70 °C) to accelerated extraction (150 °C), also using ethanol as a solvent, concluded that the extraction temperature affects the quantity of bioactive compounds obtained more than the percentage of ethanol used. [39].

On the other hand, in light of the use of green extraction technologies for cherry plant parts, data from the literature has noted the use of supercritical carbon dioxide extraction [40], a technique that can also be applied to cherry woody biomass [41] or other plant samples [42].

To optimize this method, one can also resort to coupling it with microwave-assisted extraction. The application of the two combined techniques led to the optimization of extraction under the following conditions: particle size of approximately 0.3–0.4 mm, liquid–solid ratio of 54 mL/g, and extraction time of 30 min [43].

Table 2 presents the representative extraction methods applied to the four plant sources studied.

Table 2. Extraction methods of bioactive compounds, applied to different types of plant waste from *Rubus* and *Prunus* species.

Bioactive Compound/Class of Compounds	Sources	Extraction Methods	References
		R. idaeus	
Non-extractable/bound phenolic compounds	leaves	Acid and enzymatic hydrolysis (especially for ellagic acid)	[44]
Phenolic compounds	dry, non-lignified shoots	Soxhlet, using chloroform and methanol	[23,45]
	dry leaves	Reflux extraction	[30]
	dry leaves	Aqueous extraction in a mass ratio of 3:1	[24]
	dry leaves	Extraction with acetone and trichloromethane	[32]
	lyophilized leaves	Alcoholic extraction (2 g sample in 80 mL 70% methanol) with stirring	[46]
	dried leaves and woody material	Ultrasound-assisted extraction, using 1 g of dried and ground sample, 30 mL of 80:20 ethanol–water solution	[47]

Table 2. *Cont.*

Bioactive Compound/Class of Compounds	Sources	Extraction Methods	References
Polyphenols, catechins, hydroxycinnamic acids, flavonoids	shoots	Reflux extraction (solid–liquid)	[48]
Quercetin 3-glucosid and K_2 vitamin	frozen leaves	Ultrasound-assisted extraction (solvent: methanol–acetonitrile–water solution in a volume ratio of 2:2:1)	[49]
Carotenoids	lyophilized leaves	Extraction with acetone and hexane (4:6 *v/v*)	[46]
		P. serotina	
Phenolic compounds	dry leaves lyophilized leaves	Ultrasound-assisted methanol extraction Aqueous extraction	[27] [16]
Tannins	dry bark	Reflux extraction (25 g sample + 200 mL 90% ethyl alcohol + 200 mL glacial acetic acid)	[50]
		P. avium	
Phenolic compounds	dry branches	Pressurized liquid extraction (ethanol–water) Supercritical fluid extraction (CO_2)	[26]
	lyophilized branches	Hydromethanolic extraction (80/20 *v/v*)–decoction Infusion (distilled water)	[31]
	lyophilized leaves	Extraction with water/methanol/ascorbic acid/hydrochloric acid 37% (6.8:3:0.1:0.1; *v/v/g/v*), assisted by ultrasound	[35]
	dry bark	Ultrasound-assisted extraction (solvent: 80% aqueous ethanol solution)	[51]
Fatty acids, organic and phenolic acids, aromatic aldehydes, isoprenoids	dry branches	Subcritical water extraction	[52]
Hydroxycinnamic acids	salks and leaves	Maceration Supercritical fluid extraction–CO_2	[53]
Caffeic acid	salks	Solvent extraction, maceration	[53]
Proanthocyanidin	salks	Accelerated solvent extraction	[53]
Catechin	salks	Solvent extraction, supercritical fluid extraction, ultrasound-assisted extraction	[53]
		P. cerasus	
Phenolic compounds	lyophilized leaves	Extraction with water/methanol/ascorbic acid/hydrochloric acid 37% (6.8:3:0.1:0.1; *v/v/g/v*), assisted by ultrasound	[35]
Fatty acids, organic and phenolic acids, aromatic aldehydes, isoprenoids	dry branches	Subcritical water extraction	[52]

According to the data presented in the previous table, it is observed that, at least in the case of phenolic compounds, for all four plant sources, the extraction using ethanol or methanol as a solvent is among the most commonly used, also having satisfactory yields. Even if the extraction process can be optimized by using modern green methods, the presence of the alcoholic solvent could ensure performance regardless of the nature of the plant source.

The content of ellagic acid obtained in the extract from aerial parts of *R. idaeus* varies depending on the method used, as follows: 3.24 mg/g extract for decoction (solvent: water), 3.12 mg/g extract for infusion (solvent: water), 2.45 mg/g extract for maceration (hydroalcoholic solvent), and 2.38 mg/g extract for ultrasound-assisted extraction (hydroalcoholic solvent) [47]. The same study mentions that for phenol extraction, ultrasound-assisted extraction is more efficient, while for flavonoids, infusion and maceration are recommended. Knowing that the solubility of ellagic acid in water and alcohol is influenced by temperature, probably, these results obtained, better in the case of extraction by decoction and infusion, are due to the different working conditions: the high temperature of the decoction and infusion versus UAE in an ice bath and maceration at ambient temperature, respectively. Among the natural sources of ellagic acid, some studies mention residues from the wood industry as an attractive alternative in terms of commercial exploitation. But at the same time, it is emphasized that it is necessary to find an ecological extraction methodology, knowing that currently the production of commercial ellagic acid from natural sources is based on obtaining extracts from plants rich in ellagitannins using acid–methanol mixtures as solvents, followed by their hydrolysis in a strongly acidic environment (HCl or concentrated H_2SO_4) [54].

A study conducted in 2021 by Brozdowski et al. demonstrated that in the case of phenolic compounds extracted from dried cherry leaves/flowers (*P. serotina*), the content was significantly higher when methanol was used as the solvent, compared to aqueous extraction [27]. Ademović et al. showed that the use of ethanol as a solvent led to an increase in the total content of phenols and flavonoids compared to the aqueous extraction of dried *P. avium* branches, achieving concentrations 3 and 4 times higher in the first case, respectively [18]. Taking into account the field in which these extracts are intended to be utilized, even if the extraction yield when using methanol or alcohol has proven to be more efficient than an aqueous medium, it is desirable to use eco-friendly solvents.

Regarding the chemical composition of the branches of *P. avium* and *P. cerasus*, there are no significant differences in the case of extracts obtained with subcritical water, which also supports the relatively similar biological activity [55].

4.2. Isolation

The main techniques for refining and fractionating crude extracts in order to isolate one or more groups of bioactive molecules found in *Rubus* and *Prunus* species are presented in Table 3.

Table 3. Isolation methods applicable to some representative bioactive compounds.

Bioactive Compound	Isolation Methods	Observations	References
Anacardic acid	Obtaining the extract using supercritical carbon dioxide, followed by precipitation in the form of calcium anacardate, which, after treatment with hydrochloric acid, is converted back into anacardic acid	It is a thermolabile compound, and distillation under low pressure favors the acid thermal decomposition into cardanol	[56]
Chlorogenic acid	Surface imprint polymerization based on hyper-branched amino magnetic nanoparticles	Soluble in water It is a thermosensitive compound and easily oxidized	[57,58]
Ellagic acid	The use of cotton fibers grafted with graphene oxide promotes insulation through hydrophobic interaction, serving as a stationary absorbent	It is thermally stable Slightly soluble in water, alcohol, and ether Soluble in potassium hydroxide High solubility in pyridine	[54,59,60]

Table 3. *Cont.*

Bioactive Compound	Isolation Methods	Observations	References
Apigenin	The hydroalcoholic, methanolic, or ethyl acetate fractions of the aqueous extract are subjected to column chromatography and preparative HPLC The methanolic extract is subjected to partitioning with ethyl acetate, followed by column chromatography on silica gel for separation, thin-layer chromatography for purification, and NMR spectroscopy for compound confirmation	Low solubility in lipophilic and highly hydrophilic solvents High solubility in phosphate buffers with pH 7.5 Low solubility in water	[61–63]
Astragalin	The ethyl acetate fraction is concentrated and isolated by column chromatography (TLC and HPLC) on silica gel, using a mixture of ethyl acetate, methanol, and water as the eluent	Solubility is reduced in water	[64,65]
Hydroquinone	The crude extract is loaded onto a silica gel column (ethyl acetate and hexane), followed by purification through semi-preparative HPLC (methanol-water)	Soluble in methanol, ether, and water It oxidizes in contact with air and light Significant thermal sensitivity	[66–68]
Isorhamnetin	High-speed countercurrent preparative chromatography	Low solubility in water Thermal stability	[69–71]
Juglanin	The alcoholic extract is subjected to Sephadex column chromatography on silica gel, using a mixture of chloroform, methanol, and water as the eluent	Great solubility in water	[72,73]
Kaempeferol	The alcohol is evaporated under vacuum from the methanolic extract, yielding an ethyl acetate fraction that is separated with n-hexane and subjected to vacuum liquid chromatography, followed by other chromatographic techniques (Sephadex column and TLC) until the target compound is isolated	Low solubility in water Thermal stability	[74–76]
Naringenin	Methanolic extraction followed by crystallization in water containing 14–15% dichloromethane	Low solubility in water Solubility in different solvents: ethyl acetate > isopropanol > methanol > n-butanol > petroleum ether > hexane	[77–79]
Proanthocyanidins	Sephadex column chromatography	Solubility varies directly proportionally with temperature; in alcohol, it decreases with increasing molecular weight; it exhibits shorter interaction times with tetrahydrofuran and ethyl acetate	[80,81]
Prunin	The methanolic extract is divided into several fractions, the one soluble in ethyl acetate is subjected to silica gel chromatography, a mixture of chloroform and methanol is used as the eluent, followed by a separation using Sephadex, with methanol as the solvent	Low solubility in lipophilic media	[82,83]

Table 3. *Cont.*

Bioactive Compound	Isolation Methods	Observations	References
Quercetin	The chloroform fraction of the ethanolic extract is subjected to column chromatography on silica gel, using a mixture of methanol, chloroform, and ethyl acetate as solvents. The use of a mixture of formic acid, water, and methanol in a gradient system, through the HPLC-DAD-MS/MS method. The application of column chromatography on polyamide of the ethyl acetate fraction	Insoluble in water. Stability to light in concentrations greater than 10% Unstable when exposed to atmospheric oxygen Thermal stability	[61,76,84, 85]
Rutin	Dichloromethane fractions or aqueous fractions with a higher rutin content are obtained, which are chromatographically separated on a Sephadex column with methanol as the mobile phase	Low liposolubility. Increases water solubility through glycosylation	[86–88]
Sanguiin H6	Quantification from the hydrolytic solution, by HPLC	Soluble in water Hydrolyzes in acidic or basic environments, giving rise to ellagic acid	[89]
Scopoletin	Chromatographic separation (TLC or HPLC) with elution in a mixture of methanol and other compounds (chloroform, acetonitrile, acetic acid)	It is soluble in water and stable in solution at a pH between 3 and 10, a stability that can be extended in time and pH range by the addition of methanol	[90,91]

The data presented in the previous table highlight chromatographic methods as the most frequently used in the isolation of the bioactive compounds targeted in this study. Additionally, their lack of or low affinity for water is highlighted, and thermolabile or thermostable compounds appear in the isolate (Table 3). The literature has highlighted the fact that aglycone flavonoids degrade faster under the influence of temperature, compared to glycosylated ones [92]. It is important to mention the concern for a reproducible isolation and the application of specific structural confirmation methods (^{1}H NMR, ^{13}C NMR, HMBC, HSQC, COSY, NOESY, MS, UV absorption spectroscopy, etc.), robust and accurate to preserve the quality and activity of the phytocompounds and the extracts obtained.

5. Biological Activity

5.1. Pharmacological Importance, Bioavailability, and Toxicity

The biological activity of red raspberry, sweet cherry, sour cherry, and black cherry extracts can be determined both by the presence of common bioactive compounds identified in the four plant sources described previously, as well as by those specific to each species. Table 4 summarizes the information from the literature regarding their pharmacological activity, bioavailability, and toxicity.

Table 4. Correlation of bioactive compound–pharmacological activity, bioavailability, and toxicity [17,65,67,70,75,78,87,93–250].

	Bioactive Compound	Pharmacological Activity	Ref	Bioavailability and Toxicity	Ref
			R. idaeus		
Phenols	Anacardic acid	Bactericide, anticancerogenic, fungicide, insecticide, anti-termite, and molluscicidal Tyrosinase and urease inhibition	[93,94]	Physicochemical stability and low water solubility result in limited bioavailability One of the main culprits of cashew allergy is due to the presence of the carboxyl group and the unsaturated side chain May induce allergic contact dermatitis	[93,96]
		Prevention and treatment of breast cancer	[95]		
	Sanguiin H6	Antioxidant Anticancerigenic (breast)	[97]	Low upon oral administration, being stable in the acidic environment of the stomach, hydrolysis is possible in the intestinal environment It has no adverse effects	[100,101]
		Anti-inflammatory	[98]		
		Antiangiogenic	[99]		
Flavonoids	Quercetin ramnoside	Antioxidant and liver protection	[102–104]	Higher than quercetin Does not present any potential toxicity to animals	[107,108]
		Antivirals	[105]		
		Restoring the intestinal microbiota	[106]		
	Astragalin (kaempferol 3-glucoside)	Antidepressant	[109]	Low, structural modification by enzymatic synthesis is suggested Studies conducted to date have not revealed any toxic activity of this compound	[65,115]
		Hypoglycemic	[110]		
		Anti-inflammatory, antioxidant, neuroprotective, cardioprotective, antiobesity, antiosteoporotic, anticancer, antiulcer, and antidiabetic	[111,112]		
		Analgesic, procoagulant, antibacterial, antiallergic, and antihepatotoxic	[113]		
		Neuroprotective	[114]		
Vegetal hormones	Kinetin	Antioxidant	[116]	Good oral absorption. Is not mutagenic nor cardiotoxic	[118]
		Inhibition of colorectal cancer	[117]		
	Salicylic acid	Antimicrobial and anti-inflammatory	[119]	Higher bioavailability in intravenous form compared to oral administration Topical toxicity is rare	[121,122]
		Obtaining the 4-chloro-5-chlorosulfonyl salicylic acid derivative–diuretic agent	[120]		
Vitamins	Ascorbic Acid (Vitamin C)	Antioxidant, anticancer Wound healing	[123]	Intravenous bioavailability is higher compared to oral Does not show toxicity even in higher doses	[124,125]
	Tocopherol (Vitamin E)	Antioxidant, platelet anticoagulant	[126]	The absorption efficiency can be close to 80%, but it depends on many factors (pH, presence of proteins, etc.)	[127]
			P. serotina		
Phenols	Hydroquinone (1,4 dihydroxy-benzene)	Reduces hyperpigmentation (possible side effects) May cause ochronosis	[128–130]	Improved permeability may be associated with an increase in toxicity due to poor physicochemical stability The instability of this compound can lead to the formation of potentially carcinogenic products, but skin and eye side effects can also be recorded It has high toxicity for the aquatic environment and soil In human and animal organisms, it promotes the occurrence of cancer, damages DNA, and favors allergic immune responses	[67,131,132]
		Antiphotoaging	[131]		
Flavonoids	Kaempferol	Antimicrobial, anti-inflammatory, antioxidant, antitumor, cardioprotective, neuroprotective, and antidiabetic, anticarcinogenic	[133]	Low May react with iron and decrease bioavailability May decrease the action of anticancer drugs Possible genotoxic action	[75,135]
		Antifungal and antiprotozoal, hepatoprotective, renoprotective, gastroprotective, and antimutagenic	[134]		
		Effective in treating cervical cancer	[112]		

Table 4. *Cont.*

	Bioactive Compound	Pharmacological Activity	Ref	Bioavailability and Toxicity	Ref
Flavonols	Juglanin (kaempferol 3-O-α-L-arabinofuranoside)	Anti-inflammatory, antioxidant, antifibrotic, antithrombotic, antiangiogenic, hepatoprotective, hypolipidemic, hypoglycemic	[17]	Good, especially in glycoside form. Low probability of presenting toxicity when ingested, but significant when applied topically.	[17]
		Renal protection	[136]		
		Antidepressant	[137]		
		Procoagulant effect	[138]		
	Isorhamnetin	Neuroprotective, cardioprotective, antioxidant, anti-inflammatory, and antiapoptosis	[139]	Higher than quercetin as a liver protector It has no adverse effects and reduces those associated with classic cancer treatment	[70,143]
		Antiobesity	[140]		
		Antiviral	[141]		
		Anticoagulants	[142]		
Terpen	Squalen	Antitumor, antioxidant, and emollient activity on the skin	[144]	High cutaneous availability	[146]
		Vaccine adjuvant	[145]		
Cyanogenic glycoside	Prunasin	Treating respiratory conditions (risk of toxicity–cyanide release)	[146]	Larger in the form of decoction. Cyanide can be eliminated through hydrolysis, the lethal dose of which is 0.5 – 3.5 mg/kg body weight	[151,152]
		Anticarcinogenic properties	[147]		
		Anti-inflammatory and antioxidant	[148]		
		Hepatoprotective and antifibrogenic	[149,150]		
			P. avium		
Flavonoids	Taxifolin	Anticarcinogenic (minimal adverse effects) Anti-inflammatory, hepatoprotective, antioxidant, cardioprotective, antimicrobial, antiviral, antifungal, antiangiogenic, antihyperglycemic, antipsoriatic, anti-Alzheimer	[153,154]	Low bioavailability Compared to quercetin, this compound is not phototoxic.	[155,156]
	Aroma-dendrin	Anti-inflammatory, antioxidant, antidiabetic, antiproliferative, antimicrobial, hepatoprotective, and gastroprotective	[157]	Studies suggest that it is not a mutagenic compound, but may exhibit promutagenic activity	[159]
		Antityrosinase, neuroprotective, cardioprotective, antiviral, immunomodulatory, antiacetylcholinesterase, antiapoptotic, antityrosinase, neuroprotective, cardioprotective, antiviral, immunomodulatory, antiacetylcholinesterase, antiapoptotic	[158]		
	Naringenin	Antioxidant, antitumor, antiviral, antibacterial, anti-inflammatory, antiadipogenic, anticancer, antiproliferative, and cardioprotective anti-HCV (hepatitis C virus)	[160]	Small, but still larger than that of the plum There are no adverse reactions recorded when administered to humans. In amphibian embryos, it produced mutations or death in fairly low doses.	[78,164, 165]
		Antidiabetic	[161]		
		Antifibrogenic	[162]		
		Neuroprotective, antidiabetic, antidepressant	[163]		

Table 4. *Cont.*

	Bioactive Compound	Pharmacological Activity	Ref	Bioavailability and Toxicity	Ref
Flavonoids	Apigenin	Radioprotective and radiosensitive	[166]	Oral bioavailability approaches 30% and increases with coadministration with friedelin.	[169,170]
		Neuroprotective, antidiabetic, antidepressant, anti-insomnia	[167]		
		Hepatoprotective, renoprotective, cardioprotective, antimicrobial, dermatoprotective (anti-UV, antiaging, combats dermatitis and supports wound healing), antiarthritic Supports oral and ocular health	[168]		
	Prunin	Antioxidant, anti-inflammatory, anticancer, immune regulation, antiosteoporosis, antihypoxia, and protective effects for the lungs, liver and kidneys	[171]	Exhibits selective toxicity for cancer cells, but glycosylated derivatives develop lower toxicity on human cells. Glycosylation at position 7 is responsible for increasing bioavailability	[171]
		Antiviral effect (Human Enterovirus A17)	[172]		
		Antidiabetic	[173]		
		Antianxiety	[174]		
		Broad-spectrum antibacterial activity	[175]		
Flavone	Chrysin (5,7-dihydro-xyflavone)	Anti-inflammatory, anticancer, antidiabetic, antirachitic, antiasthmatic, antidepressant, neuroprotective	[176]	Low in oral administration caused by poor absorption, metabolism and rapid elimination At a dose of 400–500 mg, it does not cause any notable adverse effects, but it is likely to induce liver toxicity at the cellular level and inhibit de novo DNA synthesis	[176]
		Antihypercholesterolemic, cardioprotective, antiepileptic, antiamyloidogenic, antiatherogenic	[177]		
		Antidiabetic, antioxidant, antihyperlipidemic	[178]		
	Genistein	Effects of reducing the risk of osteoporosis and post-menopausal symptoms, as well as anticancer, antioxidant, cardioprotective, antiapoptotic, neuroprotective, hepatoprotective, and antimicrobial activities.	[179]	It grows in glycosylated form. Minimal toxicity at doses up to 16 mg/kg body weight	[181]
		Treating thrombocytopenia	[180]		
Aldehydes	Vanillin	Neuroprotective, anti-inflammatory, antifungal, antibacterial, antiviral, and anticancer Modulates the activities of antibiotics	[182]	May pose health risks by increasing the absorption of drugs with moderate oral bioavailability.	[183]
Carboxylic acids	Cinamic acid	Antioxidant, antimicrobial, anticancer, neuroprotective, anti-inflammatory	[184]	Reduced for antidiabetic activity. Compared to some derivatives, it has reduced toxicity or no dermatological toxicity.	[186,187]
		Lipid-lowering, antiobesity, antihyperglycemic, cardioprotective, and vasorelaxant	[185]		

Table 4. *Cont.*

	Bioactive Compound	Pharmacological Activity	Ref	Bioavailability and Toxicity	Ref
			P. cerasus		
Phenols	Gallic acid	Antioxidant	[188]	Compared to other polyphenols, it has a high absorption	[196]
		Anti-inflammatory, antiobesity	[189]		
		It can be used to manage several neurological diseases and disorders, such as Alzheimer's disease, Parkinson's disease, stroke, sedation, depression, psychosis, neuropathic pain, anxiety, and memory loss, as well as neuroinflammation.	[190]		
		Anti-HIV, antiulcer, UV protection	[191]		
		Anticarcinogenic	[192]		
		Antioxidant and antineoplastic	[193]		
		Antiviral, antimicrobial, antiallergic, anti-melanogenic, neuroprotective, anti-Alzheimer's, antidiabetic, and antiobesity	[194]		
		It can be used to treat atherosclerotic cardiovascular disease, coronary artery disease, and cerebral ischemia	[195]		
Flavonoids	Phloridzin	Antigenotoxic, antioxidant, anti-inflammatory, and anticarcinogenic	[197]	Possible adverse effects on the musculoskeletal system in conditions of hyperglycemia.	[201]
		Antiaging	[198]		
		Antiarthritic effect	[199]		
		Antidiabetic, antihyperglycemic, antibacterial, cardioprotective, neuroprotective, hepatoprotective, immunomodulatory, and antiobesity	[200]		
	Galangin	Anticancer (breast, renal, lung, esophageal, laryngeal, ovarian, cervical, colon)	[202]	Very low oral bioavailability	[206]
		Strong ability to control apoptosis and inflammation	[203]		
		Antioxidant, anti-inflammatory, antiarthritic	[204]		
		Hepatoprotectors	[205]		
Coumarin	Scopoletin	Antioxidant	[207]	Low, but which can be positively influenced by encapsulation in Solupus micelles It does not present toxicity	[210,211]
		Antimicrobial, immunomodulatory, anti-inflammatory, anticarcinogenic, neuroprotective	[208]		
		Antibacterial, antifungal, antiparasitic, hepatoprotective, antihyperlipidemic, antidiabetic, antiangiogenesis, antihypertensive, analgesic, anti-immunomodropozic, antiallergic, antiaging, and antigout	[209]		

Table 4. *Cont.*

	Bioactive Compound	Pharmacological Activity	Ref	Bioavailability and Toxicity	Ref
		Common bioactive compounds (Rubus and Prunus)			
Phenolic acids	Caffeic acid	Anticancer (hepatocarcinoma)	[212]	Raised in free form. Some phenolic acids may present moderate toxicity, promoting irritation of the gastric mucosa, skin, or eyes	[229,230]
		Antidiabetic, antiobesity, antiarteriosclerotic, antidepressant, antibacterial, antiviral	[213]		
		Mild antiemetic properties	[214]		
		Antiproliferative, immunomodulatory and neuroprotective	[215]		
	p-Coumaric acid	Antioxidant, efficacy in hypopigmentation and depigmentation	[216]	Raised in free form. Some phenolic acids may present moderate toxicity, promoting irritation of the gastric mucosa, skin, or eyes	[229,230]
		Antioxidant, anticancer, antimicrobial, antiviral, anti-inflammatory, antiplatelet, anxiolytic, antipyretic, analgesic and antiarthritic	[217]		
	Ferulic acid	Dermato-protectors (UV, antipigmentation, regeneration) Used as a stabilizer in cosmetic products for vitamins C and E	[218]	Raised in free form. Some phenolic acids may present moderate toxicity, promoting irritation of the gastric mucosa, skin, or eyes	[229,230]
		Antioxidant, anti-inflammatory, antiangiogenic, antiallergic, antimicrobial, antiviral, neuroprotective, and anticancer	[219]		
		Pro-angiogenesis, antithrombosis, antiaging, analgesic, antithrombotic	[220]		
		Antidiabetic, cardioprotective, neuroprotective, and antiapoptotic	[221]		
		Hepatoprotectors	[222]		
	Chlorogenic acid	Antioxidant, antibacterial, hepatoprotective, cardioprotective, anti-inflammatory, antipyretic, neuroprotective, anti-obesity, antiviral, antimicrobial, antihypertensive, free radical scavenger, and central nervous system stimulant	[223]	Raised in free form. Some phenolic acids may present moderate toxicity, promoting irritation of the gastric mucosa, skin, or eyes	[229,230]
		Antidiabetic, antifibrotic, antimelanogenesis, antiallergic, antifungal, antiatherosclerosis, dermal protection	[224]		
	Ellagic acid	Effective in treating insomnia, fatigue, ischemia, colorectal cancer, and multiple sclerosis; improves physical endurance and lowers blood glucose levels	[225]	Raised in free form. Some phenolic acids may present moderate toxicity, promoting irritation of the gastric mucosa, skin, or eyes	[229,230]
		Antitumor, antioxidant, anti-inflammatory, antimutation, antiallergic	[226]		
		Role in treating/managing metabolic syndrome	[227]		
		Neuroprotectors, hepatoprotectors, cardioprotectors, antiphotoaging, depigmenting agent	[228]		

Table 4. *Cont.*

	Bioactive Compound	Pharmacological Activity	Ref	Bioavailability and Toxicity	Ref
Flavonols	Quercetin	Anti-inflammatory, antiviral, antioxidant, and psychostimulant, immune-supporting properties	[102–104]	Low due to partial solubility in water, but also chemical stability It is not toxic to the human body at a consumption of 3–1000 mg/day.	[238,239]
		Anticancer effect against malignant gynecological tumors May improve hyperandrogenemia and insulin resistance	[231]		
		Antioxidant and neuroprotector for Alzheimer's therapy	[232]		
		Antiatherosclerosis (increased absorption in association with lipids)	[233]		
		Liver and kidney protection	[234]		
		Antihypertensive, ability to protect low-density lipoprotein (LDL) oxidation, and ability to inhibit angiogenesis	[235]		
		Antifungal, antiasthmatic, antiallergic, antiobesity	[236]		
		Antiaging, antiviral (COVID-19)	[237]		
Flavonols	Catechin	Antioxidant, anticancer, antiobesity, (in excess, it can promote hepatitis)	[240]	Intestinal absorption and bioavailability are increased by formulations with sucrose and ascorbic acid	[243]
		Antihypertensive, anticoagulant, antiulcer, antithyroid, antihyperlipidemic, antidiabetic, antiosteoporotic, antiosteopenic, hepatoprotective, nephroprotective, neuroprotective, antiallergic, anxiolytic, antimicrobial	[241]		
		It can chelate metals essential for bacterial growth, which supports bactericidal action.	[242]		
Flavonoids	Rutin	Sedative, diuretic, analgesic, anticonvulsant, anticancer, antidepressant, antiarthritic, antidiabetic, antiulcer, antiasthmatic, anticataract, antiosteoporotic, antiosteopenic, antimicrobial, antifungal, antiviral, larvicidal, antimalarial, effective in atopic dermatitis	[244]	Limited. The lethal dose in mice is between 1.49 and 1.51 g/kg	[87,246]
		Effective in combating premenstrual dysphoric disorder	[245]		
Tannins	Proanthocyanidins (oligo- or polymers of monomeric flavan-3-ols)	Antioxidant, anticancer, antidiabetic, neuroprotective, and antimicrobial	[247]	Low in oral administration Only monomers and oligomeric procyanidins with a degree of polymerization of less than 4 are absorbed. There is no evidence of toxicity when administered orally or of potential mutagenic action at a consumption of 2% of the diet.	[247,249,250]
		Hypolipidemic, anti-inflammatory, metabolic, and intestinal flora regulation, DNA repair	[248]		

As highlighted in the previous table, the bioactive compounds from the species *R. idaeus*, *P. serotina*, *P. avium*, and *P. cerasus* exhibit multiple bioactive activities in the medical or dermato-cosmetic field. Their applicability in skincare products is highlighted by the antioxidant capacity exhibited by many compounds, but they also display more complex activities, such as anticancer or neuroprotective effects (Figure 3).

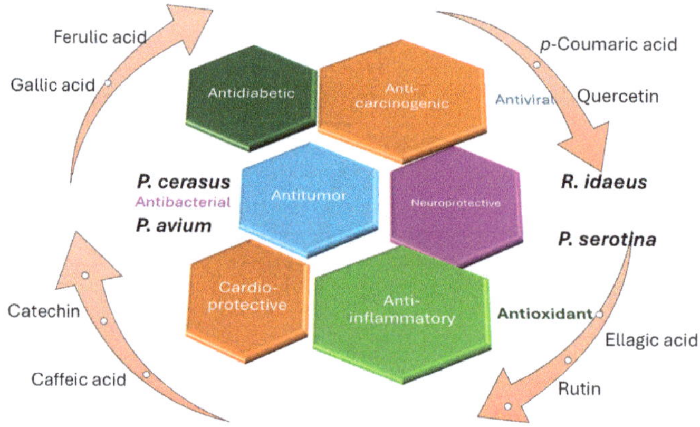

Figure 3. Pharmacological and pro-health importance of several common compounds identified in *Rubus* and *Prunus* species.

For a product containing bioactive compounds to be declared effective, it is necessary to know both its bioavailability and its toxicity [251].

Despite the biological activities possessed by the compounds identified in the *Rubus* and *Prunus* species, some exhibit toxicity to the human body, as can be seen in Table 4. This aspect of toxicity necessitates a series of additional studies to fully understand the interactions between bioactive compounds, with the aim of identifying methods to mitigate or eliminate these adverse reactions, for the maximum enhancement of pharma-cological effects.

5.2. Synergistic Activity

Compounds such as salicylic acid and astragalin from *R. idaeus* [15]; juglanin and isorhamnetin from *P. serotina* [17,139]; taxifolin, chrysin, and vanillin from *P. avium* [7,22]; phloridzin and rutin from *P. cerasus* [21,29] could exhibit synergistic action, which would enhance the individual pharmacological activities.

Interest in synergistic actions between bioactive substances has increased in recent years due to recent paradigm shifts. In this context, Table 5 presents several synergistic actions of the aforementioned bioactive compounds, based on bibliographic references consulted for this study.

Table 5. Synergistic activity of some bioactive compounds.

Chemical Compound	Synergistic Activity	References
Quercetin + vitamin C	Antiviral	[252]
Ellagic acid + gallic acid + catechin	Antibacterial	[253]
p-Coumaric acid + chlorogenic acid	Antibacterial	[254]
Proanthocyanidins + vitamin C + vitamin E	Synergistic effect for skin whitening	[248]
Catechin + quercetin	Against alcoholic liver damage	[255]
Catechin + vitamin E	Antioxidant	[256]
Ferulic acid + δ-tocotrienol (a derivative of vitamin E)	Against prostate cancer	[220]
Kaempferol + apigenin	Cytotoxic efficacy for colon cancer	[257]
Quercetin + astragalin	Anti-inflammatory	[258]
Quercetin + gallic acid + caffeic acid Quercetin + gallic acid + rutin	Antioxidant	[259]
Apigenin + naringenin	Anticarcinogenic	[260]

Table 5. *Cont.*

Chemical Compound	Synergistic Activity	References
Flavonoids + tocopherol	Inhibitors in the case of lipid peroxidation	[256]
Isorhamnetin + quercetin	Potentiation of anticancer activity and broadening of the spectrum	[261]
Isorhamnetin + caffeic acid	Increased antioxidant activity	[261]
Chrysin + apigenin	Antitumor	[262]
Kaempeferol + chrysin	Anti-inflammatory and antioxidant	[263]
Betaine-salicylic acid cocrystal	Acne treatment	[264]
Vanillin + norfloxacin (antibiotic)	Antibacterial	[265]
Juglanin + doxorubicin (antitumor drug)	High cytotoxicity	[266]
Chrysin + radiotherapy	Anticarcinogenic	[267]
Toxifolin + chemotherapy	Anticarcinogenic	[268]

These findings suggest the need to continue investigations on the possibility of using extracts obtained from the four sources, in different mixtures, in order to improve their biological activity (anticarcinogenic, anti-inflammatory, antioxidant, etc.), to enhance the effect of certain medications or medical procedures, and/or minimize the adverse effects associated with the treatments.

5.3. *Structure–Activity Relationship Study*

Considering the multiple biological activities of the compounds present in the four investigated sources, data from the literature regarding the structure-activity relationship were taken into account, which can help to understand how the chemical structures of these molecules influence their biological activities.

5.3.1. Phenolic Compounds

Phenolic compounds exhibit antioxidant activity, among other things, which is determined by their ability to donate hydrogen atoms or electrons, but it can also be attributed to the possibility of metal chelation [269]. Additionally, studies in the field have shown that the antioxidant activity of phenols is influenced by the presence and position of the hydroxyl group [269,270].

Hydroxybenzoic acids exhibit a closer relationship between their antibacterial activity and hydrophobicity compared to hydroxycinnamic acids [271]. It is worth mentioning that this activity is influenced by the presence of hydroxyl groups, as well as by that of double bonds [272].

Antioxidant capacity assessment (ORAC assay) showed that extracts rich in polyphenolic and flavanol compounds, such as those from *P. cerasus* leaves and fruits, compared to those from *P. avium*, are useful for both cosmetic and pharmaceutical use [35].

1. Simple Phenols

- Hydroquinone, in the phenolic structural form, called 1,4-dihydroxybenzene, due to the presence of the hydroxyl group in the para position, exhibits antioxidant activity [273].

2. Flavonoids

Some flavonoids have the ability to inhibit monoamine oxidase, an enzyme responsible for the onset of certain neurological disorders. An experimental study demonstrated that this inhibitory activity exhibits an ascending character for the following series of flavonoids: apigenin, luteolin, quercetin, aromadendrin, and taxifolin [274].

The presence of hydroxyl groups in the structure of flavonoids influences their antidepressant activity, specifically, the groups in positions 2 and 4 support this activity [275]. Additionally, the number of groups is particularly important; proanthocyanidins, which are polymerized monomers and therefore contain more hydroxyl groups, exhibit higher antioxidant activity, whereas the glycosylation of flavonoids reduces this activity [276]. On the other hand, methoxy or glycosidic groups attached to the flavonoid structure reduce their antioxidant activity [277].

- Quercetin, named 2-(3,4-dihydroxyphenyl)-3,5,7-trihydroxy-4H-chromen-4-one [278], whose basic structure is represented by two phenyl groups connected by three carbon atoms, can be arranged in an open form or in the form of a heterocyclic ring [279]. The antioxidant activity of this compound is determined by the presence of the hydroxyl group, which is why some quercetin derivatives exhibit lower activity. On the other hand, obtaining methylated derivatives can lead to an increase in anti-inflammatory activity, and through glycosylation reactions, compounds with higher bioavailability regarding the antiobesity effect can be obtained [280]. Of the five hydroxyl groups in the structure of quercetin, only those at positions 3, 3′, and 4′ are responsible for the antioxidant activity of this compound, also being involved in its photolability [84]. The presence of the double bond in the heterocyclic ring of quercetin determines the manner in which this compound binds to DNA, by fitting into the helix of deoxyribonucleic acid, compared to naringenin, which does not have that double bond and exhibits a groove-type DNA binding [281]. The inhibitory activity on lipase is influenced by the structure of flavonoids as follows: it decreases through the hydrogenation of the double bond in the C ring, specifically through the glycosylation reaction, and increases with the presence of the carbonyl group or the hydroxylation reaction. Quercetin, due to its chemical structure, exhibits this activity, but it is lower than that of luteolin [282].
- Astragalin is also known as kaempferol 3-*O*-*β*-d-glucopyranoside. The substitution of phenolic hydroxyl groups influences the anti-inflammatory activity of astragalin, having a stronger effect than chrysin or luteolin [115].
- Rutin, known as 3′,4′,5,7-tetrahydroxyflavone-3-rutinoside or quercetin-3-rutinoside, is a flavonoid glycoside formed from quercetin and rutin [87]. The antioxidant activity of rutin can be enhanced by complexation with cyclodextrin [283]. On the other hand, glycosylation of this compound leads to an increase in antioxidant, antibacterial, and *α*-glucosidase inhibitory activities [88].
- Aromadendrin contains four hydroxyl groups in its structure and is also called (2*R*,3*R*)-3,5,7-trihydroxy-2-(4-hydroxyphenyl)-2,3-dihydrochromen-4-one. This compound exhibits multiple pharmacological activities, but in the case of antidiabetic and anticancer actions, the 7-O methylated derivative stands out, while methylation at the 4′-O position is noted to be effective for antiulcer activity [157].
- Juglanin (kaempferol 3-*O*-*α*-L-arabinofuranoside) contains multiple hydroxyl groups in its structure. This compound exhibits a lower antiradical effect compared to quercetin, the scientific justification being the presence of a single hydroxyl group on ring B [17].
- Kaempferol, also named 3,5,7-trihydroxy-2-(4-hydroxyphenyl)-4H-1-benzopyran-4-one, has a diphenylpropane structure and can be obtained through a series of reactions applied to naringenin [134,135]. In the study conducted by Rho et al., it was highlighted that depigmentation activity and cytotoxicity are enhanced by the presence of the hydroxyl group at position 3 [284].
- Isorhamnetin is a flavonoid, considered a methylated derivative of quercetin [261]. The methoxy group at position 3′ is associated with the antitumor activity of this compound [70].
- Prunin, a flavanone glycoside, is obtained following the hydrolysis process of naringenin. In the case of prunin laurate, a strong antibacterial activity against *Porphyromonas gingivalis* was shown by Wada et al. [285]. Additionally, in another study, when examining naringenin derivatives, it was highlighted that an aliphatic chain of

10–12 carbon atoms attached to ring A has the ability to enhance antimicrobial activity, with alkylprunin being an important representative [286].

- Apigenin or 4′,5,7–trihydroxyflavone, contains a 2-phenylchromen-4-one skeleton [63]. A study aimed at comparing the biological activity of apigenin and one of its derivatives, apigenin-7-*O*-glucoside, concluded that the presence of the sugar moiety in the derivative resulted in stronger antifungal activity against *Candida albicans* and *Candida glabrata*. Additionally, in vitro, the glycosidic derivative exhibits higher cytotoxic activity against cancer cells in the case of colon cancer, compared to apigenin [287].
- Chrysin (5,7-dihydroxyflavone) is a flavone that contains hydroxyl and keto functional groups [176]. The antioxidant activity of this compound is correlated with the lack of hydroxyl in rings B and C, as well as the presence of the carbonyl group on C4 and the double bond between C2 and C3 [288]. Liu et al. highlighted that halogenated derivatives exhibit stronger anticancer activity. Additionally, an enhancement of the effect was observed when the C7-OH of ring A was linked to various hydrophilic amines. Regarding the anti-inflammatory activity, a strong effect was demonstrated in the case of the derivative containing a cyclic pyridine at position 8 [289].
- Naringenin has two hydroxyl groups missing in its chemical structure compared to quercetin, which explains its lower antioxidant activity. Quercetin, on the other hand, has an antioxidant effect comparable to that of vitamin C, and the presence of two hydroxyl groups on ring C, instead of one as in the case of naringenin, leads to the formation of a stabilized quinone structure that contributes to enhancing the effect [281]. The antibacterial activity of naringenin is lower than that of other flavones that contain fewer hydroxyl groups; additionally, the position of these groups also influences the activity, so compounds that have hydroxyl groups in ring A but not in ring B exhibit significant activity. Methylation of hydroxyl groups may contribute to the reduction of the antibacterial effect [290].
- Taxifolin exhibits inhibitory activity against certain protein structures, such as amyloid fibrils, which have been highlighted in the literature as being responsible for the onset of Alzheimer's disease. This inhibitory activity is due to the presence of the catechol group in ring B [291].
- Catechin is a flavan-3-ol, also named (2*R*,3*S*)-2-(3,4-dihydroxyphenyl)-3,4-dihydro-2H-chromene-3,5,7-triol. The position and number of hydroxyl groups influence the antibacterial activity of catechins. Additionally, the polymerization of catechin molecules enhances activity, as is the case with theaflavins [292]. The antioxidant activity is correlated with the presence of the hydroxyl group in position 3 [293].
- Genistein (4′,5,7-trihydroxyisoflavone) is a phytoestrogen that can be synthesized from naringenin in plants. It exhibits characteristics similar to those of the estrogen estradiol-17β, due to structural similarities consisting of the presence of the phenolic ring and the distance between the hydroxyl groups [294].
- Phlorizin, phloretin 2′-*β*-D-glucoside, according to Li et al., exhibits lower antioxidant activity than the parent compound because the glycosylation reaction reduces the number of phenolic hydroxyl groups [295].

Guerrero et al. investigated several flavonoids in terms of their inhibitory activity on the angiotensin-converting enzyme and highlighted the fact that at the structural level, there are some key elements underlying this activity, such as the presence of the catechol group at the B ring, the ketone group found at C4 in the C ring, and the double bond be-tween C2 and C3 of the C ring. It was concluded that this inhibitory activity has an upward trend for the following compounds:

- at a concentration of 500 μM: hesperetin, genistein, epicatechin, naringenin, apigenin, kaempferol, quercetin, and rutin;

- at a concentration of 100 μM: quercetin, rutin, kaempferol, and luteolin.

It should be mentioned that the highest activity was recorded at the minimum concentration [296].

Zhang et al. investigated the structure–activity relationship of some flavonoids responsible for inhibiting a breast cancer-resistant protein and concluded that, in this case as well, the double bond between C2 and C3 of ring C influences this interaction. Additionally, the importance of the B ring position, hydroxylation at position 5, and the absence of the hydroxyl group at position 3, as well as hydrophobic substitution at positions 6, 7, 8, or 4′, were mentioned as elements responsible for this protein–flavonoid interaction [297].

3. Tannins

- Proanthocyanidins contain significant monomeric units of flavan-3-ol, such as epicatechin or catechin, and are also referred to as condensed tannins. According to studies, these monomeric units influence biological activity, such as antioxidant or antidiabetic activity [247,298].
- Sanguiin H6, an ellagitannin derived from ellagic acid, has multiple biological activities that are influenced by the presence of hydroxyl groups and the galloyl configuration [299].

4. Phenolic Acids

A carboxyl group derived from an acid and at least one hydroxyl group that replaces hydrogen atoms in the benzene rings gives rise to phenolic acids [298].

The antioxidant activity of hydroxycinnamic acids is directly positively influenced by the presence of a double bond in the side chain, the number and position of hydroxyl groups on the aromatic ring, the esterification or amidation of the carboxyl group, as well as the presence of the catechol group [299].

- 3,4-Dihydroxycinnamic acid exhibits hepatoprotective activity that can be enhanced through methoxylation at positions 3 or 4 [300]. The esterification gives rise to derivatives that exhibit remarkable antileishmanial activity. Otero et al. highlighted in a study that the bioactivity of cinnamic acid derivatives depends on the degree of oxygenation at positions 3 and 4, the presence of a double bond in the side chain, and hydroxyl groups, as well as the length of the alkyl chain [301].
- Caffeic acid is a hydroxycinnamic acid that contains an aromatic ring and three hydroxyl groups, along with the double bond in the carbon chain, with anticancer activity [212]. Anilides and aliphatic amides of caffeic acid enhance its antioxidant activity [302]. The attachment of a naphthyl ring increases the capacity of caffeic acid to inhibit monoamine oxidase, an enzyme responsible for multiple neurological disorders [301,303].
- *p*-Coumaric acid, a phenolic acid, derived from cinnamic acid, is also known as 4-hydroxycinnamic acid [304]. Derivatives of *p*-coumaric acid exhibit higher antimicrobial activity, especially esters, anilides, and amides with bulky aromatic groups [305].
- Ferulic acid, also called 4-hydroxy-3-methoxycinnamic acid, is responsible for some biological activities [306]. The anticancer activity of some ferulic acid derivatives was investigated; thus, although some derivatives exhibit lower activity compared to caffeic acid derivatives, the phenylsulfonylfuroxan nitrates of ferulic acid stand out as having strong anticancer activity [307]. Ferulic acid, found in raspberry plant parts, has the ability to stabilize anthocyanins, but it is also recognized for its involvement in flavonoid catabolism, particularly in the spontaneous carboxylation of caffeic acid [308].
- Chlorogenic acid is derived from caffeic acid and quinic acid, and the hydroxyl groups present in its structure are responsible for the strong antioxidant effect it exhibits [58].

- Ellagic acid or 2,3,7,8-tetrahydroxy [1]-benzopyrano [5,4,3-cde] benzopyran-5,10-dione, structurally contains a hydrophilic part, represented by phenolic groups and lactone-type groups, as well as a lipophilic part represented by the four phenolic rings [50...60]. The anticancer activity of this compound is closely related to its chemical structure, specifically the presence of hydroxyl groups at positions 3 and 4, as well as the presence of lactone groups [309,310].
- Salicylic acid or 2-hydroxybenzoic acid is a plant hormone, being the main precursor of aspirin. From a structural perspective, it is notable for the *ortho* arrangement of the hydroxyl and carboxyl groups [311]. The inhibition of luciferase by salicylic acid is enhanced by the amidation of the carboxyl group or the substitution of chlorine at position 5 [312].
- Anacardic acid, a derivative of salicylic acid, has a side chain with different degrees of unsaturation, which is responsible for its varied biological activity. Regarding antioxidant activity, trienic anacardic acid (15:3) stands out, while for antifungal activity, monoenic anacardic acid (15:1) is highlighted [313]. The biological activity of anacardic acid is closely related to the structure of the side chain; thus, the presence of the trienic alkyl side chain determines a strong bactericidal activity against *Streptococcus mutans* and *Staphylococcus aureus*, while the saturated alkyl chain acts against *Propionibacterium acnes*. The antioxidant activity is synergistically influenced by the length of the alkyl chain, the presence of the salicylic acid moiety, as well as the stereochemistry of the side chain [56]. Some researchers have noted that the anticancer activity of anacardic acid largely depends on the molecular volume of the hydrophobic side chain, in addition to its metal-chelating ability and its action as a surfactant [93].

5.3.2. Coumarins

- Scopoletin, 6-methoxy-7-hydroxycoumarin, is characterized by the presence of a single hydroxyl group, a methoxy group, and a keto group [210]. Liu et al. demonstrated that derivatives containing a Δ3,4 olefinic bond, as well as naphthyl or phenyl groups with a sulfate ester at the C7 position, enhance insecticidal activity against *Tetranychus cinnabarinus* and *Artemia salina*, respectively [314].

5.3.3. Cyanogenic Glycosides

- Prunasin, the glucoside of (R)-mandelonitrile, can be glycosylated with the formation of amygdalin, and it can be converted into mandelonitrile by α-glucosidase or a hydrolase, and subsequently hydrolyzed into benzaldehyde and hydrocyanic acid [315].

5.3.4. Aldehyde

- Vanillin is an important flavor molecule, being named 4-hydroxy-3-methoxybenzaldehyde, and constitutes the major component of vanilla [316]. The aldehyde group in the structure of vanillin, as well as the position of the side group on the benzene ring, supports the antifungal activity exhibited by this compound [317]. Furthermore, this compound also exhibits antioxidant activity, stronger than that of ascorbic acid, justified by its self-dimerization in contact with free radicals [318].

5.3.5. Terpenoid

- Squalene is a precursor of cholesterol, and not only a triterpene that contains 30 carbon atoms in its structure. In the synthesis of cholesterol, the process was initially proposed to be described as a cyclization of squalene to lanosterol; later, it was demonstrated that it oxidizes to form monooxidosqualene before cyclization [319]. It exhibits a high detoxification capacity due to its ability to attach to uncharged substances, owing to its nonpolarity [320].

5.3.6. Vitamins

- Ascorbic acid, better known as vitamin C, is a compound with multiple bioactive activities, including antioxidant activity. This activity is justified on one hand by the acid's ability to donate single hydrogen atoms, and on the other hand by the interaction between radicals and the monodehydroascorbate anion [321]. It is also worth mentioning the importance of vitamin C in collagen synthesis, a compound extremely important for human health, as well as in the fixation of vitamin E or iron [322]. The structure of lactone, with two ionizable hydroxyl groups, makes this compound an excellent reducing agent. It oxidizes successively, forming ascorbate radical and then dehydroascorbic acid, a mechanism that underlies many biological activities [323].
- Tocopherol, belonging to the vitamin E family, has a chemical structure that contains a polar chromanol ring and a lipophilic phytyl chain, and its antioxidant activity is justified by its ability to form tocopherol quinone [324]. Just like in the case of vitamin C, the presence of hydroxyl groups in the chemical structure of tocopherols, which act as hydrogen donors for peroxyl radicals, reveals other biological activities, such as cellular signaling properties [325].

Research in the field has highlighted the fact that *Rubus* and *Prunus* plant waste can be used to obtain extracts with broad applicability in the medical field. The antioxidant, antimicrobial, and anti-inflammatory actions have been explored both in vitro and in vivo. It is worth noting that the identified studies, both in vitro and in vivo, mainly reported on the leaf extract [326,327].

The reviewed literature underscores the importance of woody biomass of *Prunus* and *Rubus* species as a source of bioactive compounds with multiple pharmacological and cosmetic applications [328].

6. Conclusions

Plant waste, including red raspberry stems and cherry twigs, presents significant potential for the development of a sustainable valorization model through the lens of bio-active compound content. They are predominantly applicable in the pharmaceutical and cosmetic industries, thus contributing both to the reduction of industrial waste and to the enhancement of the sustainability of economic processes.

In this analysis, recent data from the specialized literature on the biological activity of the main compounds identified in the species *R. idaeus*, *P. serotina*, *P. avium* and *P. cerasus* are presented, emphasizing the following aspects:

- presentation of the bioactive compounds representative of these species and highlighting their extraction and isolation methodology;
- correlation between biological activity and their chemical structure, with emphasis on the possible synergistic action of some compounds common to the four species.

The diversity of available extraction technologies is noteworthy, from conventional methods such as ethanol extraction, to more environmentally friendly solutions such as subcritical water extraction and supercritical CO_2 extraction that allow the obtaining of bioactive compounds with high yields.

In addition, an affinity for chromatographic methods for the isolation and purification of target compounds was observed, a fact justified both by the complexity of the chemical composition of the plant matrix and by the need to obtain high-purity products in accordance with the requirements of the pharmaceutical and cosmetic industries.

These aspects represent a starting point for in-depth research into the four plant sources rich in active phytochemical compounds, which can become a valuable source for the manufacture of pharmaceutical, cosmetic, and even food products.

7. Future Perspectives

In order to maximize the potential for valorization of plant waste, it is essential to continue exploring the correlation between the structure and biological activity, the mechanism of action, the bioavailability, and the potential toxicity of the identified compounds. It is also important to develop and improve technologies that increase the separation efficiency of bioactive compounds, applicable on an industrial scale and with low environmental impact.

In addition to these challenges, further developments are needed to increase the adoption of waste recovery technologies, economic feasibility, market potential, and policy incentives to support the superior recovery of plant waste.

Author Contributions: All the authors have equal contributions to this study.

Funding: The work was partially supported by the School of Doctoral Studies of "Vasile Alecsandri" University of Bacău through the Project SSD-0153–2025.

Institutional Review Board Statement: Not applicable.

Informed Consent Statement: Not applicable.

Data Availability Statement: Not applicable.

Conflicts of Interest: The authors declare no conflicts of interest.

References

1. Brás, I.; Silva, E.; Raimondo, R.; Saetta, R.; Mignano, V.; Fabbricino, M.; Ferreira, J. Valorisation of forest and agriculture residual biomass—The application of life cycle assessment to analyse composting, mulching, and energetic valorisation strategies. *Sustainability* **2024**, *16*, 630. [CrossRef]
2. Rousou, I.S. Importance of Reusing Wood from Pruning and Promotion of Circular Economy Principles in Agricultural Sector in Tripolis, Greece. Master Thesis, Agricultural University of Athens, Athens, Greece, 2025. Available online: http://hdl.handle.net/10329/8412 (accessed on 23 July 2025).
3. Sanoja-López, K.A.; Guamán-Marquines, C.W.; Luque, R. Advanced processes in biomass/waste valorization: A Review. *Sustain. Chem. Pharm.* **2024**, *41*, 101704. [CrossRef]
4. Syrodoy, S.V.; Yu, M.D.; Nigay, N.A.; Purin, M.V. Influence of the type of woody biomass on energy and environmental characteristics of the thermal preparation processes and ignition of bio-water-coal fuel particles. *Process Saf. Environ. Protect.* **2024**, *184*, 736–746. [CrossRef]
5. Tomlin, A.S. Air quality and climate impacts of biomass use as an energy source: A review. *Energy Fuels* **2021**, *35*, 14213–14240. [CrossRef]
6. Tran, H.; Jino, E.; Arunachalam, S. Emissions of wood pelletization and bioenergy use in the United States. *Renew. Energy* **2023**, *219*, 119536. [CrossRef]
7. Aliaño-González, M.J.; Gabaston, J.; Ortiz-Somovilla, V.; Cantos-Villar, E. Wood waste from fruit trees: Biomolecules and their applications in agri-food industry. *Biomolecules* **2022**, *12*, 238. [CrossRef]
8. Del Toro-Gipson, R.S.; Rizzo, P.V.; Hanson, D.J.; Drake, M. Sensory characterization of specific wood smoke aromas and their contributions to smoked Cheddar cheese flavor. *J. Sens. Stud.* **2020**, *35*, e12564. [CrossRef]
9. Swaney-Stueve, M.; Talavera, M.; Jepsen, T.; Severns, B.; Wise, R.; Deubler, G. Sensory and consumer evaluation of smoked pulled pork prepared using different smokers and different types of wood. *J. Food Sci.* **2019**, *84*, 640–649. [CrossRef]
10. Racovita, R.C.; Secuianu, C.; Ciuca, M.D.; Israel-Roming, F. Effects of smoking temperature, smoking time, and type of wood sawdust on polycyclic aromatic hydrocarbon accumulation levels in directly smoked pork sausages. *J. Agric. Food Chem.* **2020**, *68*, 9530–9536. [CrossRef]
11. Öncül, M.; Atagür, M.; Atan, E.; Sever, K. A preliminary evaluation of bing cherry tree (*Prunus avium* L.) pruning waste as an alternative lignocellulosic filler for lightweight composite material applications. *Polym. Compos.* **2025**, *46*, 3655–3667. [CrossRef]
12. Memete, A.R.; Sărac, I.; Teusdea, A.C.; Budău, R.; Bei, M.; Vicas, S.I. Bioactive compounds and antioxidant capacity of several blackberry (*Rubus* spp.) fruits cultivars grown in Romania. *Horticulturae* **2023**, *9*, 556. [CrossRef]

13. Buczyński, K.; Kapłan, M.; Jarosz, Z. Review of the report on the nutritional and health-promoting values of species of the *Rubus* L. genus. *Agriculture* **2024**, *14*, 1324. [CrossRef]
14. Azzini, E.; Barnaba, L.; Mattera, M.; Calina, D.; Sharifi-Rad, J.; Cho, W.C. Updated evidence on raspberries as functional foods: Anticancer bioactivity and therapeutic implications. *Food Front.* **2024**, *5*, 2351–2382. [CrossRef]
15. Ispiryan, A.; Viškelis, J.; Viškelis, P.; Urbonavičienė, D.; Raudonė, L. Biochemical and antioxidant profiling of raspberry plant parts for sustainable processing. *Plants* **2023**, *12*, 2424. [CrossRef]
16. Telichowska, A.; Kobus-Cisowska, J.; Szulc, P. Phytopharmacological possibilities of bird cherry *Prunus padus* L. and *Prunus serotina* L. species and their bioactive phytochemicals. *Nutrients* **2020**, *12*, 1966. [CrossRef]
17. Rutkowska, M.; Witek, M.; Olszewska, M.A. A comprehensive review of molecular mechanisms, pharmacokinetics, toxicology and plant sources of juglanin: Current landscape and future perspectives. *Int. J. Mol. Sci.* **2024**, *25*, 10323. [CrossRef]
18. Ademović, Z.; Hodžić, S.; Halilić-Zahirović, Z.; Husejnagić, D.; Džananović, J.; Šarić-Kundalić, B.; Suljagić, J. Phenolic compounds, antioxidant and antimicrobial properties of the wild cherry (*Prunus avium* L.) stem. *Acta Period. Technol.* **2017**, *48*, 1–13. [CrossRef]
19. Bhattacharya, S.; Chakraborty, S. A review on medicinal plants and its importance from glycosides. *Int. J. Res. Appl. Sci. Eng. Technol.* **2024**, *12*, 715–729. [CrossRef]
20. Newman, D.J.; Cragg, G.M. Natural products as sources of new drugs over the nearly four decades from 01/1981 to 09/2019. *J. Nat. Prod.* **2020**, *83*, 770–803. [CrossRef]
21. Zymonė, K.; Liaudanskas, M.; Lanauskas, J.; Nagelytė, M.; Janulis, V. Variability in the qualitative and quantitative composition of phenolic compounds and the in vitro antioxidant activity of sour cherry (*Prunus cerasus* L.) leaves. *Antioxidants* **2024**, *13*, 553. [CrossRef]
22. Tomar, O.; Akarca, G.; Gök, V.; İstek, Ö. Chemical composition and antifungal potential of apricot, sour cherry, and cherry tree bio-products (resins) against food-borne molds. *Food Biosci.* **2022**, *47*, 101627. [CrossRef]
23. Krauze-Baranowska, M.; Głód, D.; Kula, M.; Majdan, M.; Hałasa, R.; Matkowski, A.; Kozłowska, W.; Kawiak, A. Chemical composition and biological activity of *Rubus idaeus* shoots—A traditional herbal remedy of Eastern Europe. *BMC Complement. Altern. Med.* **2014**, *14*, 480. [CrossRef]
24. Cyboran-Mikołajczyk, S.; Męczarska, K.; Solarska-Ściuk, K.; Ratajczak-Wielgomas, K.; Oszmiański, J.; Jencova, V.; Bonarska-Kujawa, D. Protection of erythrocytes and microvascular endothelial cells against oxidative damage by *Fragaria vesca* L. and *Rubus idaeus* L. leaves extracts—The mechanism of action. *Molecules* **2022**, *27*, 5865. [CrossRef]
25. Raal, A.; Vahtra, A.; Koshovyi, O.; Ilina, T.; Kovalyova, A.; Püssa, T. Polyphenolic compounds in the stems of raspberry (*Rubus idaeus*) growing wild and cultivated. *Molecules* **2024**, *29*, 5016. [CrossRef]
26. Nastić, N.; Lozano-Sánchez, J.; Borrás-Linares, I.; Švarc-Gajić, J.; Segura-Carretero, A. New technological approaches for recovering bioactive food constituents from sweet cherry (*Prunus avium* L.) stems. *Phytochem. Anal.* **2020**, *31*, 119–130. [CrossRef]
27. Brozdowski, J.; Waliszewska, B.; Gacnik, S.; Hudina, M.; Veberic, R.; Mikulic-Petkovsek, M. Phenolic composition of leaf and flower extracts of black cherry (*Prunus serotina* Ehrh.). *Ann. For. Sci.* **2021**, *78*, 66. [CrossRef]
28. Jesus, F.; Gonçalves, A.C.; Alves, G.; Silva, L.R. Health benefits of *Prunus avium* plant parts: An unexplored source rich in phenolic compounds. *Food Rev. Int.* **2022**, *38*, 118–146. [CrossRef]
29. Nunes, A.R.; Gonçalves, A.C.; Alves, G.; Falcão, A.; Garcia-Viguera, C.; Moreno, D.A.; Silva, L.R. Valorisation of *Prunus avium* L. by-products: Phenolic composition and effect on Caco-2 cells viability. *Foods* **2021**, *10*, 1185. [CrossRef]
30. Costea, T.; Vlase, L.; Gostin, I.N.; Olah, N.K.; Predan, G.M.I. Botanical characterization, phytochemical analysis and antioxidant activity of indigenous red raspberry (*Rubus idaeus* L.) leaves. *Stud. Univ. Vasile Goldis Ser. Stiintele Vietii* **2016**, *26*, 463–472.
31. Bastos, C.; Barros, L.; Dueñas, M.; Calhelha, R.C.; Queiroz, M.J.R.P.; Santos-Buelga, C.; Ferreira, I.C.F.R. Chemical characterisation and bioactive properties of *Prunus avium* L.: The widely studied fruits and the unexplored stems. *Food Chem.* **2015**, *173*, 1045–1053. [CrossRef]
32. Dudzinska, D.; Luzak, B.; Boncler, M.; Rywaniak, J.; Sosnowska, D.; Podsedek, A.; Watala, C. CD39/NTPDase-1 expression and activity in human umbilical vein endothelial cells are differentially regulated by leaf extracts from *Rubus caesius* and *Rubus idaeus*. *Cell. Mol. Biol. Lett.* **2014**, *19*, 361–380. [CrossRef]
33. Jakopič, J.; Štampar, F.; Veberič, R. Influence of hail net and reflective foil on cyanidin glycosides and quercetin glycosides in 'Fuji'apple skin. *HortScience* **2010**, *45*, 1447–1452. [CrossRef]
34. Alkhudaydi, H.M.S.; Muriuki, E.N.; Spencer, J.P. Determination of the polyphenol composition of raspberry leaf using LC-MS/MS. *Molecules* **2025**, *30*, 970. [CrossRef]
35. Wojdyło, A.; Nowicka, P.; Turkiewicz, I.P.; Tkacz, K. Profiling of polyphenols by LC-QTOF/ESI-MS, characteristics of nutritional compounds and in vitro effect on pancreatic lipase, α-glucosidase, α-amylase, cholinesterase and cyclooxygenase activities of sweet (*Prunus avium*) and sour (*P. cerasus*) cherries leaves and fruits. *Ind. Crops Prod.* **2021**, *174*, 114214. [CrossRef]
36. Tian, Y.; Liimatainen, J.; Alanne, A.L.; Lindstedt, A.; Liu, P.; Sinkkonen, J.; Kallio, H.; Yang, B. Phenolic compounds extracted by acidic aqueous ethanol from berries and leaves of different berry plants. *Food Chem.* **2017**, *220*, 266–281. [CrossRef]

37. Kanoun, K.; Belyagoubi-Benhammou, N.; Ghembaza, N.; Atik Bekkara, F. Comparative studies on antioxidant activities of extracts from the leaf, stem and berry of *Myrtus communis* L. *Int. Food Res. J.* **2014**, *21*, 1957–1962.
38. Cvetanović, A.; Zengin, G.; Zeković, Z.; Švarc-Gajić, J.; Ražić, S.; Damjanović, A.; Mašković, P.; Mitić, M. Comparative in vitro studies of the biological potential and chemical composition of stems, leaves and berries *Aronia melanocarpa*'s extracts obtained by subcritical water extraction. *Food Chem. Toxicol.* **2018**, *121*, 458–466. [CrossRef]
39. Willig, G.; Brunissen, F.; Brunois, F.; Godon, B.; Magro, C.; Monteux, C.; Peyrot, C.; Ioannou, I. Phenolic compounds extracted from cherry tree (*Prunus avium*) branches: Impact of the process on cosmetic properties. *Antioxidants* **2022**, *11*, 813. [CrossRef]
40. Zhang, H.; Li, Q.; Qiao, G.; Qiu, Z.; Wen, Z.; Wen, X. Optimizing the supercritical carbon dioxide extraction of sweet cherry (*Prunus avium* L.) leaves and UPLC-MS/MS analysis. *Anal. Methods* **2020**, *12*, 3004–3013. [CrossRef]
41. Kniepkamp, K.; Errico, M.; Yu, M.; Roda-Serrat, M.C.; Eilers, J.G.; Wark, M.; van Haren, R. Lipid extraction of high-moisture sour cherry (*Prunus cerasus* L.) stones by supercritical carbon dioxide. *J. Chem. Technol. Biotechnol.* **2024**, *99*, 810–819. [CrossRef]
42. Pavlić, B.; Aćimović, M.; Sknepnek, A.; Miletić, D.; Mrkonjić, Ž.; Kljakić, A.C.; Jerković, J.; Mišan, A.; Pojić, M.; Stupar, A.; et al. Sustainable raw materials for efficient valorization and recovery of bioactive compounds. *Ind. Crops Prod.* **2023**, *193*, 116167. [CrossRef]
43. Zhang, H.; Yan, H.; Lu, C.; Lin, H.; Li, Q. Optimization of ultrasound and microwave-assisted extraction of sweet cherry tree branches and chemical component analysis by UPLC–MS/MS. *Trees—Struct. Funct.* **2021**, *35*, 1247–1256. [CrossRef]
44. Wang, L.; Lin, X.; Zhang, J.; Zhang, W.; Hu, X.; Li, W.; Li, C.; Liu, S. Extraction methods for the releasing of bound phenolics from *Rubus idaeus* L. leaves and seeds. *Ind. Crops Prod.* **2019**, *135*, 1–9. [CrossRef]
45. Hałasa, R.; Turecka, K.; Mizerska, U.; Krauze-Baranowska, M. Anti-*Helicobacter pylori* biofilm extracts from *Rubus idaeus* and *Rubus occidentalis*. *Pharmaceutics* **2024**, *16*, 501. [CrossRef]
46. Kotuła, M.; Kapusta-Duch, J.; Smoleń, S.; Doskočil, I. Phytochemical composition of the fruits and leaves of raspberries (*Rubus idaeus* L.)—Conventional vs. organic and those wild grown. *Appl. Sci.* **2022**, *12*, 11783. [CrossRef]
47. Plasencia, P.; Finimundy, T.C.; Carocho, M.; Calhelha, R.C.; Añibarro-Ortega, M.; Pires, T.C.S.P.; Barreiro, F.; Garcia, P.A.; Barros, L.; Heleno, S.A. Extraction of bioactive compounds from *Rubus idaeus* bioresidues: A full screening on phenolic composition and bioactive potential. *Waste Biomass Valor.* **2025**, *16*, 737–747. [CrossRef]
48. Maslov, O.; Komisarenko, M.; Kolisnyk, S.; Kostina, T.; Golik, M.; Moroz, V.; Tarasenko, D.; Akhmedov, E. Investigation of the extraction dynamic of the biologically active substances of the raspberry (*Rubus idaeus* L.) shoots. *Curr. Issues Pharm. Med. Sci.* **2023**, *36*, 194–198. [CrossRef]
49. Zhang, S.; Liu, Z.; Li, X.; Abubaker, M.A.; Liu, X.; Li, Z.; Wang, X.; Zhu, X.; Zhang, J.; Chen, X. Comparative study of three raspberry cultivar (*Rubus idaeus* L.) leaves metabolites: Metabolome profiling and antioxidant activities. *Appl. Sci.* **2022**, *12*, 990. [CrossRef]
50. Ruiz-Aquino, F.; Feria-Reyes, R.; Rutiaga-Quiñones, J.G.; Robledo-Taboada, L.H.; Gabriel-Parra, R. Characterization of tannin extracts derived from the bark of four tree species by HPLC and FTIR. *For. Sci. Technol.* **2023**, *19*, 38–46. [CrossRef]
51. Agarwal, C.; Hofmann, T.; Vršanská, M.; Schlosserová, N.; Visi-Rajczi, E.; Voběrková, S.; Pásztory, Z. In vitro antioxidant and antibacterial activities with polyphenolic profiling of wild cherry, the european larch and sweet chestnut tree bark. *Eur. Food Res. Technol.* **2021**, *247*, 2355–2370. [CrossRef]
52. Švarc-Gajić, J.; Clavijo, S.; Suárez, R.; Cvetanović, A.; Cerdà, V. Simultaneous dispersive liquid-liquid microextraction derivatisation and gas chromatography mass spectrometry analysis of subcritical water extracts of sweet and sour cherry stems. *Anal. Bioanal. Chem.* **2018**, *410*, 1943–1953. [CrossRef]
53. Voss, M.; Gaudino, E.C.; Tabasso, S.; Forte, C.; Cravotto, G. Current emerging green technologies for the valorization of grape and cherry wastes. *Curr. Food Sci. Technol. Rep.* **2023**, *1*, 47–61. [CrossRef]
54. Evtyugin, D.D.; Magina, S.; Evtuguin, D.V. Recent advances in the production and applications of ellagic acid and its derivatives. A review. *Molecules* **2020**, *25*, 2745. [CrossRef]
55. Švarc-Gajić, J.; Cerdà, V.; Clavijo, S.; Suárez, R.; Mašković, P.; Cvetanović, A.; Delerue-Matos, C.; Carvalho, A.P.; Novakov, V. Bioactive compounds of sweet and sour cherry stems obtained by subcritical water extraction. *J. Chem. Technol. Biotechnol.* **2018**, *93*, 1627–1635. [CrossRef]
56. Hamad, F.B.; Mubofu, E.B. Potential biological applications of bio-based anacardic acids and their derivatives. *Int. J. Mol. Sci.* **2015**, *16*, 8569–8590. [CrossRef]
57. Li, Z.; Niu, L.; Chen, Y.; Qiu, X.; Du, T.; Zhu, M.; Wang, M.; Mo, H.; Xiao, S. Recent advance in the biological activity of chlorogenic acid and its application in food industry. *Int. J. Food Sci. Technol.* **2023**, *58*, 4931–4947. [CrossRef]
58. Wang, L.; Pan, X.; Jiang, L.; Chu, Y.; Gao, S.; Jiang, X.; Zhang, Y.; Chen, Y.; Luo, S.; Peng, C. The biological activity mechanism of chlorogenic acid and its applications in food industry: A review. *Front. Nutr.* **2022**, *9*, 943911. [CrossRef]
59. Peng, R.; Wu, Q.; Chen, J.; Ghosh, R.; Chen, X. Isolation of ellagic acid from pomegranate peel extract by hydrophobic interaction chromatography using graphene oxide grafted cotton fiber adsorbent. *J. Sep. Sci.* **2018**, *41*, 747–755. [CrossRef]

60. García-Niño, W.R.; Zazueta, C. Ellagic acid: Pharmacological activities and molecular mechanisms involved in liver protection. *Pharmacol. Res.* **2015**, *97*, 84–103. [CrossRef]
61. Tomou, E.M.; Papakyriakopoulou, P.; Skaltsa, H.; Valsami, G.; Kadoglou, N.P.E. Bio-actives from natural products with potential cardioprotective properties: Isolation, identification, and pharmacological actions of apigenin, quercetin, and silibinin. *Molecules* **2023**, *28*, 2387. [CrossRef]
62. Kumar, K.S.; Sabu, V.; Sindhu, G.; Rauf, A.A.; Helen, A. Isolation, identification and characterization of apigenin from *Justicia gendarussa* and its anti-inflammatory activity. *Int. Immunopharmacol.* **2018**, *59*, 157–167. [CrossRef]
63. Cvetanović, A.; Švarc-Gajić, J.; Gašić, U.; Tešić, Ž.; Zengin, G.; Zeković, Z.; Đurović, S. Isolation of apigenin from subcritical water extracts: Optimization of the process. *J. Supercrit. Fluids* **2017**, *120*, 32–42. [CrossRef]
64. Mehdi, A.; Al-ani, W.M.K.; Raoof, A. Isolation of astragalin from IRAQI *Chenopodium album*. *Asian J. Pharm. Clin. Res.* **2018**, *11*, 530–535. [CrossRef]
65. Ruan, J.; Shi, Z.; Cao, X.; Dang, Z.; Zhang, Q.; Zhang, W.; Wu, L.; Zhang, Y.; Wang, T. Research progress on anti-inflammatory effects and related mechanisms of astragalin. *Int. J. Mol. Sci.* **2024**, *25*, 4476. [CrossRef]
66. Jeyanthi, V.; Anbu, P.; Vairamani, M.; Velusamy, P. Isolation of hydroquinone (benzene-1,4-diol) metabolite from halotolerant *Bacillus methylotrophicus* MHC10 and its inhibitory activity towards bacterial pathogens. *Bioprocess Biosyst. Eng.* **2016**, *39*, 429–439. [CrossRef]
67. Enguita, F.J.; Leitão, A.L. Hydroquinone: Environmental pollution, toxicity, and microbial answers. *BioMed Res. Int.* **2013**, *2013*, 542168. [CrossRef]
68. Raza, M.J.; Jalil, O.; Kumar, D.; Pandey, C.M. Highly sensitive electrochemical detection of hydroquinone in wastewater using ionic liquid grafted rGO-ZrO2 nanohybrid-based conducting paper. *J. Electrochem. Soc.* **2025**, *172*, 067508. [CrossRef]
69. Cao, X.; Wei, Y.; Ito, Y. Preparative isolation of isorhamnetin from *Stigma Maydis* using high speed countercurrent chromatography. *J. Liq. Chromatogr. Relat. Technol.* **2009**, *32*, 273–280. [CrossRef]
70. Mei, C.; Liu, Y.; Lyu, X.; Jiang, Z.; Liu, Z.; Zhi, Y.; Xu, X.; Wang, H. Advances in isorhamnetin treatment of malignant tumors: Mechanisms and applications. *Nutrients* **2025**, *17*, 1853. [CrossRef]
71. Duan, M.; Wang, X.; Feng, J.; Xiao, X.; Zhang, L.; He, S.; Ma, L.; Wang, X.; Yang, S.; Rao, M.J. From agricultural waste to functional tea: Optimized processing enhances bioactive flavonoid recovery and antioxidant capacity with multifaceted health benefits in loquat (*Eriobotrya japonica* Lindl.) flowers. *Horticulturae* **2025**, *11*, 766. [CrossRef]
72. Nguelefack, T.B.; Mbakam, F.H.K.; Tapondjou, L.A.; Watcho, P.; Nguelefack-Mbuyo, E.P.; Ponou, B.K.; Kamanyi, A.; Park, H.J. A dimeric triterpenoid glycoside and flavonoid glycosides with free radical-scavenging activity isolated from *Rubus rigidus* var. *camerunensis*. *Arch. Pharmacal Res.* **2011**, *34*, 543–550. [CrossRef]
73. Gajjar, N.D.; Dhameliya, T.M.; Shah, G.B. In search of RdRp and Mpro inhibitors against SARS CoV-2: Molecular docking, molecular dynamic simulations and ADMET analysis. *J. Mol. Struct.* **2021**, *1239*, 130488. [CrossRef]
74. Wahab, A.; Begum, S.; Mahmood, I.; Mahmood, T.; Ahmad, A.; Fayyaz, N. Luteolin and kaempferol from *Cassia Alata*. Antimicrobial and antioxidant activity of its methanolic extracts. *FUUAST J. Biol.* **2014**, *4*, 1–5.
75. Bangar, S.P.; Chaudhary, V.; Sharma, N.; Bansal, V.; Ozogul, F.; Lorenzo, J.M. Kaempferol: A flavonoid with wider biological activities and its applications. *Crit. Rev. Food Sci. Nutr.* **2023**, *63*, 9580–9604. [CrossRef]
76. Montenegro, I.; Pérez, C.; González, B.; Domínguez, Á.; Gómez, E. Thermal characterization and heat capacities of seven polyphenols. *Molecules* **2025**, *30*, 199. [CrossRef]
77. Sudto, K.; Pornpakakul, S.; Wanichwecharungruang, S. An efficient method for the large scale isolation of naringin from pomelo (*Citrus grandis*) peel. *Int. J. Food Sci. Technol.* **2009**, *44*, 1737–1742. [CrossRef]
78. Koirala, M.; Lee, Y.K.; Kim, M.S.; Chung, Y.C.; Park, J.S.; Kim, S.Y. Biotransformation of naringenin by *Bacillus amyloliquefaciens* into three naringenin derivatives. *Nat. Prod. Commun.* **2019**, *14*, 465–472. [CrossRef]
79. Zhang, L.; Song, L.; Zhang, P.; Liu, T.; Zhou, L.; Yang, G.; Lin, R.; Zhang, J. Solubilities of naringin and naringenin in different solvents and dissociation constants of naringenin. *J. Chem. Eng. Data* **2015**, *60*, 932–940. [CrossRef]
80. Kylli, P.; Nohynek, L.; Puupponen-Pimiä, R.; Westerlund-Wikström, B.; Leppänen, T.; Welling, J.; Moilanen, E.; Heinonen, M. Lingonberry (*Vaccinium vitis-idaea*) and European cranberry (*Vaccinium microcarpon*) proanthocyanidins: Isolation, identification, and bioactivities. *J. Agric. Food Chem.* **2011**, *59*, 3373–3384. [CrossRef]
81. Chen, S.; Song, J.; Du, L.; Ma, Y.; Ren, S.; Ren, J.; Li, S. Quantitative analysis of solubility parameters and surface properties of larch bark proanthocyanidins. *Polymers* **2020**, *12*, 2800. [CrossRef]
82. Choi, J.S.; Yokozawa, T.; Oura, H. Improvement of hyperglycemia and hyperlipemia in streptozotocin-diabetic rats by a methanolic extract of *Prunus davidiana* stems and its main component, prunin. *Planta Med.* **1991**, *57*, 208–211. [CrossRef]
83. Céliz, G.; Daz, M. Biocatalytic preparation of alkyl esters of citrus flavanone glucoside prunin in organic media. *Process Biochem.* **2011**, *46*, 94–100. [CrossRef]
84. Dall'Acqua, S.; Miolo, G.; Innocenti, G.; Caffieri, S. The photodegradation of quercetin: Relation to oxidation. *Molecules* **2012**, *17*, 8898–8907. [CrossRef]

85. Ramešová, Š.; Sokolová, R.; Degano, I.; Bulíčková, J.; Žabka, J.; Gál, M. On the stability of the bioactive flavonoids quercetin and luteolin under oxygen-free conditions. *Anal. Bioanal. Chem.* **2012**, *402*, 975–982. [CrossRef]
86. Yingyuen, P.; Sukrong, S.; Phisalaphong, M. Isolation, separation and purification of rutin from banana leaves (*Musa balbisiana*). *Ind. Crops Prod.* **2020**, *149*, 112307. [CrossRef]
87. Baldisserotto, A.; Vertuani, S.; Bino, A.; De Lucia, D.; Lampronti, I.; Milani, R.; Gambari, R.; Manfredini, S. Design, synthesis and biological activity of a novel rutin analogue with improved lipid soluble properties. *Bioorg. Med. Chem.* **2015**, *23*, 264–271. [CrossRef]
88. Choi, S.S.; Park, H.R.; Lee, K.A.A. Comparative study of rutin and rutin glycoside: Antioxidant activity, anti-inflammatory effect, effect on platelet aggregation and blood coagulation. *Antioxidants* **2021**, *10*, 1696. [CrossRef]
89. Choe, U.; Li, Y.; Yu, L.; Gao, B.; Wang, T.T.Y.; Sun, J.; Chen, P.; Yu, L. Chemical composition of cold-pressed blackberry seed flour extract and its potential health-beneficial properties. *Food Sci. Nutr.* **2020**, *8*, 1215–1225. [CrossRef]
90. Firmansyah, A.; Winingsih, W.; Manobi, J.D.Y. Review of scopoletin: Isolation, analysis process, and pharmacological activity. *Biointerface Res. Appl. Chem.* **2021**, *11*, 12006–12019. [CrossRef]
91. Galán-Pérez, J.A.; Gámiz, B.; Celis, R. Determining the effect of soil properties on the stability of scopoletin and its toxicity to target plants. *Biol. Fertil. Soils* **2021**, *57*, 643–655. [CrossRef]
92. Chaaban, H.; Ioannou, I.; Chebil, L.; Slimane, M.; Gérardin, C.; Paris, C.; Charbonnel, C.; Chekir, L.; Ghoul, M. Effect of heat processing on thermal stability and antioxidant activity of six flavonoids. *J. Food Process. Preserv.* **2017**, *41*, e13203. [CrossRef]
93. Hemshekhar, M.; Sebastin Santhosh, M.; Kemparaju, K.; Girish, K.S. Emerging roles of anacardic acid and its derivatives: A pharmacological overview. *Basic Clin. Pharmacol. Toxicol.* **2012**, *110*, 122–132. [CrossRef]
94. Rosa, M.E.P.; Rebouças, L.M.; Marques, S.P.D.; Silva, L.M.R.; Cunha, F.E.T.; Costa, P.M.S.; de Assis, D.A.; Silveira, K.B.; Muniz, C.R.; Trevisan, M.T.S.; et al. Sodium hyaluronate microcapsules to promote antitumor selectivity of anacardic acid. *Int. J. Biol. Macromol.* **2025**, *296*, 139616. [CrossRef]
95. Schultz, D.J.; Krishna, A.; Vittitow, S.L.; Alizadeh-Rad, N.; Muluhngwi, P.; Rouchka, E.C.; Klinge, C.M. Transcriptomic response of breast cancer cells to anacardic acid. *Sci. Rep.* **2018**, *8*, 8063. [CrossRef]
96. Anjum, M.M.; Patel, K.K.; Pandey, N.; Tilak, R.; Agrawal, A.K.; Singh, S. Development of anacardic acid/hydroxypropyl-β-cyclodextrin inclusion complex with enhanced solubility and antimicrobial activity. *J. Mol. Liq.* **2019**, *296*, 112085. [CrossRef]
97. Jit, T.; Deb Roy, S.; Shil, D.; Chakraborty, J.; Paul, A.; Roy, S.; De, D. The potential of tannins from medicinal plants as anti-cancer agents. *J. Med. Plants Stud.* **2024**, *12*, 414423.
98. Radha, R.; Prakash, S.; Kumari, N.; Sharma, N.; Puri, S.; Singh, J.; Thakur, M.; Kumar, M. Bioactives and bioactivities from food byproducts. *Curr. Food Sci. Technol. Rep.* **2024**, *2*, 297–308. [CrossRef]
99. Ko, H.; Jeon, H.; Lee, D.; Choi, H.K.; Kang, K.S.; Choi, K.C. Sanguiin H6 suppresses TGF-β induction of the epithelial–mesenchymal transition and inhibits migration and invasion in A549 lung cancer. *Bioorg. Med. Chem. Lett.* **2015**, *25*, 5508–5513. [CrossRef]
100. Gesek, J.; Jakimiuk, K.; Atanasov, A.G.; Tomczyk, M. Sanguiins—Promising molecules with broad biological potential. *Int. J. Mol. Sci.* **2021**, *22*, 12972. [CrossRef]
101. Park, E.J.; Lee, D.; Baek, S.E.; Kim, K.H.; Kang, K.S.; Jang, T.S.; Lee, H.L.; Song, J.H.; Yoo, J.E. Cytotoxic effect of sanguiin H-6 on MCF-7 and MDA-MB-231 human breast carcinoma cells. *Bioorg. Med. Chem. Lett.* **2017**, *27*, 4389–4392. [CrossRef]
102. Huang, Z.Q.; Chen, P.; Su, W.W.; Wang, Y.G.; Wu, H.; Peng, W.; Li, P.B. Antioxidant activity and hepatoprotective potential of quercetin 7-rhamnoside in vitro and in vivo. *Molecules* **2018**, *23*, 1188. [CrossRef]
103. Deng, D.; Zhao, B.; Yang, H.; Wang, S.; Geng, Z.; Zhou, J.; Yang, G.; Han, L. Investigating the effect and potential mechanism of rhamnetin 3-o-α-rhamnoside on acute liver injury in vivo and in vitro. *Pharmaceuticals* **2025**, *18*, 116. [CrossRef]
104. Li, L.; Lei, X.; Chen, L.; Ma, Y.; Luo, J.; Liu, X.; Xu, X.; Zhou, G.; Feng, X. Protective Mechanism of quercetin compounds against acrylamide-induced hepatotoxicity. *Food Sci. Hum. Wellness* **2024**, *13*, 225–240. [CrossRef]
105. Choi, H.J.; Song, J.H.; Park, K.S.; Kwon, D.H. Inhibitory effects of quercetin 3-rhamnoside on influenza a virus replication. *Eur. J. Pharm. Sci.* **2009**, *37*, 329–333. [CrossRef]
106. Meng, X.; Xia, C.; Wu, H.; Gu, Q.; Li, P. Metabolism of quercitrin in the colon and its beneficial regulatory effects on gut microbiota. *J. Sci. Food Agric.* **2024**, *104*, 9255–9264. [CrossRef]
107. Reinboth, M.; Wolffram, S.; Abraham, G.; Ungemach, F.R.; Cermak, R. Oral bioavailability of quercetin from different quercetin glycosides in dogs. *Br. J. Nutr.* **2010**, *104*, 198–203. [CrossRef]
108. Li, Y.; Yao, J.; Han, C.; Yang, J.; Chaudhry, M.T.; Wang, S.; Liu, H.; Yin, Y. Quercetin, inflammation and immunity. *Nutrients* **2016**, *8*, 167. [CrossRef]
109. Cao, M.M.; Guo, Z.; Wang, J.; Ma, H.Y.; Qin, X.Y.; Hu, Y.; Lan, R. Astragalin alleviates lipopolysaccharide-induced depressive-like behavior in mice by preserving blood-brain barrier integrity and suppressing neuroinflammation. *Free Radic. Biol. Med.* **2025**, *232*, 340–352. [CrossRef]

110. Li, Q.; Yang, Z.; Lu, H.; Liu, F.; Zhou, D.; Zou, Y. Astragalin Exerted hypoglycemic effect by both inhibiting α-glucosidase and modulating AMPK signaling pathway. *Nutrients* **2025**, *17*, 406. [CrossRef]
111. Riaz, A.; Rasul, A.; Hussain, G.; Zahoor, M.K.; Jabeen, F.; Subhani, Z.; Younis, T.; Ali, M.; Sarfraz, I.; Selamoglu, Z. Astragalin: A bioactive phytochemical with potential therapeutic activities. *Adv. Pharmacol. Pharm. Sci.* **2018**, *2018*, 9794625. [CrossRef]
112. Zeng, W.; Chen, L. Astragalin inhibits the proliferation of high-risk HPV-positive cervical epithelial cells and attenuates malignant cervical lesions. *Cytotechnology* **2025**, *77*, 80. [CrossRef]
113. Li, C.; Hu, M.; Jiang, S.; Liang, Z.; Wang, J.; Liu, Z.; Wang, H.M.D.; Kang, W. Evaluation procoagulant activity and mechanism of astragalin. *Molecules* **2020**, *25*, 177. [CrossRef]
114. Yang, C.Z.; Wang, S.H.; Zhang, R.H.; Lin, J.H.; Tian, Y.H.; Yang, Y.Q.; Liu, J.; Ma, Y.X. Neuroprotective effect of astragalin via activating PI3K/Akt-MTOR-mediated autophagy on APP/PS1 mice. *Cell Death Discov.* **2023**, *9*, 15. [CrossRef]
115. Chen, J.; Zhong, K.; Qin, S.; Jing, Y.; Liu, S.; Li, D.; Peng, C. Astragalin: A food-origin flavonoid with therapeutic effect for multiple diseases. *Front. Pharmacol.* **2023**, *14*, 1265960. [CrossRef]
116. Duszka, K.; Clark, B.F.C.; Massino, F.; Barciszewski, J. Biological activities of kinetin. In *Herbal Drugs: Ethnomedicine to Modern Medicine*; Ramawat, K.G., Ed.; Springer: Berlin/Heidelberg, Germany, 2009; pp. 369–380. [CrossRef]
117. Jiang, X.; Yang, L.; Chen, G.; Feng, X.; Liu, Y.; Gao, Q.; Mai, M.; Chen, C.; Yu, C.; Ye, S.; et al. Discovery of kinetin in inhibiting colorectal cancer progression via enhancing PSMB1-mediated RAB34 degradation. *Cancer Lett.* **2024**, *584*, 216600. [CrossRef]
118. Souza, T.M.L.; Pinho, V.D.; Setim, C.F.; Sacramento, C.Q.; Marcon, R.; Fintelman-Rodrigues, N.; Chaves, O.A.; Heller, M.; Temerozo, J.R.; Ferreira, A.C.; et al. Preclinical development of kinetin as a safe error-prone SARS-CoV-2 antiviral able to attenuate virus-induced inflammation. *Nat. Commun.* **2023**, *14*, 199. [CrossRef]
119. Chandorkar, Y.; Valeske, M.; Kolrosova, B.; Elbs-Glatz, Y.; Zuber, F.; Schoeller, J.; Kummer, N.; Ren, Q.; Rottmar, M.; Maniura-Weber, K. Bioactive salicylic acid containing coating for dental implants to combat infection and inflammation. *Adv. Mater. Interfaces* **2024**, *11*, 2300750. [CrossRef]
120. Miclaus, M.O.; Borodi, G.; Turza, A. Four polymorphs of the bioactive diuretic drug 4-chloro-5-chlorosulfonyl salicylic acid. *Crystals* **2025**, *15*, 136. [CrossRef]
121. Nagelschmitz, J.; Blunck, M.; Kraetzschmar, J.; Ludwig, M.; Wensing, G.; Hohlfeld, T. Pharmacokinetics and pharmacodynamics of acetylsalicylic acid after intravenous and oral administration to healthy volunteers. *Clin. Pharmacol.: Adv. Appl.* **2014**, *6*, 51–59. [CrossRef]
122. Madan, R.K.; Levitt, J. A review of toxicity from topical salicylic acid preparations. *J. Am. Acad. Dermatol.* **2014**, *70*, 788–792. [CrossRef]
123. Varvara, M.; Bozzo, G.; Celano, G.; Disanto, C.; Pagliarone, C.N.; Celano, G.V. The use of ascorbic acid as a food additive: Technical-legal issues. *Ital. J. Food Saf.* **2016**, *5*, 4313. [CrossRef]
124. Davis, J.L.; Paris, H.L.; Beals, J.W.; Binns, S.E.; Giordano, G.R.; Scalzo, R.L.; Schweder, M.M.; Blair, E.; Bell, C. Liposomal-encapsulated ascorbic acid: Influence on vitamin C bioavailability and capacity to protect against ischemia-reperfusion injury. *Nutr. Metab. Insights* **2016**, *9*, 25–30. [CrossRef]
125. Stephenson, C.M.; Levin, R.D.; Spector, T.; Lis, C.G. Phase I clinical trial to evaluate the safety, tolerability, and pharmacokinetics of high-dose intravenous ascorbic acid in patients with advanced cancer. *Cancer Chemother. Pharmacol.* **2013**, *72*, 139–146. [CrossRef]
126. Bhatt, S.C.; Naik, B.; Kumar, V.; Kumar Gupta, A.; Kumar, S.; Singh Preet, M.; Sharma, N.; Rustagi, S. Untapped potential of non-conventional *Rubus* species: Bioactivity, nutrition, and livelihood opportunities. *Plant Methods* **2023**, *19*, 114. [CrossRef]
127. Borel, P.; Preveraud, D.; Desmarchelier, C. Bioavailability of vitamin E in humans: An update. *Nutr. Rev.* **2013**, *71*, 319–331. [CrossRef]
128. Gad, S.C. Hydroquinone. In *Encyclopedia of Toxicology*, 4th ed.; Wexler, P., Ed.; Academic Press: Cambridge, MA, USA, 2024; Volume 5, pp. 425–430. [CrossRef]
129. Fabian, I.M.; Sinnathamby, E.S.; Flanagan, C.J.; Lindberg, A.; Tynes, B.; Kelkar, R.A.; Varrassi, G.; Ahmadzadeh, S.; Shekoohi, S.; Kaye, A.D. Topical hydroquinone for hyperpigmentation: A narrative review. *Cureus* **2023**, *15*, e48840. [CrossRef]
130. Banodkar, P.D.; Banodkar, K.P. History of hydroquinone. *Indian J. Dermatol. Venereol. Leprol.* **2022**, *88*, 696–699. [CrossRef]
131. Shivaram, K.; Edwards, K.; Mohammad, T.F. An update on the safety of hydroquinone. *Arch. Dermatol. Res.* **2024**, *316*, 378. [CrossRef]
132. Serrano, D.R.; Gordo, M.J.; Matji, A.; González, S.; Lalatsa, A.; Torrado, J.J. Tuning the transdermal delivery of hydroquinone upon formulation with novel permeation enhancers. *Pharmaceutics* **2019**, *11*, 167. [CrossRef]
133. Imran, M.; Salehi, B.; Sharifi-Rad, J.; Gondal, T.A.; Saeed, F.; Imran, A.; Shahbaz, M.; Fokou, P.V.T.; Arshad, M.U.; Khan, H.; et al. Kaempferol: A key emphasis to its anticancer potential. *Molecules* **2019**, *24*, 2277. [CrossRef]
134. Periferakis, A.; Periferakis, K.; Badarau, I.A.; Petran, E.M.; Popa, D.C.; Caruntu, A.; Costache, R.S.; Scheau, C.; Caruntu, C.; Costache, D.O. Kaempferol: Antimicrobial properties, sources, clinical, and traditional applications. *Int. J. Mol. Sci.* **2022**, *23*, 15054. [CrossRef]

135. Calderón-Montaño, J.M.; Burgos-Morón, E.; Pérez-Guerrero, C.; López-Lázaro, M. A review on the dietary flavonoid kaempferol. *Mini-Rev. Med. Chem.* **2011**, *11*, 298–344. [CrossRef]
136. Li, Q.; Ge, C.; Tan, J.; Sun, Y.; Kuang, Q.; Dai, X.; Zhong, S.; Yi, C.; Hu, L.F.; Lou, D.S.; et al. Juglanin protects against high fat diet induced renal injury by suppressing inflammation and dyslipidemia via regulating NF-KB/HDAC3 signaling. *Int. Immunopharmacol.* **2021**, *95*, 107340. [CrossRef]
137. Ren, Y.; Hu, S.; Pu, H.; Zhou, Y.; Jiang, M.; Li, Y.; Deng, C.; Gao, J.; Xu, M.; Ge, C. Juglanin Ameliorates depression-like behavior in chronic unpredictable mild stress-induced mice by improving AMPK signaling. *J. Funct. Foods* **2022**, *98*, 105263. [CrossRef]
138. Wang, P.; Hu, M.; Wang, L.; Qu, J.; Liu, Y.; Li, C.; Liu, Z.; Ma, C.; Kang, W. Chemical constituents and coagulation effects of the flowers of *Rosa chinensis* Jacq. *J. Future Foods* **2023**, *3*, 155–162. [CrossRef]
139. Gong, G.; Guan, Y.Y.; Zhang, Z.L.; Rahman, K.; Wang, S.J.; Zhou, S.; Luan, X.; Zhang, H. Isorhamnetin: A review of pharmacological effects. *Biomed. Pharmacother.* **2020**, *128*, 110301. [CrossRef]
140. González-Arceo, M.; Gomez-Lopez, I.; Carr-Ugarte, H.; Eseberri, I.; González, M.; Cano, M.P.; Portillo, M.P.; Gómez-Zorita, S. Anti-obesity effects of isorhamnetin and isorhamnetin conjugates. *Int. J. Mol. Sci.* **2022**, *24*, 299. [CrossRef]
141. Dayem, A.A.; Choi, H.Y.; Kim, Y.B.; Cho, S.G. Antiviral effect of methylated flavonol isorhamnetin against influenza. *PLoS ONE* **2015**, *10*, e0121610. [CrossRef]
142. Ku, S.K.; Kim, T.H.; Bae, J.S. Anticoagulant activities of persicarin and isorhamnetin. *Vascul. Pharmacol.* **2013**, *58*, 272–279. [CrossRef]
143. Scarlata, G.G.M.; Lopez, I.; Gambardella, M.L.; Milanović, M.; Milić, N.; Abenavoli, L. Preventive and therapeutic effects of baicalein, galangin, and isorhamnetin in chronic liver diseases: A narrative review. *Molecules* **2025**, *30*, 1253. [CrossRef]
144. Huang, Z.R.; Lin, Y.K.; Fang, J.Y. Biological and pharmacological activities of squalene and related compounds: Potential uses in cosmetic dermatology. *Molecules* **2009**, *14*, 540–554. [CrossRef]
145. Shalu, S.; Raveendranathan, P.K.; Vaidyanathan, V.K.; Blank, L.M.; Germer, A.; Balakumaran, P.A. Microbial squalene: A sustainable alternative for the cosmetics and pharmaceutical industry – A review. *Eng. Life Sci.* **2024**, *24*, e202400003. [CrossRef]
146. Maxim, C.; Turcov, D.; Bulgariu, A.G.; Șuteu, D. Squalene—Background and perspectives in cosmeceuticals formulas. *Bul. Inst. Polit. Iasi* **2024**, *70*, 47–57. [CrossRef]
147. Hussain, S.; Javed, M.; Abid, M.A.; Khan, M.A.; Syed, S.K.; Faizan, M.; Feroz, F. *Prunus avium* L.; Phytochemistry, nutritional and pharmacological review. *Adv. Life Sci.* **2021**, *8*, 307–314. [CrossRef]
148. Kumari, N.; Radha; Kumar, M.; Puri, S.; Zhang, B.; Rais, N.; Pundir, A.; Chandran, D.; Raman, P.; Dhumal, S.; et al. Peach (*Prunus persica* (L.) Batsch) seeds and kernels as potential plant-based functional food ingredients: A review of bioactive compounds and health-promoting activities. *Food Biosci.* **2023**, *54*, 102914. [CrossRef]
149. Kajla, V.; Singh, B.; Muskaan, S.K.D.; Sharma, P.; Vishali, M.; Sayam, A. Harnessing amygdalin in integrative medicine: Novel insights for endocrine disorders. *Rev. Argent. Clin. Psicol.* **2024**, *33*, 54–73. [CrossRef]
150. Mungamuri, S.K.; Chatterjee, N.; Ara, D. Phytotherapy for liver fibrosis: Insights from the biology of hepatic stellate cells—A narrative review. *Liver Int. Commun.* **2025**, *6*, e70015. [CrossRef]
151. Qin, Y.; Wang, S.; Wen, Q.; Xia, Q.; Wang, S.; Chen, G.; Sun, J.; Shen, C.; Song, S. Interactions between *Ephedra sinica* and *Prunus armeniaca*: From stereoselectivity to deamination as a metabolic detoxification mechanism of amygdalin. *Front. Pharmacol.* **2021**, *12*, 744624. [CrossRef]
152. EFSA Panel on Contaminants in the Food Chain (CONTAM). Acute health risks related to the presence of cyanogenic glycosides in raw apricot kernels and products derived from raw apricot kernels. *EFSA J.* **2016**, *14*, e04424. [CrossRef]
153. Das, A.; Baidya, R.; Chakraborty, T.; Samanta, A.K.; Roy, S. Pharmacological basis and new insights of taxifolin: A comprehensive review. *Biomed. Pharmacother.* **2021**, *142*, 112004. [CrossRef]
154. Liu, Y.; Shi, X.; Tian, Y.; Zhai, S.; Liu, Y.; Xiong, Z.; Chu, S. An insight into novel therapeutic potentials of taxifolin. *Front. Pharmacol.* **2023**, *14*, 1173855. [CrossRef]
155. Zu, Y.; Wu, W.; Zhao, X.; Li, Y.; Wang, W.; Zhong, C.; Zhang, Y.; Zhao, X. Enhancement of solubility, antioxidant ability and bioavailability of taxifolin nanoparticles by liquid antisolvent precipitation technique. *Int. J. Pharm.* **2014**, *471*, 366–376. [CrossRef]
156. Rajnochová Svobodová, A.; Ryšavá, A.; Psotová, M.; Kosina, P.; Zálešák, B.; Ulrichová, J.; Vostálová, J. The phototoxic potential of the flavonoids, taxifolin and quercetin. *Photochem. Photobiol.* **2017**, *93*, 1240–1247. [CrossRef]
157. Patel, K.; Patel, D.K. Biological potential of aromadendrin against human disorders: Recent development in pharmacological activities and analytical aspects. *Pharmacol. Res. Mod. Chin. Med.* **2024**, *11*, 100424. [CrossRef]
158. El-Shiekh, R.A.; Radi, M.H.; Abdel-Sattar, E. Unveiling the therapeutic potential of aromadendrin (AMD): A promising anti-inflammatory agent in the prevention of chronic diseases. *Inflammopharmacology* **2025**, *33*, 1209–1220. [CrossRef]
159. Fernandes, F.H.; Guterres, Z.D.R.; Corsino, J.; Garcez, W.S.; Garcez, F.R. Assessment of the mutagenicity of propolis compounds from the Brazilian Cerrado biome in somatic cells of *Drosophila melanogaster*. *Orbital: Electron. J. Chem.* **2019**, *11*, 307–313. [CrossRef]

160. Salehi, B.; Fokou, P.V.T.; Sharifi-Rad, M.; Zucca, P.; Pezzani, R.; Martins, N.; Sharifi-Rad, J. The therapeutic potential of naringenin: A review of clinical trials. *Pharmaceuticals* **2019**, *12*, 11. [CrossRef]
161. Orhan, I.E.; Nabavi, S.F.; Daglia, M.; Tenore, G.C.; Mansouri, K.; Nabavi, S.M. Naringenin and atherosclerosis: A review of literature. *Curr. Pharm. Biotechnol.* **2015**, *16*, 245–251. [CrossRef]
162. Hernández-Aquino, E.; Muriel, P. Beneficial effects of naringenin in liver diseases: Molecular mechanisms. *World J. Gastroenterol.* **2018**, *24*, 1679. [CrossRef]
163. Abdelkawy, Y.S.; Elharoun, M.; Sheta, E.; Abdel-Raheem, I.T.; Nematalla, H.A. Liraglutide and naringenin relieve depressive symptoms in mice by enhancing neurogenesis and reducing inflammation. *Eur. J. Pharmacol.* **2024**, *971*, 176525. [CrossRef]
164. Rebello, C.J.; Beyl, R.A.; Lertora, J.J.L.; Greenway, F.L.; Ravussin, E.; Ribnicky, D.M.; Poulev, A.; Kennedy, B.J.; Castro, H.F.; Campagna, S.R.; et al. Safety and pharmacokinetics of naringenin: A randomized, controlled, single-ascending-dose clinical trial. *Diabetes Obes. Metab.* **2020**, *22*, 91–98. [CrossRef]
165. Pérez-Coll, C.S.; Herkovits, J. Lethal and teratogenic effects of naringenin evaluated by means of an amphibian embryo toxicity test (AMPHITOX). *Food Chem. Toxicol.* **2004**, *42*, 299–306. [CrossRef]
166. Monadi, T.; Mohajer, Z.; Soltani, A.; Khazeei Tabari, M.A.; Manayi, A.; Azadbakht, M. The influence of apigenin on cellular responses to radiation: From protection to sensitization. *Biofactors* **2024**, *51*, e2113. [CrossRef]
167. Salehi, B.; Venditti, A.; Sharifi-Rad, M.; Kręgiel, D.; Sharifi-Rad, J.; Durazzo, A.; Lucarini, M.; Santini, A.; Souto, E.B.; Novellino, E.; et al. The therapeutic potential of apigenin. *Int. J. Mol. Sci.* **2019**, *20*, 1305. [CrossRef]
168. Allemailem, K.S.; Almatroudi, A.; Alharbi, H.O.A.; AlSuhaymi, N.; Alsugoor, M.H.; Aldakheel, F.M.; Khan, A.A.; Rahmani, A.H. Apigenin: A bioflavonoid with a promising role in disease prevention and treatment. *Biomedicines.* **2024**, *12*, 1353. [CrossRef]
169. DeRango-Adem, E.F.; Blay, J. Does oral apigenin have real potential for a therapeutic effect in the context of human gastrointestinal and other cancers? *Front. Pharmacol.* **2021**, *12*, 681477. [CrossRef]
170. Lee, J.A.; Ha, S.K.; Kim, Y.C.; Choi, I. Effects of friedelin on the intestinal permeability and bioavailability of apigenin. *Pharmacol. Rep.* **2017**, *69*, 1044–1048. [CrossRef]
171. Rana, J.N.; Mumtaz, S. Prunin: An emerging anticancer flavonoid. *Int. J. Mol. Sci.* **2025**, *26*, 2678. [CrossRef]
172. Gunaseelan, S.; Wong, K.Z.; Min, N.; Sun, J.; Ismail, N.K.B.M.; Tan, Y.J.; Lee, R.C.H.; Chu, J.J.H. Prunin suppresses viral IRES activity and is a potential candidate for treating enterovirus A71 infection. *Sci. Transl. Med.* **2019**, *11*, eaar5759. [CrossRef]
173. Patel, D.K.; Patel, K. Biological importance of prunin in the medicine for the treatment of diabetes related complication: Therapeutic benefit through data analysis. *Metabolism* **2022**, *128*, 155057. [CrossRef]
174. Guo, F.; Yan, D.; Qin, Z.; Bais, S. Prunin modulates the expression of cerebral serotonin induced by anxiety-like behavior in mice. *Nat. Prod. Commun.* **2021**, *16*, 1–9. [CrossRef]
175. Pan, L.; Ye, H.; Pi, X.; Liu, W.; Wang, Z.; Zhang, Y.; Zheng, J. Effects of several flavonoids on human gut microbiota and its metabolism by in vitro simulated fermentation. *Front. Microbiol.* **2023**, *14*, 1092729. [CrossRef]
176. Mani, R.; Natesan, V. Chrysin: Sources, beneficial pharmacological activities, and molecular mechanism of action. *Phytochemistry* **2018**, *145*, 187–196. [CrossRef]
177. Nabavi, S.F.; Braidy, N.; Habtemariam, S.; Orhan, I.E.; Daglia, M.; Manayi, A.; Gortzi, O.; Nabavi, S.M. Neuroprotective effects of chrysin: From chemistry to medicine. *Neurochem. Int.* **2015**, *90*, 224–231. [CrossRef]
178. Siddiqui, A.; Badruddeen; Akhtar, J.; Shahab Uddin, M.S.; Khan, M.I.; Khalid, M.; Ahmad, M. A Naturally occurring flavone (chrysin): Chemistry, occurrence, pharmacokinetic, toxicity, molecular targets and medicinal properties. *J. Biol. Act. Prod. Nat.* **2018**, *8*, 208–227. [CrossRef]
179. Islam, A.; Islam, M.S.; Uddin, M.N.; Hasan, M.M.I.; Akanda, M.R. The potential health benefits of the isoflavone glycoside genistin. *Arch. Pharmacal Res.* **2020**, *43*, 395–408. [CrossRef]
180. Tang, X.; Liao, R.; Zhou, L.; Yi, T.; Ran, M.; Luo, J.; Huang, F.; Wu, A.; Mei, Q.; Wang, L.; et al. Genistin: A novel estrogen analogue targeting ERβ to alleviate thrombocytopenia. *Int. J. Biol. Sci.* **2024**, *20*, 2236–2260. [CrossRef]
181. Jaiswal, N.; Akhtar, J.; Singh, S.P.; Ahsan, F. An overview on genistein and its various formulations. *Drug Res.* **2019**, *69*, 305–313. [CrossRef]
182. Arya, S.S.; Rookes, J.E.; Cahill, D.M.; Lenka, S.K. Vanillin: A review on the therapeutic prospects of a popular flavouring molecule. *Adv. Tradit. Med.* **2021**, *21*, 1–17. [CrossRef]
183. Huang, W.; Yang, Y.; Wen, W.; Luo, Y.; Wu, J.; Xiang, L.; Hu, Y.; Xu, S.; Chen, S.; Wang, P. Vanillin enhances the passive transport rate and absorption of drugs with moderate oral bioavailability in *vitro* and in *vivo* by affecting the membrane structure. *Food Funct.* **2020**, *11*, 700–710. [CrossRef]
184. Ruwizhi, N.; Aderibigbe, B.A. Cinnamic acid derivatives and their biological efficacy. *Int. J. Mol. Sci.* **2020**, *21*, 5712. [CrossRef]
185. Safaeian, L.; Asghari-Varzaneh, M.; Alavi, S.S.; Halvaei-Varnousfaderani, M.; Laher, I. Cardiovascular protective effects of cinnamic acid as a natural phenolic acid: A review. *Arch. Physiol. Biochem.* **2025**, *131*, 52–62. [CrossRef]
186. Adisakwattana, S. Cinnamic acid and its derivatives: Mechanisms for prevention and management of diabetes and its complications. *Nutrients* **2017**, *9*, 163. [CrossRef]

187. Bickers, D.; Calow, P.; Greim, H.; Hanifin, J.M.; Rogers, A.E.; Saurat, J.H.; Sipes, I.G.; Smith, R.L.; Tagami, H. A Toxicologic and dermatologic assessment of cinnamyl alcohol, cinnamaldehyde and cinnamic acid when used as fragrance ingredients. *Food Chem. Toxicol.* **2005**, *43*, 799–836. [CrossRef]
188. Albuquerque, C.F.B.; de Souza, D.A.A.; Figueiredo, P.L.B.; Rocha, C.Q.; Maia, J.G.S.; Kato, M.J.; Chisté, R.C.; da Silva, J.K.R. Optimization of extraction conditions for improving gallic acid and quercetin content in *Pouteria macrophylla* fruits: A promising cosmetic ingredient. *ACS Omega* **2025**, *10*, 7371–7380. [CrossRef]
189. Jiang, Y.; Pei, J.; Zheng, Y.; Miao, Y.J.; Duan, B.Z.; Huang, L.F. Gallic acid: A potential anti-cancer agent. *Chin. J. Integr. Med.* **2022**, *28*, 661–671. [CrossRef]
190. Bhuia, M.S.; Rahaman, M.M.; Islam, T.; Bappi, M.H.; Sikder, M.I.; Hossain, K.N.; Akter, F.; Al Shamsh Prottay, A.; Rokonuzzman, M.; Gürer, E.S.; et al. Neurobiological effects of gallic acid: Current perspectives. *Chin. Med.* **2023**, *18*, 27. [CrossRef]
191. Wianowska, D.; Olszowy-Tomczyk, M. A concise profile of gallic acid—From its natural sources through biological properties and chemical methods of determination. *Molecules* **2023**, *28*, 1186. [CrossRef]
192. Verma, S.; Singh, A.; Mishra, A. Gallic acid: Molecular rival of cancer. *Environ. Toxicol. Pharmacol.* **2013**, *35*, 473–485. [CrossRef]
193. Kahkeshani, N.; Farzaei, F.; Fotouhi, M.; Alavi, S.S.; Bahramsoltani, R.; Naseri, R.; Momtaz, S.; Abbasabadi, Z.; Rahimi, R.; Farzaei, M.H.; et al. pharmacological effects of gallic acid in health and diseases: A mechanistic review. *Iran J. Basic Med. Sci.* **2019**, *22*, 225. [CrossRef]
194. Hadidi, M.; Liñán-Atero, R.; Tarahi, M.; Christodoulou, M.C.; Aghababaei, F. The potential health benefits of gallic acid: Therapeutic and food applications. *Antioxidants* **2024**, *13*, 1001. [CrossRef]
195. Zhao, X.L.; Cao, Z.J.; Li, K.-D.; Tang, F.; Xu, L.-Y.; Zhang, J.-N.; Liu, D.; Peng, C.; Ao, H. Gallic acid: A dietary metabolite's therapeutic potential in the management of atherosclerotic cardiovascular disease. *Front. Pharmacol.* **2024**, *15*, 1515172. [CrossRef]
196. Kaliora, A.C.; Kanellos, P.T.; Kalogeropoulos, N. Gallic acid bioavailability in humans. In *Handbook on Gallic Acid*; Thompson, M.A., Collins, P.B., Eds.; Nova Science: New York, NY, USA, 2013; pp. 301–312.
197. Sarimahmut, M.; Vekshari, S.; Karaali, D.; Çelikler, S. In *vitro* evaluation of antigenotoxic effects of phloridzin. *Cumhur. Sci. J.* **2022**, *43*, 358–364. [CrossRef]
198. Lv, F.; Chen, Y.; Xie, H.; Gao, M.; He, R.; Deng, W.Y.; Chen, W. Therapeutic potential of phloridzin carbomer gel for skin inflammatory healing in atopic dermatitis. *Arch. Dermatol. Res.* **2025**, *317*, 352. [CrossRef]
199. Wang, L.; Wu, X.; Wan, Q.; Yang, Y.; Gao, C. Phloridzin reduces synovial hyperplasia and inflammation in rheumatoid arthritis rat by modulating MTOR pathway. *Int. Immunopharmacol.* **2024**, *133*, 111727. [CrossRef]
200. Tian, L.; Cao, J.; Zhao, T.; Liu, Y.; Khan, A.; Cheng, G. The bioavailability, extraction, biosynthesis and distribution of natural dihydrochalcone: Phloridzin. *Int. J. Mol. Sci.* **2021**, *22*, 962. [CrossRef]
201. Londzin, P.; Siudak, S.; Cegieła, U.; Pytlik, M.; Janas, A.; Waligóra, A.; Folwarczna, J. Phloridzin, an apple polyphenol, exerted unfavorable effects on bone and muscle in an experimental model of type 2 diabetes in rats. *Nutrients* **2018**, *10*, 1701. [CrossRef]
202. Rampogu, S.; Gajula, R.G.; Lee, K.W. A comprehensive review on chemotherapeutic potential of galangin. *Biomed. Pharmacother.* **2021**, *141*, 111808. [CrossRef]
203. Thapa, R.; Afzal, O.; Alfawaz Altamimi, A.S.; Goyal, A.; Almalki, W.H.; Alzarea, S.I.; Kazmi, I.; Jakhmola, V.; Singh, S.K.; Dua, K.; et al. Galangin as an inflammatory response modulator: An updated overview and therapeutic potential. *Chem. Biol. Interact.* **2023**, *378*, 110482. [CrossRef]
204. Khawaja, G.; El-Orfali, Y.; Shoujaa, A.; Abou Najem, S. Galangin: A promising flavonoid for the treatment of rheumatoid arthritis—Mechanisms, evidence, and therapeutic potential. *Pharmaceuticals* **2024**, *17*, 963. [CrossRef]
205. Zhao, Y.; Li, B.; Deng, H.; Zhang, C.; Wang, Y.; Chen, L.; Teng, H. Galangin alleviates alcohol-provoked liver injury associated with gut microbiota disorder and intestinal barrier dysfunction in mice. *J. Agric. Food Chem.* **2024**, *72*, 22336–22348. [CrossRef]
206. Chen, F.; Tan, Y.F.; Li, H.L.; Qin, Z.M.; Cai, H.D.; Lai, W.Y.; Zhang, X.P.; Li, Y.H.; Guan, W.W.; Li, Y.B.; et al. Differential systemic exposure to galangin after oral and intravenous administration to rats. *Chem. Cent. J.* **2015**, *9*, 14. [CrossRef]
207. Çakır, D.K.; Zannou, O.; Koca, I. Scopoletin contents and antioxidant properties of some edible plants of black sea regions. *Discov. Food* **2022**, *2*, 1–10. [CrossRef]
208. Antika, L.D.; Tasfiyati, A.N.; Hikmat, H.; Septama, A.W. Scopoletin: A review of its source, biosynthesis, methods of extraction, and pharmacological activities. *Z. Naturforsch. C J. Biosci.* **2022**, *77*, 303–316. [CrossRef]
209. Gao, X.Y.; Li, X.Y.; Zhang, C.Y.; Bai, C.Y. Scopoletin: A review of its pharmacology, pharmacokinetics, and toxicity. *Front. Pharmacol.* **2024**, *15*, 1268464. [CrossRef]
210. Zeng, Y.C.; Li, S.; Liu, C.; Gong, T.; Sun, X.; Fu, Y.; Zhang, Z.R. Soluplus micelles for improving the oral bioavailability of scopoletin and their hypouricemic effect in vivo. *Acta Pharmacol. Sin.* **2017**, *38*, 424–433. [CrossRef]
211. Parama, D.; Girisa, S.; Khatoon, E.; Kumar, A.; Alqahtani, M.S.; Abbas, M.; Sethi, G.; Kunnumakkara, A.B. An overview of the pharmacological activities of scopoletin against different chronic diseases. *Pharmacol. Res.* **2022**, *179*, 106202. [CrossRef]

212. Monteiro Espíndola, K.M.; Ferreira, R.G.; Mosquera Narvaez, L.E.; Rocha Silva Rosario, A.C.; Machado Da Silva, A.H.; Bispo Silva, A.G.; Oliveira Vieira, A.P.; Chagas Monteiro, M. Chemical and pharmacological aspects of caffeic acid and its activity in hepatocarcinoma. *Front. Oncol.* **2019**, *9*, 467241. [CrossRef]
213. Pavlíková, N. Caffeic acid and diseases—Mechanisms of action. *Int. J. Mol. Sci.* **2022**, *24*, 588. [CrossRef]
214. Bhuia, M.S.; Ferdous, J.; Chowdhury, R.; Ansari, S.A.; Ansari, I.A.; Al Hasan, M.S.; Sheikh, S.; Islam, M.T. Exploring the antiemetic potential of caffeic acid: A combined in *vivo* and computational approach. *Neurogastroenterol. Motil.* **2025**, *37*, e70003. [CrossRef]
215. Muhammad Abdul Kadar, N.N.; Ahmad, F.; Teoh, S.L.; Yahaya, M.F. Caffeic acid on metabolic syndrome: A review. *Molecules* **2021**, *26*, 5490. [CrossRef]
216. Boo, Y.C. p-Coumaric acid as an active ingredient in cosmetics: A review focusing on its antimelanogenic effects. *Antioxidants* **2019**, *8*, 275. [CrossRef]
217. Pei, K.; Ou, J.; Huang, J.; Ou, S. p-Coumaric acid and its conjugates: Dietary sources, pharmacokinetic properties and biological activities. *J. Sci. Food Agric.* **2016**, *96*, 2952–2962. [CrossRef]
218. Zduńska, K.; Dana, A.; Kolodziejczak, A.; Rotsztejn, H. Antioxidant properties of ferulic acid and its possible application. *Ski. Pharmacol. Physiol.* **2018**, *31*, 332–336. [CrossRef]
219. Markowska, A.; Markowska, J.; Stanisławiak-Rudowicz, J.; Kozak, K.; Roubinek, O.K.; Jasińska, M. The role of ferulic acid in selected malignant neoplasms. *Molecules* **2025**, *30*, 1018. [CrossRef]
220. Zheng, M.; Liu, Y.; Zhang, G.; Yang, Z.; Xu, W.; Chen, Q. The antioxidant properties, metabolism, application and mechanism of ferulic acid in medicine, food, cosmetics, livestock and poultry. *Antioxidants* **2024**, *13*, 853. [CrossRef]
221. Gortzi, O.; Patsios, S.I.; Pyrzynska, K. Ferulic acid—A brief review of its extraction, bioavailability and biological activity. *Separations* **2024**, *11*, 204. [CrossRef]
222. Raj, N.D.; Singh, D. A critical appraisal on ferulic acid: Biological profile, biopharmaceutical challenges and nano formulations. *Health Sci. Rev.* **2022**, *5*, 100063. [CrossRef]
223. Naveed, M.; Hejazi, V.; Abbas, M.; Kamboh, A.A.; Khan, G.J.; Shumzaid, M.; Ahmad, F.; Babazadeh, D.; FangFang, X.; Modarresi-Ghazani, F.; et al. Chlorogenic acid (CGA): A pharmacological review and call for further research. *Biomed. Pharmacother.* **2018**, *97*, 67–74. [CrossRef]
224. Nguyen, V.; Taine, E.G.; Meng, D.; Cui, T.; Tan, W. Chlorogenic acid: A systematic review on the biological functions, mechanistic actions, and therapeutic potentials. *Nutrients* **2024**, *16*, 924. [CrossRef]
225. Golmei, P.; Kasna, S.; Roy, K.P.; Kumar, S. A review on pharmacological advancement of ellagic acid. *J. Pharmacol. Pharmacother.* **2024**, *15*, 93–104. [CrossRef]
226. Lu, G.; Wang, X.; Cheng, M.; Wang, S.; Ma, K. The multifaceted mechanisms of ellagic acid in the treatment of tumors: State-of-the-art. *Biomed. Pharmacother.* **2023**, *165*, 115132. [CrossRef]
227. Naraki, K.; Ghasemzadeh Rahbardar, M.; Ajiboye, B.O.; Hosseinzadeh, H. The effect of ellagic acid on the metabolic syndrome: A review article. *Heliyon* **2023**, *9*, e21844. [CrossRef]
228. Ríos, J.L.; Giner, R.M.; Marín, M.; Recio, M.C. A Pharmacological update of ellagic acid. *Planta Med.* **2018**, *84*, 1068–1093. [CrossRef]
229. Lafay, S.; Gil-Izquierdo, A. Bioavailability of phenolic acids. *Phytochem. Rev.* **2008**, *7*, 301–311. [CrossRef]
230. Przybylska-Balcerek, A.; Stuper-Szablewska, K. The effect of phenolic acids on living organisms. *Indian J. Med. Res. Pharm. Sci.* **2019**, *6*, 1–14. [CrossRef]
231. Jian, X.; Shi, C.; Luo, W.; Zhou, L.; Jiang, L.; Liu, K. Therapeutic effects and molecular mechanisms of quercetin in gynecological disorders. *Biomed. Pharmacother.* **2024**, *173*, 116418. [CrossRef]
232. Pei, J.; Kumarasamy, R.V.; Jayaraman, S.; Kanniappan, G.V.; Long, Q.; Palanisamy, C.P. Quercetin-functionalized nanomaterials: Innovative therapeutic avenues for Alzheimer's disease management. *Ageing Res. Rev.* **2025**, *104*, 102665. [CrossRef]
233. Kasahara, K.; Kerby, R.L.; Aquino-Martinez, R.; Evered, A.H.; Cross, T.-W.L.; Everhart, J.; Ulland, T.K.; Kay, C.D.; Bolling, B.W.; Bäckhed, F.; et al. Gut microbes modulate the effects of the flavonoid quercetin on atherosclerosis. *NPJ Biofilms Microbiomes.* **2025**, *11*, 12. [CrossRef]
234. Bian, X.; Ge, Z.; Chen, X.; Zhong, S.; Li, L.; Xu, W.; Li, B.; Chen, S.; Lv, G. Protective effects and mechanisms of quercetin in animal models of hyperuricemia: A systematic review and meta-analysis. *Pharmacol. Res.* **2025**, *213*, 107665. [CrossRef]
235. Carrillo-Martinez, E.J.; Flores-Hernández, F.Y.; Salazar-Montes, A.M.; Nario-Chaidez, H.F.; Hernández-Ortega, L.D. Quercetin, a flavonoid with great pharmacological capacity. *Molecules* **2024**, *29*, 1000. [CrossRef]
236. Aghababaei, F.; Hadidi, M. Recent advances in potential health benefits of quercetin. *Pharmaceuticals* **2023**, *16*, 1020. [CrossRef]
237. Zou, H.; Ye, H.; Kamaraj, R.; Zhang, T.; Zhang, J.; Pavek, P. A review on pharmacological activities and synergistic effect of quercetin with small molecule agents. *Phytomedicine* **2021**, *92*, 153736. [CrossRef]
238. Harwood, M.; Danielewska-Nikiel, B.; Borzelleca, J.F.; Flamm, G.W.; Williams, G.M.; Lines, T.C. A critical review of the data related to the safety of quercetin and lack of evidence of in *vivo* toxicity, including lack of genotoxic/carcinogenic properties. *Food Chem. Toxicol.* **2007**, *45*, 2179–2205. [CrossRef]

239. Kandemir, K.; Tomas, M.; McClements, D.J.; Capanoglu, E. Recent advances on the improvement of quercetin bioavailability. *Trends Food Sci. Technol.* **2022**, *119*, 192–200. [CrossRef]
240. Isemura, M. Catechin in human health and disease. *Molecules* **2019**, *24*, 528. [CrossRef]
241. Ganeshpurkar, A.; Saluja, A. The pharmacological potential of catechin. *Indian J. Biochem. Biophys.* **2020**, *57*, 505–511. [CrossRef]
242. Bernal-Mercado, A.T.; Vazquez-Armenta, F.J.; Tapia-Rodriguez, M.R.; Islas-Osuna, M.A.; Mata-Haro, V.; Gonzalez-Aguilar, G.A.; Lopez-Zavala, A.A.; Ayala-Zavala, J.F. Comparison of single and combined use of catechin, protocatechuic, and vanillic acids as antioxidant and antibacterial agents against uropathogenic *Escherichia coli* at planktonic and biofilm levels. *Molecules* **2018**, *23*, 2813. [CrossRef]
243. Peters, C.M.; Green, R.J.; Janle, E.M.; Ferruzzi, M.G. Formulation with ascorbic acid and sucrose modulates catechin bioavailability from green tea. *Food Res. Int.* **2010**, *43*, 95–102. [CrossRef]
244. Ganeshpurkar, A.; Saluja, A.K. The pharmacological potential of rutin. *Saudi Pharm. J.* **2017**, *25*, 149–164. [CrossRef]
245. Wang, X.; Xia, X.; Song, X.; Zhou, Y.; Ma, M.; Ren, Y.; Chen, X.; Xia, Z.; Guo, Y.; Song, C. Therapeutic potential of rutin in premenstrual depression: Evidence from in *vivo* and in *vitro* studies. *Front. Pharmacol.* **2024**, *15*, 1525753. [CrossRef]
246. Hamid, Z.M.; Sahib, H.B. The acute toxicity of rutin in mice. *Iraqi J. Pharm. Sci.* **2021**, *30*, 231–240. [CrossRef]
247. Rauf, A.; Imran, M.; Abu-Izneid, T.; Iahtisham-Ul-Haq; Patel, S.; Pan, X.; Naz, S.; Sanches Silva, A.; Saeed, F.; Rasul Suleria, H.A. Proanthocyanidins: A comprehensive review. *Biomed. Pharmacother.* **2019**, *116*, 108999. [CrossRef]
248. Qi, Q.; Chu, M.; Yu, X.; Xie, Y.; Li, Y.; Du, Y.; Liu, X.; Zhang, Z.; Shi, J.; Yan, N. Anthocyanins and proanthocyanidins: Chemical structures, food sources, bioactivities, and product development. *Food Rev. Int.* **2023**, *39*, 4581–4609. [CrossRef]
249. Zhang, L.; Wang, Y.; Li, D.; Ho, C.T.; Li, J.; Wan, X. The absorption, distribution, metabolism and excretion of procyanidins. *Food Funct.* **2016**, *7*, 1273–1281. [CrossRef]
250. Yamakoshi, J.; Saito, M.; Kataoka, S.; Kikuchi, M. Safety evaluation of proanthocyanidin-rich extract from grape seeds. *Food Chem. Toxicol.* **2002**, *40*, 599–607. [CrossRef]
251. Rein, M.J.; Renouf, M.; Cruz-Hernandez, C.; Actis-Goretta, L.; Thakkar, S.K.; da Silva Pinto, M. Bioavailability of bioactive food compounds: A challenging journey to bioefficacy. *Br. J. Clin. Pharmacol.* **2013**, *75*, 588–602. [CrossRef]
252. Colunga Biancatelli, R.M.L.; Berrill, M.; Catravas, J.D.; Marik, P.E. Quercetin and vitamin C: An experimental, synergistic therapy for the prevention and treatment of SARS-CoV-2 related disease (COVID-19). *Front. Immunol.* **2020**, *11*, 1451. [CrossRef]
253. Ge, C.; Wei, X.; Xu, Y.; Jiang, Y.; Yang, X.; Lin, J.; Li, M.; Tian, Y.; Fan, S.; Ye, T.; et al. Natural ellagic acid-polyphenol "sandwich biscuit" self-assembled solubilizing system for formation mechanism and antibacterial synergia. *ACS Appl. Mater. Interfaces* **2025**, *17*, 27772–27787. [CrossRef]
254. Liu, Y.; Guan, L.; Yang, D.; Luo, H.; Zhang, H. Investigating the synergistic antibacterial effects of chlorogenic and p-coumaric acids on *Shigella dysenteriae*. *Food Chem.* **2025**, *462*, 141011. [CrossRef]
255. Guan, H.; Zhang, W.; Liu, H.; Jiang, Y.; Li, F.; Wang, D.; Liu, Y.; He, F.; Wu, M.; Waterhouse, G.I.N.; et al. Simultaneous binding of quercetin and catechin to FOXO3 enhances IKKα transcription inhibition and suppression of oxidative stress-induced acute alcoholic liver injury in rats. *J. Adv. Res.* **2025**, *67*, 71–92. [CrossRef]
256. Mukai, K.; Mitani, S.; Ohara, K.; Nagaoka, S.I. Structure–activity relationship of the tocopherol-regeneration reaction by catechins. *Free Radic. Biol. Med.* **2005**, *38*, 1243–1256. [CrossRef]
257. Jaramillo Carmona, S.M.; López Martín, S.; Abia, R.; Rodriguez-Arcos, R.; Jiménez Araujo, A.; Guillén Bejarano, R.; Muriana, F.J. Combination of quercetin and kaempferol enhances in vitro cytotoxicity on human colon cancer (HCT-116) cells. *Rec. Nat. Prod.* **2014**, *8*, 262–271.
258. Mok, J.Y.; Jeong, S.I.; Kim, J.H.; Jang, S.I. Synergic effect of quercetin and astragalin from mulberry leaves on anti-inflammation. *Korean J. Orient. Physiol. Pathol.* **2011**, *25*, 830–836.
259. Hajimehdipoor, H.; Shahrestani, R.; Shekarchi, M. Investigating the synergistic antioxidant effects of some flavonoid and phenolic compounds. *Res. J. Pharmacogn.* **2014**, *1*, 35–40.
260. Liu, X.; Zhao, T.; Shi, Z.; Hu, C.; Li, Q.; Sun, C. Synergism antiproliferative effects of apigenin and naringenin in NSCLC cells. *Molecules* **2023**, *28*, 4947. [CrossRef]
261. Biswas, P.; Kaium, M.A.; Islam Tareq, M.M.; Tauhida, S.J.; Hossain, M.R.; Siam, L.S.; Parvez, A.; Bibi, S.; Hasan, M.H.; Rahman, M.M.; et al. The experimental significance of isorhamnetin as an effective therapeutic option for cancer: A comprehensive analysis. *Biomed. Pharmacother.* **2024**, *176*, 116860. [CrossRef]
262. Zhang, X.; Zhang, W.; Chen, F.; Lu, Z. Combined effect of chrysin and apigenin on inhibiting the development and progression of colorectal cancer by suppressing the activity of P38-MAPK/AKT pathway. *IUBMB Life* **2021**, *73*, 774–783. [CrossRef]
263. Harasstani, O.A.; Tham, C.L.; Israf, D.A. Kaempferol and chrysin synergies to improve septic mice survival. *Molecules* **2017**, *22*, 92. [CrossRef]
264. Wang, Z.; Wang, M.; Tao, Q.; Li, Y.; Wang, H.; Zhang, M.; Liu, X.; Zhang, J. Betaine–salicylic acid cocrystal for enhanced skincare and acne treatment. *RSC Med. Chem.* **2025**, *16*, 1705–1714. [CrossRef]

265. Bezerra, C.F.; Camilo, C.J.; do Nascimento Silva, M.K.; de Freitas, T.S.; Ribeiro-Filho, J.; Coutinho, H.D.M. Vanillin selectively modulates the action of antibiotics against resistant bacteria. *Microb. Pathog.* **2017**, *113*, 265–268. [CrossRef]
266. Catanzaro, E.; Greco, G.; Potenza, L.; Calcabrini, C.; Fimognari, C. Natural products to fight cancer: A focus on *Juglans regia*. *Toxins* **2018**, *10*, 469. [CrossRef]
267. Jafari, S.; Dabiri, S.; Mehdizadeh Aghdam, E.; Fathi, E.; Saeedi, N.; Montazersaheb, S.; Farahzadi, R. Synergistic effect of chrysin and radiotherapy against triple-negative breast cancer (TNBC) cell lines. *Clin. Transl. Oncol.* **2023**, *25*, 2559–2568. [CrossRef]
268. Sarg, N.H.; Hersi, F.H.; Zaher, D.M.; Hamouda, A.O.; Ibrahim, S.I.; El-Seedi, H.R.; Omar, H.A. Unveiling the therapeutic potential of taxifolin in cancer: From molecular mechanisms to immune modulation and synergistic combinations. *Phytomedicine* **2024**, *133*, 155934. [CrossRef]
269. Materska, M. Quercetin and its derivatives: Chemical structure and bioactivity - a review. *Pol. J. Food Nutr. Sci.* **2008**, *58*, 407–413.
270. Pietta, P.G. Flavonoids as antioxidants. *J. Nat. Prod.* **2000**, *63*, 1035–1042. [CrossRef]
271. Sanchez-Maldonado, A.F. Mode of Action, Interaction and Recovery of Plant Secondary Metabolites for Potential Applications as Food Preservatives. Ph.D. Thesis, University of Alberta, Edmonton, Canada, 2014. [CrossRef]
272. Bhuyan, D.J.; Basu, A. Phenolic compounds potential health benefits and toxicity. In *Utilisation of Bioactive Compounds from Agricultural and Food Waste*, 1st ed.; Vuong, Q.V., Ed.; CRC Press: Boca Raton, FL, USA, 2017; pp. 27–59. [CrossRef]
273. Pizzimenti, S.; Muzio, G.; Barrera, G.; Giner, R.M.; Ríos, J.L.; Máñez, S. Antioxidant activity of natural hydroquinones. *Antioxidants* **2022**, *11*, 343. [CrossRef]
274. Xiang, H.H.; Seong, S.H.; Ji, S.H.; Myung, K.L.; Bang, Y.H.; Ro, J.S. Monoamine oxidase inhibitory components from *Cayratia japonica*. *Arch. Pharm. Res.* **2007**, *30*, 13–17. [CrossRef]
275. Abou Baker, D.H. An ethnopharmacological review on the therapeutical properties of flavonoids and their mechanisms of actions: A comprehensive review based on up to date knowledge. *Toxicol. Rep.* **2022**, *9*, 445–469. [CrossRef]
276. Procházková, D.; Boušová, I.; Wilhelmová, N. Antioxidant and prooxidant properties of flavonoids. *Fitoterapia* **2011**, *82*, 513–523. [CrossRef]
277. Latos-Brozio, M.; Masek, A. Structure-activity relationships analysis of monomeric and polymeric polyphenols (quercetin, rutin and catechin) obtained by various polymerization methods. *Chem. Biodivers.* **2019**, *16*, e1900426. [CrossRef]
278. Zahoor, M.; Shafiq, S.; Ullah, H.; Sadiq, A.; Ullah, F. Isolation of quercetin and mandelic acid from *Aesculus indica* fruit and their biological activities. *BMC Biochem.* **2018**, *19*, 5. [CrossRef]
279. Bentz, A.B. A review of quercetin: Chemistry, antioxidant properties, and bioavailability. *J. Young Investig.* **2009**. Available online: https://www.jyi.org/2009-april/2017/10/15/a-review-of-quercetin-chemistry-antioxidant-properties-and-bioavailability (accessed on 1 October 2024).
280. Magar, R.T.; Sohng, J.K. A review on structure, modifications and structure-activity relation of quercetin and its derivatives. *J. Microbiol. Biotechnol.* **2020**, *30*, 11–20. [CrossRef]
281. Tu, B.; Liu, Z.-J.; Chen, Z.-F.; Ouyang, Y.; Hu, Y.-J. Understanding the structure–activity relationship between quercetin and naringenin: In *vitro*. *RSC Adv.* **2015**, *5*, 106171–106181. [CrossRef]
282. Li, M.M.; Chen, Y.T.; Ruan, J.C.; Wang, W.J.; Chen, J.G.; Zhang, Q.F. Structure-activity relationship of dietary flavonoids on pancreatic lipase. *Curr. Res. Food Sci.* **2023**, *6*, 100424. [CrossRef]
283. Nguyen, T.A.; Liu, B.; Zhao, J.; Thomas, D.S.; Hook, J.M. An investigation into the supramolecular structure, solubility, stability and antioxidant activity of rutin/cyclodextrin inclusion complex. *Food Chem.* **2013**, *136*, 186–192. [CrossRef]
284. Rho, H.S.; Ghimeray, A.K.; Yoo, D.S.; Ahn, S.M.; Kwon, S.S.; Lee, K.H.; Cho, D.H.; Cho, J.Y. Kaempferol and kaempferol rhamnosides with depigmenting and anti-inflammatory properties. *Molecules* **2011**, *16*, 3338–3344. [CrossRef]
285. Wada, E.; Ito, C.; Shinohara, M.; Handa, S.; Maetani, M.; Yasugi, M.; Miyake, M.; Sakamoto, T.; Yazawa, A.; Kamitani, S. Prunin laurate derived from natural substances shows antibacterial activity against the periodontal pathogen *Porphyromonas gingivalis*. *Foods* **2024**, *13*, 1917. [CrossRef]
286. Céliz, G.; Daz, M.; Audisio, M.C. Antibacterial activity of naringin derivatives against pathogenic strains. *J. Appl. Microbiol.* **2011**, *111*, 731–738. [CrossRef]
287. Smiljkovic, M.; Stanisavljevic, D.; Stojkovic, D.; Petrovic, I.; Vicentic, J.M.; Popovic, J.; Golic Grdadolnik, S.G.; Markovic, D.; Sanković-Babić, S.; Glamoclija, J.; et al. Apigenin-7-*O*-glucoside versus apigenin: Insight into the modes of anticandidal and cytotoxic actions. *EXCLI J.* **2017**, *16*, 795–807. [CrossRef]
288. Naz, S.; Imran, M.; Rauf, A.; Orhan, I.E.; Shariati, M.A.; Iahtisham-Ul-Haq; IqraYasmin; Shahbaz, M.; Qaisrani, T.B.; Shah, Z.A.; et al. Chrysin: Pharmacological and therapeutic properties. *Life Sci.* **2019**, *235*, 116797. [CrossRef]
289. Liu, Y.; Song, X.; He, J.; Zheng, X.; Wu, H. Synthetic derivatives of chrysin and their biological activities. *Med. Chem. Res.* **2014**, *23*, 555–563. [CrossRef]
290. Shamsudin, N.F.; Ahmed, Q.U.; Mahmood, S.; Shah, S.A.A.; Khatib, A.; Mukhtar, S.; Alsharif, M.A.; Parveen, H.; Zakaria, Z.A. Antibacterial effects of flavonoids and their structure-activity relationship study: A comparative interpretation. *Molecules* **2022**, *27*, 1149. [CrossRef]

291. Sato, M.; Murakami, K.; Uno, M.; Ikubo, H.; Nakagawa, Y.; Katayama, S.; Akagi, K.; Irie, K. Structure-activity relationship for (+)-taxifolin isolated from silymarin as an inhibitor of amyloid β aggregation. *Biosci. Biotechnol. Biochem.* **2013**, *77*, 1100–1103. [CrossRef]
292. Renzetti, A.; Betts, J.W.; Fukumoto, K.; Rutherford, R.N. Antibacterial green tea catechins from a molecular perspective: Mechanisms of action and structure–activity relationships. *Food Funct.* **2020**, *11*, 9370–9396. [CrossRef]
293. Ahmadi, S.M.; Farhoosh, R.; Sharif, A.; Rezaie, M. Structure-antioxidant activity relationships of luteolin and catechin. *J. Food Sci.* **2020**, *85*, 298–305. [CrossRef]
294. Dixon, R.A.; Ferreira, D. Genistein. *Phytochemistry* **2002**, *60*, 205–211. [CrossRef]
295. Li, X.; Chen, B.; Xie, H.; He, Y.; Zhong, D.; Chen, D. Antioxidant structure–activity relationship analysis of five dihydrochalcones. *Molecules* **2018**, *23*, 1162. [CrossRef]
296. Guerrero, L.; Castillo, J.; Quiñones, M.; Garcia-Vallvé, S.; Arola, L.; Pujadas, G.; Muguerza, B. Inhibition of angiotensin-converting enzyme activity by flavonoids: Structure-activity relationship studies. *PLoS ONE* **2012**, *7*, e49493. [CrossRef]
297. Zhang, S.; Yang, X.; Coburn, R.A.; Morris, M.E. Structure activity relationships and quantitative structure activity relationships for the flavonoid-mediated inhibition of breast cancer resistance protein. *Biochem. Pharmacol.* **2005**, *70*, 627–639. [CrossRef]
298. Li, Z.; Liu, J.; You, J.; Li, X.; Liang, Z.; Du, J. Proanthocyanidin structure-activity relationship analysis by path analysis model. *Int. J. Mol. Sci.* **2023**, *24*, 6379. [CrossRef]
299. Chen, Y.; Xu, L.; Wang, Y.; Chen, Z.; Zhang, M.; Panichayupakaranant, P.; Chen, H. Study on the active polyphenol constituents in differently colored *Rubus chingii* Hu and the structure-activity relationship of the main ellagitannins and ellagic acid. *LWT* **2020**, *121*, 108967. [CrossRef]
300. Chen, J.; Yang, J.; Ma, L.; Li, J.; Shahzad, N.; Kim, C.K. Structure-antioxidant activity relationship of methoxy, phenolic hydroxyl, and carboxylic acid groups of phenolic acids. *Sci. Rep.* **2020**, *10*, 2611. [CrossRef]
301. Otero, E.; Robledo, S.M.; Díaz, S.; Carda, M.; Muñoz, D.; Paños, J.; Vélez, I.D.; Cardona, W. Synthesis and leishmanicidal activity of cinnamic acid esters: Structure-activity relationship. *Med. Chem. Res.* **2014**, *23*, 1378–1386. [CrossRef]
302. Fernandez-Martinez, E.; Bobadilla, R.A.; Morales-Rios, M.S.; Muriel, P.; Perez-Alvarez, V.M. Trans-3-phenyl-2-propenoic acid (cinnamic acid) derivatives: Structure-activity relationship as hepatoprotective agents. *Med. Chem.* **2007**, *3*, 475–479. [CrossRef]
303. Razzaghi-Asl, N.; Garrido, J.; Khazraei, H.; Borges, F.; Firuzi, O. Antioxidant properties of hydroxycinnamic acids: A review of structure- activity relationships. *Curr. Med. Chem.* **2013**, *20*, 4436–4450. [CrossRef]
304. De Armas-Ricard, M.; Ruiz-Reyes, E.; Ramírez-Rodríguez, O. Caffeates and caffeamides: Synthetic methodologies and their antioxidant properties. *Int. J. Med. Chem.* **2019**, *2019*, 2592609. [CrossRef]
305. Dhiman, P.; Malik, N.; Khatkar, A. Hybrid caffeic acid derivatives as monoamine oxidases inhibitors: Synthesis, radical scavenging activity, molecular docking studies and in silico ADMET analysis. *Chem. Cent. J.* **2018**, *12*, 112. [CrossRef]
306. Kiliç, I.; Yeşiloğlu, Y. Spectroscopic studies on the antioxidant activity of *p*-coumaric acid. *Spectrochim. Acta A Mol. Biomol. Spectrosc.* **2013**, *115*, 719–724. [CrossRef]
307. Khatkar, A.; Nanda, A.; Kumar, P.; Narasimhan, B. Synthesis, antimicrobial evaluation and QSAR studies of p-coumaric acid derivatives. *Arab. J. Chem.* **2017**, *10*, S3804–S3815. [CrossRef]
308. de Oliveira Silva, E.; Batista, R. Ferulic acid and naturally occurring compounds bearing a feruloyl moiety: A review on their structures, occurrence, and potential health benefits. *Compr. Rev. Food Sci. Food Saf.* **2017**, *16*, 580–616. [CrossRef]
309. Li, W.; Li, N.; Tang, Y.; Li, B.; Liu, L.; Zhang, X.; Fu, H.; Duan, J.A. Biological activity evaluation and structure–activity relationships analysis of ferulic acid and caffeic acid derivatives for anticancer. *Bioorg. Med. Chem. Lett.* **2012**, *22*, 6085–6088. [CrossRef]
310. Varzaru, I.; Oancea, A.G.; Vlaicu, P.A.; Saracila, M.; Untea, A.E. Exploring the antioxidant potential of blackberry and raspberry leaves: Phytochemical analysis, scavenging activity, and in *vitro* polyphenol bioaccessibility. *Antioxidants* **2023**, *12*, 2125. [CrossRef]
311. Macario, A.; López, J.C.; Blanco, S. Molecular structure of salicylic acid and its hydrates: A rotational spectroscopy study. *Int. J. Mol. Sci.* **2024**, *25*, 4074. [CrossRef]
312. Kim, J.; Kang, S.; Hong, S.; Yum, S.; Kim, Y.M.; Jung, Y. Structure–Activity relationship of salicylic acid derivatives on inhibition of TNF-α dependent NFκB activity: Implication on anti-inflammatory effect of n-(5-chlorosalicyloyl)phenethylamine against experimental colitis. *Eur. J. Med. Chem.* **2012**, *48*, 36–44. [CrossRef]
313. Morais, S.M.; Silva, K.A.; Araujo, H.; Vieira, I.G.P.; Alves, D.R.; Fontenelle, R.O.S.; Silva, A.M.S. Anacardic acid constituents from cashew nut shell liquid: NMR characterization and the effect of unsaturation on its biological activities. *Pharmaceuticals* **2017**, *10*, 31. [CrossRef]
314. Liu, C.; Zheng, P.; Wang, H.; Wei, Y.; Wang, C.; Hao, S. Design and synthesis of scopoletin sulfonate derivatives as potential insecticidal agents. *Molecules* **2023**, *28*, 530. [CrossRef]
315. Shalayel, M.H.F.; Al-Mazaideh, G.M.; Alanezi, A.A.; Almuqati, A.F.; Alotaibi, M. The potential anti-cancerous activity of *Prunus amygdalus var. amara* extract. *Processes* **2023**, *11*, 1277. [CrossRef]
316. Walton, N.J.; Mayer, M.J.; Narbad, A. Vanillin. *Phytochemistry* **2003**, *63*, 505–515. [CrossRef]

317. Fitzgerald, D.J.; Stratford, M.; Gasson, M.J.; Narbad, A. Structure-function analysis of the vanillin molecule and its antifungal properties. *J. Agric. Food Chem.* **2005**, *53*, 1769–1775. [CrossRef]
318. Tai, A.; Sawano, T.; Yazama, F.; Ito, H. Evaluation of antioxidant activity of vanillin by using multiple antioxidant assays. *Biochim. Biophys. Acta* **2011**, *1810*, 170–177. [CrossRef]
319. Chua, N.K.; Coates, H.W.; Brown, A.J. Squalene monooxygenase: A journey to the heart of cholesterol synthesis. *Prog. Lipid Res.* **2020**, *79*, 101033. [CrossRef]
320. Güneş, F.E. Medical use of squalene as a natural antioxidant. *J. Marmara Univ. Inst. Health Sci.* **2013**, *3*, 220–228. [CrossRef]
321. Njus, D.; Kelley, P.M.; Tu, Y.J.; Schlegel, H.B. Ascorbic acid: The chemistry underlying its antioxidant properties. *Free Radic. Biol. Med.* **2020**, *159*, 37–43. [CrossRef]
322. Hon, S.L. Vitamin C (ascorbic acid). In *Encyclopedia of Toxicology*, 4th ed.; Wexler, P., Ed.; Academic Press: Cambridge, MA, USA, 2024; Volume 9, pp. 805–807. [CrossRef]
323. Du, J.; Cullen, J.J.; Buettner, G.R. Ascorbic acid: Chemistry, biology and the treatment of cancer. *Biochim. Biophys. Acta* **2012**, *1826*, 443–457. [CrossRef]
324. Lushchak, V.I.; Semchuk, N.M. Tocopherol biosynthesis: Chemistry, regulation and effects of environmental factors. *Acta Physiol. Plant.* **2012**, *34*, 1607–1628. [CrossRef]
325. Rimbach, G.; Moehring, J.; Huebbe, P.; Lodge, J.K. Gene-regulatory activity of α-tocopherol. *Molecules* **2010**, *15*, 1746–1761. [CrossRef]
326. Mamoun, C.; GhanemI, F.Z.; Yelles, N.; Chenni, F.Z.; Essid, R.Y.M.; Patoli, D.; El Haci, I.A.; Benariba, K.; Rahmoun, A.; Kharoubi, O.; et al. Exploring the therapeutic potential of sour cherry leaf extract (*Prunus cerasus* L.): A comprehensive in vitro and in vivo evaluation. *Farmacia* **2025**, *73*, 2. [CrossRef]
327. Nunes, A.R.; Gonçalves, A.C.; Falcão, A.; Alves, G.; Silva, L.R. *Prunus avium* L. (sweet cherry) by-products: A source of phenolic compounds with antioxidant and anti-hyperglycemic properties—A review. *Appl. Sci.* **2021**, *11*, 8516. [CrossRef]
328. Roșcan, A.G.; Ifrim, I.-L.; Patriciu, O.-I.; Fînaru, A.-L. Bioactive Compounds from Orchard Waste: A Pharmacological Perspective on Rubus and Prunus Species. In Proceedings of the Conference Proceedings Abstracts of the 20th International Conference OPROTEH 2025, Bacău, Romania, 21–23 May 2025.

molecules

MDPI

Article

Sustainable Production and Antioxidant Activity of Bacterial Xanthan Gum

Ilona Jonuškienė [1,2,*], Erika Davicijonaitė [1], Monika Vaškevičiūtė [1], Ihsan Kala [1], Rima Stankevičienė [1], Kristina Kantminienė [3] and Ingrida Tumosienė [1]

[1] Department of Organic Chemistry, Kaunas University of Technology, Radvilėnų Pl. 19, LT-50254 Kaunas, Lithuania; erikutedavi@gmail.com (E.D.); monika.vaskeviciute99@gmail.com (M.V.); ihsan.kala13@gmail.com (I.K.); rima.stankeviciene@ktu.lt (R.S.); ingrida.tumosiene@ktu.lt (I.T.)

[2] Bioprocess Research Centre, Kaunas University of Technology, Radvilėnų Pl. 19, LT-50254 Kaunas, Lithuania

[3] Department of Physical and Inorganic Chemistry, Kaunas University of Technology, Radvilėnų Pl. 19, LT-50254 Kaunas, Lithuania; kristina.kantminiene@ktu.lt

* Correspondence: ilona.jonuskiene@ktu.lt

Abstract

One of the world's most sustainable solutions is to replace fossil-based polymers with biopolymers. The production of xanthan gum can be optimized using various renewable and cost-effective raw materials, which is a key focus in industrial biotechnology. Xanthan gum is a bioengineered thickening, stabilizing, and emulsifying agent. It has unique properties for use in many industries (food, biotechnology, petrochemicals, agricultural, cosmetics, wastewater treatment) and medical applications. It is tasteless, environmentally safe, non-toxic, and biodegradable. The biotechnological production of xanthan gum depends on several factors: bacterial strain development, culture medium preparation, carbon sources, fermentation parameters and modes, pH, temperature, recovery, purification, and quality control regulations. Bio-innovative strategies have been developed to optimize the production of xanthan gum. A variety of carbon and nitrogen sources, as well as alternative renewable sources, have been used in the production of xanthan gum. The aim of the present study was to optimize the xanthan gum yield using *Xanthomonas campestris* bacteria and different carbon (D-glucose, D-sorbitol, lactose, sucrose, D-mannitol, D-fructose, erythritol, coconut palm sugar, L-arabinose, unrefined cane sugar), various nitrogen (bacterial peptone, casein peptone, L-glutamic acid, L-arginine, L-methionine, L-tryptophan, malt extract, meat extract, L-phenylalanine, soy peptone) and alternative carbon (orange peels, tangerine peels, lemon peels, avocado peels, melon peels, apple peels, cellulose, xylose, xylitol) sources. The xanthan gum samples were analyzed using antioxidant methods. Our study showed that using L-glutamic acid as the carbon source for 72 h of bacterial fermentation of *Xanthomonas campestris* resulted in the highest xanthan gum yield: 32.34 g/L. However, using renewable resources, we achieved a very high concentration of xanthan gum in just 24 h of fermentation. According to the reducing power and DPPH methods, the highest antioxidant activities were measured for xanthan gum whose biosynthesis was based on renewable resources. Xanthan gum structures have been verified by FT-IR and ^{1}H NMR analysis. The sustainable biotechnology study has the advantage of increasing the sustainable production of xanthan gum by using renewable alternative resources compared to other production processes. Xanthan gum continues to be a valuable biopolymer with a wide range of industrial applications while promoting environmentally friendly production practices.

Keywords: biopolymers; carbon and nitrogen sources; renewable resources; antioxidant activity

1. Introduction

The replacement of fossil-based polymers with biopolymers is one of the most sustainable solutions. Biopolymers are environmentally friendly; they are produced from renewable resources, and their degradation does not increase the concentration of CO_2 in the environment. In recent decades, interest in microbial production of xanthan gum has increased due to the growing demand for high-quality bioproducts in various industries. Based on applications, the market for xanthan gum is divided into oil and gas, food and beverages, cosmetics, pharma, and others [1]. The food and beverage segment is expected to reach a volume of over 160 kilotons by 2030. Commercial xanthan gum is a thickening agent, a tasteless, dry, white to cream-colored powder used in the production of jams, puddings, sauces, canned and frozen foods, and beverages [1,2]. The valuable commercial bacterial heteropolysaccharide xanthan gum is produced by several strains of *Xanthomonas* bacteria, among which *Xanthomonas campestris* is the most widely used strain [3]. Xanthan gum is environmentally friendly, biocompatible, and biodegradable [4]. Its biological and pharmacological activities include antibacterial, antioxidant, and anticancer ones. Xanthan gum exhibits pseudoplastic properties, high viscosity, solubility, pH, and temperature stability [5].

The biotechnological production of xanthan gum depends on the choice of bacterial strain development, carbon and nitrogen sources, composition of the culture medium, fermentation parameters and modes, cell removal, isolation and recovery, purification of the final biopolymer, and regulatory approval of quality control.

The biotechnological production of xanthan gum involves the following steps: preparation of *Xanthomonas campestris* inoculum and carbon sources, aerobic and submerged fermentation, cell removal, recovery, and purification of the final product [2,6,7]. The production and properties of xanthan gum have been found to be influenced by several factors: physiological and genetic state of bacterial cells [8,9], culture medium [10–13], nutrient source [14–20], temperature [21,22], pH [23], fermentation time [24], bioreactor type [25], fermentation mode (batch or continuous), airflow [26,27], impeller type [28–30], oxygenation, upstream and downstream processes.

Various carbon sources have been reported to produce xanthan gum. In general, the concentration of the carbon source affects the conversion yield of sugar to polysaccharide [31]. The substrate is taken up from the culture medium and converted into intermediate nucleotide derivatives, which are then further converted into monomer units, polymerized into polysaccharide chains, and exported to the extracellular environment [32].

A backbone of β-(1,4)-linked D-glucose units with a trisaccharide side chain on alternating glucose residues forms the primary structure of xanthan gum. The side chain of this trisaccharide is composed of two mannose units, which are separated by a glucuronic acid. Xanthan-derived oligosaccharides are known to have antioxidant, antibacterial, and eliciting activities [33].

Due to its interactions with cations (i.e., Na^+, K^+, Ca^{2+}, and Mg^{2+}), xanthan gum can be considered an anionic polyelectrolyte, which is bound to acidic residues in varying proportions [34]. However, there are still several challenges to overcome to increase the sustainable industrial production and applications of xanthan gum. One of the disadvantages of xanthan gum is the cost of the carbon sources used in its production, the complexity of the extraction and production technologies, and, therefore, the higher cost of the resulting bioengineering product.

Xanthan gum is produced industrially using sucrose and glucose as carbon sources, but rising prices are forcing the search for alternative renewable feedstocks that can be adapted for biotechnological production of the biopolymer. The cost of carbon accounts for a third of the bioproduction of xanthan gum. Therefore, alternatives are being sought to reduce costs and increase sustainability. The use of agricultural and industrial waste as carbon sources is an important alternative to reduce production costs. However, the successful conversion of some of these nutrient sources into xanthan gum remains a challenge [35].

The aim of the present study was threefold: to optimize the production conditions of xanthan gum using the bacterium *Xanthomonas campestris* (including the use of different carbon, nitrogen and renewable resources, as well as fermentation time); to increase the yield of xanthan gum; and to evaluate the antioxidant activity of the obtained xanthan gum using the FRAP, reducing power and DPPH methods. FT-IR and ^{1}H NMR analyses were also performed.

Here, we discuss the main challenges in understanding the microbial sustainable production of xanthan gum and the current strategies to increase its yield by combining three targets (alternative carbon and nitrogen sources, fermentation time, and antioxidant activity) in biopolymer biosynthesis.

2. Results

Xanthomonas campestris inoculum requires carbon sources, micronutrients, and macronutrients for xanthan gum biosynthesis. The concentration of the carbon source affects the xanthan gum yield; a concentration of 2 $\pm$ 4% is preferred [5]. The culture medium provides nutrients for microbial growth. It plays a crucial role in the molecular structure, biosynthesis, recovery, and production yield of xanthan gum. Glucose and sucrose are commonly used and continue to be important sources of carbon for both yield and quality [34]. Therefore, costs can be reduced, and a higher quality biopolymer can be produced by optimizing the type and concentration of nutrients (mainly the carbon source) [35]. To reduce production costs, many researchers have started using alternative carbon sources to produce xanthan gum. Examples of these alternative sources are apple juice residues, date juice palm, sugar beet molasses, sugarcane molasses, crude glycerol, kitchen waste hydrolysate, orange peels, jackfruit seed powder, and cheese whey [5,36]. The minimum nutritional requirements for the biosynthesis of xanthan gum are carbon and nitrogen sources and micronutrients [36].

Bioproduction of xanthan gum using various carbon sources. In this study, the best combination of xanthan gum yield was obtained when the following parameters were applied: pH 7.0, 37 °C, and 150 rpm during fermentation for 24–72 h.

After 24–72 h of fermentation, the concentration of xanthan gum obtained by biosynthesis using different carbon sources was determined as shown in Figures 1–3.

The biosynthetic pathway to produce xanthan gum involves several steps: (1) assembly of pentasaccharide subunits attached to an inner membrane polyprenol phosphate carrier, (2) addition of acetyl and pyruvate groups, (3) polymerization of the pentasaccharide repeating units and secretion of xanthan gum [37]. It is useful to consider the chemical structure of the carbon source used when analyzing the results of the study.

It was found (Figure 1) that after 24 h of fermentation, the highest concentrations of xanthan gum were obtained with the addition of lactose (29.19 g/L) compared to D-glucose (24.37 g/L). Previous research by scientists showed that the highest concentration (28 g/L) was achieved using hydrolyzed whey lactose supplemented with sucrose and diammonium phosphate. Xanthan gum can be successfully produced using lactose as a substrate [38]. According to the literature data, the highest xanthan gum yield was 14.74 g/L with glucose [39,40]. Also, previous experiments showed that sucrose and glucose produced the best results in terms of the quality of xanthan gum, which is characterized by high viscosity and high molecular weight [41].

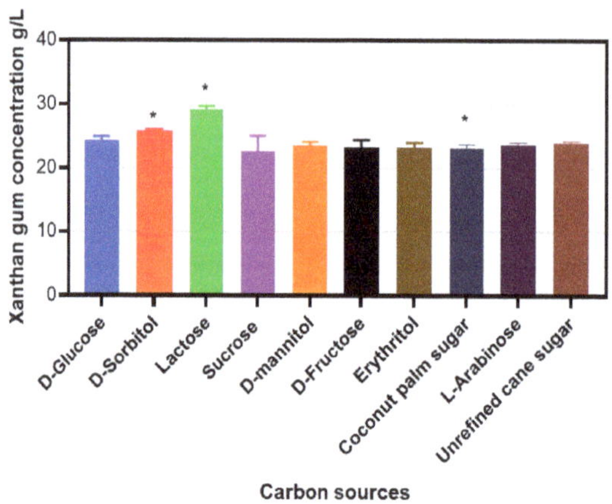

Figure 1. Xanthan gum concentration after 24 h of fermentation using carbon resources. The error bars show the mean ± SD of three experiments. Asterisks show statistically significant comparisons between D-glucose and alternative carbon sources, which were tested with an unpaired two-tailed *t*-test, with a significance level set at * $p < 0.1$.

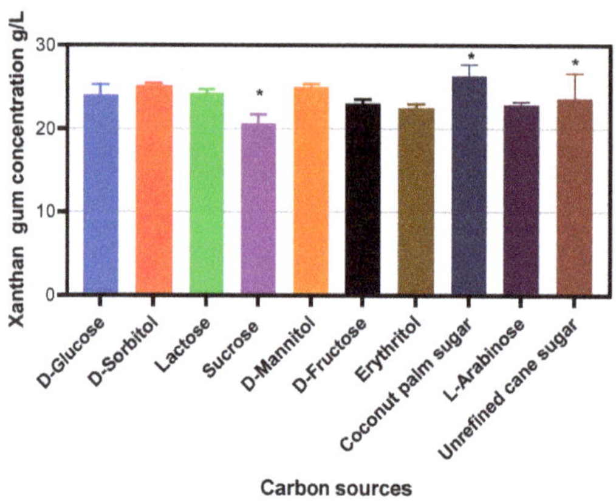

Figure 2. Xanthan gum concentration after 48 h of fermentation using carbon resources. The error bars show the mean ± SD of three experiments. Asterisks show statistically significant comparisons between D-glucose and alternative carbon sources, which were tested with an unpaired two-tailed *t*-test, with a significance level set at * $p < 0.1$.

Monosaccharide polyols, including erythritol, xylitol, and D-sorbitol, are low molecular weight carbohydrates that are commonly used as sweeteners in pharmaceutical and food applications [42]. Erythritol is used as a natural sweetener in the food and pharmaceutical industries. It has approximately 70% of the relative sweetness of sucrose and was approved by the FDA in 2001 as a low-calorie sweetener [43]. Erythritol has been shown to have oral health benefits by inhibiting the growth of oral bacteria, in addition to its sweetening properties [44].

When the results of the study were analyzed, it was found that the highest concentrations of xanthan gum (Figure 2) were obtained using coconut palm flower sugar (26.37 g/L), with D-sorbitol (25.14 g/L) and D-mannitol (24.98 g/L) as carbon sources, compared to D-glucose (24.06 g/L) after 48 h of fermentation.

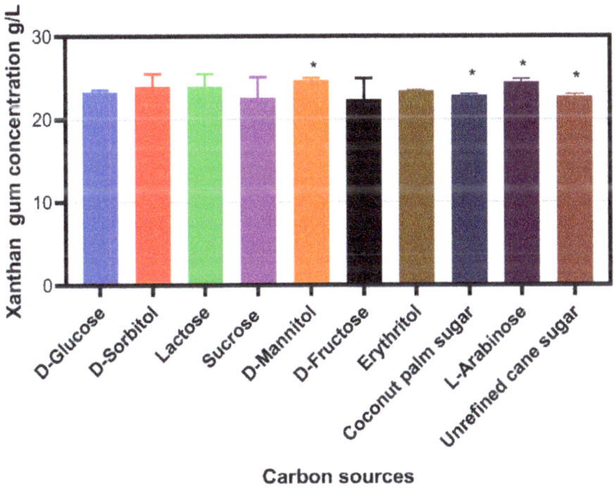

Figure 3. Xanthan gum concentration after 72 h of fermentation using carbon resources. The error bars show the mean ± SD of three experiments. Asterisks show statistically significant comparisons between D-glucose and alternative carbon sources, which were tested with an unpaired two-tailed *t*-test, with a significance level set at * $p < 0.1$.

After 72 h of fermentation, the yield of xanthan gum was using D-glucose—23.32 g/L. When analyzing the results of the study, it was found that the highest concentrations of xanthan gum (Figure 3) were obtained using D-mannitol (24.72 g/L) and L-arabinose (24.45 g/L) as carbon sources compared to D-glucose (23.32 g/L) after 72 h of fermentation.

The influence of alternative sources and renewable resources on the production of xanthan gum is described as follows. Previous research has shown that enhanced sustainable bioproduction of xanthan gum can be achieved by utilizing orange peels. Furthermore, optimized treatment in a 15 L bioreactor enabled the highest xanthan production of 30.19 g/L from orange peels to be achieved [45]. After 24–72 h of fermentation, the concentration of xanthan gum obtained by biosynthesis using different alternative carbon sources was determined as shown in Figures 4–6.

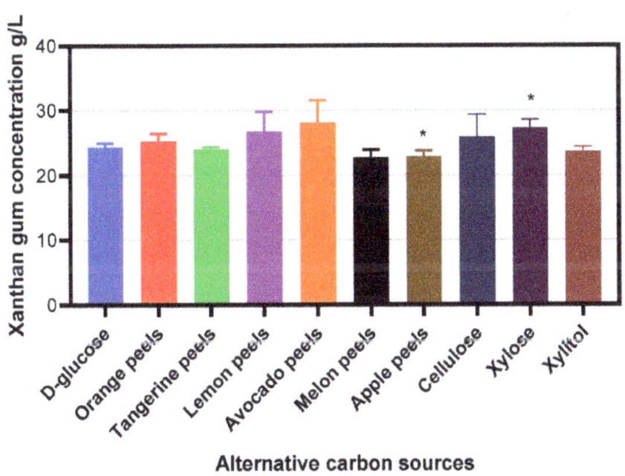

Figure 4. Xanthan gum concentration after 24 h of fermentation using alternative carbon resources. The error bars show the mean ± SD of three experiments. Asterisks show statistically significant comparisons between D-glucose and alternative carbon sources, which were tested with an unpaired two-tailed *t*-test, with a significance level set at * $p < 0.1$.

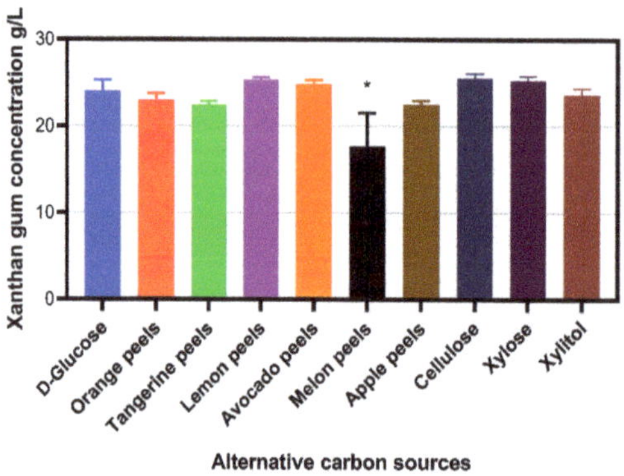

Figure 5. Xanthan gum concentration after 48 h of fermentation using alternative carbon resources. The error bars show the mean ± SD of three experiments. Asterisks show statistically significant comparisons between D-glucose and alternative carbon sources, which were tested with an unpaired two-tailed *t*-test, with a significance level set at * $p < 0.1$.

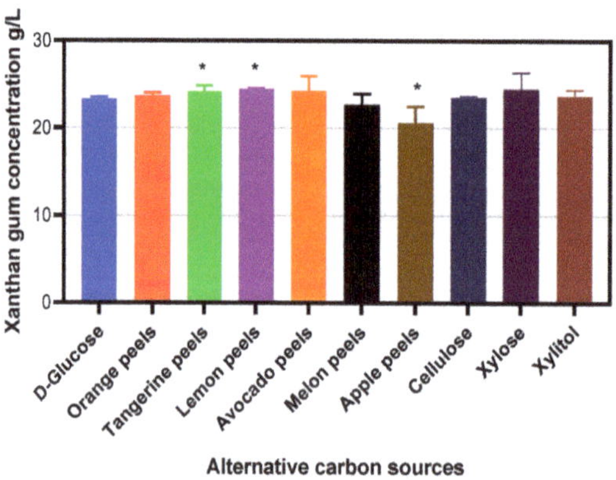

Figure 6. Xanthan gum concentration after 72 h of fermentation. The error bars show the mean ± SD of three experiments. Asterisks show statistically significant comparisons between D-glucose and alternative carbon sources, which were tested with an unpaired two-tailed *t*-test, with a significance level set at * $p < 0.1$.

After 24 h of fermentation, when analyzing the results of the study, it was found that the highest concentrations of xanthan gum (Figure 4) were obtained using avocado peels (28.09 g/L), xylose (27.20 g/L), peels of lemon (26.77 g/L) as carbon sources compared to D-glucose (24.37 g/L) after 24 h of fermentation.

After 48 h of fermentation, when analyzing the results of the study, it was found that the highest concentrations of xanthan gum (Figure 5) were obtained using cellulose (25.56 g/L), peels of lemon (25.34 g/L), xylose (25.29 g/L), as carbon sources compared to D-glucose (24.06 g/L) after 48 h of fermentation.

After 72 h of fermentation, when analyzing the results of the study, it was found that the highest concentrations of xanthan gum (Figure 6) were obtained using xylose (24.49 g/L), lemon peels (24.48 g/L), and tangerine peels (24.20 g/L) as carbon sources compared to D-glucose (23.31 g/L) after 72 h of fermentation.

Previous research has shown that sour lemon peel can be used to make a biodegradable film. The physicochemical properties of this film can be modified by adding xanthan gum and TiO_2–Ag nanoparticles [46].

The influence of nitrogen sources on xanthan gum production. Previous research has shown that amino acids such as cysteine, alanine, and histidine produce good yields of xanthan gum [38]. The concentration of xanthan gum obtained by biosynthesis using different alternative nitrogen sources was determined after 24–72 h of fermentation, as shown in Figures 7–9.

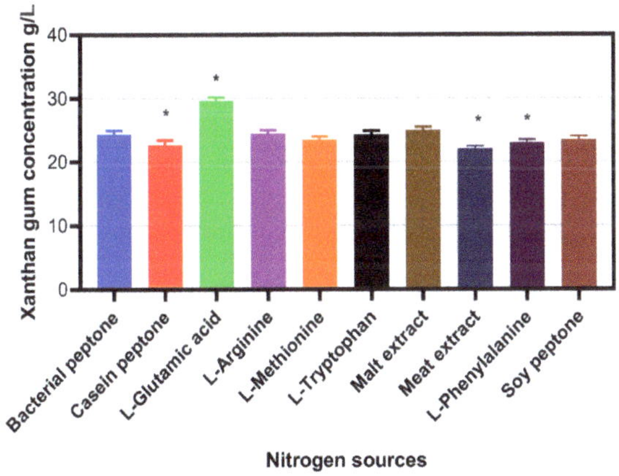

Figure 7. Xanthan gum concentration after 24 h of fermentation using nitrogen resources. The error bars show the mean ± SD of three experiments. Asterisks show statistically significant comparisons between bacterial peptone and alternative nitrogen sources, which were tested with an unpaired two-tailed t-test, with a significance level set at * $p < 0.1$.

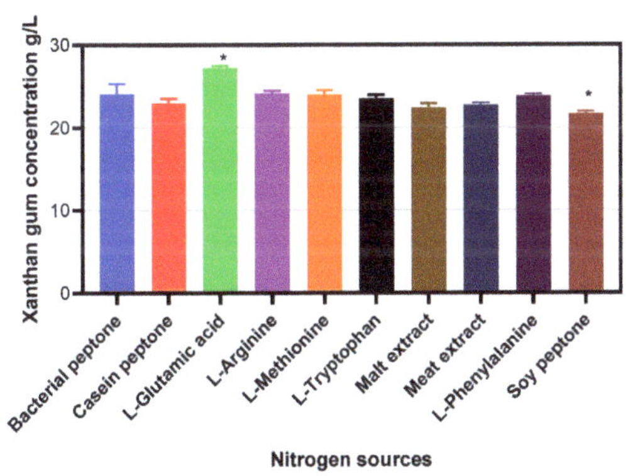

Figure 8. Xanthan gum concentration after 48 h of fermentation using nitrogen resources. The error bars show the mean ± SD of three experiments. Asterisks show statistically significant comparisons between bacterial peptone and alternative nitrogen sources, which were tested with an unpaired two-tailed t-test, with a significance level set at * $p < 0.1$.

After 24 h of fermentation, when analyzing the results of the study, it was found that the highest concentrations of xanthan gum (Figure 7) were obtained using L-glutamic acid (29.61 g/L) and malt extract (24.99 g/L) as nitrogen sources compared to bacterial peptone (24.37 g/L) after 24 h of fermentation.

After 48 h of fermentation, when analyzing the results of the study, it was found that the highest concentrations of xanthan gum (Figure 8) were obtained using L-glutamic acid (27.21 g/L), L-arginine (24.16 g/L), L-phenylalanine (23.80 g/L) as nitrogen sources compared to bacterial peptone (24.06 g/L) after 48 h of fermentation.

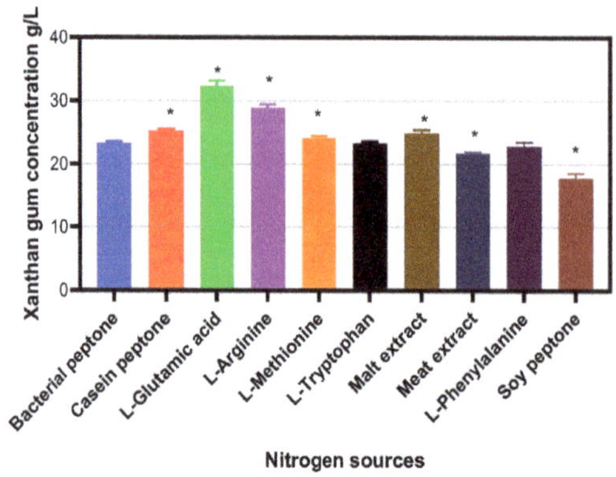

Figure 9. Xanthan gum concentration after 72 h of fermentation using nitrogen resources. The error bars show the mean ± SD of three experiments. Asterisks show statistically significant comparisons between bacterial peptone and alternative nitrogen sources, which were tested with an unpaired two-tailed *t*-test, with a significance level set at * $p < 0.1$.

After 72 h of fermentation, when analyzing the results of the study, it was found that the highest concentrations of xanthan gum (Figure 9) were obtained using L-glutamic acid (32.34 g/L), L-arginine (28.89 g/L), and casein protein (25.18 g/L) as nitrogen sources compared to bacterial peptone (23.31 g/L) after 72 h of fermentation.

Evaluation of the antioxidant activity of xanthan gum. The antioxidant activity of xanthan gum has attracted increasing attention as antioxidant health products have become popular in recent decades [47]. The biological activities of biopolymers are closely related to their structure, such as the composition of monosaccharides and the substitutions [48,49]. For example, pyruvate acid levels may reflect the association with the radical scavenging activity of xanthan oligosaccharides [50]. Furthermore, polyglucuronic oxidized xanthan and O-acetylated algal polysaccharides showed improvements in the hydroxyl radical scavenging activities [33,51,52].

Antioxidant activity according to the FRAP and reducing power assays. Xanthan gum was synthesized using different carbon and nitrogen sources, and then a study of the reducing properties was conducted using the FRAP and reducing power methods, the results of which are shown in Figures 10–15.

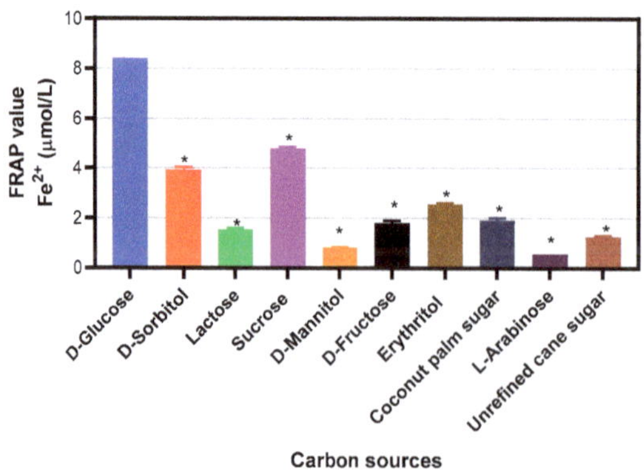

Figure 10. Antioxidant activity of extracted xanthan gum (from analyzed carbon sources) using the FRAP method. The error bars show the mean ± SD of three experiments. Asterisks show statistically significant comparisons between D-glucose and alternative carbon sources, which were tested with an unpaired two-tailed *t*-test, with a significance level set at * $p < 0.01$.

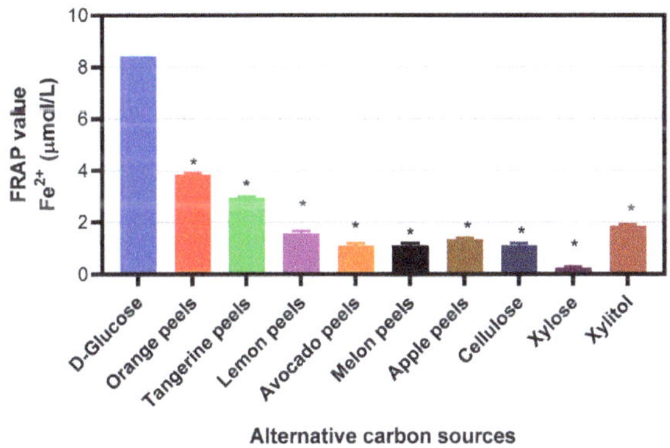

Figure 11. Antioxidant activity of extracted xanthan gum (from analyzed alternative carbon sources) using the FRAP method. The error bars show the mean ± SD of three experiments. Asterisks show statistically significant comparisons between D-glucose and alternative carbon sources, which were tested with an unpaired two-tailed *t*-test, with a significance level set at * $p < 0.01$.

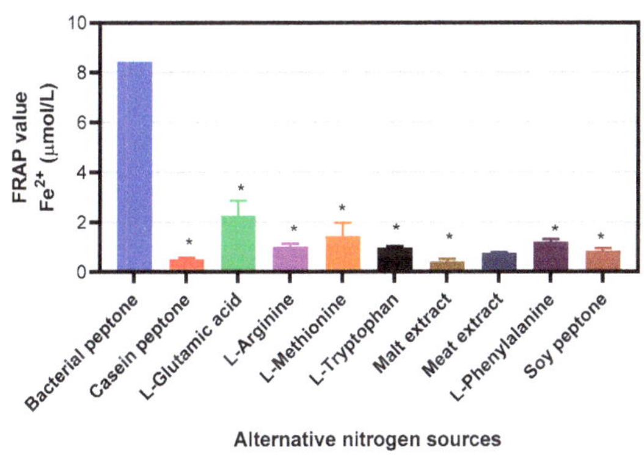

Figure 12. Antioxidant activity of extracted xanthan gum (from analyzed alternative nitrogen sources) using the FRAP method. The error bars show the mean ± SD of three experiments. Asterisks show statistically significant comparisons between bacterial peptone and alternative nitrogen sources, which were tested with an unpaired two-tailed *t*-test, with a significance level set at * $p < 0.01$.

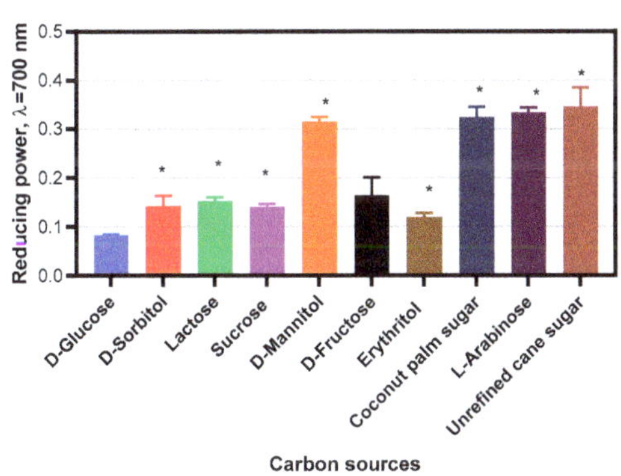

Figure 13. Antioxidant activity of extracted xanthan gum (from analyzed carbon sources) using the reducing power method. The error bars show the mean ± SD of three experiments. Asterisks show statistically significant comparisons between D-glucose and carbon sources, which were tested with an unpaired two-tailed *t*-test, with a significance level set at * $p < 0.01$.

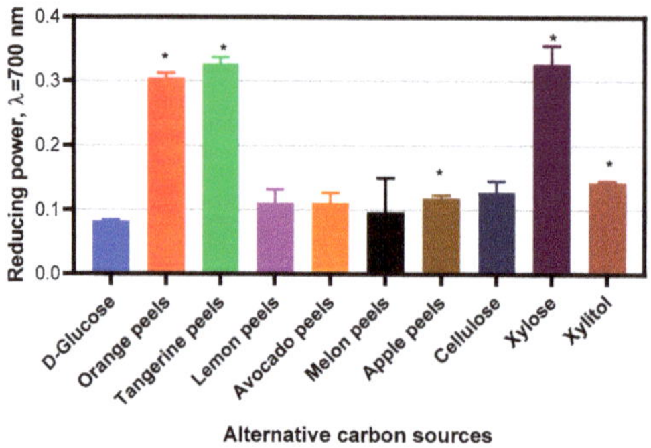

Figure 14. Antioxidant activity of extracted xanthan gum (from analyzed alternative carbon sources) using the reducing power method. The error bars show the mean ± SD of three experiments. Asterisks show statistically significant comparisons between D-glucose and alternative carbon sources, which were tested with an unpaired two-tailed *t*-test, with a significance level set at * $p < 0.01$.

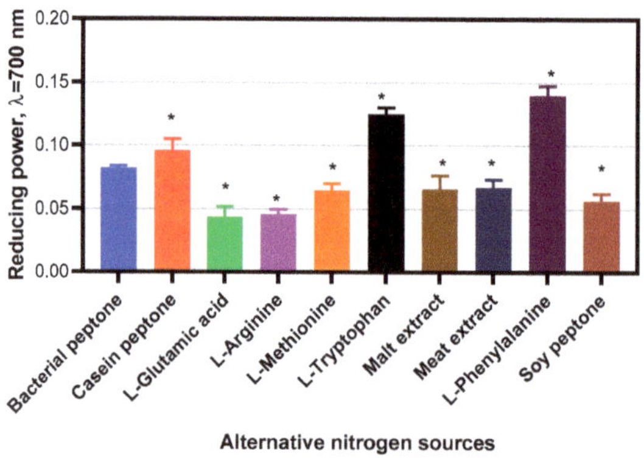

Figure 15. Antioxidant activity of extracted xanthan gum (from analyzed alternative nitrogen sources) using reducing power method. The error bars show the mean ± SD of three experiments. Asterisks show statistically significant comparisons between bacterial peptone and alternative nitrogen sources, which were tested with an unpaired two-tailed *t*-test, with a significance level set at * $p < 0.01$.

The highest antioxidant activity was measured for xanthan gum (Figure 10), whose biosynthesis was based on D-glucose (8.42 μmol/L). The results of the study showed that lower antioxidant activity of xanthan gum samples was obtained when other carbon sources were used, i.e., sucrose (4.82 μmol/L), D-sorbitol (3.95 μmol/L), and erythritol (2.55 μmol/L).

The highest antioxidant activity was measured for xanthan gum (Figure 11), whose biosynthesis was based on D-glucose (8.42 μmol/L). The results of the study showed that lower antioxidant activity of xanthan gum samples was obtained when other alternative carbon sources were used, i.e., orange peels (3.85 μmol/L), tangerine peels (2.95 μmol/L), and xylitol (1.85 μmol/L).

The highest antioxidant activity was measured for xanthan gum (Figure 12), whose biosynthesis was based on bacterial peptone (8.42 μmol/L). The results of the study showed that lower antioxidant activity of xanthan gum samples was obtained when other alternative nitrogen sources were used, i.e., L-glutamic acid (2.27 μmol/L), L-methionine (1.44 μmol/L), and L-phenylalanine (1.21 μmol/L).

The highest antioxidant activities were measured for xanthan gum (Figure 13), whose biosynthesis was based on unrefined cane sugar (0.35 o.u.), L-arabinose (0.33 o.u.), and coconut palm sugar (0.32 o.u.), in comparison with D-glucose (0.082 o.u.).

The highest antioxidant activities according to reducing power method and using renewable resources were measured for xanthan gum (Figure 15), whose biosynthesis was based on tangerine peels (0.33 o.u.), xylose (0.33 o.u.), orange peels (0.3 o.u.), in comparison with D-glucose (0.082 o.u.).

The highest antioxidant activities were measured for xanthan gum (Figure 14), whose biosynthesis was based on L-phenylalanine (0.14 o.u.), L-tryptophan (0.12 o.u.), casein peptone (0.1 o.u.), in comparison with bacterial peptone (0.082 o.u.).

Antioxidant activity according to the DPPH assay. Xanthan gum has a protective effect against the hydroxyl radical (*OH), which is the reactive oxygen species (ROS) that is most harmful to biological tissues [51]. The antioxidant capacity of the main components of xanthan gum (glucose and mannose) is very similar, although it is known that monosaccharide content plays an important role in the ability to scavenge hydroxyl radicals [52].

The antioxidant activity of xanthan gum samples obtained from different carbon sources was tested by DPPH assay. The results obtained are shown in Figure 16.

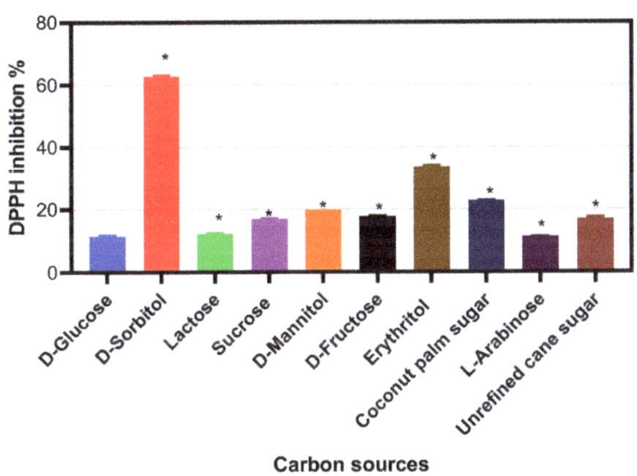

Figure 16. Antioxidant activity of xanthan gum according to the DPPH method (from analyzed carbon sources). The error bars show the mean ± SD of three experiments. Asterisks show statistically significant comparisons between D-glucose and alternative carbon sources, which were tested with unpaired two-tailed *t*-test, with a significance level set at * $p < 0.01$.

The highest antioxidant activity according to the DPPH was obtained for xanthan gum, for which a biosynthesis of D-sorbitol (62.67%) was used as the carbon source. The high antioxidant activities of xanthan gum were also obtained using erythritol supplement (33.75%) and coconut palm flower sugar (22.83%) compared to D-glucose (11.44%) (Figure 16).

The highest antioxidant activity according to the DPPH was obtained for xanthan gum, for which a biosynthesis of melon peels (19.36%) was used as the carbon source. The high antioxidant activities of xanthan gum were also obtained using lemon peels (14.83%) and peels of avocado (14.64%) compared to D-glucose (11.44%) (Figure 17).

The highest antioxidant activity according to the DPPH was obtained for xanthan gum, for which a biosynthesis of L-glutamic acid (22.14%) was used as the carbon source. The high antioxidant activities of xanthan gum were also obtained using malt extract (15.68%) and soy peptone (15.38%) compared to bacterial peptone (7.96%) (Figure 18).

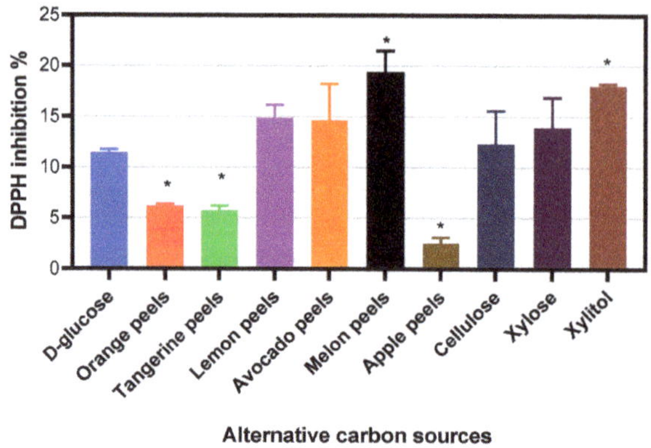

Figure 17. Antioxidant activity of xanthan gum according to the DPPH method (from analyzed alternative carbon sources). The error bars show the mean ± SD of three experiments. Asterisks show statistically significant comparisons between D-glucose and alternative carbon sources, which were tested with unpaired two-tailed *t*-test, with a significance level set at * $p < 0.01$.

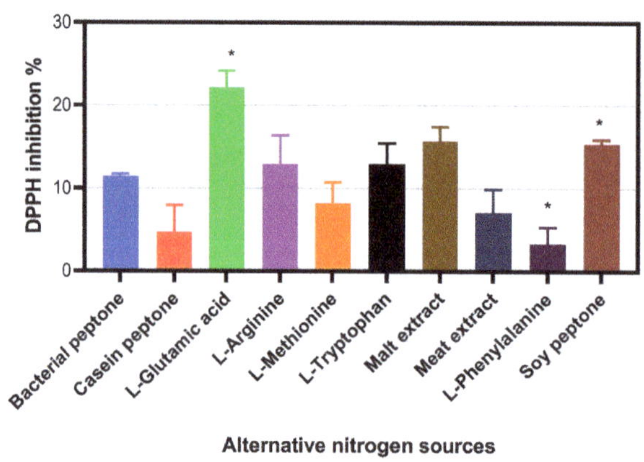

Figure 18. Antioxidant activity of extracted xanthan gum (from analyzed alternative nitrogen sources) using DPPH method. The error bars show the mean ± SD of three experiments. Asterisks show statistically significant comparisons between bacterial peptone and alternative nitrogen sources, which were tested with an unpaired two-tailed *t*-test, with a significance level set at * $p < 0.01$.

FT-IR spectra: The FT-IR spectrum was recorded for a sample of biosynthesized xanthan gum using D-glucose as the carbon source (Figure 19) and coconut palm sugar as the carbon source (Figure 20).

The broad absorption bands (Figures 19 and 20) observed at approximately 3438.76–3435.98 cm^{-1} have been ascribed to O-H stretching, while those at 2925.37–2925.50 cm^{-1} are due to C-H stretching. The absorption band at approximately 1738.47 cm^{-1} is related to the carboxyl group in xanthan gum, while the absorptions at approximately 1633.16–1634.91 cm^{-1} are due to C=O stretching in the pyruvate group of xanthan gum. Peaks at approximately 1400 cm^{-1} correspond to C-H stretching. Absorption bands in the 500 cm^{-1}–1000 cm^{-1} range have been attributed to the stretching vibrations of =C-H, C-O, O-H, and C-C bonds [53].

^{1}H NMR analysis: The ^{1}H NMR results of biosynthesized xanthan gum using D-glucose and coconut palm sugar as carbon sources are shown in the Supplementary Materials (Figures S1 and S2). The signals at 1.3 ppm and 2.0 ppm were assigned to the methyl protons of the pyruvate and acetyl groups, respectively. The protons from the hydroxyl groups in xanthan gum were found around 4.0 ppm [54]. The apparent peaks at around 4.7 ppm were due to D_2O.

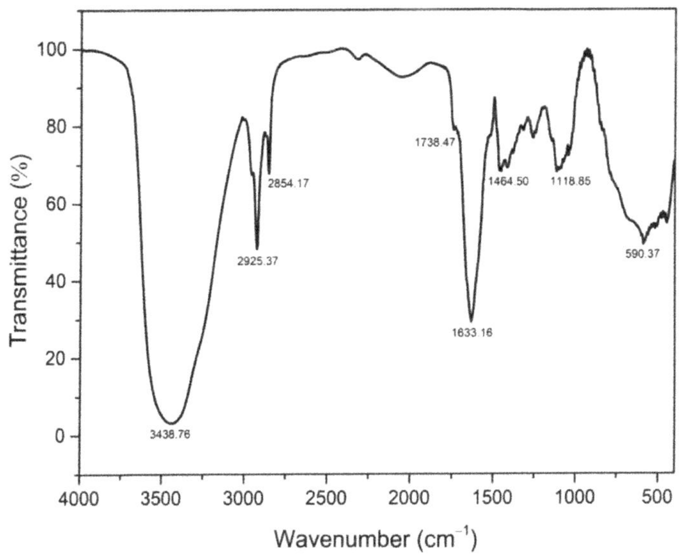

Figure 19. FT-IR spectra of biosynthesized xanthan gum using D-glucose as the carbon source.

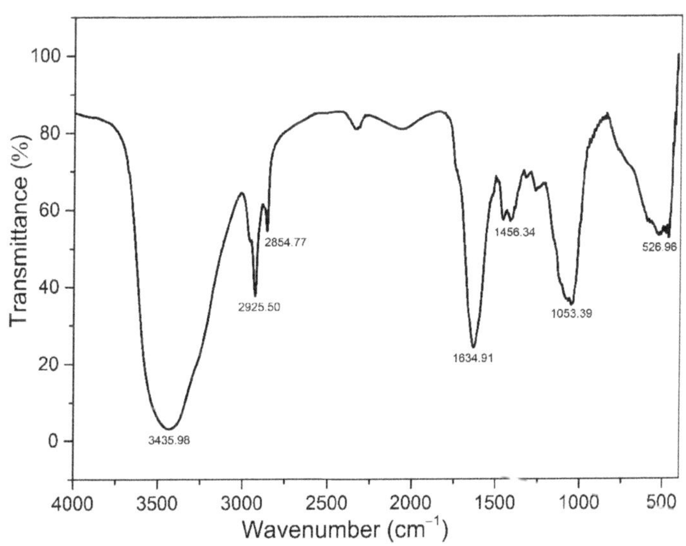

Figure 20. FT-IR spectra of biosynthesized xanthan gum using coconut palm sugar as the carbon source.

3. Discussion

It is important to understand the production of xanthan gum by integrating key parameters for its biosynthesis using different carbon sources, fermentation duration, and the determination of antioxidant activities. It is known that glucose concentrations below 2–5% are not effective for the maximal growth of bacterial cells. On the other hand, high concentrations of glucose have no significant effect on bacterial growth as well [55].

According to the literature, the highest efficiencies have been obtained using glucose, sucrose, maltose, and starch to produce xanthan gum. For example, a yield of 13.23 g/L of xanthan gum was obtained using sucrose, 12.32 g/L maltose, 5.23 g/L fructose, 1 g/L lactose as carbon sources [40]. Polyol sugars, such as inositol and D-sorbitol, were not good carbon sources for biopolymer production. According to the literature, a yield of 1.40 g/L xanthan gum was obtained using D-sorbitol [40].

Therefore, recent studies have focused on the use of natural alternatives as substrates to produce xanthan gum. As an example, the potential of various materials as alternatives to traditional substrates for xanthan gum production was assessed. These materials included green coconut shells, passion fruit peel, straw, and corn cobs, as well as agro-industrial waste. Previous research has shown that a medium based on jackfruit seed powder is useful for the economical production of xanthan gum on low-cost substrates, thereby reducing environmental impact [56–58].

In this study, we investigated the relationship between the different carbon sources, their concentration, the yield of xanthan gum, and its antioxidant activity. The bioproduction of xanthan gum should also be based on the elucidation of the chemical structure of the carbon source and the biological activity relationship. The results have shown that carbon sources and renewable resources are critical components of the bacterial media for biopolymer production.

Based on the results obtained, we can conclude that after 24 h of fermentation, the highest concentrations of xanthan gum were obtained using lactose (29.19 g/L) compared to D-glucose (24.37 g/L).

After 24 h of fermentation, when analyzing the results of the study, it was found that the highest concentrations of xanthan were obtained using hydrolyzates of renewable resources, such as avocado peels (28.09 g/L), xylose (27.20 g/L), peels of lemon (26.77 g/L), as carbon sources compared to D-glucose (24.37 g/L).

After 24 h of fermentation, when analyzing the results of the study, it was found that the highest concentrations of xanthan gum were obtained using L-glutamic acid (29.61 g/L), malt extract (24.99 g/L) as nitrogen sources compared to bacterial peptone (24.37 g/L) after 24 h of fermentation. Summarizing the results of the study, it was found that the highest concentrations of xanthan gum were obtained using L-glutamic acid (32.34 g/L) and L-arginine (28.89 g/L) after 72 h of fermentation.

The highest antioxidant activities according to reducing power activity were measured for xanthan gum, whose biosynthesis was based on unrefined cane sugar, L-arabinose, and coconut palm sugar, in comparison with D-glucose.

The highest antioxidant activity according to the DPPH was obtained for xanthan gum, for which a biosynthesis of D-sorbitol (62.67%) was used as the carbon source compared to D-glucose (11.44%).

The use of cheaper and more sustainable carbon sources for xanthan gum production can reduce production costs and, therefore, improve the economic effect of the process. Future work can focus on finding new renewable substrates (apple juice residue, sugar beet pulp waste, carrot and potato peel) to produce high-value biopolymers [56].

4. Materials and Methods

Carbon sources were used in the production of xanthan gum. (1) D-glucose anhydrous ($C_6H_{12}O_6$, Sigma-Aldrich, St. Louis, MO, USA, CAS 50-99-7) is a monosaccharide containing six carbon atoms and an aldehyde group and is, therefore, called aldohexose. (2) D-sorbitol ($C_6H_{14}O_6$, Sigma-Aldrich, St. Louis, MO, USA, CAS 50-70-4) is a polyhydric alcohol with about half the sweetness of sucrose. (3) Lactose ($C_{12}H_{22}O_{11}$, Sigma-Aldrich, St. Louis, MO, USA, CAS 63-42-3) is a disaccharide composed of glucose and galactose in human and cow milk. (4) Sucrose ($C_{12}H_{22}O_{11}$, Sigma-Aldrich, St. Louis, MO, USA, CAS 57-50-1) is a glycosyl glycoside composed of glucose and fructose units linked by an acetal oxygen bridge from the hemiacetal of glucose to the hemiketal of fructose. It acts as an osmolyte, a sweetener, and a human metabolite. (5) D-mannitol ($C_6H_{14}O_6$, Sigma-Aldrich, St. Louis, MO, USA, CAS 69-65-8) is the D-enantiomer of mannitol. (6) D-fructose ($C_6H_{12}O_6$, Sigma-Aldrich, St. Louis, MO, USA, CAS 57-48-7) is a monosaccharide found in sweet fruits and honey that is soluble in water, alcohol, or ether. It is used as a preservative and in intravenous infusions for parenteral feeding. (7) Erythritol ($C_4H_{10}O_4$, purchased from supermarket) is the meso-diastereomer of butane-1,2,3,4-tetrol. (8) Coconut palm sugar (purchased from supermarket) consists of sucrose (70–79%), glucose (3–9%), and fructose (3–9%). (9) L-Arabinose ($C_5H_{10}O_5$, Sigma-Aldrich, St. Louis, MO, USA, CAS 5328-37-0) is a metabolite found in or produced by *Saccharomyces cerevisiae*. (10) Unrefined cane sugar consists of sucrose and a small amount (3.5 to 6.5%) of molasses. The following carbon sources were used at 20 g/L in YPD broth media instead of D-glucose: D-sorbitol, lactose, sucrose, D-mannitol, D-fructose, erythritol, and L-arabinose [59].

Nitrogen sources were used in the production of xanthan gum: (1) Casein peptone (Sigma-Aldrich, St. Louis, MO, USA, CAS 91079-40-2) is a peptone derived from casein. (2) L-glutamic acid ($C_5H_9NO_4$, Sigma-Aldrich, St. Louis, MO, USA, CAS 56-86-0) is a proteinogenic amino acid. (3) L-arginine ($C_6H_{14}N_4O_2$, Sigma-Aldrich, St. Louis, MO, USA, CAS 74-79-3) is an L-alpha-amino acid and the L-isomer of arginine. It acts as a nutraceutical, a biomarker, and a micronutrient. (4) L-methionine ($C_5H_{11}NO_2S$, Sigma-Aldrich, St. Louis, MO, USA, CAS 63-68-3) is the L-enantiomer of methionine. (5) L-tryptophan ($C_{11}H_{12}N_2O_2$, Sigma-Aldrich, St. Louis, MO, USA, CAS 73-22-3) is the L-enantiomer of tryptophan. It has a role as an antidepressant, a nutraceutical, a micronutrient, and a plant metabolite. (6) Malt extract (Sigma-Aldrich, St. Louis, MO, USA, CAS 8002-48-0) and (7) meat extract (Sigma-Aldrich, St. Louis, MO, USA, CAS 68990-09-0) were also used. (8) L-phenylalanine ($C_9H_{11}NO_2$, Sigma-Aldrich, St. Louis, MO, USA, CAS 63-91-2) was also used, as well as (9) soy peptone (Sigma-Aldrich, St. Louis, MO, USA, CAS 91079-46-8). These sources were added to the YPD medium instead of bacterial peptone.

Xanthan gum was produced using alternative carbon sources: orange peels, tangerine peels, lemon peels, avocado peels, melon peels, apple peels, cellulose, xylose, and xylitol.

Xanthomonas campestris inoculation: The bacterial strain *Xanthomonas campestris*, obtained from DSMZ (DSM 1526), was used. *X. campestris* was inoculated onto Luria–Bertani (LB) agar plates. The LB agar medium consisted of peptone (10.0 g/L), yeast extract (5.0 g/L), NaCl (5.0 g/L), and agar (15.0 g/L). The plate was then incubated at 37 °C for 24 h, after which a culture colony was harvested using a sterile sampling tip. This was then transferred to a 50 mL flask containing a modified YPD broth medium consisting of bacterial peptone (25.0 g/L), yeast extract (10.0 g/L), and D-glucose (20.0 g/L). The flask was then incubated in a shaking incubator set at 37 °C at 150 rpm for 72 h. An aliquot (7 mL) of the inoculated medium was added to each 250 mL flask containing 150 mL of YPD broth. The fermentation was carried out at pH 7.0, 37 °C, and 150 rpm for 24–72 h [59].

Determination of dry bacterial biomass and xanthan gum production. The bacterial biomass and the xanthan gum were collected after 24, 48, and 72 h. To determine the biomass mass (n = 3), an aliquot of the medium culture of the *Xanthomonas campestris* was transferred to a pre-weighed tube. The tube was then centrifuged at 10,000× g for 10 min at 4 °C using a centrifuge Universal 320R (Andreas Hettich GmbH & Co. KG, Tuttlingen, Germany). After discarding the supernatant, the tube was incubated at 45 °C for 24 h in an incubator (Memmert IN55, GmbH & Co. KG, Schwabach, Germany) to dry the biomass. A solution of KCl (5 mL, at 5% *w/v* based on the final mixture) was stirred into a pre-weighed tube containing the supernatant. After adding isopropanol (35 mL), the mixture was shaken on a thermoshaker (Shaker-Incubator ES-20, Riga, Latvia) for three hours, after which the sample was refrigerated overnight. After overnight storage, the precipitated xanthan gum was centrifuged at 10,000× *g* for 10 min at 4 °C using a Universal 320R centrifuge (Andreas Hettich GmbH & Co. KG, Tuttlingen, Germany), then dried at 45 °C for 48 h in an incubator (Memmert IN55, GmbH & Co. KG, Schwabach, Germany) [59].

Production of hydrolyzates from renewable resources. The renewable resources (peels) were hydrolyzed by cellulases. The reaction was carried out in a 0.1 M citrate buffer, at pH 4.8, with a solid loading of 3% *w*/*w* and 3% *w*/*w* cellulase (CelluStar, Dyadic International, Inc., Jupiter, FL, USA) enzymes [60].

Measurement of Antioxidant Activities

Ferric reducing antioxidant power (FRAP) assay: The FRAP reagent contained 2.5 mL of 10 mM TPTZ (2,4,6-tripyridyl-*s*-triazine) solution in 40 mM HCl, 2.5 mL of $FeCl_3$ (20 mM), and 25 mL of acetate buffer (0.3 M, pH 3.6). To analyze xanthan gum samples (1 mg/mL), 50 µL were mixed with 1.5 mL of the FRAP reagent. The absorbance of the reaction mixture was measured spectrophotometrically (UV-1280 spectrophotometer (Shimadzu Corporation, Kyoto, Japan)) at 593 nm. To construct the calibration curve, five concentrations of $FeSO_4 \cdot 7H_2O$ (5, 10, 15, 20, and 25 µM) were used. Each experiment was repeated three times [61].

Ferric ion (Fe^{3+}) reducing antioxidant power (Fe^{3+}-Fe^{2+} transformation assay). Xanthan gum samples at a concentration of (1 mg/mL) 0.5 mL were mixed with phosphate buffer (1.25 mL, 0.2 M, pH 6.6) and potassium ferricyanide [$K_3Fe(CN)_6$] (1.25 mL, 1%). The mixture was then incubated at 50 °C for 20 min. Aliquots (1.25 mL) of trichloroacetic acid (10%) were then added to the mixture, which was then centrifuged for 10 min at 9000 rpm using a centrifuge Universal 320R (Andreas Hettich GmbH & Co. KG, Tuttlingen, Germany). The upper layer of the solution (1.25 mL) was mixed with distilled water (1.25 mL) and $FeCl_3$ (0.25 mL, 0.1%), and the absorbance was measured at 700 nm using a UV-1280 spectrophotometer (Shimadzu Corporation, Kyoto, Japan) [61]. Each experiment was repeated three times.

1,1-Diphenyl-2-picrylhydrazyl (DPPH) radical scavenging assay: The free radical scavenging activity of xanthan gum was measured using this method. First, a 1 mg/mL solution of xanthan gum in water was prepared. Then, a 0.1 mM solution of DPPH in ethanol was prepared, and 1 mL of this solution was added to the solutions of the analyzed xanthan gum samples. The mixture was stirred vigorously and left to stand at room temperature. After 20 min, the absorbance of the reaction mixture was measured at 517 nm using a UV-1280 spectrophotometer (Shimadzu Corporation, Kyoto, Japan). Each experiment was repeated three times [62].

FT-IR spectra analysis: IR spectra (n, cm^{-1}) were recorded on a Perkin–Elmer Spectrum BX FT–IR spectrometer (Perkin–Elmer Inc., Waltham, MA, USA) using KBr pellets.

^1H NMR analysis: Proton nuclear magnetic resonance (^1H NMR) spectra were obtained using a Bruker Avance III ^1H 700 MHz spectrometer (Billerica, MA, USA).

Statistical analysis: The results of three experiments are expressed as the mean ± SD. Statistically significant comparisons between glucose and alternative carbon sources were tested using an unpaired two-tailed *t*-test with a significance level set at $p < 0.1$. GraphPad Prism version 8.0.2 for Windows (San Diego, CA, USA) was used for the statistical analysis.

5. Conclusions

Xanthan gum is an important biodegradable, biocompatible, and renewable biopolymer that is widely used in food, biotechnology, biomedical, cosmetic, food bio-packaging, and 3D printing industries [63]. Creation and development of xanthan gum with bioactive additives in composite films for the preservation of fresh-cut vegetables and fruits is one of many examples [64,65]. Xanthan gum has attracted a great deal of attention in food packaging applications due to its extreme pseudoplastic behavior and rheological properties that enhance film-forming properties [66]. One of the most sustainable solutions is to replace fossil-based polymers with biopolymers. It is also important to find alternatives to D-glucose as a carbon source in the production medium and to use renewable resources to increase the sustainability of xanthan gum production.

Our study shows that using L-glutamic acid as the carbon source for 72 h bacterial fermentation of *Xanthomonas campestris* resulted in the highest xanthan gum yield. However, a very high concentration of xanthan gum is produced in just 24 h of fermentation using hydrolyzates of avocado and lemon peels. According to the reducing power method, xanthan gum synthesized using renewable resources exhibits the highest antioxidant activity.

The results obtained are of great importance for identifying new alternative carbon sources, as well as being an attractive approach for the potential biotechnological application of biopolymers. Understanding the influence of carbon sources and various renewable resources on biopolymer production provides opportunities for future research into new biomanufacturing routes. It is estimated that the global market for xanthan gum will grow by 15% by 2027, reaching a value of approximately USD 455.9 million [67]. However, scaling up xanthan gum production from laboratory to industrial levels using new sustainable technologies and bioeconomic strategies remains challenging [68–70].

Supplementary Materials: The following supporting information can be downloaded at: https://www.mdpi.com/article/10.3390/molecules30132734/s1, Figure S1: ^{1}H NMR spectra of biosynthesized xanthan gum using glucose as the carbon source; Figure S2: ^{1}H NMR spectra of biosynthesized xanthan gum using coconut palm sugar as the carbon source.

Author Contributions: Conceptualization, I.J., E.D., M.V., I.K., R.S., K.K. and I.T.; methodology, I.J., E.D., M.V., I.K., R.S., K.K. and I.T.; formal analysis I.J., E.D., M.V. and I.K.; investigation, I.J., E.D., M.V., I.K., R.S., K.K. and I.T.; resources, I.J., E.D., M.V., I.K., R.S., K.K. and I.T.; data curation, I.J. and E.D.; writing—original draft preparation I.J., E.D., K.K. and I.T.; writing—review and editing, I.J., K.K. and I.T. All authors have read and agreed to the published version of the manuscript.

Funding: This research received no external funding.

Institutional Review Board Statement: Not applicable.

Informed Consent Statement: Not applicable.

Data Availability Statement: Data is contained within the article.

Conflicts of Interest: The authors declare no conflicts of interest.

References

1. Xanthan Gum Market Size, Share | Forecasts Report 2022–2030. Available online: https://www.gminsights.com/ (accessed on 20 January 2025).
2. GarcõÂa-Ochoa, F.; Santosa, V.E.; Casasb, J.A.; GoÂmez, E. Xanthan gum: Production, recovery, and properties. *Biotechnol. Adv.* **2000**, *18*, 549. [CrossRef]
3. Rana, S.; Upadhyay, L.S.B. Microbial exopolysaccharides: Synthesis pathways, types and their commercial applications. *Int. J. Biol. Macromol.* **2020**, *157*, 577–583. [CrossRef]
4. Petri, D.F.S. Xanthan gum: A versatile biopolymer for biomedical and technological applications. *J. Appl. Polym. Sci.* **2015**, *132*, 2–13. [CrossRef]
5. Bhat, I.M.; Wani, S.M.; Mir, S.A.; Masoodi, F.A. Advances in xanthan gum production, modifications and its applications. *Biocatal. Agric. Biotechnol.* **2022**, *42*, 102328. [CrossRef]
6. Rosalan, S.; England, R. Review of xanthan gum production from unmodified starches by *Xanthomonas campestris* sp. *Enzym. Microb. Technol.* **2006**, *39*, 197–207. [CrossRef]

7. Dey, R.; Chatterji, B.P. Sources and methods of manufacturing xanthan by fermentation of various carbon sources. *Biotechnol. Prog.* **2023**, *39*, e3379. [CrossRef] [PubMed]
8. Steffens, T.; Vorhölter, F.J.; Teckentrup, J.; Hublik, G.; Walhorn, V.; Anselmetti, D.; Pühler, A.; Niehaus, K.; Ortseifen, V. Two Flagellar mutants of *Xanthomonas campestris* are characterized by enhanced xanthan production and higher xanthan viscosity. *J. Biotechnol.* **2022**, *347*, 9–17. [CrossRef]
9. Moreira, A.S.; Vendruscolo, J.L.S.; Gil-Turnes, C.; Vendruscolo, C.T. Screening among 18 novel strains of *Xanthomonas campestris* pv pruni. *Food Hydrocoll.* **2001**, *15*, 469–474. [CrossRef]
10. Kalogiannis, S.; Iakovidou, G.; Liakopoulou-Kyriakides, M.; Kyriakidis, D.A.; Skaracis, G.N. Optimization of xanthan gum production by *Xanthomonas campestris* grown in molasses. *Process Biochem.* **2003**, *39*, 249–256. [CrossRef]
11. Chaitali, M.; Kapadi, M.; Suraishkumar, G.K.; Gudi, R.D. Productivity improvement in xanthan gum fermentation using multiple substrate optimization. *Biotechnol. Progr.* **2003**, *19*, 1190–1198. [CrossRef]
12. Sun, H.; Ni, J.; Yang, G.; Liu, Z.; Wang, Z.; Zhu, S.; Li, Z.; Jiang, Y.; Zhan, X.; Wang, Y.; et al. A novel coupled fermentation system for low-molecular-weight xanthan gum with diverse biological activities. *Int. J. Biol. Macromol.* **2024**, *279*, 135283. [CrossRef] [PubMed]
13. Letisse, F.; Chevallereau, P.; Simon, J.L.; Lindley, N.D. Kinetic analysis of growth and xanthan gum production with *Xanthomonas campestris* on sucrose, using sequentially consumed nitrogen sources. *Appl. Microbiol. Biotechnol.* **2001**, *55*, 417–422. [CrossRef]
14. Silva, M.F.; Fornari, R.C.G.; Mazutti, M.A.; de Oliveira, D.; Padilha, F.F.; Cichoski, A.J.; Cansian, R.L.; Di Luccio, M.; Treichel, H. Production and characterization of xantham gum by *Xanthomonas campestris* using cheese whey as sole carbon source. *J. Food Eng.* **2009**, *90*, 119–123. [CrossRef]
15. Demirci, A.S.; Palabiyik, I.; Apaydın, D.; Mirik, M.; Gumus, T. Xanthan gum biosynthesis using *Xanthomonas* isolates from waste bread: Process optimization and fermentation kinetics. *LWT* **2019**, *101*, 40–47. [CrossRef]
16. Psomas, S.K.; Liakopoulou-Kyriakides, M.; Kyriakidis, M. Optimization study of xanthan gum production using response surface methodology. *Biochem. Eng. J.* **2007**, *35*, 273–280. [CrossRef]
17. Oliveira, D.B.; Kundlastsch, G.E.; Cruz, R.D.; Batista, B.; de Arruda Ribeiro, M.P.; Novo-Mansur, M.T.M.; da Silva, A.J. Xanthan gum production in *Xanthomonas campestris* is increased by favoring the biosynthesis of its monomers. *Bioresour. Technol.* **2025**, *416*, 131808. [CrossRef]
18. Lopez, M.J.; Moreno, J.; Ramos, A.C. *Xanthomonas campestris* strain selection for xanthan production from olive mill wastewaters. *Water Res.* **2001**, *35*, 1828–1830. [CrossRef]
19. Lopez, M.J.; Vargas-Garcia, M.C.; Suarez-Estrella, F.; Moreno, J. Properties of xanthan obtained from agricultural wastes acid hydrolysates. *J. Food Eng.* **2004**, *63*, 111–115. [CrossRef]
20. Lopes, B.M.; Lessa, V.L.; Silva, B.M.; Filho, M.A.S.C.; Schnitzler, E.; Lacerda, L.G. Xanthan gum: Properties, production conditions, quality and economic perspective. *J. Food Nutr. Res.* **2015**, *54*, 185–194.
21. Mudoi, P.; Bharali, P.; Konwar, B.K. Study on the Effect of pH, temperature and aeration on the cellular growth and xanthan production by *Xanthomonas campestris* using waste residual molasses. *J. Bioprocess. Biotech.* **2013**, *3*, 135. [CrossRef]
22. Palaniraj, A.; Jayaraman, V. Production, recovery and applications of xanthan gum by *Xanthomonas campestris*. *J. Food Eng.* **2011**, *106*, 1–12. [CrossRef]
23. Brunchi, C.E.; Bercea, M.; Morariu, S.; Dascalu, M. Some properties of xanthan gum in aqueous solutions: Effect of temperature and pH. *J. Polym. Res.* **2016**, *23*, 123. [CrossRef]
24. Cacik, F.; Dondo, R.G.; Marques, D. Optimal control of a batch bioreactor for the production of xanthan gum. *Comput. Chem. Eng.* **2001**, *25*, 409–418. [CrossRef]
25. Rehm, B.H.A. Bacterial polymers: Biosynthesis, modifications, and applications. *Nat. Rev. Microbiol.* **2010**, *8*, 578–592. [CrossRef]
26. de Jesus, A.D.; Brandão, L.V.; de Sousa, C.L.A.; Figueiredo, T.V.; Sousa, L.S.; Padilha, F.F.; Druzian, J.I. A study of the effects of aeration and agitation on the properties and production of xanthan gum from crude glycerin derived from biodiesel using the response surface methodology. *Appl. Biochem. Biotechnol.* **2014**, *172*, 2769–2785. [CrossRef]
27. Garcia-Ochoa, F.; Gomez, E. Bioreactor scale-up and oxygen transfer rate in microbial processes: An overview. *Biotechnol. Adv.* **2009**, *27*, 153–176. [CrossRef] [PubMed]
28. Sadino-Riquelme, M.C.; Rivas, J.; Jeison, D.; Donoso-Bravo, A.; Hayes, R.E. Investigating a stirred bioreactor: Impact of evolving fermentation broth pseudoplastic rheology on mixing mechanisms. *Fermentation* **2022**, *8*, 102. [CrossRef]
29. Xie, M.-h.; Xia, J.-y.; Zhou, Z.; Zhou, G.-z.; Chu, J.; Zhuang, Y.-p.; Zhang, S.-l.; Noorman, H. Power consumption, local and average volumetric mass transfer coefficient in multiple-impeller stirred bioreactors for xanthan gum solutions. *Chem. Eng. Sci.* **2014**, *106*, 144–156. [CrossRef]
30. Chachi, M.; Kamla, Y.; Alhaffar, M.T.; Bouzit, M.; Meliani, M.H.; Al-Badour, F.A.; Rahman, M.M.; Suleiman, R.K. Quantitative assessment of agitator performance in an anchor-stirred tank: Investigating the impact of geometry, eccentricity, and rheological characteristics. *Arab. J. Sci. Eng.* **2024**, *49*, 13885–13895. [CrossRef]

31. Woiciechowski, A.L.; Soccol, C.R.; Rocha, S.N.; Pandey, A. Xanthan gum production from cassava bagasse hydrolysate with *Xanthomonas campestris* using alternative sources of nitrogen. *Appl. Biochem. Biotechnol.* **2004**, *118*, 305–312. [CrossRef]
32. Habibi, H.; Khosravi-Daranib, K. Effective variables on production and structure of xanthan gum and its food applications: A review. *Biocatal. Agric. Biotechnol.* **2017**, *10*, 130–140. [CrossRef]
33. Wu, S.J.; Wu, J.H.; Xia, L.Z.; Chu, C.; Liu, D.; Gong, M. Preparation of xanthan-derived oligosaccharides and their hydroxyl radical scavenging activity. *Carbohydr. Polym.* **2013**, *92*, 1612–1614. [CrossRef] [PubMed]
34. Klaic, P.M.A.; Vendruscolo, C.T.; Furlan, L.; Moreira, A.S. Ion exchange as post-fermentative process enhancer of viscosity of xanthan produced by *Xanthomonas arboricola* pv pruni. *Food Hydrocoll.* **2016**, *56*, 118–126. [CrossRef]
35. da Silva, L.C.C.; Brenda, N.T.; Furtado, M.M.; de Oliveira Pinto, M.A.; Rodarte, M.P.; Hungaro, H.M. Xanthan: Biotechnological production and applications. In *Microbial Production of Food Ingredients and Additives*; Elsevier: Oxford, UK, 2017; pp. 385–422. [CrossRef]
36. Chilakamarry, C.T.; Sakinah, A.M.M.; Zularisam, A.W.; Sirohi, R.; Khilji, I.A.; Ahmad, N.; Pandey, A. Advances in solid-state fermentation for bioconversion of agricultural wastes to value-added products: Opportunities and challenges. *Bioresour. Technol.* **2022**, *343*, 126065. [CrossRef]
37. Barcelos, M.C.S.; Vespermann, K.A.C.; Pelissari, F.M.; Molina, G. Current status of biotechnological production and applications of microbial exopolysaccharides. *Crit. Rev. Food Sci. Nutr.* **2020**, *60*, 1475–1495. [CrossRef]
38. Murad, H.A.; Mohamed, S.H.; Abu-El-Khair, A.G. Impact of amino acids, nitrogen source and buffering system on xanthan yield produced on hydrolysed whey lactose. *Biotechnology* **2017**, *16*, 69–76. [CrossRef]
39. Rončević, Z.Z.; Bajić, B.Ž.; Grahovac, J.A.; Dodić, S.N.; Dodić, J.M. Effect of the initial glycerol concentration in the medium on the xanthan biosynthesis. *APTEFF* **2014**, *45*, 239–246. [CrossRef]
40. Leela, K.J.; Sharma, G. Studies on xanthan production from *Xanthomonas campestris*. *Bioprocess Eng.* **2000**, *23*, 687–689. [CrossRef]
41. Mohsin, A.; Akyliyaevna, K.A.; Zaman, W.Q.; Hussain, M.H.; Mohsin, M.Z.; Al-Rashed, S.; Tan, X.; Tian, X.; Aida, K.; Tariq, M.; et al. Kinetically modelled approach of xanthan production using different carbon sources: A study on molecular weight and rheological properties of xanthan. *Int. J. Biol. Macromol.* **2021**, *193*, 1226–1236. [CrossRef] [PubMed]
42. Rico, M.; Rodríguez-Lamazares, S.; Barral, L.; Bouza, R.; Montero, B. Processing and characterization of polyols plasticized-starch reinforced with microcrystalline cellulose. *Carbohydr. Polym.* **2016**, *149*, 83–93. [CrossRef]
43. Rzechonek, D.A.; Dobrowolski, A.; Rymowicz, W.; Mirończuk, A.M. Recent advances in biological production of erythritol. *Crit. Rev. Biotechnol.* **2018**, *38*, 620–633. [CrossRef] [PubMed]
44. Mensi, M.; Scotti, E.; Sordillo, A.; Dalè, M.; Calza, S. Clinical evaluation of air polishing with erythritol powder followed by ultrasonic calculus removal versus conventional ultrasonic debridement and rubber cup polishing for the treatment of gingivitis: A split-mouth randomized controlled clinical trial. *Int. J. Dent. Hyg.* **2022**, *20*, 371–380. [CrossRef] [PubMed]
45. Mohsin, A.; Zhang, K.; Hu, J.; Salim-ur-Rehman; Tariq, M.; Zaman, W.Q.; Khan, I.M.; Zhuang, Y.; Guo, M. Optimized biosynthesis of xanthan via effective valorization of orange peels using response surface methodology: A kinetic model approach. *Carbohydr. Polym.* **2018**, *181*, 793–800. [CrossRef] [PubMed]
46. Meydanju, N.; Pirsa, S.; Farzi, J. Biodegradable film based on lemon peel powder containing xanthan gum and TiO_2–Ag nanoparticles: Investigation of physicochemical and antibacterial properties. *Polym. Test.* **2022**, *106*, 107445. [CrossRef]
47. Gawlik-Dziki, U. Changes in the antioxidant activities of vegetables as a consequence of interactions between active compounds. *J. Funct. Foods* **2012**, *4*, 872–882. [CrossRef]
48. Chen, Y.; Zhang, H.; Wang, Y.; Nie, S.; Li, C.; Xie, M. Acetylation and carboxymethylation of the polysaccharide from *Ganoderma atrum* and their antioxidant and immunomodulating activities. *Food Chem.* **2014**, *156*, 279–288. [CrossRef]
49. Wang, Z.; Wu, J.; Zhu, L.; Zhan, X. Characterization of xanthan gum produced from glycerol by a mutant strain *Xanthomonas campestris* CCTCC M2015714. *Carbohydr. Polym.* **2017**, *157*, 521–526. [CrossRef]
50. Xiong, X.; Li, M.; Xie, J.; Jin, Q.; Xue, B.; Sun, T. Antioxidant activity of xanthan oligosaccharides prepared by different degradation methods. *Carbohydr. Polym.* **2013**, *92*, 1166–1171. [CrossRef]
51. Delattre, C.; Pierre, G.; Gardarin, C.; Traikia, M.; Elboutachfaiti, R.; Isogai, A.; Michaud, P. Antioxidant activities of a polyglucuronic acid sodium salt obtained from TEMPO-mediated oxidation of xanthan. *Carbohydr. Polym.* **2015**, *116*, 34–41. [CrossRef]
52. Spasojević, I.; Mojović, M.; Blagojević, D.; Spasić, S.D.; Jones, D.R.; Nikolić-Kokić, A.; Spasić, M.B. Relevance of the capacity of phosphorylated fructose to scavenge the hydroxyl radical. *Carbohydr. Res.* **2009**, *344*, 80–84. [CrossRef]
53. Hu, X.; Wang, K.; Yu, M.; He, P.; Qiao, H.; Zhang, H.; Wang, Z. Characterization and antioxidant activity of a low-molecular-weight xanthan gum. *Biomolecules* **2019**, *9*, 730. [CrossRef] [PubMed]
54. Kang, Y.; Li, P.; Zeng, X.; Chen, X.; Xie, Y.; Zeng, Y.; Zhang, Y.; Xie, T. Biosynthesis, structure and antioxidant activities of xanthan gum from *Xanthomonas campestris* with additional furfural. *Carbohydr. Polym.* **2019**, *216*, 369–375. [CrossRef] [PubMed]
55. Niknezhad, S.V.; Asadollahi, M.A.; Zamani, A.; Biria, D.; Doostmohammadi, M. Optimization of xanthan gum production using cheese whey and response surface methodology. *Food Sci. Biotechnol.* **2015**, *24*, 453–460. [CrossRef]

56. Swami, S.B.; Thakor, N.J.; Haldankar, P.M.; Kalse, S.B. Jackfruit and its many functional components as related to human health: A review. *Compr. Rev. Food Sci. Food Saf.* **2012**, *11*, 565–576. [CrossRef]
57. Dos Santos, F.P.; Jr, A.M.O.; Nunes, T.P.; De Farias Silva, C.E.; De Souza Abud, A.K. Bioconversion of agro-industrial wastes into xanthan gum. *Chem. Eng. Trans.* **2016**, *49*, 145–150. [CrossRef]
58. Katherine, R.F.; Muthukumaran, C.; Sharmila, G.; Kumar, N.M.; Tamilarasan, K.; Jaiganesh, R. Xanthan gum production using jackfruit-seed-powder-based medium: Optimization and characterization. *3 Biotech* **2017**, *7*, 248. [CrossRef]
59. Nejadmansouri, M.; Razmjooei, M.; Safdarianghomsheh, R.; Shad, E.; Delvigne, F.; Khalesi, M. Semi-continuous production of xanthan in biofilm reactor using *Xanthomonas campestris*. *J. Biotechnol.* **2021**, *328*, 1–11. [CrossRef]
60. Pereira, M.A.F.; Monteiro, C.R.M.; Pereira, G.N.; Júnior, S.E.B.; Zanella, E.; Ávila, P.F.; Stambuk, B.U.; Goldbeck, R.; de Oliveira, D.; Poletto, P. Deconstruction of banana peel for carbohydrate fractionation. *Bioprocess Biosyst. Eng.* **2021**, *44*, 297–306. [CrossRef]
61. Jonuškienė, I.; Stankevičienė, R.; Kantminienė, K.; Tumosienė, I. The influence of phytohormones on antioxidative and antibacterial activities in callus cultures of *Hypericum perforatum* L. *Agriculture* **2023**, *13*, 1543. [CrossRef]
62. Minickaitė, R.; Grybaitė, B.; Vaickelionienė, R.; Kavaliauskas, P.; Petraitis, V.; Petraitienė, R.; Tumosienė, I.; Jonuškienė, I.; Mickevičius, V. Synthesis of novel aminothiazole derivatives as promising antiviral, antioxidant and antibacterial candidates. *Int. J. Mol. Sci.* **2022**, *23*, 7688. [CrossRef]
63. Virzì, N.F.; Diaz-Rodriguez, P.; Concheiro, A.; Pittalà, V.; Alvarez-Lorenzo, C. Xanthan gum/Guar gum-based 3D-printed scaffolds for wound healing: Production, characterization, and biocompatibility screening. *Carbohydr. Polym. Technol. Appl.* **2024**, *7*, 100523. [CrossRef]
64. Revin, V.V.; Liyaskina, E.V.; Parchaykina, M.V.; Kurgaeva, I.V.; Efremova, K.V.; Novokuptsev, N.V. Production of bacterial exopolysaccharides: Xanthan and bacterial cellulose. *Int. J. Mol. Sci.* **2023**, *24*, 14608. [CrossRef] [PubMed]
65. Chen, J.; Zheng, M.; Tan, K.B.; Lin, J.; Chen, M.; Zhu, Y. Development of xanthan gum/hydroxypropyl methyl cellulose composite films incorporating tea polyphenol and its application on fresh-cut green bell peppers preservation. *Int. J. Biol. Macromol.* **2022**, *201*, 198–206. [CrossRef]
66. Kumar, N.; Pratibha; Upadhyay, A.; Petkoska, A.T.; Gniewosz, M.; Kieliszek, M. Extending the shelf life of mango (*Mangifera indica* L.) fruits by using edible coating based on xanthan gum and pomegranate peel extract. *J. Food Meas. Charact.* **2023**, *17*, 1300–1308. [CrossRef]
67. Guo, J.; Ge, L.; Li, X.; Mu, C.; Li, D. Periodate oxidation of xanthan gum and its crosslinking effects on gelatin-based edible film. *Food Hydrocoll.* **2014**, *39*, 243–250. [CrossRef]
68. Furtado, I.F.S.P.C.; Sydney, E.B.; Rodrigues, S.A.; Sydney, A.C.N. Xanthan gum: Applications, challenges, and advantages of this asset of biotechnological origin. *Biotechnol. Res. Innov.* **2022**, *6*, e202204. [CrossRef]
69. de Mello, A.F.M.; de Souza Vandenberghe, L.P.; Herrmann, L.W.; Letti, L.A.J.; Burgos, W.J.M.; Scapini, T.; Manzoki, M.C.; de Oliveira, P.Z.; Soccol, C.R. Strategies and engineering aspects on the scale-up of bioreactors for different bioprocesses. *Syst. Microbiol. Biomanuf.* **2023**, *4*, 365–385. [CrossRef]
70. Piccinno, F.; Hischier, R.; Seeger, S.; Som, C. From laboratory to industrial scale: A scale-up framework for chemical processes in life cycle assessment studies. *J. Clean. Prod.* **2016**, *135*, 1085–1097. [CrossRef]

molecules

MDPI

Article

Antibacterial and Antibiofilm Efficacy of Phenyllactic Acid Against Foodborne Pathogens *Salmonella enterica* Serotype Derby and *Escherichia coli* O26

Angela Maione [1], Annalisa Buonanno [1], Marianna Imparato [1], Giuseppe Maglione [2], Cristina Rossetti [2], Angela Michela Immacolata Montone [3], Marco Guida [1,4], Emilia Galdiero [1,*] and Paola Zinno [2]

1 Department of Biology, University of Naples "Federico II", 80126 Naples, Italy; angela.maione@unina.it (A.M.); annalisa.buonanno@unina.it (A.B.); marianna.imparato@unina.it (M.I.); marco.guida@unina.it (M.G.)

2 Institute for the Animal Production System in the Mediterranean Environment (ISPAAM), National Research Council, Piazzale Enrico Fermi 1, 80055 Portici, Italy; giuseppe.maglione@cnr.it (G.M.); cristina.rossetti@cnr.it (C.R.); paola.zinno@cnr.it (P.Z.)

3 Department of Food Inspection, Istituto Zooprofilattico Sperimentale del Mezzogiorno, Via Salute 2, 80055 Portici, Italy; angela.montone@izsmportici.it

4 BAT Center-Interuniversity Center of Studies on Bioinspired Agro-Environmental Technology, University of Naples Federico II, 80055 Portici, Italy

* Correspondence: egaldier@unina.it

Abstract: Nowadays, the spread of foodborne diseases and the growing concerns about antibiotic resistance have shifted the focus of researchers towards the use of substances of natural origin. Phenyllactic acid (PLA), a naturally produced compound, has already demonstrated antimicrobial properties against pathogenic microorganisms and those responsible for food spoilage. This study examines the antibacterial and antibiofilm properties of PLA against foodborne pathogens such as *Salmonella enterica* Derby and *Escherichia coli* O26. The study showed that PLA effectively inhibited both biofilm formation and bacterial planktonic growth, with minimal inhibitory concentrations (MICs) ranging from 2 to 2.75 mg mL^{-1}. A dose-dependent inhibition of biofilm formation was observed, reaching approximately 90% for *Salmonella* strains and 50% for *E. coli* at 1.5 mg mL^{-1}. The cytotoxicity evaluation on Caco-2 cells showed that PLA was well-tolerated at concentrations up to 2 mg mL^{-1}. PLA's effectiveness was also demonstrated in real food matrices, where its application in minced beef stored at 4 °C significantly reduced microbial populations, unlike in untreated samples where bacterial counts increased. PLA showed a good ability to inhibit biofilm formation and eradicate a mature biofilm, measuring the total bacterial biofilm biomass. Additionally, PLA was found to be biocompatible in Caco-2 cells, confirming that it poses no health risk at the tested concentrations. The study also observed that PLA reduced bacterial adhesion to intestinal cells, suggesting its potential in preventing intestinal bacterial colonization. These results highlight PLA as a promising natural antimicrobial agent for food preservation, with potential applications in sustainable packaging and controlling microbial contamination in food processing. Future studies should further explore PLA's long-term stability and its interactions in complex food environments.

Keywords: phenyllactic acid; antibacterial agent; biofilm; natural products; foodborne illness pathogens; food safety

https://doi.org/10.3390/molecules30081738

1. Introduction

The prevalence of foodborne diseases is a significant global health concern, with an estimated 600 million individuals (approximately 10% of the global population) falling ill from consuming contaminated food annually [1].

Salmonella enterica and shigatoxigenic *Escherichia coli* (STEC) are still emerging pathogens responsible for most cases of foodborne illness. The actual number of cases of foodborne illness is likely to be higher due to unrecognized or unreported outbreaks, leading to an increase in statistics. In 2021, Shiga toxin-producing *E. coli* (STEC) cases rose to over 6500, with Germany, Denmark, and Ireland reporting the most cases. Common *E. coli* serogroups included O157, O26, O103, and O145, which caused outbreaks linked to various food items such as raw milk and pre-cut vegetables [2,3].

In February 2024, a major outbreak of *E. coli* O26 was identified in France. The outbreak was traced to the consumption of raw milk cheese [4].

In 2022, salmonellosis was the second most frequently reported gastrointestinal infection from food in the European Union and significantly contributed to foodborne outbreaks across both EU member states and non-member state nations. The latest annual EU One Health Zoonoses Report published by the European Food Safety Authority (EFSA) and the European Centre for Disease Prevention and Control (ECDC) shows 65,208 cases, which is the same rate of notification as in 2021. The distribution of the top five *Salmonella* serovars acquired within the European Union and implicated in human infections was as follows: *Salmonella* Enteritidis, *Salmonella* Typhimurium, *Salmonella* Typhimurium monophasic variant, *Salmonella* Infantis, and *Salmonella* Derby. These serovars, as described for *S.* Infantis, may exhibit diverse genetic characteristics, including the presence of antimicrobial resistance genes, tolerance to heavy metals, mobile virulence genes, and the capacity to form biofilms. These characteristics could bolster their epidemiological resilience and confer additional virulence and persistence attributes within the food supply chain [5]. Monitoring *Salmonella* strains is of paramount importance, particularly in instances where these bacteria have acquired adaptations that enable them to thrive in challenging environmental settings [6]. A wide range of foodstuffs have been identified as potential vectors for *Salmonella* outbreaks. Poultry remains a significant contributor to the dissemination of this pathogen, but other animal-derived foods, such as beef and seafood, also play a role [7]. While beef products are less commonly linked to human infections compared to pork, they have been implicated in significant outbreaks caused by multidrug-resistant *Salmonella* in both Europe and North America [8,9].

Although pre-harvest interventions implemented at the farm level and during livestock transport aim to minimize the introduction, persistence, and transmission of *Salmonella* on farms [10], meat safety is significantly influenced by the bacterial load of animals upon arrival at the slaughterhouse and by procedures to mitigate cross-contamination during slaughter and meat processing [11]. Furthermore, *Salmonella* can adhere, proliferate, and establish biofilms in food matrices or on the surfaces of meat or meat products and their processing equipment, thereby resulting in persistent contamination [12]. The ability of foodborne strains to form biofilms on various surfaces increases their persistence in different environments by enhancing their resistance to physical and chemical stresses. Biofilm-forming bacteria can adhere to a variety of surfaces, including stainless steel, plastic, glass, and even food. This adhesion process takes only a few minutes, and mature biofilms can develop within hours or days, posing significant challenges for the food industry [13].

It has been observed that certain antimicrobial agents employed in food production to extend shelf life and enhance hygiene standards are now less efficacious than before due to the emergence of microorganisms resistant to these substances [14]. Consequently, there is a pressing need to discover novel antimicrobials capable of combating microorganisms that have developed resistance to conventional treatments. Furthermore, consumers today seek food free from artificial substances, such as antimicrobial agents and chemically synthesized preservatives, as these are viewed as potentially harmful to health. The growing demand for products without synthetic preservatives has driven the search for natural antimicrobial compounds. Extensive research has been conducted on natural food additives with a wide range of antimicrobial properties, capable of enhancing the microbiological quality and extending the shelf life of perishable foods [15].

Phenyllactic acid (PLA), a natural organic acid derived directly from phenylpyruvic acid, can be synthesized by specific strains of lactic acid bacteria using lactate dehydrogenase [16,17].

PLA is known for its effective antimicrobial properties, rendering it a crucial resource for food preservation, particularly in the context of biopreservation. This natural compound is produced by certain lactic acid bacteria (LAB) during the fermentation process. It has been demonstrated to be effective in combating a range of harmful microorganisms, including bacteria and fungi [18,19].

PLA has been demonstrated to be effective in prolonging the shelf life of food products by preventing microbial spoilage. Although the precise mechanism of action of PLA is not yet fully elucidated, studies have suggested that it may compromise the cell wall integrity of exposed bacteria [20,21]. This makes PLA particularly efficacious in the preservation of products such as dairy, meat, and bakery products, where microbial contamination is a common occurrence. Furthermore, the compound is being investigated for its potential use in active food packaging systems, which can create antimicrobial barriers on packaging surfaces. The use of PLA by the food industry is intended to mitigate the risk of foodborne diseases and extend the shelf life of products. This aligns with consumer demand for preservation solutions that utilize naturally derived ingredients as an alternative to synthetic additives.

The prevalence of foodborne pathogens such as *S. enterica* and *E. coli* in combination with their increasing resistance to conventional antimicrobial agents underscores the need for novel and sustainable solutions. PLA, a natural compound with potent antimicrobial and antibiofilm properties, is a promising candidate for enhancing food safety and preservation.

In this context, the present study aims to evaluate the in vitro antibacterial effects of PLA against important and common pathogens of foodborne infections. Although PLA is well-known for its ability to inhibit the growth of both Gram-negative and Gram-positive bacteria, there may be significant variability in its antibacterial efficacy due to the differential susceptibility of microbial isolates. This study expands on previous research by not only assessing the efficacy of PLA against these pathogens in both planktonic and biofilm forms, but also exploring its impact at the host–pathogen interface. Specifically, we investigated the ability of PLA to inhibit biofilm formation, reduce microbial viability, and ensure safety through cytotoxicity assessments. Additionally, we examined its effects on bacterial adhesion to intestinal epithelial cells and its potential role in preserving intestinal barrier integrity by modulating membrane junction permeability in Caco-2 cells. Exploring its applications in food matrices and its interactions with host cells will contribute to establishing PLA as an effective and sustainable alternative to traditional antimicrobial strategies, with promising implications for food preservation, microbial control, and food safety along the entire food chain.

2. Results

2.1. Phenotypic Antimicrobial Resistance Characterization

Antimicrobial susceptibility testing revealed notable differences in resistance profiles between *Salmonella enterica* serovar Typhimurium DSMZ 18,522 (S4), *Salmonella enterica*

Derby (S1), and *Escherichia coli* O26 (Table 1). In particular, S1 and S4 showed resistance to ampicillin (AMP), with MIC values of 64 μg mL^{-1} and greater than 512 μg mL^{-1}, respectively, both exceeding the European Committee on Antimicrobial Susceptibility Testing (EUCAST) resistance threshold (R > 8 μg mL^{-1}). This widespread resistance to ampicillin highlights the potential challenge of treating infections caused by these serovars. Conversely, both S1 and S4 exhibited continued sensitivity to kanamycin (KANA), chloramphenicol (CHL), and tetracycline (TET). The minimum inhibitory concentrations (MICs) for these antibiotics were consistently low, with kanamycin and tetracycline documented at 4 μg mL^{-1}, and chloramphenicol MICs also at 4 μg mL^{-1}. These findings suggest that these antibiotics may still be viable treatment options against these Salmonella serovars. The E2 strain, however, exhibited a distinct multidrug-resistant profile, with resistance to all the four tested antibiotics, and an ampicillin minimum inhibitory concentration (MIC) of 16 μg mL^{-1}, which exceeded the resistance threshold. Moreover, kanamycin and chloramphenicol MICs were exceptionally high, each greater than or equal to 512 μg mL^{-1}, clearly indicating resistance. The MIC for tetracycline was elevated at 16 μg mL^{-1}, which is greater than the EUCAST cut-off value. This pronounced multidrug resistance observed in E2 underscores its clinical significance and raises concerns about its role in difficult-to-treat infections.

Table 1. Antimicrobial susceptibility profiles of *S. enterica* Derby (S1), *S. enterica* Typhimurium DSMZ 18,522 (S4), and *E. coli* O26 (E2) against four antibiotics ampicillin (AMP), kanamycin (KANA), chloramphenicol (CHL), and tetracycline (TET). MIC values are interpreted based on EUCAST resistance cut-offs.

Strain	Antibiotic	Cut-Off R (EUCAST)	MIC	R/S
		(μg mL^{-1})		
S1	AMP	R > 8	>512	R
	KANA	R > 16	4	S
	CHL	R > 8	-	S
	TET	R > 8	4	S
S4	AMP	R > 8	128	R
	KANA	R > 16	4	S
	CHL	R > 8	4	S
	TET	R > 8	4	S
E2	AMP	R > 8	16	R
	KANA	R > 16	S ≥ 512	R
	CHL	R > 8	S ≥ 512	R
	TET	R > 8	16	R

Note: R: resistant; S: susceptible.

2.2. *Antibacterial Activity of PLA*

The in vitro antibacterial activity of PLA was determined using quantitative assays. Table 2 shows the minimum inhibitory concentrations (MICs) and the minimum bactericidal concentrations (MBCs). The MIC was determined by using the microdilution method, and the results reported in Table 2 show MIC values of 2 and 2.5 μg mL^{-1} observed for the two *Salmonella* strains and 2.75 μg mL^{-1} for E2. The MBC of PLA was 5 mg mL^{-1} for S1 and S4 and 5.5 mg mL^{-1} for E2, demonstrating a bactericidal effect against all the three strains, with an MBC/MIC ratio < 4.

Considering the importance of *Salmonella* in foodborne infections, PLA could be considered a good green alternative.

Table 2. Minimum inhibitory concentrations and minimum bactericidal concentrations of PLA against *S. enterica* Derby (S1), *S. enterica* Typhimurium DSMZ 18,522 (S4), and *E. coli* O26 (E2).

	MIC (μg mL^{-1})	MBC (μg mL^{-1})	MBC/MIC Ratio	
S1	2.0 ± 0.5	5.0 ± 0.5	2.5	bactericide
S4	2.5 ± 0.2	5.0 ± 0.5	2.0	bactericide
E2	2.75 ± 0.35	5.5 ± 0.25	1.81	bactericide

2.3. Challenge Test

The study evaluated the antimicrobial effect of PLA (1 μg mL^{-1}) on S1, S4, and E2 in minced beef stored under refrigeration at 4 °C for up to seven days. The results, summarized in the graphs, highlight consistent trends for the pathogens and the impact of the PLA treatment over time (Figure 1). In untreated samples (inoculated with the indicator pathogen but not treated with PLA), the bacterial populations of all the three pathogens remained relatively stable throughout the storage period, with minimal fluctuations. For E2, the population consistently varied between 5 and 6 log CFU g^{-1}, while S1 showed a similar trend, stabilizing around 5 log CFU g^{-1} with minimal fluctuations. In contrast, the samples treated with PLA exhibited a significant decrease in bacterial populations for all the tested pathogens. For E2, a notable decline was observed as early as day 1 (T1), with levels dropping to approximately 4 log CFU g^{-1} and maintaining stability until day 7. A comparable trend was observed in the case of S1, where PLA treatment led to a significant reduction in counts by T1, with levels dropping below 4 log CFU g^{-1} by T2 and remaining at low levels thereafter. The antimicrobial activity of PLA was consistent across pathogens. In the untreated samples, refrigeration alone was insufficient to suppress bacterial growth, as evidenced by stable or slightly increasing populations during storage. However, PLA treatment clearly demonstrated its efficacy in reducing bacterial counts and maintaining lower levels throughout the seven-day period. The control samples, which were neither inoculated nor treated with PLA, exhibited no bacterial growth, thereby confirming the absence of contamination by *Salmonella* and *Escherichia* bacteria in the minced meat utilized for the experiment. This further validates the efficacy of the prior thermal treatment in achieving complete inactivation of *E. coli*, ensuring the microbiological integrity of the samples. According to the USDA Food Safety and Inspection Service, ground meat should be cooked to a minimum internal temperature of 71 °C to ensure the elimination *of E. coli* [22].

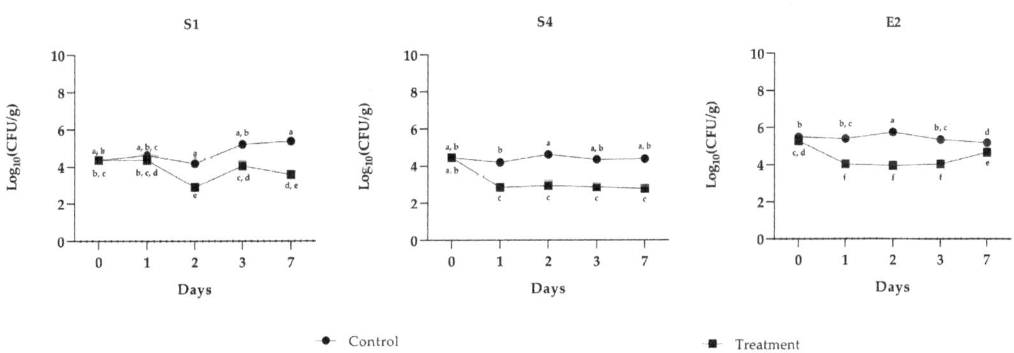

Figure 1. Challenge test of PLA against *S. enterica* Derby (S1), *S. enterica* Typhimurium DSMZ 18,522 (S4), and *E. coli* O26 (E2). The assay was performed in minced cow meat artificially contaminated with pathogens with or without the addition of PLA. The meat was stored at 4 °C for up to 7 days. Bacterial cell viability is expressed as the geometric mean of CFU g^{-1} SD of one experiment carried out in triplicate. Means without a common letter significantly differ, $p < 0.05$ (Tukey's test).

2.4. Antibiofilm Activity of PLA

The ability of the collection strain and the two foodborne isolates to assemble biofilms in vitro after 24 h of incubation at 37 °C was evaluated. All the strains were considered biofilm producers according to Stepanovic's classification [23]. S1 was considered a moderate biofilm producer, while S4 and E2 were classified as strong biofilm producers, as shown in Table 3.

Table 3. Biomass in *S. enterica* Derby (S1), *S. enterica* Typhimurium DSMZ 18,522 (S4), and *E. coli* O26 (E2) biofilms (n = 3, mean ± SD) quantified by crystal violet staining and expressed as OD570. ODc = OD570 control + (3× SD control) = 0.06. Negative (OD ≤ ODc), weak (ODc ≤ OD ≤ 2× ODc), moderate (2× ODc < OD ≤ 4× ODc), and strong biofilm production (4× ODc < OD), according to Stepanović's definition [23].

	Means (OD_{570}) ± SD	Classification
S1	0.243 ± 0.011	Moderately forming biofilm
S4	1.904 ± 0.136	Strongly forming biofilm
E2	1.561 ± 0.282	Strongly forming biofilm

The inhibition of biofilm formation by PLA was evaluated at different concentrations ranging from 0.25 to 3 mg mL^{-1} against strains S1, S4, and E2. As shown in Figure 2, a dose-dependent inhibitory effect was observed for all the strains. At the sub-MIC of 1.5 mg mL^{-1}, an inhibition of biofilm formation of about 90% for *Salmonella* strains (S1 and S4) and of about 50% for E2 was observed.

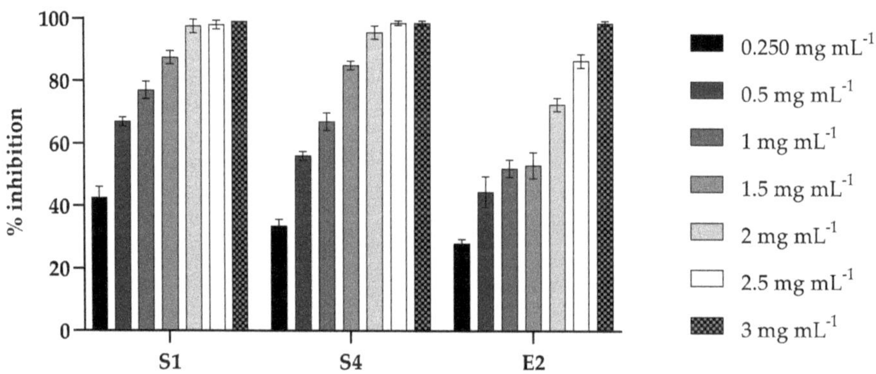

Figure 2. Inhibition effect of PLA on microbial biofilm formation in 96-well microplates. *S. enterica* Derby (S1), *S. enterica* Typhimurium DSMZ 18,522 (S4), and *E. coli* O26 (E2) were co-incubated with various concentrations (0.2, 0.5, 1, 1.5, 2, 2.5, and 3 mg mL^{-1}) of PLA for 24 h and their biofilm production was compared to that of the cells incubated without PLA (CV assay). Values obtained are given as the percentage of biofilm formation. The results shown represent the means and standard deviations (error bars) of three independent experiments.

The effect of PLA was also tested on the mature biofilm (48 h) of S1, S4, and E2 at the same concentration. The results, shown in Figure 3, exhibit moderate activity in eradicating the biofilm of the three strains, reaching approximately 50% at the highest concentration tested.

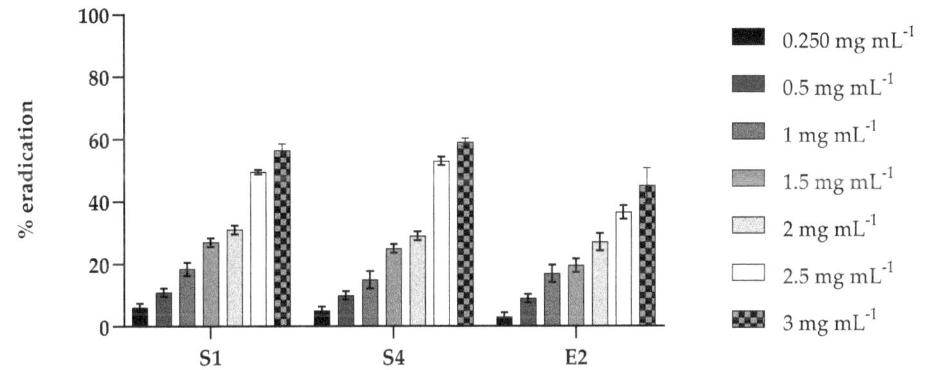

Figure 3. Eradication effect of PLA on mature biofilms in 96-well microtiter plates. Mature biofilms of *S. enterica* Derby (S1), *S. enterica* Typhimurium DSMZ 18,522 (S4), and *E. coli* O26 (E2) were treated with various concentrations (0.2, 0.5, 1.0, 1.5, 2, 2.5, and 3 mg mL^{-1}) of PLA for 24 h. Values obtained are given as the percentage of biofilm eradication. The results shown represent the means and standard deviations (error bars) of three independent experiments.

2.5. Cytotoxicity Assays

The cytotoxicity of PLA was evaluated at concentrations of 0.25, 0.5, 1, and 2 mg mL^{-1} (Figure 4). Cell viability persisted, indicating no cytotoxicity at low concentrations. However, at 3 mg mL^{-1}, a significant reduction in cell viability was observed (****, $p < 0.0001$), suggesting a cytotoxic effect at higher concentrations.

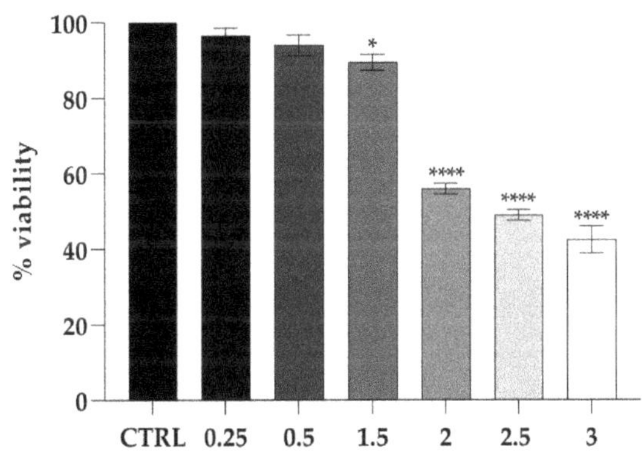

Figure 4. Viability of the CaCo-2 cell line challenged by PLA shown as the percent cell viability of the cells treated with different concentrations for 24 h. Untreated cells were used as the control. The assays were performed in three independent experiments. One-way ANOVA, followed by Dunnett's test, was performed to determine statistically significant results. Note: * = $p < 0.05$, **** = $p < 0.0001$.

2.6. Adhesion of Enteric Bacteria to Caco-2 Cells with PLA Treatments

The ability of PLA to inhibit the adhesion of S1, S4, and E2 bacteria to intestinal cells was evaluated by pre- and post-treating CaCo-2 with 1 mg mL^{-1} of PLA. As shown in Figure 5 (panel A), the pre-treatment with PLA significantly reduced the adhesion of S1, S4, and E2 by about 2 log. An adhesion reduction of 2 log was also observed for the post-treatment of S1 and S4 with PLA, and of only about 1 log for E2 (Figure 5B). Altogether, these data suggest that PLA is nontoxic and shows potential for preventing enteric bacterial interaction with intestinal cells at the tested doses.

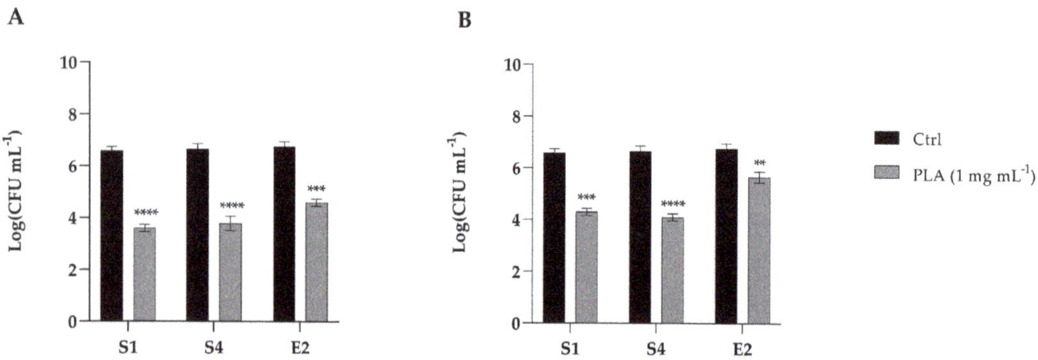

Figure 5. Inhibition of the adhesion of *S. enterica* Derby (S1), *S. enterica* Typhimurium DSMZ 18,522 (S4), and *E. coli* O26 (E2) to CaCo2 cells pre-treated (**A**) or post-treated (**B**) with PLA at a concentration of 1 mg mL^{-1}. Data reported are the means of three independent experiments ± SD. The statistical significance with respect to the corresponding controls is indicated by ** $p < 0.001$, *** $p < 0.0001$, and **** $p < 0.00001$ (Tukey's test).

2.7. Effects of PLA on Caco-2 Cell Permeability

In this study, the integrity of the intestinal barrier of differentiated Caco-2 cells, treated with different concentrations of PLA (0.25, 0.5, 1.5 mg mL^{-1}) was studied by TEER measurement. TEER values at 1, 2, 3, 5, 7, and 24 h post-treatment remained higher than the control value, except for the 0.5 mg mL^{-1} concentration, where TEER values were 92% of the control (Figure 6).

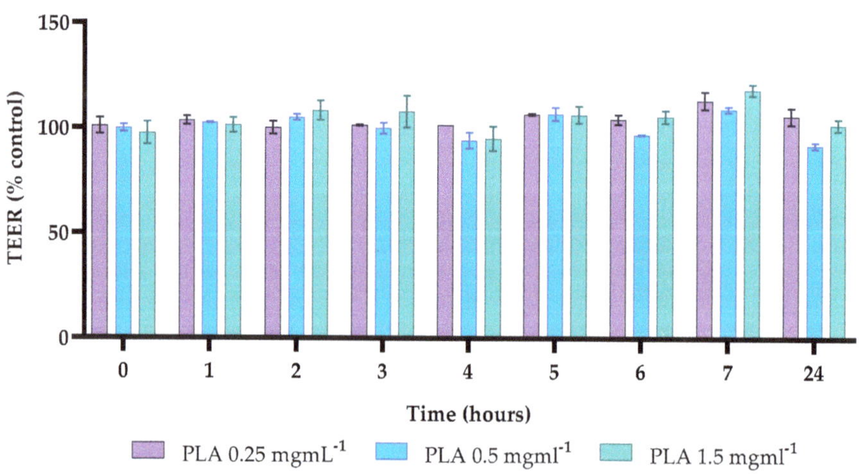

Figure 6. Transepithelial electrical resistance (TEER). TEER values for different concentrations of PLA, recorded for up to 24 h, were calculated as the percentage of C for each timepoint.

The obtained data indicate that PLA does not induce any damage to the integrity of the intestinal barrier of Caco-2 cells at the concentrations and times tested.

3. Discussion

This study investigated the antibacterial and antibiofilm activity of PLA, a naturally occurring organic acid, against foodborne pathogens, including a collection strain *Salmonella enterica* serovar Typhimurium and two isolates belonging to *Salmonella enterica* Derby and *Escherichia coli* O26 [24]. Salmonellosis remains the second most common foodborne zoonotic disease in the EU, with *S. typhimurium* strains primarily originating from various sources, including broilers, pigs, laying hens, turkeys, and cattle [25]. Similarly, *E. coli* serogroup O26 has been identified as the second most prevalent STEC-related foodborne disease in a number of European countries, including Ireland, Italy, France, and Denmark [26]. The results obtained in this work are particularly relevant considering the increasing prevalence of foodborne diseases and the rise of antimicrobial resistance among these pathogens. Tests conducted on these isolates exhibited resistance profiles and strong biofilm-forming capabilities. For instance, the *Salmonella* Derby isolate demonstrated a strong ability to form a biofilm, which can facilitate its persistence on food processing surfaces and within the food matrix. Similarly, the *E. coli* O26 isolate presented a multidrug-resistant phenotype, raising significant public health concerns. Application of PLA resulted in a marked reduction in both planktonic and biofilm-associated bacterial growth for these isolates. A salient finding of this study is the inhibitory effect of PLA on planktonic cells and biofilm formation. In vitro assays demonstrated that the minimum inhibitory concentrations (MICs) for the tested strains ranged from 2 to 2.75 mg mL^{-1}, exhibiting comparable minimum bactericidal concentrations (MBCs). These findings suggest that PLA has a broad spectrum of activity, which is consistent with previous studies that have highlighted its antimicrobial properties against both Gram-positive and Gram-negative bacteria [16,17]. Furthermore, PLA's ability to reduce biofilm formation and act on mature biofilms indicates its potential use for controlling persistent microbial contamination, a relevant aspect in food processing and preservation. Recent studies have shown PLA's strong anti-biofilm properties against microorganisms such as *Enterobacter cloacae, Pseudomonas aeruginosa, Listeria monocytogenes,* and *Enterococcus faecalis.* In particular, PLA has been shown to reduce biofilm formation even at subinhibitory concentrations and disrupt biofilms by damaging cell membranes and causing intracellular leakage. PLA also demonstrates synergy with slightly acid-electrolyzed water to enhance its effects against bacteria such as *Klebsiella oxytoca.* Additionally, PLA has been shown to interfere with the quorum-sensing system of bacteria and inhibit the expression of virulence factors, such as pyocyanin and protease, which are involved in biofilm formation [27]. The challenge test performed on minced beef stored at 4 °C provided practical indications on the applicability of PLA in realistic food matrices. In contrast to the untreated samples, in which the bacterial count remained stable or even slightly increased during cold storage, the PLA-treated samples showed a significant reduction in microbial populations over a seven-day period. As a case in point, the load of E2 decreased to approximately 4 log CFU g^{-1} at T1, while S1 decreased below 4 log CFU g^{-1} at T1 and remained consistently low throughout the 7-day storage period. A similar result was reported in [28], where PLA was used to reduce the presence of Gram-positive bacteria. The authors reported that the addition of PLA at a concentration of 3 mgL^{-1} to UHT and pasteurized whole milk effectively inhibited the growth of *L. monocytogenes* for a 14-day storage period at 4 °C. Furthermore, the study showed a reduction in the *L. monocytogenes* load on the surface of spiced beef treated with PLA at concentrations $\geq$3 mgL^{-1} during the storage period. By evaluating PLA when used to treat Gram-negative bacteria, our study expands its potential antimicrobial spectrum. Despite employing an approach divergent to that adopted in our study, further evidence of the effectiveness of PLA in ensuring food safety is provided in [29], which describes the development of an innovative food packaging based on an antibacterial hydrogel of gelatin, chitosan, and 3-phenyllactic acid, called GCP-1, designed to extend the shelf life of chilled chicken. The GCP-1 antibacterial formulation exhibited effective antimicrobial activity against both *Staphylococcus aureus* and *Escherichia coli*, thereby significantly extending the shelf life of the product. Since high concentrations of PLA have been shown to result in the production of a pungent odor, the concentration that was tested in the present study may be considered optimal in order to achieve the desired antimicrobial effect while maintaining the organoleptic properties of the food. This decrease in the pathogenic load not only validates the antimicrobial effectiveness of PLA, but also indicates that its incorporation into storage methodologies could potentially extend the shelf life of perishable products, contributing to enhanced food safety. The composition of ground beef necessitates consideration of its substantial fat content; this can result in the potential for enhanced bacterial resistance, thereby mitigating the effect of stress on bacterial populations. Consequently, the employment of a combination of diverse antibacterial agents within food applications can serve to counterbalance this effect, thereby achieving a more pronounced decontamination outcome. The antimicrobial mechanism of PLA, although not fully elucidated in this study, is likely to be related to its ability to disrupt bacterial cell membranes and interfere with key cellular processes. It is well-established that PLA exhibits antimicrobial properties; however, the precise mechanism through which it functions remains to be elucidated. Ning et al. [30] proposed that the amphiphilic nature of PLA enables its interaction with membrane lipids and proteins, thereby affecting their permeability and integrity. This mechanism is analogous to that observed in other phenolic acids [20]. However, future investigations should aim to further elucidate these mechanisms, particularly in the context of complex food matrices where interactions with other components may occur.

PLA represents a promising agent for the control of pathogenic biofilms in food processing environments, although its efficacy may vary depending on the target microorganism. The study by Liu et al. [31] showed high activity of PLA as a sanitizer against *Listeria monocytogenes*, an efficacy that appears to be higher than that found in our study against *Salmonella* and *E. coli*. This difference could be attributed to the distinct composition of the biofilm extracellular matrix among the bacterial species, which may influence the efficacy of PLA in penetrating and disrupting the biofilm structure.

Safety assessments were conducted on Caco-2 cells, a highly used model in part due to their ability to reproduce in vitro the intestinal mucosa environment and as such provide useful data on both the possible inflammatory state or alteration generated by pathogens [32]. Indeed, the intestinal lining acts as a protective barrier, due to the presence of tight junctions (TJs) located in the apical region of the epithelial cells' lateral membrane. This barrier is capable of protecting the organism from pathogens or allergens, yet allowing the passage of water and ions. Damage to the integrity of this barrier determines an alteration of the normal functions of the intestinal barrier [24]. In this study, cytotoxicity assays showed that PLA, even at concentrations up to 2 mg mL^{-1}, does not adversely affect cell viability. Furthermore, transepithelial electrical resistance (TEER) measurements confirmed that exposure to PLA at three different concentrations (0.25, 0.5, and 1.5 mg mL^{-1}) did not determine any alteration of the integrity of the intestinal barrier, a crucial factor in ensuring the safe interaction of food packaging materials with the human digestive system. These results are significant, as they indicate that PLA can be safely incorporated into food systems and active packaging without posing a health risk to consumers. Given the growing demand for sustainable and biodegradable packaging solutions, the proven biocompatibility of PLA reinforces its validity as a sustainable alternative to conventional strategies adopted in the food industry.

The inhibitory effect of PLA is also shown on the adhesion of enteric bacteria (S1, S4, and E1) to intestinal epithelial cells, both before and after treatment with 1 mg mL^{-1} PLA. These results suggest that PLA may serve as an effective antimicrobial agent to reduce bacterial colonization in the intestinal environment. This suggests that PLA could potentially create a protective barrier or induce changes in the cell surface, reducing bacterial attachment. Potential mechanisms could include modulation of host cell receptors or the formation of a protective layer by interacting with the cell microenvironment, thereby changing the physicochemical properties of the epithelial surface and rendering it less hospitable for bacterial adhesion [17].

Jiang et al. reported that, despite its strong antibiofilm properties, PLA did not significantly affect *L. monocytogenes* adhesion and invasion in Caco-2 cells. In contrast, our study demonstrated that PLA effectively reduced the adhesion of *Salmonella enterica* and *E. coli* O26 to Caco-2 cells, suggesting that its antimicrobial interactions may vary depending on the bacterial species. The observed discrepancy could be ascribed to variations in bacterial surface structures, adhesion strategies, or PLA's capacity to interfere with specific virulence factors in Gram-negative versus Gram-positive bacteria.

4. Materials and Methods

4.1. Strain and Culture Conditions

The microorganisms used were *Salmonella enterica* serovar Typhimurium DSMZ 18,522 (DSMZ; Braunschweig, Germany) (S4), while the isolates of *Salmonella enterica* Derby (S1) from chicken samples and *Escherichia coli* O26 (E2) provided by the Istituto Zooprofilattico Sperimentale del Mezzogiorno (Portici, Naples, Italy). *Salmonella* strains were routinely grown in tryptone soy broth (TSB; Oxoid, Basingstoke, UK) while *E. coli* O26 (E2) was grown in Luria–Bertani (LB) broth, Miller (DIFCO, Rodano (MI), Italy) at their optimal growth temperature, 37 °C.

4.2. Antibiotic Susceptibility Test

Antibiotic susceptibility test was performed for a selected panel of antibiotics, namely ampicillin, kanamycin, erythromycin, chloramphenicol, and tetracycline chosen as representatives of the most used pharmacological classes of antimicrobials.

The minimum inhibitory concentration (MIC) evaluation was performed using the broth microdilution method in accordance with internationally recognized standard protocols from the Clinical and Laboratory Standards Institute (CLSI) and ISO standards. The antibiotic concentrations tested ranged from 1 to 512 mg L^{-1} for all the antibiotics and from 2 to 512 mg L^{-1} for tetracycline. The antibiotics were provided by Sigma-Aldrich (Milan, Italy). Resistance profiles were generated, with isolates classified as multidrug-resistant (MDR) if they showed non-susceptibility to one antimicrobial agent in three or more antimicrobial classes [33,34].

4.3. Determination of the Minimum Inhibitory Concentration (MIC) and of the Minimum Bactericidal Concentration (MBC) of PLA

The MIC of PLA was determined according to the CLSI guidelines [34]. PLA (Sigma-Aldrich, Saint Louis, MO, USA) was dissolved in DMSO 5% v/v to prepare a 50 mg mL^{-1} stock solution. Briefly, the bacterial culture was diluted to a final concentration of 1×10^6 cells mL^{-1} in TSB (Oxoid, Basingstoke, UK) at 37 °C for 24 h together with PLA ranging from 0.625 to 10 mg mL^{-1}, and growth was determined at the 590 nm wavelength with a microplate reader (Varioskan LUX Multimode Microplate Reader; Thermofisher Scientific, Waltham, MA, USA). The MIC was defined as the lowest drug concentration that resulted in a $\geq$90% inhibition of growth compared to the growth control.

Following the MIC assay, the minimum bactericidal concentration (MBC) of PLA was determined. Ten µL of the sample from each well without visible growth were plated on tryptone soy agar plates (TSA; Oxoid, Basingstoke, UK) and incubated at 37 °C for 24 h. The MBC was defined as the lowest concentration of PLA that completely inhibited bacterial growth after plating. The compound was considered bactericidal if the MBC/MIC ratio was $\leq$4, and bacteriostatic if the ratio was $\geq$4.

4.4. Challenge Test

The challenge test used minced beef from a supermarket. Meat portions (100 g each), previously heat-treated at 72 °C for 20 s, were inoculated with an S1, S4, or E2 inoculum (approximately 1×10^4 CFU g^{-1}), as described in Serio 2010 [35].

To ensure effective pathogen distribution, the inoculated samples were homogenized using Stomacher bags (Bag Mixer-400; Interscience, Saint-Nom-la-Bretèche, France) for 2 min at room temperature. After homogenization, the inoculated meat was divided into two equal portions (50 g each), one of which was treated with PLA at a concentration of 1 mg mL^{-1}. In addition, one meat portion was neither inoculated nor PLA-treated (control). The Stomacher bags were sealed and stored under aerobic conditions at 4 °C for up to seven days.

Microbiological analysis of the populations of the S1, S4, and E2 isolates was carried out after 0–1–2–3 and 7 days of refrigerated storage. At each sampling time, the aliquots of minced meat were aseptically diluted 10-fold in 0.9% NaCl and homogenized for 2 min at room temperature in Stomacher bags. The resulting slurries were serially diluted and plated in duplicate on a selective xylose lysine deoxycholate (XLD) agar (Merck, Darmstadt, Germany). The populations of bacteria were determined and quantified by means of colony counting, after incubation for 24 h.

Before inoculation with the pathogens, the minced meat was also examined for the presence of any bacteria by means of estimating the total viable counts (TVCs) on plate count agar (PCA; Oxoid, Basingstoke, UK) after 72 h of incubation at 25 °C.

4.5. Biofilm Formation

The biofilm-forming potential of the strains used in this study was investigated using our previous protocol [36]. Briefly, to form biofilms, a 96-well sterile flat-bottomed microplate was seeded with a 10^6 CFU mL^{-1} inoculum of the test organisms (100 µL per well) and incubated for 24 h at 37 °C. The total biofilm mass was detected using the crystal violet (CV; Sigma-Aldrich, Saint Louis, MO, USA) staining methodology. After incubation, the plate was washed three times with phosphate-buffered saline (PBS; Oxoid, Basingstoke, UK), and the biofilm was fixed at 37 °C for 1 h. The CV solution (0.2% v/v) was added to each well (200 µL), and after 15 min of incubation at room temperature, the excess was washed with PBS. The bound CV was solubilized with 300 µL of 30% (v/v) acetic acid, and absorbance was measured at 570 nm using a microplate reader [37]. OD cut-off (ODc) was calculated to classify the ability of bacteria to form biofilm using the following formula: OD_{570} mean of the negative control plus three times the standard deviation (SD). The classification was as follows: non-biofilm formers (OD $\leq$ ODc), weak producers (ODc $\leq$ OD $\leq$ 2× ODc), moderate producers (2× ODc < OD), or strong producers (OD $\geq$ 4× ODc).

4.6. Antibiofilm Activity

The efficacy of PLA in inhibiting biofilm formation and eradicating pre-formed biofilms was evaluated using a previously described methodology [38].

The inhibition of biofilm formation was evaluated by adding increasing concentrations of PLA (ranging from 0.2 to 3 mg mL^{-1}) to 96-well microplate wells containing 10^6 CFU mL^{-1} of each bacterium, and after incubating plates at 37 °C for 24 h. After incubation, the staining method with crystal violet was performed, followed by microplate reading at the wavelength of 600 nm. The results were indicated as the percentage of biofilm formation inhibition as follows:

$$Biofilm\ formation\ inhibition\ \% = \left(\frac{ODcontrol - ODassay}{ODcontrol}\right) \times 100 \quad (1)$$

where ODcontrol corresponds to the mean optical density measured for bacterial biofilms grown in the absence of PLA, while ODassay is the mean optical density measured for bacterial biofilms grown in the presence of PLA.

The minimum biofilm inhibition concentration (MBIC) was defined as the lowest concentration of PLA capable of bacterial biofilm inhibition.

The influence of PLA on mature biofilms was assessed as follows: 24 h biofilms were treated with different concentrations of PLA (range, 0.2–3 mg mL^{-1}), and the plates were further incubated at 37 °C for another 24 h. The supernatant was removed, and the total cell biomass was quantified by CV staining. The percentage of biofilm reduction was calculated using the following equation:

$$Biofilm\ reduction\ \% = \frac{(AbsControl - AbsPLA)}{AbsControl} \times 100 \quad (2)$$

The minimum eradication concentration (MBEC) was defined as the lowest concentration of PLA capable of eradicating mature bacterial biofilm.

4.7. Cytotoxicity Assays

The cytotoxicity of PLA was assessed in Caco-2 cells (Human Caucasian colon adenocarcinoma, ATCC collection) using the MTT assay. The cells were grown in Dulbecco's modified Eagle's medium (DMEM; Sigma-Aldrich, Saint Louis, MO, USA), supplemented with 1% penicillin–streptomycin, 1% L-glutamine, and 10% fetal bovine serum (Sigma-Aldrich, Saint Louis, MO, USA) at 37 °C with 5% CO_2 in a humid environment. Cells were seeded at a density of 2×10^5 cells per well in 96-well plates and incubated for 24 h. A concentration ranging between 0.25 and 2 mg mL^{-1} of PLA was used for cell treatment. Untreated cells were used as a negative control. After 24 h of treatment, 3-[4,5-dimethylthiazol-2-yl]-3,5 diphenyl tetrazolium bromide (MTT) solution was added to each well for 4 h at 37 °C. The resulting formazan crystals were solubilized with DMSO, and the absorbance was measured at 570 nm using a microplate reader.

4.8. Adhesion of Enteric Bacteria to Caco-2 Cells with PLA Treatments

To evaluate the ability of PLA to reduce the adhesion to cells, Caco-2 cells were seeded (2×10^5 cells mL^{-1}) onto 24-well plates and incubated for 24 h at 37 °C in 5% CO_2 overnight. The cells were then treated with three different strains (10^8 CFU mL^{-1}) at a multiplicity of infection (MOI) of 100. The assays of adhesion on human cells were performed under pre-inoculation and post-inoculation conditions as reported previously [39].

In the pre-inoculation condition, the cells were treated with 1 mg mL^{-1} of PLA for 1.5 h and subsequently infected with each strain for 2 h; in the displacement assay, the cells were first infected with S1, S4, and E2, respectively, for 2 h, then treated with PLA at the same concentration, and further incubated for an additional 1.5 h. For both experiments, at the end of incubation, the infected monolayers were rinsed three times with PBS, serially diluted, plated on TSA agar plates and incubated for 24 h at 37 °C. The results were expressed as the percentage inhibition of the adhesion, with respect to controls performed in the same condition without the inoculation of PLA.

4.9. Transepithelial Electrical Resistance (TEER)

Caco-2 cells, grown as previously described, were seeded in the apical compartment of a transwell system (Falcon™ 6.4 mm diameter, 0.4 m pore size polyethylene terephthalate permeable Transwell filters, Corning) at a density of 3×10^5/filter, and the medium was changed every 2 days. The cells were cultured for 21 days to ensure complete differentiation. Before the experimental phase, the monolayer integrity was evaluated by measuring the transepithelial electrical resistance (TEER) with a Millicell-ERS 3 voltohmmeter (Merck Millipore, Darmstadt, Germany) considering only those with the TEER higher than 300 Ohm cm^2. Three different concentrations of PLA were tested (0.25, 0.5, and 1.5 mg mL^{-1}) each in triplicate, and the measurement of the TEER was performed every hour for the first 3 h, and at the following 5–7–24 h from the treatment.

5. Conclusions

In conclusion, together with these results, PLA produced by lactic acid bacteria has shown strong antibacterial and antibiofilm activity against such foodborne pathogens as *Salmonella enterica* serotype Derby and *Escherichia coli* O26, which are known to form biofilms that enhance their persistence and resistance to treatments. It not only inhibits bacterial growth at low concentrations, but also disrupts biofilm formation, helping to reduce contamination and prevent infection spread. PLA's non-toxic nature, especially toward human cells, makes it a promising option for food safety. Its ability to target both planktonic and biofilm-associated bacteria positions it as a valuable tool in managing foodborne illnesses. Overall, PLA offers a sustainable, natural solution for foodborne pathogen control, though further research is needed to fully understand its mechanisms and optimize its use, and future research should explore the long-term stability of PLA in different environmental conditions, as well as its efficacy in complex food matrices.

Author Contributions: Conceptualization, E.G. and P.Z.; methodology, G.M.; software, A.M.; validation, E.G., P.Z. and A.M.; formal analysis, A.B. and M.I.; investigation, C.R.; resources, M.G.; data curation, A.B.; writing—original draft preparation, P.Z.; writing—review and editing, E.G.; visualization, A.M.; supervision, A.M.I.M.; project administration, M.G.; funding acquisition, E.G. All authors have read and agreed to the published version of the manuscript.

Funding: This research received no external funding.

Institutional Review Board Statement: Not applicable.

Informed Consent Statement: Not applicable.

Data Availability Statement: The data presented in this study are available herein.

Conflicts of Interest: The authors declare no conflict of interest.

References

1. World Health Organization. *Estimating the Burden of Foodborne Diseases: A Practical Handbook for Countries*; World Health Organization: Geneva, Switzerland, 2021.
2. European Centre for Disease Prevention and Control. Salmonellosis. In *ECDC. Annual Epidemiological Report for 2022*; ECDC: Solna, Sweden, 2024.
3. European Centre for Disease Prevention and Control. Chlamydia infection. In *ECDC. Annual Epidemiological Report for 2021*; ECDC: Solna, Sweden, 2022.
4. Zavišić, G.; Ristić, S.; Petričević, S.; Janković, D.; Petković, B. Microbial Contamination of Food: Probiotics and Postbiotics as Potential Biopreservatives. *Foods* **2024**, *13*, 2487. [CrossRef] [PubMed]
5. Alba, P.; Carfora, V.; Feltrin, F.; Diaconu, E.L.; Sorbara, L.; Dell'Aira, E.; Cerci, T.; Ianzano, A.; Donati, V.; Franco, A.; et al. Evidence of structural rearrangements in ESBL-positive pESI(like) megaplasmids of S.Infantis. *FEMS Microbiol. Lett.* **2023**, *370*, fnad014. [CrossRef]
6. Chousalkar, K.K.; Willson, N.L. Nontyphoidal *Salmonella* infections acquired from poultry. *Curr. Opin. Infect. Dis.* **2022**, *35*, 431–435. [CrossRef]
7. Ferrari, R.G.; Rosario, D.K.A.; Cunha-Neto, A.; Mano, S.B.; Figueiredo, E.E.S.; Conte-Junior, C.A. Worldwide Epidemiology of *Salmonella* Serovars in Animal-Based Foods: A Meta-analysis. *Appl. Environ. Microbiol.* **2019**, *85*, e00591-19. [CrossRef]
8. Mindlin, M.J.; Lang, N.; Maguire, H.; Walsh, B.; Verlander, N.Q.; Lane, C.; Taylor, C.; Bishop, L.A.; Crook, P.D. Outbreak investigation and case-control study: Penta-resistant *Salmonella* Typhimurium DT104 associated with biltong in London in 2008. *Epidemiol. Infect.* **2013**, *141*, 1920–1927. [CrossRef]

9. Gieraltowski, L.; Higa, J.; Peralta, V.; Green, A.; Schwensohn, C.; Rosen, H.; Libby, T.; Kissler, B.; Marsden-Haug, N.; Booth, H.; et al. National Outbreak of Multidrug Resistant Salmonella Heidelberg Infections Linked to a Single Poultry Company. *PLoS ONE* **2016**, *11*, e0162369. [CrossRef] [PubMed]
10. Pessoa, J.; Rodrigues da Costa, M.; Nesbakken, T.; Meemken, D.; on behalf of the RIBMINS Cost Action. Assessment of the Effectiveness of Pre-harvest Meat Safety Interventions to Control Foodborne Pathogens in Broilers: A Systematic Review. *Curr. Clin. Microbiol. Rep.* **2021**, *8*, 21–30. [CrossRef]
11. Salines, M.; Lazou, T.; Gomez-Luengo, J.; Holthe, J.; Nastasijevic, I.; Bouwknegt, M.; Dadios, N.; Houf, K.; Blagojevic, B.; Antic, D. Risk categorisation of abattoirs in Europe: Current state of play. *Food Control* **2023**, *152*, 109863. [CrossRef]
12. Harrell, J.E.; Hahn, M.M.; D'Souza, S.J.; Vasicek, E.M.; Sandala, J.L.; Gunn, J.S.; McLachlan, J.B. *Salmonella* Biofilm Formation, Chronic Infection, and Immunity Within the Intestine and Hepatobiliary Tract. *Front. Cell. Infect. Microbiol.* **2020**, *10*, 624622. [CrossRef]
13. Alvarez-Ordóñez, A.; Coughlan, L.M.; Briandet, R.; Cotter, P.D. Biofilms in Food Processing Environments: Challenges and Opportunities. *Annu. Rev. Food Sci. Technol.* **2019**, *10*, 173–195. [CrossRef]
14. Coban, H.B. Organic acids as antimicrobial food agents: Applications and microbial productions. *Bioprocess Biosyst. Eng.* **2020**, *43*, 569–591. [CrossRef]
15. Ghosh, D.; Gupta, P.K.; Rath, D. A critical review on food adulteration and its risk on health. *IJNRD-Int. J. Nov. Res. Dev.* **2022**, *7*, 353–356.
16. Debonne, E.; Vermeulen, A.; Bouboutiefski, N.; Ruyssen, T.; Van Bockstaele, F.; Eeckhout, M.; Devlieghere, F. Modelling and validation of the antifungal activity of DL-3-phenyllactic acid and acetic acid on bread spoilage moulds. *Food Microbiol.* **2020**, *88*, 103407. [CrossRef]
17. Rajanikar, R.V.; Nataraj, B.H.; Naithani, H.; Ali, S.A.; Panjagari, N.R.; Behare, P.V. Phenyllactic acid: A green compound for food biopreservation. *Food Control* **2021**, *128*, 108184. [CrossRef]
18. Shao, L.; Xi, Y.; Weng, Y. Recent Advances in PLA-Based Antibacterial Food Packaging and Its Applications. *Molecules* **2022**, *27*, 5953. [CrossRef]
19. Ponzio, A.; Rebecchi, A.; Zivoli, R.; Morelli, L. Reuterin, Phenyllactic Acid, and Exopolysaccharides as Main Antifungal Molecules Produced by Lactic Acid Bacteria: A Scoping Review. *Foods* **2024**, *13*, 752. [CrossRef] [PubMed]
20. Sorrentino, E.; Tremonte, P.; Succi, M.; Iorizzo, M.; Pannella, G.; Lombardi, S.J.; Sturchio, M.; Coppola, R. Detection of Antilisterial Activity of 3-Phenyllactic Acid Using Listeria innocua as a Model. *Front. Microbiol.* **2018**, *9*, 1373. [CrossRef]
21. Ji, Q.Y.; Wang, W.; Yan, H.; Qu, H.; Liu, Y.; Qian, Y.; Gu, R. The Effect of Different Organic Acids and Their Combination on the Cell Barrier and Biofilm of *Escherichia coli*. *Foods* **2023**, *12*, 3011. [CrossRef]
22. Industry Guideline for Minimizing the Risk of Shiga Toxin-Producing Escherichia coli (STEC) in Beef (Including Veal) Slaughter Operations 2021 Guideline. 2021. Available online: https://www.fsis.usda.gov/sites/default/files/media_file/2021-08/FSIS-GD-2021-0008.pdf (accessed on 10 September 2024).
23. Stepanović, S.; Vuković, D.; Hola, V.; Di Bonaventura, G.; Djukić, S.; Cirković, I.; Ruzicka, F. Quantification of biofilm in microtiter plates: Overview of testing conditions and practical recommendations for assessment of biofilm production by staphylococci. *Apmis* **2007**, *115*, 891–899. [CrossRef]
24. Maqoud, F.; Orlando, A.; Tricarico, D.; Antonacci, M.; Di Turi, A.; Giannelli, G.; Russo, F. Anti-Inflammatory Effects of a Novel Acetonitrile–Water Extract of Lens Culinaris against LPS-Induced Damage in Caco-2 Cells. *Int. J. Mol. Sci.* **2024**, *25*, 3802. [CrossRef]
25. European Food Safety Authority (EFSA); European Centre for Disease Prevention and Control (ECDC). The European Union One Health 2023 Zoonoses report. *EFSA J.* **2024**, *22*, e9106. [CrossRef]
26. Alharbi, M.G.; Al-Hindi, R.R.; Esmael, A.; Alotibi, I.A.; Azhari, S.A.; Alseghayer, M.S.; Teklemariam, A.D. The "Big Six": Hidden Emerging Foodborne Bacterial Pathogens. *Trop. Med. Infect. Dis.* **2022**, *7*, 356. [CrossRef]
27. Shakya, S.; Danshiitsoodol, N.; Noda, M.; Inoue, Y.; Sugiyama, M. 3-Phenyllactic acid generated in medicinal plant extracts fermented with plant-derived lactic acid bacteria inhibits the biofilm synthesis of *Aggregatibacter actinomycetemcomitans*. *Front. Microbiol.* **2022**, *13*, 991144. [CrossRef] [PubMed]
28. Jiang, X.; Jiang, C.; Yu, T.; Jiang, X.; Kang, R.; Ren, S.; Chen, H.; Zhang, Y.; Li, Y.; Meng, H.; et al. Phenyllactic acid application to control *Listeria monocytogenes* biofilms and its growth in milk and spiced beef. *Int. J. Food Microbiol.* **2022**, *381*, 109910. [CrossRef]
29. Liu, Y.; Wang, R.; Wang, D.; Sun, Z.; Liu, F.; Zhang, D.; Wang, D. Development of a food packaging antibacterial hydrogel based on gelatin, chitosan, and 3-phenyllactic acid for the shelf-life extension of chilled chicken. *Food Hydrocoll.* **2022**, *127*, 107546. [CrossRef]
30. Ning, Y.; Yan, A.; Yang, K.; Wang, Z.; Li, X.; Jia, Y. Antibacterial activity of phenyllactic acid against *Listeria monocytogenes* and *Escherichia coli* by dual mechanisms. *Food Chem.* **2017**, *228*, 533–540. [CrossRef]
31. Liu, F.; Du, L.; Zhao, T.; Zhao, P.; Doyle, M.P. Effects of phenyllactic acid as sanitizing agent for inactivation of *Listeria monocytogenes* biofilms. *Food Control* **2017**, *78*, 72–78. [CrossRef]

32. Verhoeckx, K.; Cotter, P.; Lopez-Exposito, I.; Kleiveland, C.; Lea, T.; Mackie, A.; Requena, T.; Swiatecka, D.; Wichers, H. (Eds.) *The Impact of Food Bioactives on Health In Vitro and Ex Vivo Models*; Springer: Cham, Switzerland, 2015; p. 338.
33. Magiorakos, A.P.; Srinivasan, A.; Carey, R.B.; Carmeli, Y.; Falagas, M.E.; Giske, C.G.; Harbarth, S.; Hindler, J.F.; Kahlmeter, G.; Olsson-Liljequist, B.; et al. Multidrug-resistant, extensively drug-resistant and pandrug-resistant bacteria: An international expert proposal for interim standard definitions for acquired resistance. *Clin. Microbiol. Infect.* **2012**, *18*, 268–281. [CrossRef]
34. *CLSI M100*; Performance Standards for Antimicrobal Susceptibility Testing. Clinical and Laboratory Standards Institute: Malvern, PA, USA, 2022.
35. Serio, A.; Chiarini, M.; Tettamanti, E.; Paparella, A. Electronic paramagnetic resonance investigation of the activity of *Origanum vulgare* L. essential oil on the Listeria monocytogenes membrane. *Lett. Appl. Microbiol.* **2010**, *51*, 149–157. [CrossRef]
36. Maione, A.; Buonanno, A.; Galdiero, M.; de Alteriis, E.; Petrillo, F.; Reibaldi, M.; Guida, M.; Galdiero, E. A Re-Purposing Strategy: Sub-Lethal Concentrations of an Eicosanoid Derived from the Omega-3-Polyunsaturated Fatty Acid Resolvin D1 Affect Dual Species Biofilms. *Int. J. Mol. Sci.* **2023**, *24*, 12876. [CrossRef]
37. Stepanovic, S.; Vukovic, D.; Dakic, I.; Savic, B.; Svabic-Vlahovic, M. A modified microtiter-plate test for quantification of staphylococcal biofilm formation. *J. Microbiol. Methods* **2000**, *40*, 175–179. [CrossRef] [PubMed]
38. Maione, A.; La Pietra, A.; de Alteriis, E.; Mileo, A.; De Falco, M.; Guida, M.; Galdiero, E. Effect of Myrtenol and Its Synergistic Interactions with Antimicrobial Drugs in the Inhibition of Single and Mixed Biofilms of Candida auris and Klebsiella pneumoniae. *Microorganisms* **2022**, *10*, 1773. [CrossRef] [PubMed]
39. Maione, A.; Imparato, M.; Buonanno, A.; Galdiero, M.; de Alteriis, E.; Guida, M.; Galdiero, E. Protective and immunomodulatory effects of the novel probiotic yeast Pichia kudriavzevii isolated from a home-made kefir during infection in human colon epithelial cells: An exploratory study. *J. Funct. Foods* **2025**, *125*, 106666. [CrossRef]

molecules

MDPI

Article

Kujigamberol Inhibits IFN-γ and IL-2 mRNA Expression and NFATc2 Binding to Their Promoters in Response to a Phorbol Ester and Ionomycin Stimulation

Tanpitcha Yodweerapong [1], Yuto Ueno [1], Rikako Yamaguchi [1], Piimwara Yarangsee [1], Ken-ichi Kimura [2] and Takao Kataoka [1,3,*]

1 Department of Applied Biology, Kyoto Institute of Technology, Matsugasaki, Sakyo-ku, Kyoto 606-8585, Japan
2 The United Graduate School of Agricultural Sciences, Iwate University, 3-18-8 Ueda, Morioka 020-8550, Japan
3 Center for Social and Biomedical Engineering, Kyoto Institute of Technology, Matsugasaki, Sakyo-ku, Kyoto 606-8585, Japan
* Correspondence: takao.kataoka@kit.ac.jp

Abstract: Kujigamberol, a dinorlabdane compound isolated from Kuji amber, exerts multiple biological effects, including anti-allergic and anti-inflammatory activities. The present study demonstrated that kujigamberol inhibited cytokine production by T cells. In response to a phorbol 12-myristate 13-acetate (PMA) and ionomycin (IM) stimulation, kujigamberol suppressed interferon-γ (IFN-γ) and interleukin-2 (IL-2) mRNA expression in murine T-cell lymphoma BW5147 cells stably transfected with the T-box transcription factor eomesodermin. IL-4 and Fas ligand mRNA expression was also inhibited by kujigamberol. In the murine cytotoxic T-cell line CTLL-2, kujigamberol more strongly decreased IFN-γ mRNA expression induced by IM alone than that induced by the combination of PMA and IM. A luciferase reporter assay showed that kujigamberol preferentially reduced nuclear factor of activated T cell (NFAT)-dependent transcription in human embryonic kidney 293T cells. Unlike the calcineurin inhibitor FK506, kujigamberol did not markedly affect NFATc2 protein levels in BW5147 cells but interfered with the binding of NFATc2 to the IFN-γ and IL-2 promoters. These results indicate that kujigamberol inhibited IFN-γ and IL-2 mRNA expression by preventing the binding of NFATc2 to their promoters; therefore, it has potential as an immunosuppressive agent.

Keywords: kujigamberol; NFAT; T cells; interferon γ; interleukin-2; interleukin-4; Fas ligand; eomesodermin

1. Introduction

T cells play a critical role in the adaptive immune system by responding and adapting to various biomechanical signals in order to regulate adhesion, migration, and trafficking and elicit immune functions [1]. T cells differentiate into distinct subsets that produce different sets of cytokines [2,3]. Cytokines are essential for the regulation of immune responses in a wide variety of target cells; however, excessive levels of cytokines cause inflammatory and allergic diseases [4,5].

Interleukin-2 (IL-2) is a primary cytokine that is predominantly produced by helper T cells, but it is also secreted by other cell types [6,7]. IL-2 has fundamental functions, such as supporting T-cell proliferation and survival and the differentiation of naïve T cells into effector and memory T cells [8,9]. IL-2 transcription is regulated by the proximal IL-2 promoter, which interacts with transcription factors, such as nuclear factor of activated T cell (NFAT), nuclear factor κB (NF-κB), and activated protein-1 (AP-1) [10,11]. Previous studies demonstrated that T-cell receptor stimulation induced increases in Ca^{2+} levels and activated protein kinases, which led to transcriptional activation mediated by NFAT, NF-κB, and AP-1 [12,13]. In addition to IL-2, T cells produce other cytokines, including interleukins, interferons, and members of the tumor necrosis factor superfamily [4,5].

Interferon-γ (IFN-γ) is a proinflammatory cytokine that plays a critical role in the regulation of immune responses, including antigen presentation and cytokine production [14,15]. It is mainly produced by T helper type 1 (Th1) cells, cytotoxic T cells, and natural killer (NK) cells [16,17]. NFAT and NF-κB were shown to be essential for IFN-γ transcription by interacting with the IFN-γ promoter [18]. In addition to these conventional transcription factors, lineage-specifying transcription factors are required to promote IFN-γ transcription through the epigenetic modification of the IFN-γ locus [18–20].

The NFAT family of transcription factors are regulated by Ca^{2+} signaling and are highly phosphorylated in the regulatory domain, which is a prerequisite for their sequestration in the cytosol [21,22]. Calcineurin, a serine/threonine phosphatase, is capable of directly dephosphorylating NFAT [21,22]. An increase in intracellular Ca^{2+} promotes the interaction of Ca^{2+}-calmodulin with calcineurin and its phosphatase activity [23]. Upon dephosphorylation, NFAT is transcriptionally activated and translocates to the nucleus [24]. As a NFAT member, NFATc2 (also known as NFAT1) has been shown to play a critical role in the transcription of IFN-γ [25–27].

The T-box family member eomesodermin (Eomes) is regarded as a lineage-specifying transcription factor and consists of a T-box (DNA binding) domain and a transactivation domain [28,29]. Eomes plays an essential role in the differentiation and function of Th1 cells, cytotoxic T cells, and NK cells, including IFN-γ production [28,29]. Consistent with this notion, we reported that Eomes-transfected murine T-cell lymphomas acquired the ability to produce IFN-γ, even though their parental cell lines did not express detectable IFN-γ [30,31].

Kujigamberol (15,20-dinor-5,7,9-labdatrien-18-ol) (Figure 1) is a dinorlabdane compound that was originally identified in Kuji amber using screening based on mutant yeast hypersensitive to Ca^{2+}-dependent signal transduction [32]. Previous studies demonstrated that kujigamberol exerted several biological effects, including anti-tumor activity against human leukemia HL-60 cells [32], anti-inflammatory activity in human vascular endothelial cells [33], and anti-allergic activity in rat basophilic leukemia RBL-2H3 cells and an in vivo rhinitis model using guinea pigs [34]. Our evaluation of the biological activity of kujigamberol in T cells showed that it suppressed IFN-γ and IL-2 expression in Eomes-transfected BW5147 cells. In the present study, we investigated the mechanisms by which kujigamberol inhibits T-cell cytokine expression.

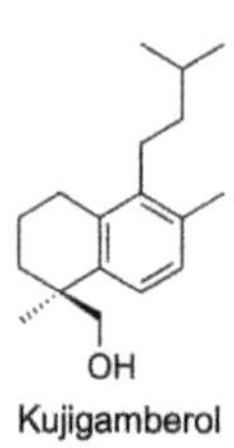

Figure 1. Structure of kujigamberol.

2. Results

2.1. Kujigamberol Inhibited IFN-γ and IL-2 mRNA Expression in Murine T-Cell Lymphoma BW5147 Cells

Murine T-cell lymphoma BW5147 cells are capable of producing IL-2, but only a trace amount of IFN-γ, in response to phorbol 12-myristate 13-acetate (PMA) and A23187, which mimic T-cell receptor stimulation [35]. We previously showed that the T-box transcription factor Eomes enabled BW5147 cells to produce high levels of IFN-γ in response to PMA and ionomycin (IM) [30,31]. In the present study, we used Eomes-transfected BW5147 cells as a T-cell model to examine the effects of kujigamberol on cytokine production by T cells.

Eomes-transfected BW5147 cells were treated with kujigamberol for 6 h. Kujigamberol did not significantly affect cell viability at concentrations up to 40 μM (Figure 2A). Under these conditions, cytokine production at the mRNA level was assessed by reverse transcription-quantitative PCR (RT-qPCR). IFN-γ and IL-2 mRNA expression was up-regulated when Eomes-transfected BW5147 cells were stimulated with PMA and IM (Figure 2B,C). Kujigamberol decreased IFN-γ and IL-2 mRNA expression in a dose-dependent manner and at concentrations higher than 20 and 10 μM, respectively (Figure 2B,C). These results showed that kujigamberol inhibited IFN-γ and IL-2 mRNA up-regulated by PMA and IM.

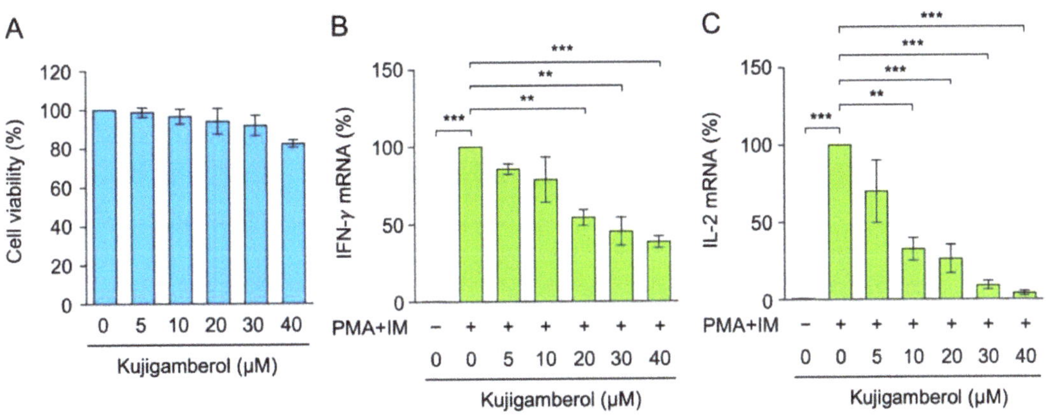

Figure 2. Kujigamberol inhibited IFN-γ and IL-2 mRNA expression in murine T-cell lymphoma BW5147 cells transfected with Eomes. (**A**) Eomes-transfected BW5147 cells were treated with (+) or without (−) serial dilutions of kujigamberol for 6 h at the indicated concentrations. Cell viability was evaluated by the MTT assay. Cell viability (%) is shown as the mean ± S.E. of three independent experiments. No significant differences were observed. (**B**,**C**) Eomes-transfected BW5147 cells were pretreated with (+) or without (−) serial dilutions of kujigamberol for 1 h and were then incubated with (+) or without (−) PMA (100 nM) plus IM (1 μM) for 6 h in the presence of kujigamberol at the indicated concentrations. IFN-γ and IL-2 mRNA expression was evaluated by RT-qPCR. IFN-γ mRNA (%) (**B**) and IL-2 mRNA (%) (**C**) are shown as the mean ± S.E. of three independent experiments. ** $p < 0.01$ and *** $p < 0.001$.

2.2. Kujigamberol Inhibited IL-4 and Fas Ligand mRNA Expression in Eomes-Transfected BW5147 Cells

We further investigated the effects of kujigamberol on the production of other T-cell cytokines. The results obtained showed that IL-4 and Fas ligand mRNA expression was highly up-regulated in Eomes-transfected BW5147 cells stimulated with PMA and IM (Figure 3A,B). Kujigamberol markedly inhibited the up-regulation of IL-4 and Fas ligand mRNA expression (Figure 3A,B). Collectively, these results demonstrate that kujigamberol exerted potent inhibitory effects on cytokine mRNA expression in BW5147 cells.

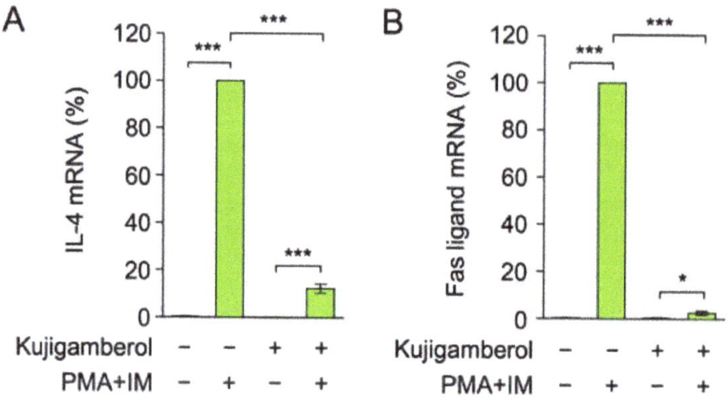

Figure 3. Kujigamberol inhibited IL-4 and Fas ligand mRNA expression in Eomes-transfected BW5147 cells. (**A**,**B**) Eomes-transfected BW5147 cells were pretreated with (+) or without (−) kujigamberol for 1 h, followed by stimulation with (+) or without (−) PMA (100 nM) plus IM (1 μM) for 6 h in the continued presence (+) or absence (−) of kujigamberol (40 μM). IL-4 and Fas ligand mRNA expression was evaluated by RT-qPCR. IL-4 mRNA (%) (**A**) and Fas ligand mRNA (%) (**B**) are shown as the mean ± S.E. of three independent experiments. * $p < 0.05$ and *** $p < 0.001$.

2.3. Kujigamberol Inhibited IFN-γ mRNA Expression in the Murine Cytotoxic T-Cell Line CTLL-2

In addition to helper T cells, IFN-γ is one of the cytokines produced by cytotoxic T cells and NK cells [16,17]. The murine cytotoxic T-cell line CTLL-2 has been reported to produce IFN-γ [36,37]. To investigate the effects of kujigamberol on cell viability, CTLL-2 cells were treated with serial dilutions of kujigamberol for 6 h. Kujigamberol did not affect CTLL-2 cell viability at concentrations up to 50 μM (Figure 4A). CTLL-2 cells were stimulated with PMA, IM, or both for 6 h. In contrast to BW5147 cells, IM alone was sufficient to up-regulate IFN-γ mRNA expression by approximately 20-fold (Figure 4B). Furthermore, the combination of PMA and IM up-regulated IFN-γ mRNA expression to a lesser extent than IM alone (Figure 4B). This may be due to the influence of PMA-induced AP-1 and NF-κB on IFN-γ transcription by competing with IM-induced NFAT as a major transcription factor in CTLL-2 cells. These results demonstrate that IM was the most suitable stimulation to promote IFN-γ expression in CTLL-2 cells.

CTLL-2 cells were treated with kujigamberol for 1 h and then stimulated with IM alone or the combination of PMA and IM. The pretreatment with kujigamberol suppressed IFN-γ mRNA expression by more than 80% in IM-stimulated CTLL-2 cells (Figure 4C). In contrast, kujigamberol inhibited IFN-γ mRNA expression by approximately 40% in PMA- and IM-stimulated CTLL-2 cells (Figure 4D), which was less than that in IM-stimulated CTLL-2 cells (Figure 4C). These results show that kujigamberol inhibited IFN-γ mRNA expression up-regulated by IM alone or PMA plus IM in CTLL-2 cells.

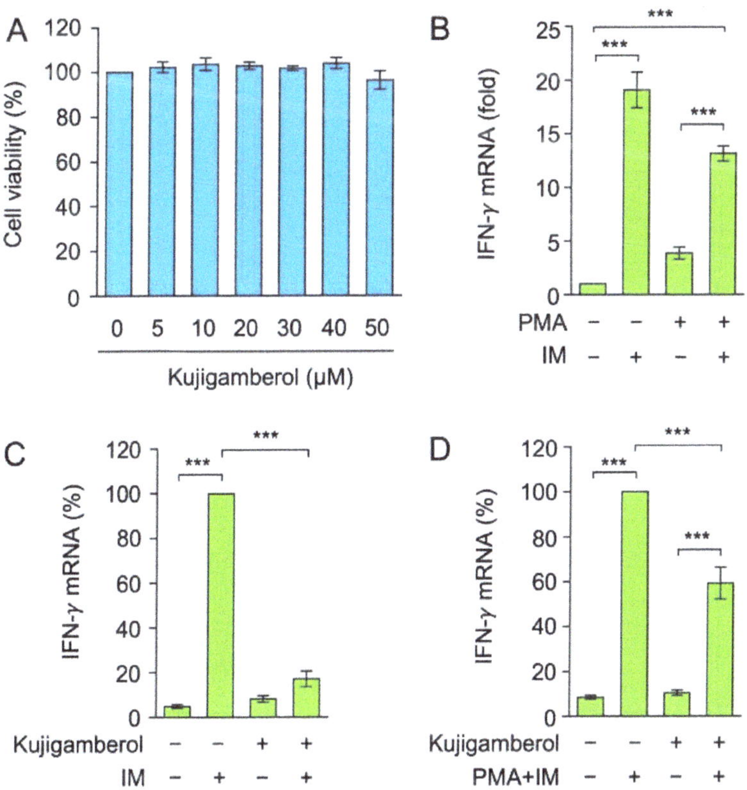

Figure 4. Kujigamberol inhibited IFN-γ mRNA expression in the murine cytotoxic T-cell line CTLL-2. (**A**) CTLL-2 cells were incubated with serial dilutions of kujigamberol for 6 h. Cell viability was evaluated by the MTT assay. Cell viability (%) is shown as the mean ± S.E. of three independent experiments. No significant differences were observed. (**B–D**) CTLL-2 cells were incubated with (+) or without (−) PMA (100 nM) and IM (1 μM) for 6 h (**B**). CTLL-2 cells were pretreated with (+) or without (−) kujigamberol for 1 h and were then incubated with (+) or without (−) IM (1 μM) (**C**) or PMA (100 nM) plus IM (1 μM) (**D**) for 6 h in the presence (+) or absence (−) of kujigamberol (50 μM). IFN-γ mRNA expression was evaluated by RT-qPCR. IFN-γ mRNA (fold) (**B**) and IFN-γ mRNA (%) (**C**,**D**) are shown as the mean ± S.E. of three independent experiments. *** $p < 0.001$.

2.4. Kujigamberol Suppressed NFAT-Dependent Transcriptional Activity in Human Embryonic Kidney 293T Cells

We previously used human embryonic kidney 293T cells in a luciferase reporter assay on the IFN-γ promoter [30] because of their higher transfection efficiency for transient expression. To examine the effects of kujigamberol on cell viability, 293T cells were pretreated with kujigamberol for 1 h and then stimulated with PMA and IM for 6 h. The pretreatment with kujigamberol did not affect 293T cell viability at concentrations up to 50 μM (Figure 5A).

T-cell receptor stimulation or PMA and IM stimulation have been shown to activate transcription factors, such as AP-1, NF-κB, and NFAT, which then promote the transcription of cytokine genes, including IFN-γ and IL-2 [12,13]. To investigate the effects of kujigamberol on the transcription factors involved in cytokine production, 293T cells were transiently transfected with plasmid vectors encoding luciferase reporters responsive to AP-1, NFAT, and NF-κB. In transfected 293T cells, the PMA and IM stimulation up-regulated luciferase reporter activities for AP-1 and NFAT to high levels, but to a lesser extent for

NF-κB (Figure 5B–D). Kujigamberol decreased AP-1-dependent luciferase activity by approximately 25%, whereas it inhibited NFAT-dependent luciferase activity by more than 65% (Figure 5B,C). In contrast, kujigamberol did not reduce NF-κB-dependent luciferase activity (Figure 5D). These results suggest that kujigamberol preferentially inhibited NFAT-dependent transcriptional activity over AP-1 or NF-κB.

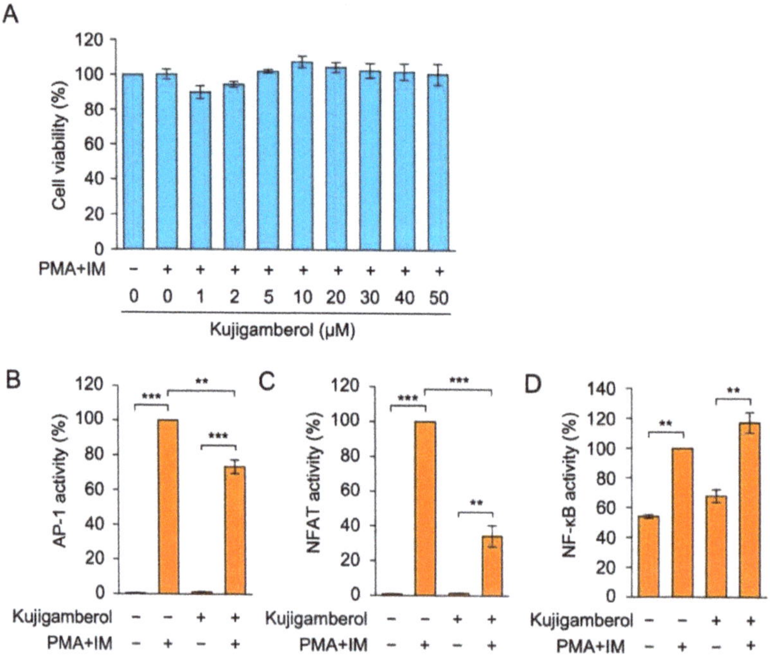

Figure 5. Kujigamberol inhibited NFAT-dependent luciferase reporter activity in human embryonic kidney 293T cells. (**A**) 293T cells were pretreated with (+) or without (−) serial dilutions of kujigamberol for 1 h and were then incubated with PMA (100 nM) plus IM (1 μM) for 6 h in the presence of kujigamberol at the indicated concentrations. Cell viability was evaluated by the MTT assay. Cell viability (%) is shown as the mean ± S.E. of three independent experiments. No significant differences were observed. (**B–D**) 293T cells were transfected with plasmid vectors encoding firefly luciferase reporters responsive to AP-1 (**B**), NFAT (**C**), and NF-κB (**D**), together with the *Renilla* luciferase reporter driven by the cytomegalovirus promoter. Transfected 293T cells were pretreated with (+) or without (−) kujigamberol (50 μM) for 1 h and were then treated with (+) or without (−) PMA (100 nM) and IM (1 μM) for 6 h. Firefly luciferase activity was normalized to *Renilla* luciferase activity. Luciferase activity (%) is shown as the mean ± S.E. of three independent experiments. ** $p <$ 0.01 and *** $p < 0.001$.

2.5. Kujigamberol Did Not Affect NFATc2 Protein Expression in Eomes-Transfected BW5147 Cells

NFATs are dephosphorylated by the Ca^{2+}- and calmodulin-dependent serine/threonine protein phosphatase calcineurin, leading to their activation and promotion of cytokine gene transcription [21,22]. The immunosuppressant FK506 (also known as tacrolimus) interacts with FK506-binding protein 12 (FKBP12), and the FK506–FKBP12 complex potently inhibits calcineurin activity and subsequent NFAT-dependent transcription [38]. We previously reported that FK506 inhibited the production of IFN-γ and IL-2 in Eomes-transfected BW5147 cells [30], indicating that NFAT plays an essential role in IFN-γ and IL-2 expression.

NFATc2 is one of five NFAT isoforms and is responsible for IFN-γ expression in T cells [25–27]. Eomes-transfected BW5147 cells have been shown to express the NFATc2 protein [31]. The luciferase reporter assay revealed that kujigamberol preferentially inhibited NFAT transcriptional activity (Figure 5C). Based on these results, we investigated the NFAT signaling pathway. Eomes-transfected BW5147 cells were pretreated with or without kujigamberol or FK506 for 1 h and then treated with PMA plus IM for 2 h. Whole-cell lysates were then prepared and analyzed via Western blotting. The mouse NFATc2 protein is composed of 927 amino acids and is estimated to be approximately 100 kDa. Consistent with this information, the NFATc2 protein was observed as a main band migrating near the 130 kDa marker (Figure 6). FK506 converted the NFATc2 protein to a band with a larger molecular weight (Figure 6), which may correspond to the phosphorylated form by preventing calcineurin-dependent dephosphorylation. The total amount of the NFATc2 protein was not affected by kujigamberol, whereas it was markedly decreased by FK506 (Figure 6). These results suggest that the mode of action of kujigamberol on the NFATc2 protein differed from that of FK506.

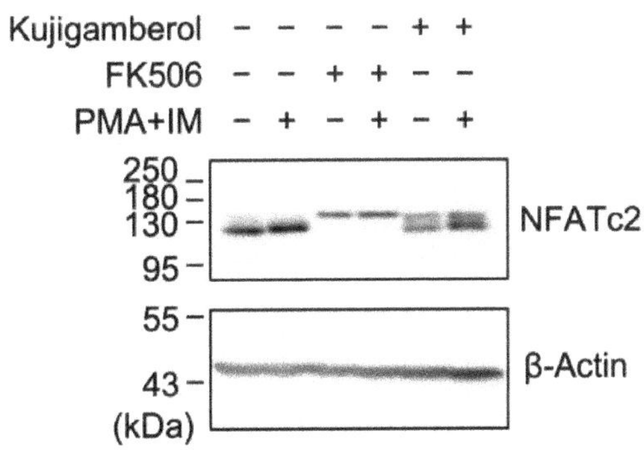

Figure 6. Kujigamberol did not markedly affect the NFATc2 protein in Eomes-transfected BW5147 cells. Eomes-transfected BW5147 cells were pretreated with (+) or without (−) kujigamberol or FK506 for 1 h and were then treated with (+) or without (−) PMA (100 nM) plus IM (1 μM) for 2 h in the presence of kujigamberol (40 μM) or FK506 (100 nM). Whole-cell lysates were prepared in at least two independent experiments. Blots were probed with anti-NFATc2 antibody and re-probed with β-actin antibody.

2.6. *Kujigamberol Interfered with the Binding of NFATc2 to IFN-γ and IL-2 Promoters in Eomes-Transfected BW5147 Cells*

We previously demonstrated that NFATc2 bound to the IFN-γ promoter in response to PMA and IM stimulation [31]. The JASPAR 2024 database [39] revealed that the IFN-γ promoter contains four consensus NFAT binding sites within −500 bp of the mouse IFN-γ promoter (Figure 7A and Figure S1), whereas six consensus NFAT binding sites exist within −500 bp of the IL-2 promoter (Figure 7B and Figure S2). Therefore, we investigated whether kujigamberol affected the binding of NFATc2 to the IFN-γ and IL-2 promoters using a chromatin immunoprecipitation (ChIP) assay. Eomes-transfected BW5147 cells were pretreated with kujigamberol and then stimulated with PMA and IM for 6 h. The PMA and IM stimulation markedly increased the binding of NFATc2 to the IFN-γ and IL-2 promoters (Figure 7C–E). The pretreatment with kujigamberol inhibited the binding of NFATc2 to the IFN-γ and IL-2 promoters in PMA- and IM-stimulated BW5147 cells (Figure 7C–E). These results show that kujigamberol inhibited the interaction of NFATc2 with the IFN-γ and IL-2 promoters.

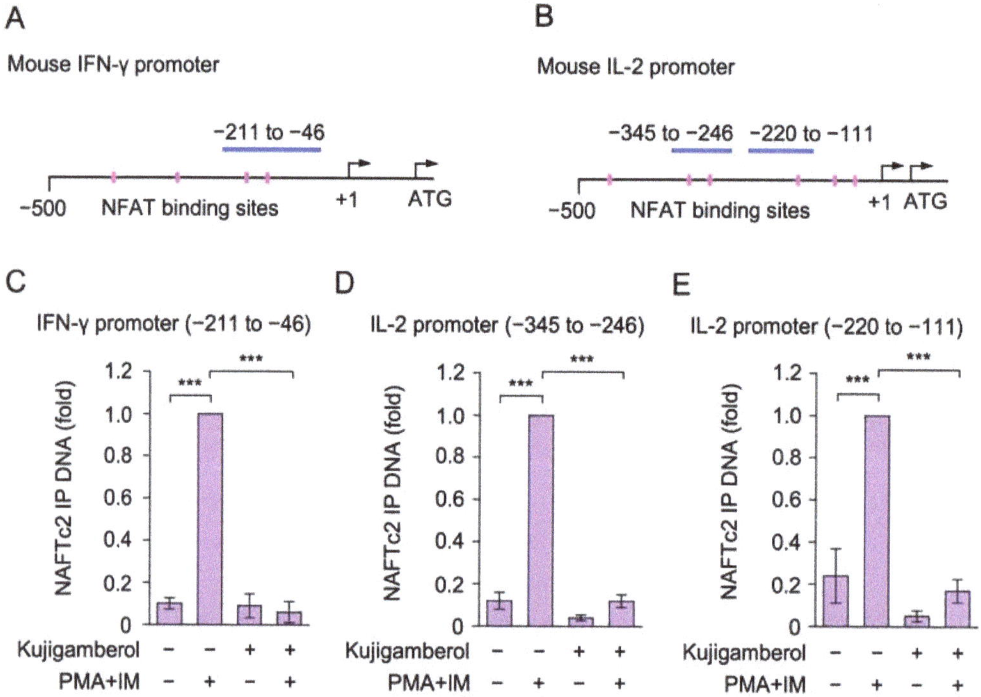

Figure 7. Kujigamberol reduced NFATc2 binding to IFN-γ and IL-2 promoters in Eomes-transfected BW5147 cells. (**A**,**B**) Consensus NFATc2 binding sites on the mouse IFN-γ promoter (**A**) and mouse IL-2 promoter (**B**) (magenta squares) are represented based on the JASPAR 2024 database. DNA regions amplified for the ChIP assay (blue lines) are shown. (**C**–**E**) Eomes-transfected BW5147 cells were pretreated with (+) or without (−) kujigamberol for 1 h and were then treated with (+) or without (−) PMA (100 nM) plus IM (1 μM) for 6 h in the presence (+) or absence (−) of kujigamberol (30 μM). The ChIP assay was performed using an anti-NFATc2 antibody. The amount of immunoprecipitated (IP) DNA for the IFN-γ promoter (−211 to −46) (**C**), IL-2 promoter (−345 to −246) (**D**), and IL-2 promoter (−220 to −111) (**E**) was measured by qPCR. NFATc2 IP DNA (fold) is shown as the mean ± S.E. of three independent experiments. *** $p < 0.001$.

3. Discussion

Kujigamberol is a major bioactive compound derived from Kuji amber [32]. It has been shown to exert anti-tumor effects on human leukemia HL-60 cells [32], anti-inflammatory activity in human vascular endothelial cells [33], and anti-allergic activity in rat basophilic leukemia RBL-2H3 cells and an in vivo rhinitis model [34]. In the present study, we revealed a novel biological effect of kujigamberol, namely the inhibition of cytokine expression by T cells. In Eomes-transfected BW5147 cells, kujigamberol inhibited the mRNA expression of IFN-γ, IL-2, IL-4, and the Fas ligand. IFN-γ mRNA expression was also suppressed by kujigamberol in CTLL-2 cells. Kujigamberol inhibited the binding of NFATc2 to the IFN-γ and IL-2 promoters in Eomes-transfected BW5147 cells. Previous studies reported that NFATc2 was indispensable for IFN-γ expression, while NFATc1 and NFATc2 were both required for IL-2 expression [25–27]. These findings show that kujigamberol inhibits IFN-γ transcription by preventing NFATc2 binding to the IFN-γ promoter.

IL-2 is a fundamental growth factor produced by T cells [8,9]. T cells differentiate into distinct subsets, including Th1 cells that produce IFN-γ and Th2 cells that secrete IL-4 [2,3]. Parental BW5147 cells are murine T-cell lymphoma cells that produce high levels of IL-2 and no or trace levels of IL-4 and IFN-γ, respectively [35]. Consistent with these findings, we previously demonstrated that BW5147 cells did not produce detectable levels of IFN-γ, whereas IFN-γ was clearly generated by Eomes-transfected BW5147 cells [30,31]. In contrast, BW5147 cells have been shown to express the Fas ligand in response to the calcium ionophore A23187 [40]. Eomes was previously found to up-regulate IFN-γ and Fas ligand expression in T cells [41,42]. It was previously shown that enforced expression of Eomes did not reduce IL-4 production in Th2 cells [43,44], whereas Eomes suppressed the IL-5 expression through inhibition of GATA3 in Th2 cells [44]. Our present results showed that Eomes-transfected BW5147 cells up-regulated the transcription of IFN-γ, IL-2, IL-4, and the Fas ligand in response to PMA and IM stimulation. However, it is currently unclear whether IL-4 expression is enhanced by Eomes in BW5147 cells or whether the present stimulation condition by PMA and IM is more potent in inducing IL-4 expression than that used in the previous study [35]. Using Eomes-transfected BW5147 cells as a T-cell model, we demonstrated that kujigamberol inhibited the mRNA expression of IFN-γ, IL-2, IL-4, and the Fas ligand as T-cell cytokines.

The results of the luciferase reporter assay showed that kujigamberol preferentially inhibited NFAT reporter activity over AP-1 reporter activity, whereas NF-κB reporter activity was unaffected. Previous studies reported that the binding sites for NFAT, NF-κB, and AP-1 were located in the IFN-γ promoter [45,46], IL-2 promoter [47,48], IL-4 promoter [49], and Fas ligand promoter [50]. Therefore, among the three types of transcription factors, NFAT appears to be the main target of kujigamberol. NFATc2 is one of five members of the NFAT family. Its role in the transcription of IFN-γ, IL-2, IL-4, and the Fas ligand has been demonstrated using gene knockout mice. Using NFATc2-deficient mice, NFATc2 was found to be indispensable for IFN-γ, IL-4, and Fas ligand expression in T cells, whereas IL-2 expression was not affected [25,26]. Furthermore, IL-2 expression was completely reduced in T cells deficient for NFATc1 and NFATc2 [51], suggesting that NFATc1 and NFATc2 have redundant roles in IL-2 expression. Consistent with these findings, FK506, which blocks the calcineurin–NFAT pathway, markedly inhibited the expression of IFN-γ and IL-2 in Eomes-transfected BW5147 cells [30]. Based on these findings, we focused on NFATc2 and investigated the effects of kujigamberol on NFATc2 protein and function.

The JASPAR 2024 database revealed the presence of four NFATc2 binding sites in the mouse IFN-γ promoter (−500 to −1) and six NFATc2 binding sites in the mouse IL-2 promoter (−500 to −1). We previously showed that PMA and IM stimulation increased the binding of NFATc2, the NF-κB subunit RelA, and Eomes to the IFN-γ promoter in Eomes-transfected BW5147 cells [30,31]. It has also been reported that T-cell receptor stimulation or PMA and IM stimulation up-regulated NFATc2 binding to the IL-2 promoter in T cells [52,53]. By using the same primers as those in ChIP assays in these studies, we demonstrated that kujigamberol inhibited the binding of NFATc2 to the IFN-γ and IL-2 promoters in Eomes-transfected BW5147 cells. However, unlike FK506, kujigamberol did not affect the total amount of the NFATc2 protein or its apparent molecular weight, suggesting that the phosphorylation status of the NFATc2 protein remained unchanged. Therefore, the mechanism by which kujigamerol inhibits NFATc2 binding activity differs from that of FK506, which inactivates calcineurin.

In our previous study, kujigamberol inhibited degranulation and Ca^{2+} mobilization in rat basophilic leukemia RBL-2H3 cells in response to A23187 [34]. The kujigamberol derivative 8-labden-15-oic acid also suppressed degranulation and Ca^{2+} mobilization in RBL-2H3 cells [54]. Kujigamberol did not inhibit calcineurin, even at 200 μM [32], whereas 8-labden-15-oic acid suppressed calcineurin at an IC_{50} value of 34.2 μM [54]. Collectively, these findings suggest that kujigamberol does not affect calcineurin but inhibits Ca^{2+}-dependent cellular processes. Consistent with this notion, we demonstrated herein that the inhibitory mechanisms of kujigamberol and FK506 are different. In T cells, PMA mimics diacylglycerol and thereby activates protein kinases (e.g., protein kinase C and protein kinase θ), leading to the activation of the NF-κB and AP-1 pathways, whereas IM increases cytoplasmic Ca^{2+} through direct ionophore activity and the activation of calcium channels, which triggers the calcineurin–NFAT pathway [12]. Therefore, the Ca^{2+}-dependent NFAT pathway appears to be more sensitive to kujigamberol than the protein-kinase-dependent NF-κB and AP-1 pathways. However, it is currently unclear whether kujigamberol reduced AP-1 reporter activity in 293T cells and inhibited IFN-γ mRNA expression in CTLL-2 cells induced by IM alone to a greater extent than the combination of PMA plus IM. Further experiments are needed to elucidate the molecular mechanisms by which kujigamberol inhibits cytokine production in T cells.

4. Materials and Methods

4.1. Cells

Murine T-cell lymphoma BW5147 cells (JCRB9002) were obtained from the National Institutes of Biomedical Innovation, Health and Nutrition JCRB Cell Bank (Osaka, Japan). BW5147 cells transfected with the pEF pGK puro expression vector encoding FLAG-Eomes (Eomes #2 BW5147 transfectant) were established and used in our previous studies [30,31]. The murine cytotoxic T-cell line CTLL-2 (RCB0637) and human embryonic kidney 293T cells (RCB2202) were obtained from the RIKEN BioResource Research Center (Tsukuba, Japan). Eomes-transfected BW5147 cells were maintained in RPMI 1640 medium (Thermo Fisher Scientific, Grand Island, NY, USA) supplemented with heat-inactivated fetal bovine serum (FBS) (Sigma-Aldrich, St. Louis, MO, USA) and penicillin–streptomycin mixed solution (stabilized) (Nacalai Tesque, Kyoto, Japan). CTLL-2 cells were maintained in RPMI 1640 medium supplemented with heat-inactivated FBS, penicillin–streptomycin mixed solution, and recombinant human IL-2 (100 U/mL) (PeproTech, Cranbury, NJ, USA). The 293T cells were maintained in DMEM medium supplemented with heat-inactivated FBS and penicillin–streptomycin mixed solution. All cells were incubated in a CO_2 incubator at 37 °C and under 5% CO_2 conditions.

4.2. Reagents

Kujigamberol was prepared as previously described [32]. FK506 (Cayman Chemical, Ann Arbor, MI, USA), IM (Merck Millipore, Darmstadt, Germany), and PMA (Wako Pure Chemical Industries, Osaka, Japan) were commercially purchased.

4.3. Antibodies

Primary antibodies reactive to NFATc2 (4G6-G5; Santa Cruz Biotechnology, Dallas, TX, USA) and β-actin (AC-15; Sigma-Aldrich) and a peroxidase-conjugated anti-mouse IgG (H+L) antibody (115-035-146; Jackson Immuno Research Laboratories, West Grove, PA, USA) were used. An anti-NFATc2 antibody (4G6-G5) was used for both Western blotting and immunoprecipitation.

4.4. Plasmid Vectors

Plasmid vectors encoding firefly luciferase reporters responsive to AP-1, NF-κB, and NFAT (kindly provided by Prof. Ralph C. Budd) were used as previously described [55]. A plasmid vector encoding a cytomegalovirus promoter-driven *Renilla* luciferase reporter was employed as previously described [56].

4.5. Cell Viability Assay

Cells (5×10^4 cells/well for BW5147 cells, 5×10^4 cells/well for CTLL-2 cells, and 2×10^4 cells/well for 293T cells) were seeded on 96-well plates and preincubated overnight. Cell viability was assessed by the formazan formation of 3-(4,5-dimethyl-2-thiazolyl)-2,5-diphenyltetrazolium bromide (MTT). Cells were treated with reagents and then incubated with MTT (500 μg/mL) for the last 2 h. MTT formazan was solubilized with sodium dodecyl sulfate overnight at the final concentration of 5%. Absorbance at 570 nm was measured using an iMark microplate reader (Bio-Rad Laboratories, Hercules, CA, USA).

4.6. RT-qPCR

Cells (6×10^5 cells/dish for BW5147 cells and 5×10^5 cells/dish for CTLL-2 cells) were seeded on 35 mm dishes and preincubated overnight. Cells were treated with reagents, harvested by centrifugation (800× *g*, 5 min), and treated with Sepasol RNA I Super G (Nacalai Tesque) according to the manufacturer's protocol. Total RNA was purified and solubilized with DEPC water (Nacalai Tesque). Total RNA was converted into cDNA using ReverTra Ace® (TOYOBO, Osaka, Japan) and oligo $(dT)_{20}$. mRNA levels were measured by the Thermal Cycler Dice® Real Time System Lite (Takara Bio, Kusatsu, Japan) using primer pairs [57–59] (Table S1). Primer-specific standard curves were used for the quantification of initial DNA. The PCR conditions were 94 °C for 3 min, followed by 45 cycles at 95 °C for 20 s, 58 °C for 30 s, and 72 °C for 30 s.

4.7. Reporter Assay

The 293T cells (5×10^4 cells/well) were seeded on 24-well plates and preincubated overnight. Cells were transfected with plasmid vectors encoding firefly luciferase reporters responsive to AP-1, NF-κB, and NFAT, together with a plasmid vector encoding a cytomegalovirus promoter-driven *Renilla* luciferase reporter using the calcium phosphate method. Transfected cells were treated with reagents, harvested by centrifugation (800× *g*, 5 min), and washed with phosphate-buffered saline (PBS). Cells were lysed with digitonin lysis buffer consisting of 1% Triton X-100, 50 mM Tris-HCl (pH 7.4), 2 mM dithiothreitol, 2 mM sodium vanadate, and the cOmplete™ Protease Inhibitor Cocktail (Sigma-Aldrich) and incubated on ice for 15 min, followed by centrifugation (15,300× *g*, 5 min) to collect the supernatants. Luciferase activities were measured using Lumitester C-110 (Kikkoman Biochemifa, Tokyo, Japan). Firefly luciferase activities were normalized to *Renilla* luciferase activities.

4.8. Western Blotting

The preparation of whole-cell lysates and Western blotting were performed as previously described [30]. In brief, BW5147 cells (6×10^5 cells/dish) were seeded on 35 mm dishes and preincubated overnight. Cells were treated with reagents, harvested by centrifugation (800× *g*, 5 min), and washed with PBS. Cells were then lysed using Triton X-100 lysis buffer consisting of 50 mM Tris-HCl (pH 7.4), 1% Triton X-100, 2 mM dithiothreitol, 2 mM sodium orthovanadate, and the protease inhibitor cocktail cOmplete™ (Sigma-Aldrich) and treated via sonication to prepare whole-cell lysates. The anti-NFATc2 antibody (4G6-G5) was used for Western blotting. Blots were visualized and captured using Amersham Imager 680 (GE Healthcare Japan, Tokyo, Japan). Membranes were treated with stripping solution (Fujifilm Wako Pure Chemical Corporation, Richmond, VA, USA) and were then subjected to additional Western blotting using the anti-β-actin antibody (AC-15).

4.9. ChIP Assay

BW5147 cells (5×10^6 cells/dish) were seeded on 100 mm dishes and preincubated overnight. Cells were treated with reagents and fixed via the direct addition of formaldehyde to the culture medium. The ChIP assay was performed as previously described [30]. Immunoprecipitation was conducted with the anti-NFATc2 antibody (4G6-G5) (2 μg). Control IgG was not used in this study because the specificity of the anti-NFATc2 antibody (mouse IgG2a) used for the ChIP assay was validated in our previous study using mouse IgG2a (MOPC-173) as a negative control [60]. Immunoprecipitated DNA and input DNA were analyzed by qPCR using primers for the mouse IFN-γ promoter and mouse IL-2 promoter [52,53,61] (Table S2).

4.10. Statistical Analysis

Experiments were repeated to confirm reproducibility. Regarding quantification, means ± standard errors were evaluated based on at least three independent experiments. Each figure caption indicates the number of experiments. One-way ANOVA followed by Tukey's test were used to assess the significance of the differences (KaleidaGraph software version 4.5.1; Hulinks, Tokyo, Japan). p-values less than 0.05 were considered to be significant.

5. Conclusions

The present study demonstrated that kujigamberol reduced the mRNA expression of IFN-γ, IL-2, IL-4, and the Fas ligand in T cells. Kujigamberol preferentially suppressed the transcriptional activity of NFAT and interfered with the DNA binding activity of NFATc2. The NFAT signaling pathway is activated by Ca^{2+}- and calmodulin-dependent calcineurin [21,22]. The calcineurin inhibitor FK506 has been used clinically as an immunosuppressant in organ transplantation [62,63]. In a mechanistic manner distinct from FK506, the present study showed that kujigamberol inhibited IFN-γ and IL-2 mRNA expression by preventing NFATc2 binding to their promoters. Therefore, kujigamberol is expected to be a potential lead for the development of immunosuppressive agents.

Supplementary Materials: The following supporting information can be downloaded at: https://www.mdpi.com/article/10.3390/molecules30102214/s1, Figure S1: NFATc2 binding sites of the mouse IFN-γ promoter; Figure S2: NFATc2 binding sites of the mouse IL-2 promoter; Figure S3: Original blots in Figure 6; Table S1: Primers used for RT-qPCR; Table S2: Primers used for the ChIP assay.

Author Contributions: Conceptualization, T.Y., Y.U., R.Y., P.Y., K.-i.K. and T.K.; formal analysis, T.Y., Y.U., R.Y., P.Y. and T.K.; investigation, T.Y., Y.U., R.Y. and P.Y.; resources, K.-i.K.; writing—original draft preparation, T.Y.; writing—review and editing, K.-i.K. and T.K.; visualization, T.Y. and T.K.; supervision, T.K.; funding acquisition, T.K. All authors have read and agreed to the published version of the manuscript.

Funding: This work was supported in part by the Japan Society for the Promotion of Science (JSPS) KAKENHI grant to T.K. (grant number: 19H02885) and the JSPS Core-to-Core Program (grant number: JPJSCCB20230005).

Institutional Review Board Statement: Not applicable.

Informed Consent Statement: Not applicable.

Data Availability Statement: Data will be made available upon reasonable request.

Acknowledgments: We thank Ralph C. Budd for providing the reagents. We also thank Riho Tanigaki and Yukina Higashi for their help in performing this study.

Conflicts of Interest: The authors declare no conflicts of interest.

References

1. Chen, W.; Zhu, C. Mechanical regulation of T-cell functions. *Immunol. Rev.* **2013**, *256*, 160–176. [CrossRef] [PubMed]
2. Raphael, I.; Nalawade, S.; Eagar, T.N.; Forsthuber, T.G. T cell subsets and their signature cytokines in autoimmune and inflammatory diseases. *Cytokine* **2015**, *74*, 5–17. [CrossRef] [PubMed]
3. Dong, C. Cytokine Regulation and Function in T Cells. *Annu. Rev. Immunol.* **2021**, *39*, 51–76. [CrossRef]
4. Turner, M.D.; Nedjai, B.; Hurst, T.; Pennington, D.J. Cytokines and chemokines: At the crossroads of cell signalling and inflammatory disease. *Biochim. Biophys. Acta.* **2014**, *1843*, 2563–2582. [CrossRef]
5. Liu, C.; Chu, D.; Kalantar-Zadeh, K.; George, J.; Young, H.A.; Liu, G. Cytokines: From clinical significance to quantification. *Adv. Sci.* **2021**, *8*, e2004433. [CrossRef]
6. Rosenberg, S.A. IL-2: The first effective immunotherapy for human cancer. *J. Immunol.* **2014**, *192*, 5451–5458. [CrossRef]
7. Damoiseaux, J. The IL-2—IL-2 receptor pathway in health and disease: The role of the soluble IL-2 receptor. *Clin. Immunol.* **2020**, *218*, 108515. [CrossRef]
8. Liao, W.; Lin, J.X.; Leonard, W.J. IL-2 family cytokines: New insights into the complex roles of IL-2 as a broad regulator of T helper cell differentiation. *Curr. Opin. Immunol.* **2011**, *23*, 598–604. [CrossRef]
9. Shouse, A.N.; LaPorte, K.M.; Malek, T.R. Interleukin-2 signaling in the regulation of T cell biology in autoimmunity and cancer. *Immunity* **2024**, *57*, 414–428. [CrossRef]
10. Bunting, K.; Wang, J.; Shannon, M.F. Control of interleukin-2 gene transcription: A paradigm for inducible, tissue-specific gene expression. *Vitam. Horm.* **2006**, *74*, 105–145.
11. Crispín, J.C.; Tsokos, G.C. Transcriptional regulation of IL-2 in health and autoimmunity. *Autoimmun. Rev.* **2009**, *8*, 190–195. [CrossRef] [PubMed]
12. Shah, K.; Al-Haidari, A.; Sun, J.; Kazi, J.U. T cell receptor (TCR) signaling in health and disease. *Signal Transduct. Target Ther.* **2021**, *6*, 412. [CrossRef] [PubMed]
13. Hermann-Kleiter, N.; Baier, G. NFAT pulls the strings during CD4$^+$ T helper cell effector functions. *Blood* **2010**, *115*, 2989–2997. [CrossRef] [PubMed]
14. Schroder, K.; Hertzog, P.J.; Ravasi, T.; Hume, D.A. Interferon-γ: An overview of signals, mechanisms and functions. *J. Leukoc. Biol.* **2004**, *75*, 163–189. [CrossRef] [PubMed]
15. Jorgovanovic, D.; Song, M.; Wang, L.; Zhang, Y. Roles of IFN-γ in tumor progression and regression: A review. *Biomark. Res.* **2020**, *8*, 49. [CrossRef]
16. Rožman, P.; Švajger, U. The tolerogenic role of IFN-γ. *Cytokine Growth Factor Rev.* **2018**, *41*, 40–53. [CrossRef]
17. Burke, J.D.; Young, H.A. IFN-γ: A cytokine at the right time, is in the right place. *Semin. Immunol.* **2019**, *43*, 101280. [CrossRef]
18. Balasubramani, A.; Mukasa, R.; Hatton, R.D.; Weaver, C.T. Regulation of the *Ifng* locus in the context of T-lineage specification and plasticity. *Immunol. Rev.* **2010**, *238*, 216–232. [CrossRef]
19. Wilson, C.B.; Rowell, E.; Sekimata, M. Epigenetic control of T-helper-cell differentiation. *Nat. Rev. Immunol.* **2009**, *9*, 91–105. [CrossRef]
20. Aune, T.M.; Collins, P.L.; Collier, S.P.; Henderson, M.A.; Chang, S. Epigenetic activation and silencing of the gene that encodes IFN-γ. *Front. Immunol.* **2013**, *4*, 112. [CrossRef]
21. Li, H.; Rao, A.; Hogan, P.G. Interaction of calcineurin with substrates and targeting proteins. *Trends Cell Biol.* **2011**, *21*, 91–103. [CrossRef]
22. Qin, J.J.; Nag, S.; Wang, W.; Zhou, J.; Zhang, W.D.; Wang, H.; Zhang, R. NFAT as cancer target: Mission possible? *Biochim. Biophys. Acta.* **2014**, *1846*, 297–311. [CrossRef] [PubMed]
23. Dewenter, M.; von der Lieth, A.; Katus, H.A.; Backs, J. Calcium signaling and transcriptional regulation in cardiomyocytes. *Circ. Res.* **2017**, *121*, 1000–1020. [CrossRef] [PubMed]
24. Fric, J.; Zelante, T.; Wong, A.Y.W.; Mertes, A.; Yu, H.B.; Ricciardi-Castagnoli, P. NFAT control of innate immunity. *Blood* **2012**, *120*, 1380–1389. [CrossRef]
25. Hodge, M.R.; Ranger, A.M.; Charles de la Brousse, F.; Hoey, T.; Grusby, M.J.; Glimcher, L.H. Hyperproliferation and dysregulation of IL-4 expression in NF-ATp-deficient mice. *Immunity* **1996**, *4*, 397–405. [CrossRef]
26. Kiani, A.; García-Cózar, F.J.; Habermann, I.; Laforsch, S.; Aebischer, T.; Ehninger, G.; Rao, A. Regulation of interferon-γ gene expression by nuclear factor of activated T cells. *Blood* **2001**, *98*, 1480–1488. [CrossRef]
27. Teixeira, L.K.; Fonseca, B.P.F.; Vieira-de-Abreu, A.; Barboza, B.A.; Robbs, B.K.; Bozza, P.T.; Viola, J.P. IFN-γ production by CD8$^+$ T cells depends on NFAT1 transcription factor and regulates Th differentiation. *J. Immunol.* **2005**, *175*, 5931–5939. [CrossRef]
28. Zhang, J.; Marotel, M.; Fauteux-Daniel, S.; Mathieu, A.L.; Viel, S.; Marçais, A.; Walzer, T. T-bet and Eomes govern differentiation and function of mouse and human NK cells and ILC1. *Eur. J. Immunol.* **2018**, *48*, 738–750. [CrossRef]

29. Pritchard, G.H.; Kedl, R.M.; Hunter, C.A. The evolving role of T-bet in resistance to infection. *Nat. Rev. Immunol.* **2019**, *19*, 398–410. [CrossRef]
30. Fukuoka, N.; Harada, M.; Nishida, A.; Ito, Y.; Shiota, H.; Kataoka, T. Eomesodermin promotes interferon-γ expression and binds to multiple conserved noncoding sequences across the *Ifng* locus in mouse thymoma cell lines. *Genes Cells* **2016**, *21*, 146–162. [CrossRef]
31. Harada, M.; Vo, N.T.; Nakao, A.; Tanigaki, R.; Fukuoka, N.; Nishida, A.; Kataoka, T. Eomesodermin promotes interaction of RelA and NFATc2 with the *Ifng* promoter and multiple conserved noncoding sequences across the *Ifng* locus in mouse lymphoma BW5147 cells. *Immunol. Lett.* **2020**, *225*, 33–43. [CrossRef] [PubMed]
32. Kimura, K.; Minamikawa, Y.; Ogasawara, Y.; Yoshida, J.; Saitoh, K.; Shinden, H.; Ye, Y.Q.; Takahashi, S.; Miyakawa, T.; Koshino, H. Kujigamberol, a new dinorlabdane diterpenoid isolated from 85 million years old Kuji amber using a biotechnological assay. *Fitoterapia* **2012**, *83*, 907–912. [CrossRef]
33. Fukuhara, S.; Tanigaki, R.; Kimura, K.; Kataoka, T. Kujigamberol interferes with pro-inflammatory cytokine-induced expression of and N-glycan modifications to cell adhesion molecules at different stages in human umbilical vein endothelial cells. *Int. Immunopharmacol.* **2018**, *62*, 313–325. [CrossRef]
34. Maruyama, M.; Kobayashi, M.; Uchida, T.; Shimizu, E.; Higashio, H.; Ohno, M.; Uesugi, S.; Kimura, K. Anti-allergy activities of Kuji amber extract and kujigamberol. *Fitoterapia* **2018**, *127*, 263–270. [CrossRef]
35. Hagiwara, H.; Yokota, T.; Luh, J.; Lee, F.; Arai, K.; Arai, N.; Zlotnik, A. The AKR thymoma BW5147 is able to produce lymphokines when stimulated with calcium ionophore and phorbol ester. *J. Immunol.* **1988**, *140*, 1561–1565. [CrossRef]
36. Li, Y.Q.; Kobayashi, M.; Yuan, L.; Wang, J.; Matsushita, K.; Hamada, J.; Kimura, K.; Yagita, H.; Okumura, K.; Hosokawa, M. Protein kinase C mediates the signal for interferon-γ mRNA expression in cytotoxic T cells after their adhesion to laminin. *Immunology* **1998**, *93*, 455–461. [CrossRef]
37. Lv, S.; Yi, P.F.; Shen, H.Q.; Zhang, L.Y.; Dong, H.B.; Wu, S.C.; Xia, F.; Guo, X.; Wei, X.B.; Fu, B.D. Ginsenoside Rh2-B1 stimulates cell proliferation and IFN-γ production by activating the p38 MAPK and ERK-dependent signaling pathways in CTLL-2 cells. *Immunopharmacol. Immunotoxicol.* **2014**, *36*, 43–51. [CrossRef]
38. Sieber, M.; Baumgrass, R. Novel inhibitors of the calcineurin/NFATc hub–Alternatives to CsA and FK506? *Cell Commun. Signal.* **2009**, *7*, 25. [CrossRef]
39. Rauluseviciute, I.; Riudavets-Puig, R.; Blanc-Mathieu, R.; Castro-Mondragon, J.A.; Ferenc, K.; Kumar, V.; Lemma, R.B.; Lucas, J.; Chèneby, J.; Baranasic, D.; et al. JASPAR 2024: 20th anniversary of the open-access database of transcription factor binding profiles. *Nucleic Acids Res.* **2024**, *52*, D174–D182. [CrossRef]
40. Benbijja, M.; Mellouk, A.; Bobé, P. Sensitivity of leukemic T-cell lines to arsenic trioxide cytotoxicity is dependent on the induction of phosphatase B220/CD45R expression at the cell surface. *Mol. Cancer.* **2014**, *13*, 251. [CrossRef]
41. Pearce, E.L.; Mullen, A.C.; Martins, G.A.; Krawczyk, C.M.; Hutchins, A.S.; Zediak, V.P.; Banica, M.; DiCioccio, C.B.; Gross, D.A.; Mao, C.A.; et al. Control of effector $CD8^+$ T cell function by the transcription factor Eomesodermin. *Science* **2003**, *302*, 1041–1043. [CrossRef]
42. Eshima, K.; Chiba, S.; Suzuki, H.; Kokubo, K.; Kobayashi, H.; Iizuka, M.; Iwabuchi, K.; Shinohara, N. Ectopic expression of a T-box transcription factor, eomesodermin, renders $CD4^+$ Th cells cytotoxic by activating both perforin- and FasL-pathways. *Immunol. Lett.* **2012**, *144*, 7–15. [CrossRef]
43. Yagi, R.; Junttila, I.S.; Wei, G.; Urban, J.F., Jr.; Zhao, K.; Paul, W.E.; Zhu, J. The transcription factor GATA3 actively represses RUNX3 protein-regulated production of interferon-γ. *Immunity* **2010**, *23*, 507–517. [CrossRef]
44. Endo, Y.; Iwamura, C.; Kuwahara, M.; Suzuki, A.; Sugaya, K.; Tumes, D.J.; Tokoyoda, K.; Hosokawa, H.; Yamashita, M.; Nakayama, T. Eomesodermin controls interleukin-5 production in memory T helper 2 cells through inhibition of activity of the transcription factor GATA3. *Immunity* **2011**, *35*, 733–745. [CrossRef]
45. Aune, T.M.; Penix, L.A.; Rincón, M.R.; Flavell, R.A. Differential transcription directed by discrete gamma interferon promoter elements in naive and memory (effector) CD4 T cells and CD8 T cells. *Mol. Cell. Biol.* **1997**, *17*, 199–208. [CrossRef]
46. Sica, A.; Dorman, L.; Viggiano, V.; Cippitelli, M.; Ghosh, P.; Rice, N.; Young, H.A. Interaction of NF-κB and NFAT with the interferon-γ promoter. *J. Biol. Chem.* **1997**, *272*, 30412–30420. [CrossRef]
47. Rooney, J.W.; Sun, Y.L.; Glimcher, L.H.; Hoey, T. Novel NFAT sites that mediate activation of the interleukin-2 promoter in response to T-cell receptor stimulation. *Mol. Cell. Biol.* **1995**, *15*, 6299–6310. [CrossRef]
48. Walters, R.D.; Drullinger, L.F.; Kugel, J.F.; Goodrich, J.A. NFATc2 recruits cJun homodimers to an NFAT site to synergistically activate interleukin-2 transcription. *Mol. Immunol.* **2013**, *56*, 48–56. [CrossRef]
49. Li-Weber, M.; Giaisi, M.; Baumann, S.; Pálfi, K.; Krammer, P.H. NF-κB synergizes with NF-AT and NF-IL6 in activation of the IL-4 gene in T cells. *Eur. J. Immunol.* **2004**, *34*, 1111–1118. [CrossRef]
50. Kavurma, M.M.; Khachigian, L.M. Signaling and transcriptional control of Fas ligand gene expression. *Cell Death Differ.* **2003**, *10*, 36–44. [CrossRef]

51. Peng, S.L.; Gerth, A.J.; Ranger, A.M.; Glimcher, L.H. NFATc1 and NFATc2 together control both T and B cell activation and differentiation. *Immunity* **2001**, *14*, 13–20. [CrossRef]
52. Wu, Y.; Borde, M.; Heissmeyer, V.; Feuerer, M.; Lapan, A.D.; Stroud, J.C.; Bates, D.L.; Guo, L.; Han, A.; Ziegler, S.F.; et al. FOXP3 controls regulatory T cell function through cooperation with NFAT. *Cell* **2006**, *126*, 375–387. [CrossRef]
53. Ishihara, S.; Schwartz, R.H. Two-step binding of transcription factors causes sequential chromatin structural changes at the activated IL-2 promoter. *J. Immunol.* **2011**, *187*, 3292–3299. [CrossRef]
54. Abe, T.; Kobayashi, M.; Okawa, Y.; Inui, T.; Yoshida, J.; Higashio, H.; Shinden, H.; Uesugi, S.; Koshino, H.; Kimura, K. Yeast Ca^{2+}-signal transduction inhibitors isolated from Dominican amber prevent the degranulation of RBL-2H3 cells through the inhibition of Ca^{2+}-influx. *Fitoterapia* **2016**, *113*, 188–194. [CrossRef]
55. Dohrman, A.; Kataoka, T.; Cuenin, S.; Russell, J.Q.; Tschopp, J.; Budd, R.C. Cellular FLIP (long form) regulates $CD8^+$ T cell activation through caspase-8-dependent NF-κB activation. *J. Immunol.* **2005**, *174*, 5270–5278. [CrossRef]
56. Matsuda, I.; Matsuo, K.; Matsushita, Y.; Haruna, Y.; Niwa, M.; Kataoka, T. The C-terminal domain of the long form of cellular FLICE-inhibitory protein ($c\text{-}FLIP_L$) inhibits the interaction of the caspase 8 prodomain with the receptor-interacting protein 1 (RIP1) death domain and regulates caspase 8-dependent nuclear factor κB (NF-κB) activation. *J. Biol. Chem.* **2014**, *289*, 3876–3887.
57. Casteels, K.M.; Mathieu, C.; Waer, M.; Valckx, D.; Overbergh, L.; Laureys, J.M.; Bouillon, R. Prevention of type I diabetes in nonobese diabetic mice by late intervention with nonhypercalcemic analogs of 1,25-dihydroxyvitamin D_3 in combination with a short induction course of cyclosporin A. *Endocrinology* **1998**, *139*, 95–102. [CrossRef]
58. Orsatti, C.L.; Missima, F.; Pagliarone, A.C.; Sforcin, J.M. Th1/Th2 cytokines' expression and production by propolis-treated mice. *J. Ethnopharmacol.* **2010**, *129*, 314–318. [CrossRef]
59. Pinhu, L.; Qin, Y.; Xiong, B.; You, Y.; Li, J.; Sooranna, S.R. Overexpression of Fas and FasL is associated with infectious complications and severity of experimental severe acute pancreatitis by promoting apoptosis of lymphocytes. *Inflammation* **2014**, *37*, 1202–1212. [CrossRef]
60. Tanaka, Y.; Nakao, A.; Miyake, Y.; Higashi, Y.; Tanigaki, R.; Kataoka, T. Small molecule inhibitors targeting nuclear factor κB activation markedly reduce expression of interleukin-2, but not interferon-γ, induced by phorbol esters and calcium ionophores. *Int. J. Mol. Sci.* **2021**, *22*, 13098. [CrossRef]
61. Chang, S.; Aune, T.M. Dynamic changes in histone-methylation "marks" across the locus encoding interferon-γ during the differentiation of T helper type 2 cells. *Nat. Immunol.* **2007**, *8*, 723–731. [CrossRef] [PubMed]
62. Dheer, D.; Jyoti; Gupta, P.N.; Shankar, R. Tacrolimus: An updated review on delivering strategies for multifarious diseases. *Eur. J. Pharm. Sci.* **2018**, *114*, 217–227. [CrossRef]
63. Ong, S.C.; Gaston, R.S. Thirty years of tacrolimus in clinical practice. *Transplantation* **2021**, *105*, 484–495. [CrossRef] [PubMed]

MDPI AG
Grosspeteranlage 5
4052 Basel
Switzerland
Tel.: +41 61 683 77 34

Molecules Editorial Office
E-mail: molecules@mdpi.com
www.mdpi.com/journal/molecules

www.ingramcontent.com/pod-product-compliance
Lightning Source LLC
Chambersburg PA
CBHW061605220926
51850CB00005B/425
9783725864904